Blackwell's Five-Minute Veterinary Consult: Reptile and Amphibian

BLACKWELL'S FIVE-MINUTE VETERINARY CONSULT

Reptile and Amphibian

First Edition

Edited by
Javier G. Nevarez, DVM, PhD, DACZM, DECZM (Herpetology)
Louisiana State University
Baton Rouge, Louisiana, USA

Five Minute Veterinary Consult

Wiley Blackwell

This edition first published 2022

Registered Office
John Wiley & Sons, Inc., 111 River Street, Hoboken, NJ 07030, USA

Editorial Office
111 River Street, Hoboken, NJ 07030, USA

For details of our global editorial offices, customer services, and more information about Wiley products visit us at www.wiley.com.

Wiley also publishes its books in a variety of electronic formats and by print-on-demand. Some content that appears in standard print versions of this book may not be available in other formats.

Library of Congress Cataloging-in-Publication Data

Names: Nevarez, Javier G., 1976– editor.
Title: Blackwell's five-minute veterinary consult. Reptile and amphibian / edited by Javier G. Nevarez.
Other titles: Five-minute veterinary consult. Reptile and amphibian
Description: First edition. | Hoboken, NJ : Wiley-Blackwell, 2022. | Includes bibliographical references and index.
Identifiers: LCCN 2020050273 (print) | LCCN 2020050274 (ebook) | ISBN 9781119233725 (cloth) | ISBN 9781119233855 (adobe pdf) | ISBN 9781119233862 (epub)
Subjects: MESH: Reptiles | Amphibians | Animal Diseases | Handbook
Classification: LCC SF997.5.R4 (print) | LCC SF997.5.R4 (ebook) | NLM SF 997.5.R4 | DDC 639.3/9–dc23
LC record available at https://lccn.loc.gov/2020050273
LC ebook record available at https://lccn.loc.gov/2020050274

Cover Design: Wiley
Cover Images: © Che_Tina_Plant/Getty Images, © filo/Getty Images, Wiley

Set in 9/10pt Adobe Garamond by Straive, Pondicherry, India
Printed and bound by CPI Group (UK) Ltd, Croydon, CR0 4YY
C064266_310821

I dedicate this book to my wife, Leslie, and my daughters, Emma, Evi, and Peeps, for reminding me what is important in life and keeping me grounded. I also dedicate it to all the reptiles and amphibians that have afforded me the opportunity to learn from them in a clinical and research setting.

CONTENTS

SECTION III: LIZARDS

SECTION V: CROCODILIANS

SECTION VI: AMPHIBIANS

Contributors

VOLUME EDITOR

JAVIER G. NEVAREZ, DVM, PHD, DACZM, DECZM (HERPETOLOGY)
Professor of Zoological Medicine
School of Veterinary Medicine-
Veterinary Clinical Sciences
Louisiana State University
Baton Rouge, LA
USA

CONTRIBUTORS

MADS F. BERTELSEN, DVM, DVSC, DACZM, DECZM (ZOO HEALTH MANAGEMENT)
Zoological Director
Copenhagen Zoo
Frederiksberg
Denmark

THOMAS H. BOYER, DVM, DABVP, REPTILE AND AMPHIBIAN PRACTICE
Pet Hospital of Peñasquitos
San Diego, CA
USA

ELSBURGH O. CLARKE III DVM, DACZM
Senior Staff Veterinarian
SeaWorld San Diego, CA
USA

ROB L. COKE, DVM, DACZM, DABVP (REPTILE & AMPHIBIAN), CVA
Director of Veterinary Care
San Antonio Zoo
Animal Health Center
San Antonio, TX
USA

NICOLA DI GIROLAMO, DMV, MSC (EBHC), PHD, DECZM (HERPETOLOGY)
Center for Veterinary Health Sciences
Oklahoma State University
Stillwater, OK
USA

GRAYSON DOSS, DVM, DACZM
Clinical Assistant Professor, Zoological Medicine
School of Veterinary Medicine
University of Wisconsin-Madison
Madison, WI
USA

CHRISTOPHER S. HANLEY, DVM, DACZM
Assistant Director
Department of Animal Health
Saint Louis Zoo
Saint Louis, MO
USA

JOANNA HEDLEY BVM&S, DZOOMED (REPTILIAN), DECZM (HERPETOLOGY), MRCVS
Royal Veterinary College
London
UK

ERIC KLAPHAKE, DVM, DACZM
Associate Veterinarian
Cheyenne Mountain Zoo
Colorado Springs, CO
USA

TAMARA KRUSE, DVM, MS
Assistant Director of Veterinary Care
San Antonio Zoo
Animal Health Center
San Antonio, TX
USA

STACEY LEONATTI WILKINSON, DVM, DABVP (REPTILE AND AMPHIBIAN)
Owner and Head Veterinarian
Avian and Exotic Animal Hospital of Georgia
Pooler, GA
USA;
Adjunct Assistant Professor
Companion Animal
North Carolina State University College of Veterinary Medicine
Raleigh, NC
USA

CHRISTOPH MANS, DR. MED. VET., DACZM
School of Veterinary Medicine
University of Wisconsin-Madison
Madison, WI
USA

RACHEL E. MARSCHANG, PD, DR. MED. VET., DECZM (HERPETOLOGY), FTÄ MIKROBIOLOGIE
Laboklin GmbH & Co. KG
Bad Kissingen, Germany

ALBERT MARTÍNEZ-SILVESTRE, DVM, MSC, PHD, DECZM (HERPETOLOGY), EBVS EUROPEAN VETERINARY SPECIALIST IN HERPETOLOGICAL MEDICINE AND SURGERY, ACRED. AVEPA (EXOTIC ANIMALS)
Scientific Director
Catalonian Reptile and Amphibian Rescue Center (CRARC)
Masquefa, Barcelona
Spain

KARINA A. MATHES, DVM, DR. MED. VET., DECZM (HERPETOLOGY), EUROPEAN VETERINARY SPECIALIST IN ZOOLOGICAL MEDICINE (HERPETOLOGY), CERTIFIED SPECIALIST IN REPTILES (FACHTIERAERZTIN FUER REPTILIEN), CERTIFIED SPECIALIST IN REPTILES AND AMPHIBIANS (ZB REPTILIEN UND AMPHIBIEN)
Head of the Department of Reptiles and Amphibians
Clinic for Small Mammals, Reptiles and Birds
University of Veterinary Medicine Hannover
Hannover
Germany

MARK A. MITCHELL, DVM, MS, PHD, DECZM (HERPETOLOGY)
Louisiana State University
Baton Rouge, LA
USA

FRANCESCO C. ORIGGI DVM, PHD, DACVM (VIROLOGY), DACVP, DECZM (HERPETOLOGY)
Vetsuisse Faculty
University of Bern
Bern
Switzerland

JORGE ORÓS, DVM, PHD, DECZM
Veterinary Faculty
University of Las Palmas de Gran Canaria
Las Palmas
Spain

JEAN A. PARÉ, DMV, DVSC, DACZM, DECZM (ZOO HEALTH MANAGEMENT)
Senior Veterinarian
Zoological Health Program
Wildlife Conservation Society
Bronx, New York, NY
USA

SEAN M. PERRY, DVM, PHD
Associate Veterinarian
Mississippi Aquarium
Gulfport, MS
USA

PAUL RAITI, DVM, DABVP (REPTILE AND AMPHIBIAN PRACTICE)
Beverlie Animal Hospital
Mt. Vernon, New York, NY
USA

DRURY R. REAVILL, DVM, DABVP (AVIAN AND REPTILE & AMPHIBIAN PRACTICE), DACVP
Zoo/Exotic Pathology Service
Carmichael, CA
USA

SAM RIVERA, DVM, MS, DABVP (AVIAN), DACZM, DECZM (ZOO HEALTH MANAGEMENT)
Senior Director of Animal Health
Zoo Atlanta
Atlanta, GA
USA

T. FRANCISCUS SCHEELINGS, BVSC, MVSC, PHD, MANZCVSC (WILDLIFE HEALTH), DECZM (HERPETOLOGY)
Monash University
School of Biological Sciences
Clayton, Victoria
Australia

LIONEL SCHILLIGER, DVM, DECZM (HERPETOLOGY), DABVP (REPTILE & AMPHIBIAN PRACTICE)
Clinique Vétérinaire du Village d'Auteuil
Paris
France

PAOLO SELLERI, DMV, PHD, SPECPACS, DECZM (HERPETOLOGY & SMALL MAMMALS)
Clinica per Animali Esotici
Rome
Italy

JACQUELINE SERIO, DVM
Animal Emergency and Specialty Center of Brevard
Melbourne, FL
USA

KURT K. SLADKY, MS, DVM, DACZM, DECZM (ZOO HEALTH MANAGEMENT & HERPETOLOGY)
Clinical Professor
Zoological Medicine/Special Species Health
Department of Surgical Sciences
School of Veterinary Medicine
University of Wisconsin-Madison
Madison, WI
USA

TREVOR T. ZACHARIAH, DVM, MS, DACZM
Director of Veterinary Programs
Brevard Zoo
Melbourne, FL
USA

PREFACE

Herpetological medicine has been an important part of my professional career and has provided me with the opportunity to travel the world and broaden my horizons. These experiences have shown me that, as with many aspects of life, we are all more similar than we are different and veterinary medicine is no exception.

This book has contributions from authors working around the world, most of whom are specialists in herpetological medicine or have a keen interest in the field. This was a conscious approach when starting this project to ensure that the information contained in the text was from the most reliable sources while also not being a strictly academic approach. As a result, this book provides a combination of accepted scientific data combined with clinical and practical experience and advice on various subjects in herpetological medicine. It serves as a quick reference to learn new information or as a refresher of previously learned material in a concise manner.

The needs of our patients and the basic principles of how we approach their care are the same around the world. As you read the information, my hope is that you come to the realization that we ultimately practice one medicine in one world. I hope this book inspires you to continue to learn more about herpetological medicine and be a lifelong learner. I believe that veterinary students, practitioners, and others will find it a useful resource for navigating through cases in quick manner that fits our busy lives.

Javier G. Nevarez

Acknowledgments

I have been fortunate in my professional career to have mentors and individuals support my goals and ambitions. Specifically, I would like to thank Drs. Thomas Tully and Mark Mitchell, two of the best mentors anyone could have, for their unwavering support and dedication. To the LSU zoological medicine team: Jordan Padlo, interns, residents, and veterinary students, thank you for keeping me honest and serving as an inspiration to stay current on the most up to date literature. I would also like to thank all the authors who answered the call and agreed to contribute to this book. It was truly overwhelming to see your positive responses and willingness to work on this project.

About the Companion Website

The book is accompanied by a website:

www.wiley.com/go/nevarez/reptileamphibian

The website includes the contents listed below:

REPTILES

HISTORY
- History form

PHYSICAL EXAM
- Chelonian physical exam form
- Crocodilian physical exam form
- Lizard physical exam form
- Snake physical exam form

SEXING
- Figures 1–6

VENIPUNCTURE SITES
- Figures 1–23

AMPHIBIANS

HISTORY
- History form

PHYSICAL EXAM
- Anuran physical exam form
- Salamander physical exam

VENIPUNCTURE SITES
- Figures 1 and 2

SUPPLEMENTARY CONTENT FOR MAIN TEXT

SECTION I
- Reptile Anatomy and Physiology
- UVB Lighting Principles for Captive Reptiles
- Anatomy and Physiology of Amphibians
- UVB Lighting Principles for Captive Amphibians
- Equipment and Medications Useful for Treating Reptile Patients
- Figures 1 and 2

SECTION II: CHELONIANS
- Figures 1–12

SECTION III: LIZARDS
- Figures 1–6

SECTION IV: SNAKES
- Figure 1

SECTION V: CROCODILIANS
- Figures 1 and 2

SECTION I

INTRODUCTION

INTRODUCTION TO REPTILE MEDICINE

Captive reptiles can be found in zoological institutions, the pet trade, commercial farming, universities, and laboratory animal facilities. Along with the prevalence of captive reptiles, there is a higher demand for improved welfare and veterinary care. As veterinarians, it is our duty not only to provide high-quality medicine but also to serve as a source of reliable information and education for reptile owners and keepers. Veterinary care of reptiles must include education on proper husbandry and nutrition, two critical factors that influence the health of reptile patients. To be successful in this endeavor, we must understand the reptile market and the demographics of reptile owners and keepers. According to a 2019–2020 report by the American Pet Products Association, reptiles comprise approximately 4.5% of the pets owned by households in the United States. The Federation of British Herpetologists claims that the number of pet reptiles in the United Kingdom may surpass that of dogs and cats, but it is difficult to find supporting data for these claims across European countries. Nonetheless, it is well known that the reptile trade is strong and thriving in Europe as well as in the United States. Of interest is the age distribution of reptile owners in the United States. Fifty-three percent of reptile owners are in the "gen Y" (1994–1980) generation followed by 26% "gen X" (1979–1965), 19% "baby boomers" (1964–1946) and 2% "builders" (1945–1920).

Not surprisingly, the majority of reptile owners rely on the internet to obtain information about reptile care. The second most common source of information is pet store employees, while only 21% rely on veterinarians. This should be a clear indication that veterinarians need to be more proactive in reaching out a to the reptile-owning generations in ways that they can relate to so they can build up clientele and improve the welfare of captive reptiles. This requires a paradigm shift in which veterinarians seek out promoting and advertising opportunities to make the public aware of their services. Many reptile-owning individuals are not even aware of all the veterinary services available for reptile species. If these individuals were more aware and developed a relationship with veterinarians, we would be more likely to have a positive impact on the captive care and welfare of reptiles. While there may be varying degrees of the bond that humans form with reptiles, most reptile owners are very appreciative of veterinarians willing and able to care for their pets. Veterinarians should offer the same standard of care to reptiles as they do to other species and charge accordingly for their time and services.

With over 10,000 species of reptiles, it is impossible to know the proper care for all species. Instead, the focus should be placed on becoming knowledgeable about the more common species that one will be working with in the course of practice. The commonality of species may vary with geographical location; nonetheless, some species such as bearded dragons, ball pythons, and sulcata tortoises are overrepresented in the pet trade.

The first approach to learning about reptiles is to think in terms of their biology. Reptiles are not domesticated species and still retain many of the behaviors observed in their natural environment. Being familiar with their natural history and biology will facilitate their captive care and treatment. In order to understand reptiles, one must be able to correctly identify the species and be familiar with their country of origin, climate, habitat, dietary scheme, photoperiod, and natural behaviors. Field guides and books have an abundance of information to help identify species and their environment.

Knowing the country and climate in which reptiles live will help to differentiate tropical from temperate and desert species. This information will directly influence their temperature requirements and photoperiod. Tropical and desert species will require higher environmental temperatures and will have longer photoperiods as compared with temperate species. Their habitat can also be divided into arboreal, aquatic, terrestrial, and fossorial (live underneath leaves and shallow layer of soil). Many species cross between habitats but will have a preference for one and feel most comfortable in it. For example, green iguanas are an arboreal species but spend time on the ground searching for food and during the breeding season. When they are done foraging and at the end of the day, they roost in trees where they feel more comfortable high off the ground away from predators.

An important consideration is the natural patterns of activity according to photoperiod. Diurnal species are active during the day and should be fed during the day to allow ample time to ingest food. Nocturnal species should be fed at dusk, dawn, or during the night, when they are more active and likely to be on the search for food. Knowing their dietary scheme is another important aspect of reptile biology. Reptiles can be omnivores, herbivores, insectivores, or carnivores. Providing high quality nutrition according to their dietary scheme is essential for good health and a primary challenge in captivity. Omnivores should be fed high-quality commercial diets in combination with fresh produce. Carnivores should be fed whole, pre-killed prey items of appropriate size. Herbivores should be fed a variety of fresh produce, grasses, and hays, in addition to a high-quality commercial diet. Insectivores should be fed a high-quality commercial diet in addition to a variety of invertebrates. In Europe, there is a wider variety of commercially available invertebrates compared to the United States. In order to offer a wide variety of invertebrates in the United States, owners are primarily restricted to purchasing through online retailers.

Finally, one must also be aware of the behavior and personalities of different reptile species. Green iguanas are very gregarious animals living in large groups under constant struggle for territory. Therefore, iguanas maintained alone will show similar behaviors expressed as a willingness to share space and time with the owner but also establishing clear territory demarcations. Adult male iguanas can become very aggressive and territorial during the breeding season. Snakes, on the other hand, tend to be solitary and show aggressiveness as a sign of defense and fear, not as an effort to establish territory. Turtles and tortoises can be solitary or gregarious and, for the most part, are very timid. Being familiar with these aspects about each group of reptiles will help you design a plan for restraint as well as make appropriate husbandry and dietary recommendations.

A thorough knowledge of the anatomy of reptiles is essential for interpretation of physical exam, diagnostic tests, and during surgical procedures. The skin of most reptiles is covered with scales; in some species there are osteoderms, or bony plates under the scales. The mucous membranes of reptiles are usually lighter in color than mammals and can be somewhat tacky, making assessment of hydration status more challenging. In addition, some species have pigmentation of the oral mucosa. For example, bearded dragons have a yellow coloration of the mucosa in their oral cavity. The position of the eyes may help in assessing hydration status, but some species (e.g., chameleons) are able to voluntarily retract their eyes, which negates eye position as an indication of dehydration. Some reptiles have eyelids, while others rely on spectacles (a skin layer covering the eye) to protect the cornea. Reptiles may have pleurodont, acrodont, or thecodont teeth. Pleurodont teeth have no socket, attach on the lateral aspect of the mandible, and are replaced throughout life (e.g., green iguanas). Acrodont teeth have firm attachments via sockets and are not replaced. Extra care must therefore be taken when examining the oral cavity of reptiles with acrodont teeth (e.g., chameleons and agamids). Thecodont teeth have a socket and are replaced throughout life (e.g., crocodilians). The tongues of reptiles range from a moveable structure (e.g., snakes, monitor lizards) to a fixed structure (e.g., crocodilians). Green iguanas have a red to purple coloration on the tip of their tongue, which is normal and must not be confused with trauma or necrosis. The musculoskeletal system is also very different, with some having no limbs (e.g., snakes) while some have additional adaptations such as prehensile tails (e.g., chameleons) and tail autotomy (e.g., green iguanas).

Reproduction of reptiles occurs primarily as vivipary (give birth to live young) or ovipary (lay eggs). Some species are parthenogenic (asexual reproduction, species are females only). It is important to know that intact reptiles may show reproductive behaviors even in the absence of a mate. This is especially important in oviparous species, which can develop and lay infertile eggs, to the surprise of the owner. It is important to ensure proper calcium intake in these species to prevent dystocia problems. Some species will also decrease their activity and will eat less or become anorectic during certain times of the year, all associated with reproductive activity.

Knowledge of internal anatomy is critical for surgery and radiographic interpretation. Reptiles do not have a diaphragm, so the viscera and the lungs are found within the same cavity, the coelomic cavity. Radiographically, the lungs may be observed to occupy over 50% of the coelomic cavity, especially during inspiration. The detail of the viscera is usually less rewarding, and the goal is to identify any well-demarcated masses that may appear out of place within the cavity. In females, follicles and/or eggs may be observed if they are reproductively active. The bony opacity should appear similar to that observed in mammals. Reduced bone opacity may be an indication of metabolic disease. Mineralization of the kidneys, joints, or other viscera is indicative of salt/mineral deposits, usually composed of calcium and causing pseudo gout. Uric acid is radiolucent, so gout does not manifest itself radiographically. In some cases of gout there is a combination of uric acid and calcium crystals, which are visible on radiographs.

Radiographs are also rewarding for identifying fracture of the long bones. Spinal and pelvic fractures may be more challenging to visualize. Ultrasound, fluoroscopy, contrast studies, computed tomography, and magnetic resonance imaging can all be useful in the reptiles, but interpretation is challenging for those unfamiliar with normal anatomy. Some reptile species have a dark pigmentation of their internal mucosa and connective tissues. This pigmentation is normal but can make visualization of organs and tissues difficult during coelioscopy or surgery. Herbivorous reptiles will have a large cecum, which must be avoided during incision of the coelomic cavity. In lizards, there is a ventral abdominal vessel that runs on the ventral midline superficially underneath the skin. For this reason, it is recommended that, in lizards, a paramedian incision be made cranial to the umbilicus, to avoid lacerating this vessel. The vessel splits into a left and right branch at the umbilicus, so a midline incision can be made caudal to this point.

Metabolic activity is the key feature in maintaining health and homeostasis in reptiles. The body temperature of reptiles is primarily regulated by environmental temperature. Reptiles in captivity therefore rely on their caregivers to provide the appropriate temperature for support of normal body functions. All body systems are regulated and stimulated by temperature. Appropriate environmental temperature will lead to a more active metabolism, stronger immune system, and better ability to resist and cope with diseases. Inadequate, low temperature is one of the most common husbandry mistakes when housing reptiles. These colder temperatures can contribute to impaired immunity, respiratory infections, decreased appetite and gut motility, and can eventually lead to a catabolic state that predisposes to disease and even death.

The medical care of the sick reptile is an important consideration if one decides to see them as patients in practice. The first step is to have all the appropriate equipment to care for these patients. While some equipment may be shared by all species, other is more specialized. Box 1 presents a list of equipment and medications that are commonly used for treating reptiles in practice. It is also important to note that the environment provided in a veterinary clinic or hospital is aimed at short-term housing that will temporarily provide the reptile with appropriate temperature, lighting and nutrition. In the meantime the owner must correct any husbandry issues and prepare the enclosure for when the animal is discharged.

Box 1. Equipment and medications useful for treating reptile patients

EQUIPMENT

Gram scale (capacity of 3–4 kg)
Oral speculums (rubber, plastic, and/or wood)
Welding gloves
22-g, 25-g, 26-g needles
1-cc, 3-cc syringes
U-100 30-unit (0.3-cc) insulin syringes (BD Consumer Healthcare, NJ, 07417)
BD Microtainer™ tubes for blood collection (0.5 ml capacity) (BD Vacutainer Systems, NJ, 07417)
22-g, 24-g, 26-g intravenous catheters
Glass capillary tubes (with and without heparin) and clay for packed cell volume
1-inch bandaging material
Sexing probes
Metal feeding tubes with ball tip
Assorted red rubber tubes
Sizes 1–6 cuffed or uncuffed endotracheal tubes
Doppler
Flexible temperature probe and thermometer
Respiratory monitor
Heat lamps
Heating pads and/or forced air warmers (Bair Hugger™, Augustine Medical, Inc., Eden Prairie, MN)
Incubators with temperature control
Thermometer and hygrometer for cages
Food/water bowls and accessories that can be easily disinfected
Appropriate food for the species
UVB lights
Surgical pack with micro-instruments (ophthalmic instruments)
Otoscope and ophthalmoscope

DRUGS AND MEDICATIONS

Topical antibiotics (silver sulfadiazine, SilvaSorb®, Medline Industries, Inc., Mundelein, IL)
Ceftazidime
Ceftiofur crystalline free acid
Ciprofloxacin
Enrofloxacin
Metronidazole
Trimethoprim sulfa drugs
Tetracycline
Fenbendazole
Ivermectin (toxic to chelonians)
Alfaxalone
Ketamine
Medetomidine and atipamezole
Midazolam and flumazenil
Morphine/hydromorphone
Propofol
Tiletamine–zolazepam
Dextrose
Balanced crystalloid fluids (Normosol™ R, Hospira, Inc., Lake Forest, IL)
Lactated Ringer's solution
0.9% NaCl

ANATOMY AND PHYSIOLOGY OF REPTILES

Taxonomy (over 10,000 species)

Order	Sub-order	# of species
Squamata	Sauria (lizards)	6,512
	Serpentes (snakes)	3,709
	Amphisbaenia (worm lizards)	196
Chelonia	Cryptodira (turtles and tortoises)	351 (sub-orders combined)
	Pleurodira (side-necked turtles)	
Crocodylia (crocodilians)		24
Rhynchocephalia (tuataras)		1

METABOLISM

Reptiles have one-fifth to one-seventh of a mammal's metabolism at 37 degrees C (98.6 degrees F) and one-tenth of the food requirements compared with birds and mammals. The digestive efficiency of herbivores is 30–85% and that of carnivores is 70–95%. Reptiles are capable of switching to anaerobic metabolism to satisfy physiological needs during diving, fast sprints, etc., but this causes a significant drain of energy reserves.

Reptiles are ectothermic, but some species are capable of generating or retaining large amounts of heat. Some pythons can generate heat by muscle contractions to maintain the temperature of their eggs. Leatherback turtles (*Dermochelys coriacea*) have large amounts of body fat, which allows them to retain heat. Thermoregulation is primarily controlled by the preoptic nucleus of the hypothalamus but the pineal gland and parietal eye may also play a role. Most reptiles regulate their temperature by heliothermy or thigmothermy. Heliotherms absorb heat from radiant sources such as the sun. Thigmotherms absorb heat via conduction by being in contact with hot surfaces. Because of a greater ability to regulate heart rate, reptiles can heat up faster that they cool down. Right to left blood shunts allow reptiles to bypass the lungs and decrease evaporative losses. Vasodilation and constriction of peripheral vessels also aid in thermoregulation. During the day, the extremities will warm up first and peripheral vasodilation occurs. At night, peripheral vasoconstriction combined with a slower heart rate allows retention of core body heat. The heating and cooling of larger reptiles occurs more slowly. In general terms, the majority of common reptile species cared for in captivity typically have a preferred optimal temperature zone of 20–38 degrees C (68–100.4 degrees F) for most species. However, due to the wide array of natural habitats from which reptiles originate, the preferred optimal temperature zone can be quite varied.

BRUMATION

Brumation is the process by which a reptile reduces its metabolism and becomes dormant during the winter. As opposed to hibernation in mammals, brumating reptiles may retain a low level of activity, wake up to drink water and then go back into dormancy. The stimulus for and emergence from brumation is primarily influenced by temperature, but other factors, including reproduction and food availability, may also play a role. There are four stages of brumation:

1. A decrease in temperature leads to inhibition of appetite.
2. Reptiles seek a hibernaculum that provides insulation against freezing and enough moisture. Oxygen availability is less important.
3. Fat stores (liver, fat bodies, tail) are used as energy source, especially when emergence occurs in the spring.
4. Emergence from brumation is triggered by an increase in temperature with photoperiod having little to no influence since most brumate underground. During this period a reptile should not lose more than 10% of their body weight.

Captive reptiles undergoing brumation should be weighed on a bi-monthly schedule to monitor their weight. It is critical that water be available during brumation in captivity to avoid dehydration. Brumating reptiles can be soaked weekly to every other week.

Estivation is a period of inactivity during the dry season, mostly used by desert species in an effort to conserve water. Some turtles may leave the water during periods of drought and bury themselves on land until the conditions are favorable again. This is less likely to occur in captivity since a constant water source is available.

INTEGUMENT

The epidermis consists of the stratum corneum with an outer keratin layer, an intermediate lipid-rich layer and the stratum germinatum with cuboidal cells. Two types of keratin—alpha and beta—are present. Alpha keratin is flexible and is found in hinge regions of the skin, while the more rigid beta keratin provides strength and hardness, as in the shell of chelonians. The wide ventral scales of snakes are called gastropeges. The dermis is composed of connective tissue, blood vessels, lymphatics, and nerves.

Chromatophores are pigment-containing cells that lie between the epidermis and dermis. They may also occur in the peritoneum. Chromatophores function in camouflage, sexual display, thermoregulation, and behavior. Melanophores are located deep in the sub-epidermal layer and produce melanins, black, brown, yellow, or gray in color. Carotenoids can be found beneath the epidermis but above melanophores and produce yellow, red, and orange pigments. Iridophores located within the dermis contain guanine (a breakdown product of uric acid), which reflects light in the blue wavelength (Tyndall scattering). The combination of the iridophores' blue reflection and carotenoid yellow pigmentation create the green coloration common in many reptiles.

Ecdysis is the process by which reptiles shed their skin. Ecdysis is under pituitary and thyroid control. Continuous ecdysis occurs in chelonians and crocodilians while discontinuous ecdysis occurs in snakes, lizards, and tuataras. For simplicity, the ecdysis cycle can be split into a resting phase and a renewal phase, which has up to five stages. During the beginning of the renewal phase, the skin begins to appear duller, as regeneration of cells and enzymatic separation of the skin layers becomes activated. This period lasts approximately 5 ± 2 days. Afterwards, the skin becomes even duller and the spectacles turn opaque in what is commonly described as snakes being in "blue". This appearance is in large part due to lymphatic fluid accumulation that helps separate the old and new skin layers. This second period lasts 5 ± 2 days, followed by the last stage, during which lymphatic fluid resorption occurs leading to a clearing of the skin and spectacle. At this time, the skin regains some of its sheen and shedding typically occurs 5 ± 2 days after that. Hydration is critical for proper ecdysis and dehydration is a common cause of dysecdysis. The frequency of shedding will vary with environmental temperature, food intake, and growth of the animal.

SKELETAL SYSTEM

Unlike mammals, the bone epiphyses do not close in chelonians, snakes, and crocodilians. Epiphyses close later in life in lizards.

Reptiles have intervertebral bodies rather than disks. These intervertebral bodies are softer and form convexities in the anterior or posterior aspect to allow for additional flexibility and decreased pressure on the spinal cord. This arrangement allows reptiles the ability to tolerate and recover from spinal trauma better than mammals.

Reptile orders are classified based on the presence or absence of fenestrae in the temporal region of the skull. Anapsids lack temporal openings (e.g., chelonians). Diapsids have two openings in the temporal region behind the orbit, one superior (dorsal) and one inferior (e.g., tuataras and crocodilians). Squamates are modified diapsids, with lizards having only a dorsal opening while snakes have lost the upper temporal arch between the two openings. The quadrate bone articulates between the maxilla and mandible allowing increased movement of the skull, including the maxilla, a feature critical for some reptile species. Streptostyly is the ability of the quadrate bone to move back and forth in snakes due to their modified diapsid skull. Lizards and crocodilians have powerful snapping jaws due to the adductor muscles that arise from the temporal fossae and insert at right angles to close the jaw.

The vertebral column of reptiles can be divided into three sections: presacral (24 in lizards, 18 in chelonians, over 200 in snakes), sacral, and caudal. The atlas and axis are more rigidly connected than in mammals, so primary neck movement is between the single occipital condyle and the vertebral column. The number of cervical vertebrae varies across species, with crocodilians and varanids having nine, chelonians, tuataras, and most lizards eight, and chameleons three to five. There is no subarachnoid space but a subdural space between the leptomeninges and the dura mater is present.

CARDIOVASCULAR

The heart of crocodilians has four chambers (two atria and two ventricles) while that of all other reptile species has three chambers (two atria and one ventricle). The ventricle of non-crocodilian reptile hearts is divided into three chambers separated by incomplete muscular ridges. The cavum venosum receives blood from the right atrium dorsally and the paired aortas ventrally. The cavum arteriosum receives blood from the left atrium. The cavum pulmonale opens into the pulmonary artery and is equivalent to right ventricle in mammals. The admixture of oxygenated and deoxygenated blood varies across species and is influenced by the presence of a muscular ridge separating the three areas of the ventricle. The right and left cranial vena cava and the left hepatic vein supply blood to the sinus venosus. Reptiles have two aortas, with the left aorta giving rise to the celiac, cranial mesenteric, and left gastric arteries before joining the right aorta caudal to the heart. The blood flow through a non-crocodilian heart is outlined in Figure 1 (see web image supplementary content for section I).

RESPIRATORY SYSTEM

Nasal conchae are absent in chelonians but are present in other reptiles. Crocodilians and chelonians have complete tracheal rings, while they are incomplete in snakes and lizards. The lung anatomy is one of three basic types. Unicameral lungs are simple, single-chambered structures found in most snakes and some lizards, including tuataras. Paucicameral or transitional lungs have some internal divisions, but these are mostly incomplete and do not split the lung into separate chambers. They also lack intrapulmonary bronchus. Most iguanids, chameleons, and agamids have paucicameral lungs. Multicameral lungs are more complex with internal divisions and multiple bronchi. These lungs can be found in varanids, helodermatids, chelonians, and crocodilians. Chelonians have an exception as they possess a single, unbranched bronchus running the entire length of the lungs, with all lung chambers opening into this single bronchus.

In snakes, the lungs transform into an air sac structure caudally near the liver. In terrestrial species, the lung air sac terminates near the gallbladder, while in some aquatic species it terminates near the cloaca. In boids and colubrids, the respiratory portion is located between the heart and the cranial pole of the liver, while in most viperids and elapids there is a respiratory portion cranial to the heart. The right lung is always larger than the left. The left lung is well developed in boids and vestigial in colubrids. Multichambered lungs are found in the snake families Anomalepididae (primitive blind snakes), Typhlopidae (blind snakes), and Acrochordidae (primitive aquatic snakes from Australia and Indonesia).

Instead of alveoli, reptiles have faveolae (deeper than they are wide) and ediculae (wider than they are deep), which are air exchange chambers that have a similar function to alveoli. Both are present in the lung tissue but absent in the air sacs. Reptiles have a large lung volume but only 10–20% of the surface area when compared with mammals of similar size. Ventilation is triphasic with a cycle of expiration, inspiration, and relaxation (breath holding) that creates a constant fluctuation of oxygen concentration in the lungs. Oxygen tension and temperature have a significant role in ventilation/respiration. At higher temperatures, there is an increased demand for oxygen, which leads to an increase in tidal volume. Respiratory rate increases at low oxygen tensions and decreases at high oxygen tension.

DIGESTIVE SYSTEM

Reptilian teeth are composed of enamel, dentine, and cement, but lack a periodontal membrane. There are three types of dentition. Acrodont teeth attach to the surface of the bone and are not replaced. These are present in many lizards (bearded dragons, chameleons, water dragons). Pleurodont teeth attach to the labial aspect of the bone and are replaced. Pleurodont teeth can be found in snakes and iguanid lizards. Thecodont teeth attach via deep bony sockets and are continuously replaced, often throughout life. Thecodont teeth are present in crocodilians and some consider snake teeth as modified thecodonts.

Snakes and lizards hatched out of eggs possess an egg tooth, a modified premaxillary tooth to help break through the egg and its membranes. Chelonians and crocodilians have an egg caruncle—a horny tissue in that serves the function of the egg tooth.

Snake dentition is further classified based on presence or absence of fangs. Aglyphous snakes lack fangs (boids). Opisthoglyphous species are rear fanged. Some Colubridae, have modified parotid glands (hognose and boomslangs). Solenoglyphous species (Viperidae, i.e., copperheads, pit vipers, etc.) have rotating front fangs. Proteroglyphous snakes (Elapidae, i.e., cobras, sea snakes) have fixed front fangs. The venom glands are located behind the eyes.

Oral secretory glands (palatine, sublingual, mandibular) are present in many species for lubrication of prey items. In some snakes, these are modified into venom glands like the Duvernoy's gland in colubrids. Duvernoy's glands are posterior to the eye and some think they are analogous to venom glands in vipers and elapids while others consider them to be distinct glands. Helodermatids (Gila monsters and beaded lizards) have labial venom glands in the mandible, while snakes have maxillary venom glands.

Gastroliths may be seen radiographically and are thought to be functionally ingested only in crocodilians, with other species having accidental ingestion. Insectivorous species are thought to secrete chitinase by the stomach and pancreas to help digestion of the exoskeleton of insects.

As in birds, the cloaca is composed of the coprodeum, urodeum, and proctodeum. The colon empties into the coprodeum, while the genital and urinary openings enter

ANATOMY AND PHYSIOLOGY OF REPTILES (CONTINUED)

the urodeum. The proctodeum is the most caudal common chamber, which receives feces and urine before an evacuation occurs.

HEPATIC SYSTEM

The liver is surrounded by a Glisson's capsule and is a paler color in young and neonates. The right lobe is significantly larger in chelonians, which leads to the majority of urinary bladder stones being left sided, as the larger lobe pushes them to the left. The gallbladder is found within the right lobe. Biliverdin reductase is thought to be absent in most species, but may be present in crocodilians. Kupffer cells serve as sinusoidal macrophages.

Melanomacrophages may be numerous in some species and function as macrophages and free radical scavengers. Their brown pigment (as seen with hematoxylin and eosin stain) consists of iron and melanin granules. These cells may increase in size and number during disease states. Ito cells for storage of vitamin A may also be numerous in some species.

URINARY SYSTEM

Reptilian kidneys are metanephric, lack loop of Henle, renal pelvis, and pyramids. The nephron is composed of glomerulus, long and thick proximal convoluted tubule, short and thin intermediate segment, and a short distal tubule. The sexual segment, a terminal segment of the kidney in male snakes and lizards, becomes pale and enlarged during reproduction.

Osmoregulation in reptiles presents unique challenges. A reptile's body mass is approximately 70% water, similar to mammals but lower than amphibians (75–80%). Total sodium and potassium is similar to mammals but variation exists in larger species. Because of the lack of a loop of Henle, reptiles are unable to concentrate urine beyond their plasma osmolality. Methods of water conservation include the secretion of uric acid, presence of salt glands, fluid reabsorption from the cloaca, the renal portal system, and the ability to tolerate decreases in glomerular filtration rate. All reptiles produce and excrete uric acid, but some may also excrete ammonia and/or urea. Uric acid is the primary or only excretory product of terrestrial species. Uric acid is excreted via the renal tubules, so dehydration does not stop its excretion. It precipitates out of solution in the bladder or cloaca to form urates, which can be composed of potassium salts (herbivores) or sodium salts (carnivores). Uric acid is not a sensitive indicator of renal disease because over 60% of renal function must be lost in order to cause hyperuricemia; thus, dehydration is a more common cause of hyperuricemia. Ammonia and urea excretion occurs primarily in aquatic species. Crocodilians are ammoniotelic while freshwater turtles are ureotelic. Sea turtles excrete variable amounts of urea and ammonia. The cloaca, colon, and urinary bladder are significant sites of osmoregulation and allow active ion transport and passive water absorption through their walls. The bladder actively absorbs sodium while secreting potassium and urates.

The renal portal system is an afferent blood supply from the renal artery to the glomerulus. The renal portal vein (arising near epigastric and iliac veins) bypasses the glomerulus and enters at the tubules; thus, during dehydration the renal portal system perfuses the tubules to prevent necrosis. For this reason, the effects of the renal portal system on drug metabolism is of primary consideration for pharmaceuticals excreted by the tubules and not as critical for those excreted by glomerular filtration. Effects of the renal portal system on drug metabolism and excretion are variable according to the metabolic status of the animal and the pharmacokinetics of the drug.

REPRODUCTION

Reproduction is regulated by the pineal gland, hypothalamus, and pituitary glands, which process environmental stimuli into hormonal changes. In temperate species, gonadal stimulation occurs by increased temperature and longer days while in tropical species increased food availability and rainfall provide gonadal stimulation.

Sex determination may be genotypic (ZZ are males, ZW are female) or temperature dependent. Temperature sex determination is not reported or well known in snakes but occurs in all the other reptile groups. In chelonians, high temperatures yield mostly females while low temperatures yield a majority of males. In most the lizards, temperature sex determination is opposite to chelonians. Some turtles and lizards will have a predominance of females at high and low temperatures and males at intermediate temperatures. For crocodilians, females occur at low temperature (28–30 degrees C) in all species. At higher temperatures, different ratios of males and females occur across species.

The right gonad is located close to vena cava and connected to it by small vessels, while the left is associated with the left adrenal and has its own blood supply. In some male lizards, there is a single urodeum opening for the ureter and vas, while in other reptiles there are two separate openings.

The oviducts are responsible for egg transport and secretion of albumin, proteins, and calcium. The oviduct is divided from proximal to distal into the infundibulum, uterine tube, isthmus, uterus, and vagina. There is a three-phase ovarian cycle comprising:

1. Quiescent stage—no follicular development.
2. Vitellogenic phase—rapid hypertrophy of the ovary and oviduct, yolk production, increased estrogen, and calcium mobilization.
3. Gravidity/pregnancy—during which fertilization and oviposition occur. Many species have a pre-lay and/or a pre-ovulatory shed.

Reptiles may be oviparous or viviparous. All chelonians and crocodilians, most lizards (iguanids, monitors, geckos), all pythons, and most colubrids are oviparous. Oviparous reptiles produce two to three clutches per season, with the yolk being the only source of nutrients for the embryo. All boas and vipers, some skinks and chameleons, the European lizard, and garter snakes are viviparous. Viviparous species maintain the corpus luteum for longer, and produce one clutch per year with a longer gestation time. Viviparous species have a more drastic decrease in body condition of the females because they provide direct nutrition to the embryos.

IMMUNE SYSTEM

The lymphatic system is a wide network of lymphatic ducts, which are pumped by lymph hearts (smooth muscle dilations in lymphatic channels). Their primary connection with the venous system is at the base of the neck where a precardiac sinus transfers lymph to the venous system. A number of lymphatic trunks are described in mammals. The jugular trunk drains the head and neck regions. The subclavian trunk drains the forelimbs. The lumbar trunk drains the hind limbs, and the thoracic trunk drains the trunk and coelom. The lumbar and thoracic trunks form a dilation known as the cisterna chili. Some version of this system is suspected to exist in reptiles, but its specific anatomy and species variability are unknown.

The thymus of reptiles does not involute but does decrease in weight and size over time. In some species, such as crocodilians, there can be well-defined and widespread gut-associated lymphoid tissue. Well-defined lymphoid aggregates may also be found in other tissues such as the lungs.

SPECIAL SENSES

The eyes of reptiles can be quite varied. Reptiles have avascular retinas. Scleral ossicles are present in lizards and chelonians but absent in other reptiles. Reptiles have a conus papillary that is analogous to the pecten of birds. Most lizards have a nasolacrimal duct, but eyelids may be absent, as in the case of some gecko species. Chelonians lack a nasolacrimal duct and have a predominance of cones. Snakes have a nasolacrimal duct that drains the subspectacular space, but they lack a nasolacrimal gland. They are the only group to have scleral cartilage. The number of rods and cones in snakes will vary by species. Although it looks transparent, the spectacle of snakes is very vascular.

A vomeronasal organ is present in tuataras, lizards, and snakes, but absent in crocodilians. Its presence is debated in chelonians. Pit organs are openings in the maxillary and/or mandible of boas, pythons, and pit vipers, which serve to provide infrared detection of environmental cues. There are free nerve endings within the pits or scales, and this is thought to be a very sensitive system.

Suggested Reading

O'Malley, B. *Clinical Anatomy and Physiology of Exotic Species*. Edinburgh, NY: Elsevier Saunders, 2005.

Jacobson, ER. Overview of Reptile Biology, Anatomy, and Histology. In: Jacobson ER, ed. *Infectious Diseases and Pathology of Reptiles: Color Atlas and Text*. Boca Raton, FL: CRC Press; 2007: 1–130.

Fowler ME, Miller RE. Fowler's Zoo and Wild Animal Medicine, *Volume 8. St. Louis, MO: Elsevier*, 2015: Part II: Reptile Groups.

Mader DR. *Reptile Medicine and Surgery*. 2nd ed. St. Louis, MO: Saunders/ Elsevier; 2006.

Pet Industry Market Size & Ownership Statistics. The 2019–2020 American Pet Products Association National Pet Owners Survey © American Pet Products Association, Inc. https://www. american-petproducts.org/press_industrytrends.asp.

UVB LIGHTING PRINCIPLES FOR CAPTIVE REPTILES

Exposure to ultraviolet B (UVB) light is a critical aspect of reptile husbandry. UVB light supplementation is an absolute requirement for diurnal, herbivorous or omnivorous reptiles. While it is not an absolute requirement for nocturnal and carnivorous species, some may benefit from it. Unfortunately, this is an essential husbandry component that is still lacking in some captive reptiles and its omission contributes to the occurrence of secondary nutritional hyperparathyroidism. One challenge is the difficulty of obtaining easy to follow and accurate information on how to choose and use UVB lights properly. The abundance of misinformation on internet sites and the lack of training of pet store employees are further contributors to this problem. It is therefore essential that veterinarians working with reptiles are able to properly educate clients and provide easy to follow instructions on the use of UVB lights.

UVB LIGHT AND VITAMIN D3

Ultraviolet light is electromagnetic radiation that exists in three main bands: UVA, UVB, and UVC. Each band is characterized by a specific wavelength. UVA has the longest wavelength at 320–400nm while UVB has a wavelength of 290–320nm. Both UVA and UVB have low tissue penetration with most light being absorbed at the epidermis. UVA has a wavelength of less than 290nm, the deepest penetration, and is the most harmful. These wavelengths place ultraviolet somewhere between visible light (369–769nm) and X-rays (0.01–10nm). The ozone layer is responsible for filtering the majority of UV radiation hence protecting living organisms from its harmful exposure. UVC is considered germicidal and can have significant harmful effects to living animals while both UVA and UVB have therapeutic and physiologic applications. Still, as we know from human medicine, too much sun/ultraviolet exposure has a slew of negative implications ranging from sunburn to premature aging, and cancer.

UVB light is essential for the synthesis of vitamin D3. Although commonly referred to as a vitamin, D3 is actually a hormone. UVB light from the sun stimulates conversion of 7-dehydrocholesterol to cholecalciferol (D3) in the skin. Cholecalciferol is then transported to the liver via the blood stream and hydroxylated into 25-hydroxycholecalciferol (calcidiol), which is then transported to the kidneys for hydroxylation into 1,25-dihydroxycholecalci ferol(calcitriol), the active form of D3. The 25-hydroxycholecalciferol in the liver is the storage form of D3 and is a natural source of D3 for animals fed whole prey. Plants are a source of ergocalciferol or ergosterol (D2), which is not readily bioavailable to most reptiles and is therefore not an appropriate source of D3 supplementation. Calcidiol, an animal source of D3, is more bioavailable for reptiles.

There are two main sources of UVB, natural sunlight and UVB bulbs. Exposure to natural sunlight is the most efficient way for reptiles to produce adequate levels of D3. However, this is often not possible year round, outside the tropics and some subtropical regions, necessitating the use of artificial UVB light sources.

CHOOSING UVB LIGHTING

There has been a long-standing debate about the effectiveness and even potential harmful effects of artificial UVB lights. Like the application of any treatment or therapeutic, the use of UVB lights must be in accordance with certain parameters for it to be effective and safe. Nowadays there are high-quality bulbs in the market that provide adequate UVB while also being safe when used appropriately. UVB bulbs can be further divided into linear fluorescent, compact fluorescents, and mercury vapor. In the future, commercial LED UVB lights may also become available. Fluorescent UVB bulbs provide light in the required wavelength for D3 synthesis but no heat. Mercury vapor bulbs provide both heat and UVB.

There are six main aspects to consider when selecting a UVB bulb:

1. Size/type of the enclosure.
2. Type of material between the bulb and the reptile.
3. Type of bulb.
4. Effective distance of the bulb.
5. Bulb longevity.
6. Species of reptile.

Another consideration is the type of fixture used for the bulb. There are a number of reptile-specific fixtures that offer the advantage of having reflective materials to increase light reflection and decrease scattered light emission (radiation). Some also have a ceramic base and are more tolerant of higher temperatures produced by mercury vapor bulbs. Reptile-specific light fixtures or those that reflect light away from the bulb and towards the animal are preferred over plastic fixtures or those without reflective properties.

T8 LINEAR FLUORESCENT TUBES

T8 bulbs (25-mm or 1-inch diameter) are available in different lengths and fit into standard aquarium or reptile hoods. Some manufacturers further classify their bulbs by a number system ranging from 2.0 to 10.0. This number represents the percentage of light that is emitted in the UVB spectrum. A 5.0 has 5% of the emitted light in the UVB spectrum; a 10.0 has 10% UVB emission, and so on. Arcadia® has simplified the process by simply stating the percentage of UVB emission with their bulbs ranging from 6% to 14%.

Being a longer bulb also means there is more scattered radiation so the UVB exposure is not as focused. One recommendation is that the longest bulb possible be used to cover a wide area of the enclosure. An alternative is to use a shorter bulb in combination with a heat lamp while leaving the rest of the cage shaded. These bulbs emit UVB light at an average effective distance of 12–20 inches, depending on the brand and percentage of emitted UVB. It is generally recommended that animals should not be abe to get any closer than within 3–4 inches of bulb's surface. Bulbs need to be replaced every 6–12 months according to manufacturer's recommendations.

T5 HIGH OUTPUT LINEAR FLUORESCENTS

A high-output light is a T5 bulb (16-mm or 0.6-inch diameter) that requires a hood with a T5 fixture. T5 bulbs are more efficient and provide a higher amount of UVB than T8 or compact fluorescent bulbs. In theory a T5 10.0 bulb produces a higher amount of UVB than a T8 10.0 or compact fluorescent. It is worth mentioning that Zoo Med Laboratories Inc. produces a T8 10.0 bulb labeled high output but their T5 10.0 bulb is actually a much stronger bulb and is considered as a true high output for our purposes. These bulbs emit UVB light at an effective distance of 12–36 inches, depending on the brand and percent of emitted UVB. While it is generally recommended that animals should not have the ability to get any closer than within 3–4 inches of bulb's surface, this distance may actually need to be longer for high output bulbs. They must be replaced every 9–12 months according to manufacturer's recommendations.

COMPACT FLUORESCENT

Compact fluorescent bulbs can be fitted into any incandescent fixture that would fit a household bulb but a reflective or reptile-specific fixture is preferred. The light is focused over a smaller area so there is less scattered radiation. For this reason, it is possible that a 10.0 compact fluorescent may actually emit a higher UVB output than a 10.0 linear fluorescent over the same area. It is usually recommended to place these bulbs next to the heat lamp so the reptile gets UVB exposure while basking. All other properties are similar to the linear fluorescent bulbs although some may think of these as being less effective and being "weaker" in the UVB spectrum.

MERCURY VAPOR BULBS

Mercury vapor bulbs have been successfully used by breeders and zoological institutions for decades but have just recently made it into the mainstream exotic pet market. Their external appearance is that of a floodlight and they are commonly found as a self-ballasted variety in the pet trade. Self-ballasted bulbs can be fitted into an incandescent fixture that would fit a household bulb but a reflective or reptile-specific fixture is preferred. A fixture with a ceramic base is also recommended because of the high amount of heat the bulbs produce. The light is focused over a shorter area so there is less scattered radiation. Their UVB output is based on the wattage of the bulb and the fixture should accommodate the appropriate wattage. Their effective distance is 12–36 inches. There are also some high-output bulbs with an effective distance of up to 8 feet. A major advantage is the production of heat and a stronger UVB output compared with all other bulb types. In the hands of inexperienced individuals, however, these bulbs could be detrimental to reptiles. If placed too close to the animal, they could cause thermal damage. There is also a concern about overexposure to UVB, which could cause eye damage and even neoplasias. It is imperative that these bulbs are used properly; the author only recommends them for zoological institutions and advanced hobbyist who understand the principles of UVB exposure in reptiles. They must be replaced every 3—12 months, depending on manufacturer, model, and use.

METAL HALIDE BULBS

Metal halide bulbs are becoming more commonly available. They produce heat, UVB, and infrared light. Their beam is very narrow compared to all other bulb types which means that they can provide very high UVB levels but over a narrow area, which may be a positive feature in some enclosures (e.g., tall enclosures) but dangerous in others (e.g., short enclosures). These bulbs require external ballast and a properly rated fixture for operation and safety. Their use is best reserved for advanced hobbyist familiar with the principles of UVB lighting.

UVB REDUCTION

As previously mentioned, the type of material present between the bulb and the animal is an important consideration when selecting a UVB bulb. Most glass and plastics are known to block or filter out UVB radiation and are not recommended. The ideal scenario is one of an open-topped enclosure with no material present between the bulb and the animal. While this is a possible application for chelonians, it is not feasible when housing snakes and some lizard species. A study by Burger et. al. revealed the UVB attenuating effects of common materials used in reptile enclosures and provides a sobering insight into the use of UVB bulbs (Burger et al, 2007).

The type of material, aperture of the openings, thickness, and reflective properties can all influence UVB attenuation and can significantly decrease the UVB exposure of reptiles. Most reptile enclosures have a screen or wire mesh top to keep the animals from escaping. Some of these screens may reduce the UVB light exposure to the animal by as much as 50%. To put this in perspective, if a reptile had a 10.0 linear fluorescent bulb, the effectiveness of that bulb might be reduced to that of a 5.0 by the time the light passes the screen and reaches the animal. This is why knowing the type of screen material is critical when selecting a bulb. A general recommendation is to select a screen with the largest aperture possible and with a mat or painted finish that will reflect less light.

SELECTING BULBS BASED ON SPECIES

There is a common trend toward making recommendations of bulbs based on the species with which it will be used. The principle behind this makes sense but in practice it is flawed. The thought is that tropical, desert or diurnal species require higher UVB exposure and therefore a stronger UVB bulb, while more temperate, or forest species require a lower UVB exposure and therefore a weaker bulb. These principles would hold true in open-topped enclosures without a lid or when the bulb is placed inside the enclosure. However as mentioned previously, when the bulb is placed atop a screen, it can block a significant portion of the UVB reaching the animal. Therefore the author recommends selecting a bulb not simply based on the species but rather a combination of the species and the specific enclosure set-up for the particular animal. There have been some cases in which animals where overexposed to UVB due to manufacturing errors in some UVB bulbs. As a consequence, some people believe that 10.0 bulbs are too strong and harmful for reptiles. This is not the case. In fact, it is difficult to replicate the natural UVB exposure from the sun and most bulbs cannot replace natural sunlight. It is rather the erroneous use of UVB bulbs that can lead to problems. Even a 2.0 bulb could cause problems if the reptile is allowed to come in direct contact with the bulb, as this is not the intended use. Buying a UVB bulb from a reputable manufacturer that provides clear guidance as to how to use the bulbs is the first step in the safe use of UVB bulbs. The second aspect is ensuring that the owners and caretakers are indeed using the bulbs in the safest, most efficient manner for the particular species.

MEASURING UVB

Another challenge in selecting the proper UVB bulb is the fact that bulb strength or percentage UVB emission does not directly translate to its effectiveness in stimulating vitamin D3 synthesis in the body. There are in vitro models to assess the efficiency of UVB light (Burger et al, 2007) but these are impractical in a clinical setting. We must rely on the reputation of the manufacturer to ensure the bulb is of good enough quality. How much UVB a particular reptile species requires is another question, without a clear answer. In general terms, reptiles should have exposure to a minimum of 13–20 $\mu W/cm^2$ UVB irradiance with tropical species needing as much as 30–40 $\mu W/cm^2$, and desert species requiring as much as 150 $\mu W/cm^2$. Much research is needed to confirm this information, but it is a starting reference point. In nature, UVB exposure will vary with time of day, cloud covering, and so on, but in captivity the exposure level will be fairly constant while the bulb is turned on. Providing hiding places and a gradient of UVB light can help to reduce UVB overexposure although in practice overexposure is not as common of an event.

One practical option is to measure the UVB irradiance using a hand-held radiometer. While expensive (approximately $250.00) these units are available to the general public. Their accuracy has been questioned, but they remain a good tool for the average reptile owner. A radiometer can be used to measure UVB irradiance of a bulb at any distance to determine how much UVB is being emitted and to record the decay of transmission over time. For example a 10.0 linear fluorescent bulb may emit 50 $\mu W/cm^2$ at 12 inches when first purchased but after 6 months, the irradiance at 12 inches may have decreased to 25 $\mu W/cm^2$. While this may still be acceptable exposure, it certainly indicates decrease in the bulb's effectiveness over time. This decay is normal but if one desires to provide a more constant UVB exposure year round, it may be time to purchase a new bulb. They can also be used to evaluate the effect of the screen or mesh cover on the effectiveness of a bulb to help clients select the most appropriate bulb for their set-up. Some newer radiometers measure ultraviolet index providing scale from minimum to very high while others provide readout based on the

UVB LIGHTING PRINCIPLES FOR CAPTIVE REPTILES (CONTINUED)

Ferguson zones to help determine the UVB exposure. These radiometers are advertised as being able to measure the appropriate UVB dose for vitamin D3 synthesis although that claim has not been verified.

CALCIUM SUPPLEMENTATION

All animals need a source of calcium and a calcium to phosphorus ratio of 1.5 to 2. Carnivorous animals eating adult whole prey items have the advantage of obtaining calcium form the prey's bones. However herbivorous and omnivorous reptiles often lack an appropriate source of calcium. Young carnivores being fed immature prey items or carnivores not being offered whole prey items should also be supplemented with calcium. Most plant materials and invertebrates have a negative calcium to phosphorus ratio, so animals must find other sources of calcium. In their natural environment, these animals will travel to clay and mineral deposits or select particular feedstuffs to supplement their calcium intake. In captivity, reptiles do not have the opportunity to seek calcium sources but rather rely on it being supplemented in their diet. All herbivorous, omnivorous, and insectivorous reptiles require calcium supplementation.

Various commercial sources of calcium are available, but some are better than others. First off, it is recommended that calcium supplements be purely calcium with no phosphorus or vitamin D3. While many see a benefit of adding a D3 supplement, there are serious and real concerns about over supplementation with vitamin D3. Adding a calcium supplement that also contains phosphorus does not make sense because the reptiles are already in a negative calcium to phosphorus imbalance. Adding more phosphorus would not help solve this imbalance in an effective manner. The author prefers calcium only supplements including calcium powders sold for reptiles, cuttle bones, and crushed oyster shells. Another alternative is the use of fruit-flavored calcium carbonate antacid tablets. These tables are more palatable than other products. They can be pulverized or fed in small pieces.

Regardless of the type of supplement, calcium is best offered daily to account for variations in intake. The supplement is mixed with the vegetables or by coating prey items. However, it must be noted that when insects are coated with a powdered supplement, the powder will fall off within 10–20 minutes. Insects should therefore be dusted immediately before feeding. There are some products that advertise calcium in a spray or gel cubes. These have not been proven to be effective and should be avoided until research to support their effectiveness is available. There are also some multivitamin products advertised for reptiles, and many of these include calcium as well as D3. Given that we do not know the nutritional requirement of most reptile species, the use of multivitamins is questionable. While it may be beneficial in some species it could be detrimental in others that may be over supplemented by certain minerals or vitamins. Finally, earthworms and hornworms (Manduca sp.) are two excellent sources of nutrition for carnivores and invertebrates because they tend to have a positive calcium to phosphorus ratio. However, this ratio can also vary with the conditions in which they are reared and maintained.

SUMMARY

All this information can be overwhelming to veterinarians and clients alike. It is important to understand the basics of UVB requirements and the factors that affect UVB supplementation. All six factors must be considered when selecting a bulb, as there is no single best bulb for every situation. There are new studies and products available every year, so it is also important to stay current on the literature and technological advances in order to provide better recommendations to clients. Proper calcium supplementation together with UVB light exposure is critical to prevent secondary nutritional hyperparathyroidism. The absence of either or both of these elements from the history of a reptile's case should prompt veterinarians to include nutritional secondary hyperparathyroidism as a differential diagnosis.

GENERAL RECOMMENDATIONS FOR UVB LIGHTING IN REPTILE ENCLOSURES

For open-topped enclosures or when there is no material between the bulb and the animal:

1. Use a T8 5–12% bulb at distances up to 15 inches between the bulb and the animal; for distances over 15 inches, a T8 12–14% or T5 10% bulb may be required.
2. Provide a UVB and heat gradient with the UVB bulb covering one-third to three-quarters of the cage length/depth.
3. Turn UVB light on for 10–12 hours daily.

For enclosures with a screen/mesh between the bulb and the animal:

1. Use a T8 10–12% bulb at distances up to 15 inches between the bulb and the animal; for distances over 15 inches, a T8 12–14% or T5 10% bulb may be required.
2. Provide a UVB and heat gradient with the UVB bulb covering one-third to three-quarters of the cage length/depth.
3. Turn UVB light on for 10–12 hours daily.

Note: Depending on the type of mesh, there may be a 30–50% reduction in UVB, which must be taken into consideration when selecting the bulb. The use of a UVB radiometer is more critical when the bulb is placed above a mesh to determine the actual UVB exposure.

Suggested Reading

Acierno MJ, Mitchell MA, Zachariah TT, et al. Effects of ultraviolet radiation on plasma 25-hydroxyvitamin D3 concentrations in corn snakes (*Elaphe guttata*). *Am J Vet Res* 2008;69(2):294–297.

Burger RM, Gehrmann WH, Ferguson GW. Evaluation of UVB reduction by materials commonly used in reptile husbandry. *Zoo Biol.* 2007;26:417–423.

ANATOMY AND PHYSIOLOGY OF AMPHIBIANS

Amphibians are a group of vertebrates with significant conservation challenges. They have a worldwide distribution, but most species occur in tropical climates. There are over 8,000 amphibian species distributed among three orders: Anura, Cuadata, and Gymnophiona.

The order Anura includes frogs and toads and comprises the majority of amphibians with over 7,200 known species. In general terms, frogs live in or near water while toads are more terrestrial. As such, frogs have thinner more permeable skin while toads have thicker skin to protect against dehydration. The vast majority of anurans are oviparous but a few ovoviviparous to viviparous species exist.

The order Caudata includes salamanders and newts, with over 700 species. Salamanders are primarily terrestrial while newts are aquatic to semiaquatic. Sirens and amphiumas are primarily aquatic. Amphibians in this order are mostly oviparous and are capable of neoteny, which is the retention of juvenile characteristics in fully mature animal. As such, neotenic amphibians can reproduce despite the retention of juvenile features like gills. There are three types of neoteny described—obligate, inducible, and facultative. Obligate neotenic species are not able to metamorphose either in nature or through experimental stimulation. The families Amphiumidae (amphiumas), Sirenidae (sirens), Proteidae (mudpuppies, waterdogs, European blind cave salamander), and Cryptobranchidae (giant salamanders) are all known to express obligate neoteny. Inducible obligate neotenic species do not metamorphose in nature but can be induced to metamorphose through the administration of thyroxine or thyroid-stimulating hormone. Perhaps the best-known neotenic species, the axolotl (*Ambystoma mexicanum*) is an inducible obligate neotenic species, although many specimens are reported to have a shorter lifespan after metamorphosis. Some members of the family Plethodontidae (lungless salamanders) are also inducible obligate neotenic species. Metamorphosis in the facultative neotenic species occurs according to environmental conditions, most commonly associated with the lack of development of the thyroid gland. Facultative neotenic species can be found in the families Ambystomatidae, Salamandridae (true salamanders, newts), and Hynobiidae (Asiatic salamanders). The tiger salamander (*Ambystoma tigrinum*) is the best-known facultative neotenic species.

The order Gymnophiona includes caecilians, which are a lesser known and studied group with over 200 species. Caecilians resemble earthworms and have reduced or absent eyes and limbs. There are both aquatic and terrestrial species that are mostly found in tropical lowlands. New world species are primarily viviparous while those from the old-world are oviparous.

METABOLISM

When housed in captivity, providing an appropriate temperature and thermal gradient is critical for amphibian health. Amphibians may show a variety of clinical signs at extreme temperatures (Figure 2– see web image supplementary content for section I).

Amphibians are sensitive to desiccation and have developed techniques for regulating body temperature and retaining moisture. Changes in posture, locomotion, and skin color can be used to regulate temperature. Cooling can be accomplished by standing away from the ground and changing to a pale body color to decrease heat absorption. Peripheral vasodilation or constriction can also regulate the rate at which they dissipate or absorb heat. Some amphibians, anurans in particular, can produce glandular secretions that allow them to cover part of their bodies in a waxy substance to protect against desiccation. These secretions are usually limited to the dorsal skin only, as ventral skin must remain thin to allow water uptake via the pelvic drink patch. Up to 80% of the total water uptake may occur through this pelvic patch. Dried mucus may also be used to cover the skin. Finally, they have iridophores that provide high skin reflectivity near the infrared spectrum (700–900 μm) to decrease solar heat exposure.

Some amphibians have developed specialized methods for surviving cold temperatures through a technique known as super cooling. Super cooling lowers the freezing point of tissues through a combination of physiological adaptations: higher amount of fibrinogen, glucose-transporting proteins and ice-nucleating proteins in blood, low molecular weight carbohydrates (glycerol or glucose) in blood and tissues, and increasing plasma osmolarity by dehydration. These adaptations also promote ice growth in extracellular compartments while sparing the cells. In addition, they have good anoxia tolerance for freeze-induced ischemia.

ANATOMY

Anurans can range from 1 cm to 30 cm in length and have glandular skin that may be smooth or have protuberances. Adults lack gills and claws are absent except in *Xenopus* sp. While anurans lack tails, frogs in the genus *Ascaphus* are referred to as tailed frogs due to the presence of a cloacal protrusion resembling a tail, which is actually an organ used by the males for copulation and internal fertilization.

Salamanders range from 4 cm to 1.5 m in length, have glandular skin and lack claws. Most have four legs except sirens, which lack pelvic limbs.

Caecilians range from 7.5 cm to 75 cm in length and lack limbs. A short tail is present in some species. A unique feature is the presence of small olfactory and sensory tentacles in the nasolabial groove.

Skeleton

Order	Features
Anurans	4 legs with 4 toes on the front and 5 toes on the back Fused vertebrae—presacral, sacral, postsacral Lack sacrum Pelvic girdle is fused Forelimb—scapula, humerus, radioulnar joint, carpals, metacarpals, phalanges Hind limb—femur, tibiofibular joints, tarsals, metatarsal, phalanges Urostyle—fused caudal vertebrae
Caudata	4 legs but hind reduced in mud eels and missing in sirens 4 toes on the front and 5 toes on the back Capable of limb and toe regeneration Tail autotomy
Caecilians	Lack pectoral/pelvic girdle and sacrum

CARDIOVASCULAR

Amphibians have a three-chambered heart with two atria and one ventricle. There is an interatrial septum that is complete in anurans but fenestrated in caecilians and most salamanders. This septum may allow for some mixture of oxygenated and deoxygenated blood. A renal portal system is also present. A unique adaptation of amphibians is the presence of an extensive lymphatic system with lymph hearts, lymph sac dilations surrounded by muscle, which allows them to beat independently of the heart. The lymph hearts provide unidirectional flow of lymph to the heart and can beat at a rate of up to 60 beats/minute. The lymph contains all blood components except red cells.

ANATOMY AND PHYSIOLOGY OF AMPHIBIANS (CONTINUED)

VENIPUNCTURE SITES

Venipuncture can be challenging in many species but there are various sites where blood can be accessed. Sedation or anesthesia may be required to successfully collect blood, especially if attempting cardiac puncture. Venipuncture sites include the femoral vein, ventral abdominal vein, lingual vein/plexus, tail vein, maxillary/facial vein, musculocutaneous vein, and the heart.

IMMUNE SYSTEM

The blood of amphibians is composed of erythrocytes, thrombocytes, monocytes, lymphocytes, eosinophils, basophils, and neutrophils. Morphology of the white blood cells can be quite variable, so obtaining accurate white cell counts can be challenging when working with laboratories not familiar with their cell morphology. Their function is presumed to be similar to other species, but further research is still needed in this area.

Some amphibians lack a truly functional bone marrow, so hematopoiesis can occur in the spleen, liver, and kidneys, according to age and species. The spleen is composed of a red pulp responsible for erythropoiesis and white pulp responsible for myelopoiesis. The thymus produces T-lymphocytes and is functional through life. The size of the spleen and thymus are affected by seasons, nutritional status, and stress. A well-developed gut associated lymphoid tissue is present instead of lymph nodes.

RESPIRATORY SYSTEM

Amphibians have unique adaptations for respiration. In addition to traditional lung (pulmonic) respiration, they can also exchange gas via buccopharyngeal respiration, which allows exchange at the level of the oral and pharyngeal cavity. Cutaneous respiration may comprise up to 80% of the gas exchange, especially in aquatic species. Lateral folds, costal grooves, or cutaneous hairs may be present to increase surface area of the skin and improve the efficiency of cutaneous respiration. Finally, branchial/gill respiration occurs in juvenile stages and in neotenic species.

Amphibians have short tracheas with complete rings and single chambered lungs without alveoli. Instead there are a series of infoldings of the lungs that increase surface area. Lungs are absent in Plethodontidae and reduced or absent in the Hynobiidae.

Anuran larvae have small, simple gills covered by an operculum similar to fish. In contrast, salamander larvae have external gills without an operculum. The gills of caecilians are resorbed before birth/hatch. In anurans, they are resorbed during stages of metamorphosis. Salamanders resorb their gills during metamorphosis but they are retained in neotenic species.

INTESTINAL TRACT

The majority of adult amphibians are carnivores, but larvae may be herbivores. Sirens may also remain omnivorous into adulthood. Caecilians rely on olfaction to find prey while anurans and urodeles rely primarily on sight. Amphibians have jointed pediceled teeth in which the crown is loosely attached to the base (pedicel) of the tooth. The tooth itself attaches to the jaw. Teeth are used for holding prey in place rather than chewing, so they are often angled backward toward the pharynx. Teeth are shed and replaced through life. There are one or two rows of maxillary and mandibular teeth in most species. However, ranid frogs lack mandibular teeth and bufonid toads have no teeth. Anurans and salamanders have well-developed moveable tongues commonly used for prey apprehension. Caecilians have fixed tongues. Frogs in the family Pipidae (clawed frogs and Surinam toads) lack tongues and vocal cords.

LIVER

Liver anatomy varies among amphibian species. Anurans have a more traditional bilobed liver while in Caudates and Caecilians it is elongated and marginated. The gall bladder is usually well developed and intimately associated with the liver. A bile duct connects to the duodenum or pancreatic duct in some species. The liver is a significant erythropoietic center and also contributes to leukocyte production during metamorphosis. A large amount of pigmented melanomacrophages and non-pigmented Kupffer cells can be found and contribute to immune function. The amount of these cells present at any given time is influenced by seasonality. They also increase in numbers with age and antigenic stimulation. Melanomacrophages are commonly identified in aspirates of animals with coelomitis.

URINARY SYSTEM

Amphibians have mesonephric kidneys that cannot concentrated urine above plasma osmolality. A single or bilobed urinary bladder is present in most species. Larvae and aquatic species are primarily ammoniotelic while terrestrial species are primarily ureotelic. There is a lesser number of primary uricotelic species (waxy tree frogs). Clawed frogs have the ability to be ammoniotelic or ureotelic depending on water availability.

REPRODUCTION

The amphibian reproductive tract consists of either testes – Wolffian duct – cloaca, or ovaries – coelom – infundibulum – oviduct.

The Bidder's organ is a remnant of ovarian tissue in male bufonid frogs and does not indicate hermaphroditism. Salamanders have internal fertilization but lack an intromittent organ. Instead, sperm packets are deposited on the environment to be picked up by the female. The exceptions are the Asiatic salamanders and giant salamander, which deposit sperm on egg masses. Caecilians have internal copulation and fertilization with a phallodeum for intromission and 75% are viviparous.

Examples of sexual dimorphism:

- bullfrogs—males have large tympanic membranes
- White's tree frogs—males have nuptial pads during breeding season
- dyeing arrow frogs—males have large triangular toes, females have small, round toes
- red-eyed tree frogs—males are smaller.

NERVOUS SYSTEM

The spinal cord in anurans ends in the lumbar vertebrae and a cauda equina is present. In caecilians and salamanders, the spinal cord extends to the tip of the tail. A lateral line similar to that in fish is present in larvae and aquatic species.

UVB Lighting Principles for Captive Amphibians

Exposure to ultraviolet B (UVB) light is a critical aspect of reptile husbandry, but there is less information available about its requirement for amphibian species. As in reptiles, UVB and/or calcium deficiencies are suspected to contribute to the development of nutritional secondary hyperparathyroidism in amphibians. However, it is more difficult to make specific recommendations on UVB use in amphibians due to the lack of information on this subject. Some background information and general guidelines are provided here to assist in the decision-making process when selecting UVB sources for amphibians.

UVB LIGHT AND VITAMIN D3

Ultraviolet light (UV) is electromagnetic radiation that exists in three main bands: UVA, UVB, and UVC. Each band is characterized by a specific wavelength. UVA has the longest wavelength at 320–400 nm while UVB has a wavelength of 290–320 nm. Both UVA and UVB have low tissue penetration with most being absorbed at the epidermis. UVA has a wavelength of less than 290 nm, the deepest penetration, and is the most harmful. These wavelengths place ultraviolet somewhere between visible light (369–769 nm) and x-rays (0.01–10 nm). The ozone layer is responsible for filtering the majority of ultraviolet radiation hence protecting living organisms from its harmful exposure. UVC is considered germicidal and can have significant harmful effects to living animals while both UVA and UVB have therapeutic and physiologic applications. Still, as we know from human medicine, too much sun/ultraviolet exposure, has a slew of negative implications ranging from sunburn to premature aging, and cancer.

UVB light is essential for the synthesis of vitamin D3. Although commonly referred to as a vitamin, D3 is actually a hormone. UVB light from the sun stimulates conversion of 7-dehydrocholesterol to cholecalciferol (D3) in the skin. Cholecalciferol is then transported to the liver via the blood stream and hydroxylated into 25-hydroxycholecalciferol (calcidiol), which is then transported to the kidneys for hydroxylation into 1,25-dihydroxycholecalciferol (calcitriol), the active form of D3. The 25-hydroxycholecalciferol in the liver is the storage form of D3 and is a natural source of D3 for animals fed whole prey. Plants are a source of ergocalciferol or ergosterol (D2), which is not readily bioavailable to most animals and is therefore not an appropriate source of D3 supplementation. Calcidiol, an animal source of D3, is more bioavailable for most animal species, and is suspected to be the same for amphibians.

There are two main sources of UVB, natural sunlight and UVB bulbs. Exposure to natural sunlight is likely the most efficient way for amphibians to synthesize adequate levels of D3. However, there is a high degree of variability in the lifestyle of amphibians from cryptic species that barely get sunlight exposure to those that may display basking behaviors similar to reptiles. This variability makes it nearly impossible to provide blanket recommendations for UVB supplementation for amphibians. Instead, we must rely on knowledge of the natural behaviors of the species, their geographical location, and expected UVB exposures at that location to make extrapolations about the use of UVB light supplementation in captivity. One thing that most can agree on is the fact that amphibians should be exposed to lower levels of UVB than reptiles.

CHOOSING UVB LIGHTING

UVB bulbs can be divided into linear fluorescent, compact fluorescents, and mercury vapor. In the future, commercial LED UVB lights may also become available. Fluorescent UVB bulbs provide light in the required wavelength for D3 synthesis, but no heat. Mercury vapor bulbs provide both heat and UVB. Mercury vapor bulbs can provide very high levels of UVB exposure and their use should be avoided in amphibians. There are six main aspects to consider when selecting a UVB bulb:

1. Size/type of the enclosure.
2. Type of material between the bulb and the amphibian.
3. Type of bulb.
4. Effective distance of the bulb.
5. Bulb longevity.
6. Species of amphibian.

Another consideration is the type of fixture used for the bulb. There are a number of fixtures that offer the advantage of having reflective materials to increase light reflection and decrease scattered light emission (radiation). Reptile/amphibian-specific light fixtures or those that reflect light away from the bulb and towards the animal are preferred over plastic fixtures or those without reflective properties.

T8 Linear Fluorescent Tubes

The T8 bulbs (25-mm or 1-inch diameter) are available in different lengths and fit into standard aquarium or reptile hoods. Some manufacturers further classify their bulbs by a number system ranging from 2.0 to 10.0. This number represents the percentage of light that is emitted in the UVB spectrum. A 5.0 has 5% of the emitted light in the UVB spectrum, a 10.0 has 10% UVB emission, and so on. Arcadia® has simplified the process by simply stating the percentage of UVB emission with their bulbs ranging from 6% to 14%. For amphibians, bulbs emitting less than 5% UVB are likely the best option to avoid the possibility of overexposure.

Being a longer bulb also means that there is more scattered radiation, so the UVB exposure is not as focused. This may actually be of benefit for amphibian enclosures. The use of a shorter bulb, while leaving the rest of the cage shaded, is a preferred setup for amphibians. These bulbs emit UVB light at an average effective distance of 12–20 inches depending on the brand and percent of emitted UVB. It is generally recommended that animals should not have the ability to get any closer than within 3–4 inches of bulb's surface. They must be replaced every 6–12 months according to manufacturer's recommendations.

T5 High-Output Linear Fluorescents

A high-output light is a T5 bulb (16-mm or 0.6-inch diameter) that requires a hood with a T5 fixture. T5 bulbs are more efficient and provide a higher amount of UVB than T8 or compact fluorescent bulbs. In theory, a T5 10.0 bulb produces a higher amount of UVB than a T8 10.0 or compact fluorescent. It is worth mentioning that Zoo Med Laboratories Inc. produces a T8 10.0 bulb labeled high output but their T5 10.0 bulb is actually a much stronger bulb and is considered as a true high output for our purposes. These bulbs emit UVB light at an effective distance of 12–36 inches depending on the brand and percentage of emitted UVB. While it is generally recommended that animals should not be able to get any closer than within 3–4 inches of bulb's surface, this distance may actually need to be longer for high output bulbs. They must be replaced every 9–12 months, according to manufacturer's recommendations. T5 bulbs likely produce more UVB than most amphibians should be exposed to, and should be avoided or only used under extreme caution while monitoring UVB exposure levels. As with the T8 bulbs, only those with 5% UVB or less should be used.

Compact Fluorescent

Compact fluorescent bulbs can be fitted into any incandescent fixture that would fit a household bulb but a reflective or reptile-specific fixture is preferred. The light is focused over a smaller area so there is less scattered radiation. For this reason, it is possible that a 10.0 compact fluorescent may actually emit a higher UVB output than a 10.0 linear fluorescent over the same area. It is usually recommended to place these bulbs next to the heat lamp, so the amphibian gets UVB exposure while basking. All other properties are similar to the linear

UVB LIGHTING PRINCIPLES FOR CAPTIVE AMPHIBIANS (CONTINUED)

fluorescent bulbs although some may think of these as being less effective and being "weaker" in the UVB spectrum. As with the linear fluorescent bulb, animals should not have the ability to get any closer than within 3–4 inches of bulb's surface. A 5% or lower should be used for amphibians.

UVB REDUCTION

As previously mentioned, the type of material present between the bulb and the animal is an important consideration when selecting a UVB bulb. Most glass and plastics are known to block or filter out UVB radiation and are not recommended. The ideal scenario is one of an open-topped enclosure with no material present between the bulb and the animal. While this is a possible application for salamanders and some aquatic species, it is not feasible when housing anurans and other species. A study by Burger et al revealed the UVB attenuating effects of common materials used in reptile enclosures and provides a sobering insight into the use of UVB bulbs (Burger et al, 2007). The type of material, aperture of the openings, thickness, and reflective properties can all influence UVB attenuation and can significantly decrease the UVB exposure of reptiles. Most amphibian enclosures have a screen or wire mesh top to keep the animals from escaping. Some of these screens may reduce the UVB light exposure to the animal by as much as 50%. To put this in perspective, if an amphibian had a 5% linear fluorescent bulb, the effectiveness of that bulb might be reduced to that of a 2.5% by the time the light passes the screen and reaches the animal. This is why knowing the type of screen material is critical when selecting a bulb. A general recommendation is to select a screen with the largest aperture possible and with a mat or painted finish that will reflect less light.

SELECTING BULBS BASED ON SPECIES

There is a common trend toward make recommendations of bulbs based on the species with which it will be used. The principle behind this makes sense but in practice it is flawed. The thought is that certain species require higher UVB exposure and therefore a stronger UVB bulb while others require a lower UVB exposure and therefore a weaker bulb according to their biology and behavior. These principles would hold true in open-topped enclosures without a lid or when the bulb is placed inside the enclosure. However as mentioned previously, when the bulb is placed atop a screen, it can block a significant portion of the UVB reaching the animal. The author therefore recommends selecting a bulb not simply based on the species but rather a combination of the species and the specific enclosure setup of the particular animal. Buying a UVB bulb from a reputable manufacturer that provides clear guidance as to how to use the bulbs is the first step in safe use of UVB bulbs. The second aspect is ensuring that the owners and caretakers are indeed using the bulbs in the safest, most efficient manner for the particular species.

MEASURING UVB

Another challenge in selecting the proper UVB bulb is the fact that bulb strength or percentage UVB emission does not directly translate to its effectiveness in stimulating vitamin D3 synthesis in the body. There are in vitro models to assess the efficiency of UVB light (Burger et al, 2007) but these are impractical in a clinical setting. We must rely on the reputation of the manufacturer to ensure that the bulb is of good enough quality. How much UVB a particular amphibian species requires is unknown at this time. In nature, UVB exposure will vary with time of day, cloud covering, and so on, but in captivity the exposure level will be fairly constant while the bulb is turned on. Providing hiding places and a gradient of UVB light can help to reduce UVB overexposure for amphibians. An additional consideration is to only turn the UVB lights on for 2–4 hours of daily or every other day exposure.

RADIOMETERS

UVB irradiance cab be measured using a hand-held radiometer. While expensive (approximately $250.00) these units are available to the general public. Their accuracy has been questioned, but they remain a good tool. A radiometer can be used to measure UVB irradiance of a bulb at any distance to determine how much UVB is being emitted and to record the decay of transmission over time. For example a 5% linear fluorescent bulb may emit 25 $\mu W/cm^2$ at 12 inches when first purchased but, after 6 months, the irradiance at 12 inches may have decreased to 12 $\mu W/cm^2$. While this may still be acceptable exposure, it certainly indicates decrease in the bulb's effectiveness over time. This decay is normal but if one desires to provide a more constant UVB exposure year round, it may be time to purchase a new bulb. They can also be used to evaluate the effect of the screen or mesh cover on the effectiveness of a bulb to help clients select the most appropriate bulb for their setup. Some newer radiometers measure ultraviolet index providing scale from minimum to very high while others provide readout based on the Ferguson zones to help determine the UVB exposure. These radiometers are advertised as being able to measure the appropriate UVB dose for vitamin D3 synthesis although that claim has not been verified. Most amphibians should be exposed to a Ferguson zone of 1 or 2 maximum.

CALCIUM SUPPLEMENTATION

All animals need a source of calcium and a calcium to phosphorus ratio of 1.5 to 2. Most invertebrates have a negative calcium to phosphorus ratio, so animals must find other sources of calcium. In their natural environment, these animals will seek out mineral deposits or particular feedstuffs to supplement their calcium intake. In captivity, amphibians do not have the opportunity to seek calcium sources but rather rely on it being supplemented in their diet. Various commercial sources of calcium are available, but some are better than others. First, it is recommended that calcium supplements be purely calcium with no phosphorus or vitamin D3. While many see a benefit of adding a D3 supplement, there are serious and real concerns about oversupplementation of vitamin D3. Adding a calcium supplement that also contains phosphorus does not make sense because the amphibians are already in a negative calcium to phosphorus imbalance. Adding more phosphorus would not help solve this imbalance in an effective manner. The author prefers calcium only supplements including calcium powders sold for reptiles, cuttle bones, and crushed oyster shells. Another alternative is the use of fruit-flavored calcium carbonate antacid tablets. These tables are more palatable than other products. They can be pulverized or fed in small pieces.

Regardless of the type of supplement, calcium is best offered daily to account for variations in intake. The supplement can be provided by coating prey items. However, it must be noted that when insects are coated with a powdered supplement, it will fall off within 10–20 minutes. Insects should therefore be dusted immediately before feeding. There are some products that advertise calcium in a spray or gel cubes. These have not been proven to be effective and should be avoided until research to support their effectiveness is available. There are also some multivitamin products advertised for reptile and many of these include calcium as well as D3. Given that we do not know the nutritional requirement of most amphibian species, the use of multivitamins is questionable. While it may be beneficial in some species it could be detrimental in others that may be over supplemented by certain minerals or

(CONTINUED) UVB LIGHTING PRINCIPLES FOR CAPTIVE AMPHIBIANS

vitamins. Finally, earthworms and hornworms (*Manduca* spp.) are two excellent sources of nutrition because they tend to have a positive calcium to phosphorus ratio. However this ratio can also vary with the conditions in which they are reared and maintained.

SUMMARY

All this information can be overwhelming to veterinarians and clients alike. It is important to understand the basics of UVB requirements and the factors that affect UVB supplementation. All six factors must be considered when selecting a bulb, as there is no single best bulb for every situation. There are new studies and product available every year, so it is also important to stay up to date with the literature and technological advances to provide better recommendations to clients. Proper calcium supplementation, together with UVB light exposure, is critical to prevent secondary nutritional hyperparathyroidism. The absence of either or both of these elements from the history of an amphibian case should prompt veterinarians to include secondary nutritional hyperparathyroidism as a differential diagnosis.

GENERAL RECOMMENDATIONS FOR UVB LIGHTING IN AMPHIBIAN ENCLOSURES

A. For open top enclosures or when there is no material between the bulb and the animal:

1. Use a T8 2–6% bulb at distances up to 15 inches between the bulb and the animal; for distances over 15 inches, a T8 10–12% or T5 6% bulb may be required.
2. Provide a UVB and heat gradient so animals are not constantly exposed to UVB light.
3. Turn UVB light on for 2–4 hours daily to every other day, especially for cryptic or fossorial species that are naturally exposed to low levels of UVB.

For enclosures with a screen/mesh between the bulb and the animal:

1. Use a T8 6–12% bulb at distances up to 15 inches between the bulb and the animal; for distances over 15 inches, a T8 12% or T5 6% bulb may be required.
2. Provide a UVB and heat gradient so animals are not constantly exposed to UVB light.
3. Turn UVB light on for 2–4 hours daily to every other day, especially for cryptic or fossorial species that are naturally exposed to low levels of UVB.

Note: depending on the type of mesh, there may be a 30–50% reduction in UVB, which must be taken into consideration when selecting the bulb. The use of a UVB radiometer is more critical when the bulb is placed above a mesh in order to determine the actual UVB exposure.

Suggested Reading

Acierno MJ, Mitchell MA, Zachariah TT, Roundtree MK, Kirchgessner MS, Guzman D. Effects of ultraviolet radiation on plasma 25-hydroxyvitamin D3 concentrations in corn snakes (*Elaphe guttata*). *Am J Vet Res* 2008;69(2):294–297.

Burger RM, Gehrmann WH, Ferguson GW. Evaluation of UVB reduction by materials commonly used in reptile husbandry. *Zoo Biol* 2007;26:417–423.

Section II

Chelonians

ABSCESSES

BASICS

DEFINITION/OVERVIEW

Abscesses are non-fluctuating hard masses of variable size, formed by concentric layers of purulent material in which the outermost layer has the most liquid consistency. All purulent material is contained in a fibrous capsule. Coloration ranges from brown to yellow. Adhesions occasionally occur with adjacent tissues. There are no general symptoms if the abscess does not result from a systemic infection (salmonellosis, pseudomonas, microsporidiosis, etc.). Dermal abscesses in reptiles evolve from external wounds, ectoparasites or contamination by direct contact with feces or water with a high bacterial population, all of which may be exacerbated by immunosuppression.

ETIOLOGY/PATHOPHYSIOLOGY

- Can be a result of local or systemic infections.
- Local infections typically isolated to the skin—contamination of wounds with environmental, fecal, or normal flora leading to abscess formation.
- Existence of local infections in the skin is very frequent.
- Cultures show a high causative flora, including bacteria, fungi, and viruses.
- Systemic infections may also lead to abscess formation particularly in internal organs.
- Some local abscesses may spread and become systemic if environmental conditions are favorable.
- Systemic mycosis has been described by *Penicillium griseofulvum* in *Dypsochelys (Geochelone) gigantea*, or sepsis by *Serratia marcescens* in *Gopherus agasizii.*
- In tortoises, not unusual to find proliferations of fibrous connective tissue, which form hard, subcutaneous, adherent but sometimes mobile structures, comprised of a dense fibrin network that captures inflammatory cells—fibriscess.
- Fibriscess grows constantly and becomes fully visible—should not be confused with a fibroid or benign connective tissue neoplasia.

SIGNALMENT/HISTORY

- No specific signalment.
- Main focus should be on obtaining a thorough history of the husbandry and social interactions of the reptiles.
- A history of aggression in a group of reptiles may contribute to the appearance of abscesses.
- Poor cleanliness and hygiene of the enclosure can lead to increase environmental bacterial load, which can contribute to skin lesions and abscess formation.

CLINICAL PRESENTATION

- Reptiles may present with cutaneous abscesses ranging in size from a few millimeters to centimeters in diameter. These can either be freely moveable or firmly attached to the underlying tissues.
- Some abscesses become chronic and expel a malodorous, purulent discharge. The content of the abscess is mostly caseous in nature.
- Sometimes abscesses can affect nearby bones, and animals may present with lameness. Dysecdysis may also be observed in association with the abscess or through the animals' body.
- In aquatic chelonians, the most affected parts are the hindquarters and the neck.
- Although they can occur throughout the body of the animal, there is a greater frequency of cutaneous abscesses in the parotid, maxillary, interdigital, limbs, neck, and costal wall.

RISK FACTORS

Husbandry

- Poor hygiene and overpopulation can lead to increased bacterial load in the enclosure and possibly stress and immunosuppression.
- Rough substrate or surfaces in the terrarium can lead to cuts or abrasions that may become infected.
- Inappropriate diet and/or UVB exposure may also lead to a weakened immune status.

Others

N/A

DIAGNOSIS

DIFFERENTIAL DIAGNOSIS

- Chronic dysecdysis
- Blister disease
- Limb fractures can occur with symptoms similar to osteolytic abscesses at the same extremities (limb malposition, lameness, etc.).

DIAGNOSTICS

Cytology

- Cytology can be used as the first screening tool to identify whether a mass is an abscess either via an aspirate or an impression smear of the material within.
- Abscesses usually reveal a large number of leukocytes, cellular detritus, tissue remnants, and desquamation of cells.
- Infectious organisms may also be observed, but their absence does not rule out an infection.

Microbiology

- Bacterial culture and sensitivity are essential for identification of the existing bacterial population and the best antibiotic treatment to follow.
- Obtaining bacterial growth from abscesses can be difficult.
- Samples must be obtained not only from the abscess material but also from the wall of the abscess, to maximize the possibility of bacterial growth.
- Anaerobic cultures must be considered, especially when there is no aerobic growth and in cases of malodorous discharge. 16s rRNA PCR is another tool that is becoming more readily available for bacterial identification.
- Fungal cultures can also be considered, especially if hyphae are observed in the cytologic exam.

Hematology and Biochemistry

- Some changes that may be observed include leukocytosis, heterophilia, and eosinophilia.
- The heterophils may appear reactive (toxic granulation).
- Thrombocytes are also activated
- Mitosis may be observed in many leukocytes.
- Total protein values (gamma globulins and alpha globulins), and the enzymes AST, CPK, and alkaline phosphatase may be elevated.
- The majority of these changes are not consistent and may vary according to the nature of the abscess and how well encapsulated the abscess is.

Histology

Histopathologic exam of a suspected abscess can more definitively confirm the diagnosis and help identify the presence of infectious organisms.

Imaging

- Radiographs—in cases where an abscess is firmly attached to underlying bone, radiographs can help determine whether there is bony involvement and osteomyelitis.
- Ultrasound—abscesses (regardless of their location) have a hyperechogenic capsule that creates intense acoustic shadowing with a hypoechogenic interior, especially when they still have a liquid content (the first stage of internal caseum formation). In advanced stages, there is a thin layer of fibrin that surrounds the abscess and under it the inflammatory liquid that forms the internal caseum.

PATHOLOGICAL FINDINGS

Histologically, necrotic cell layers and a thin layer of phagocytic mononuclear cells in palisade are observed delimiting the core of the abscess. Organisms may be visible on numerous sections. A correct differential diagnosis of diseases such as mycosis, neoplasia, or myiasis must be carried out.

TREATMENT

APPROPRIATE HEALTH CARE

- Treatment often requires a combination of medical and surgical therapy for best results.
- Any suspected or confirmed bacteria should be treated with appropriate systemic antibiotics until results of sensitivity panel confirm its effectiveness.
- For suspected fungal infections, systemic therapy may not be necessary, as long as the infection is restricted to the abscess.
- In conjunction with medical therapy, surgery to either remove or debride the abscess must be performed.
- Complete removal of the whole abscess and capsule is preferred but often not possible due to size limitations for skin closure or involvement of underlying tissues. A debridement is more commonly performed.
- The abscess should be opened to extract the purulent material and as much of the capsule as possible. It can then be irrigated with a disinfectant solution (iodine, clorhexidine, etc.) and left open to heal by secondary intention.
- Daily flushing and cleaning should be performed until no more purulent material is observed.
- Topical antibiotic ointments can also be applied within the abscess cavity. An additional treatment is the placement of antibiotic (amikacin, cephalosporins) impregnated beads, or dental antibiotic gels, such as doxycycline hyclate (DOXIROBE® gel, Zpetis, USA), or clindamycin hydrochloride 1% (ClinzGard®, VEDCO Inc, USA) especially in non-responsive cases, fractious animals, or those that cannot be easily treated on a daily basis
- Most abscesses will take between 2 weeks and 1 month to heal. In some cases, once the caseous material has been completely removed and there is certainty that only healthy tissue remains, then the wound can be sutured.

NUTRITIONAL SUPPORT

- Proper nutrition is key for the prevention and treatment of anemia.
- Diet should be as varied as possible and adapted to each species.
- Nutritional support via gavage feeding should be implemented in very ill and/or anorectic animals.

CLIENT EDUCATION/HUSBANDRY RECOMMENDATIONS

- Correct any husbandry deficiencies with special attention to hygiene, temperature, humidity, and ventilation.
- Isolate animal from others in collection during treatment.
- Important to ensure a full course of treatment to avoid recurrence.

MEDICATIONS

DRUG(S) OF CHOICE

- Broad-spectrum antibiotics (e.g., fluoroquinolones, aminoglycosides, sulfamides)
- Some penicillins (e.g., carbenicillin or ampicillin)

PRECAUTIONS/INTERACTIONS

- Fluid therapy should be considered when administering systemic antimicrobials, especially aminoglycoside antibiotics (gentamicin, streptomycin, amikacin, kanamycin) due to their nephrotoxic potential.
- Systemic antifungals should also be used and monitored cautiously.

FOLLOW-UP

PATIENT MONITORING

- Abscesses should not grow out again 1 month after treatment.
- If there is recurrence, a more aggressive approach is needed.
- Scarring and pigmentation changes may be observed at the site of the healed abscess.

EXPECTED COURSE AND PROGNOSIS

- Generally, abscesses heal well, are not complicated, and have a good prognosis.
- If allowed to become chronic they can become systemic, affect the internal viscera and compromise the life of the reptile. At this point, the prognosis would be guarded to grave.

MISCELLANEOUS

COMMENTS

Figure 1—see web image supplementary content for section II (Chelonians).

ZOONOTIC POTENTIAL

- Zoonotic potential will depend on the type of bacteria associated with the abscess.
- Appropriate precautions must be taken when working with reptile abscesses to minimize exposure to zoonotic organisms.

SYNONYMS

- Purulent dermatitis
- Subcutaneous abscesses
- Superficial pyoderma

ABBREVIATIONS

- AST = aspartate aminotransferase
- CPK = creatine phosphokinase
- PCR = polymerase chain reaction
- UVB = ultraviolet B

INTERNET RESOURCES

- Kaplan M. Treating Abscesses in Reptiles. Melissa Kaplan's Herp Care Collection. 1996, last updated January 1, 2014. www.anapsid.org/abscess.html
- Negron V. 4 Diseases Your Pet Reptile Can Give You. May 1, 2015. www.petmd.com/reptile/care/diseases-your-pet-reptile-can-give-you
- PetMD Editorial. Internal Abscesses in Reptiles. July 28, 2008. www.petmd.com/reptile/conditions/skin/c_rp_internal_abscesses

Suggested Reading

Huchzermeyer FW, Cooper JE. Fibriscess, not abscess, resulting from a localized inflammatory response to infection in reptiles and birds. *Vet Record* 2000;147:515–517.

Mayer J, Pizzirani S, DeSena R. Bilateral exophtalmos in an adult iguana (*Iguana iguana*) caused by an orbital abscess. *J Herp Med Surg* 2010;20:5–10.

Williams SR, Sims M, Roth-Jonson L, Wickes B. Surgical removal of an abscess associated with Fusarium solani from a Kemp's ridley sea turtle (*Lepidochelys kempii*). *J Zoo Wildl Med* 2012;43:402–406.

Author Albert Martínez-Silvestre, DVM, MSc, PhD, DECZM (Herpetology), EBVS European Veterinary Specialist in Herpetological Medicine and Surgery, Acred. AVEPA (Exotic Animals)

ADENOVIRUS

BASICS

DEFINITION/OVERVIEW

- Adenoviruses have been found to infect all classes of bony vertebrates and most appear to have co-evolved with their hosts.
- Adenoviral infections in reptiles have ranged from clinically inapparent to enteritis, necrotizing hepatitis, esophagitis, splenitis, and encephalopathy.

ETIOLOGY/PATHOPHYSIOLOGY

- Adenoviruses are double stranded non-enveloped DNA viruses.
- They fall in the family Adenoviridae, which is further classified into five currently accepted genera:
  - Mastadenovirus isolated from mammals
  - Aviadenovirus in birds
  - Atadenovirus isolated from squamates
  - Siadenovirus found in some chelonians, amphibians and birds
  - Ichtadenovirus isolated from a sturgeon
- A sixth genus, Testadenovirus, isolated from tortoises, has been proposed.
- AdV infections have been identified in wild-caught and captive lizards, snakes, chelonians, and crocodiles.
- Disease is often a combination of other disease agents and/or stress and the viral infection.

SIGNALMENT/HISTORY

- The listing below is of the species reported with an adenovirus isolate.
  - Chelonians: Sulawesi tortoises, red-footed tortoise, pancake tortoise, Eastern box turtle, ornate box turtle, red eared slider.
- With molecular diagnostics, more affected species are expected to be identified.
- There is no sex predilection.
- Juvenile and/or stressed animals are more frequently reported with disease.

CLINICAL PRESENTATION

- Non-specific; often the animal is found dead.
- Sulawesi tortoises had severe systemic disease and high mortality rate; however, these animals suffered multiple stressors.
- Clinical signs included anorexia, lethargy, oral cavity ulcerations, nasal and ocular discharge, and diarrhea.
- Subclinical disease has been reported in other tortoises.

RISK FACTORS

Husbandry

- Adenoviruses are very stable in the environment and commonly spread through fecal–oral transmission.
- Poor biosecurity can help disseminate the virus throughout a collection.

Others

- Stressors such as capture, substandard housing, nutritional inadequacies or underlying disease play a role in the development of clinical infection.
- Concurrent disease and/or immunosuppression increases the likelihood of severe systemic disease.
- Sulawesi tortoises had concurrent amoebiasis, nematodiasis, and/or bacterial sepsis.

DIAGNOSIS

DIFFERENTIAL DIAGNOSIS

Intranuclear coccidiosis, mycoplasmosis, and tortoise herpesvirus 1.

DIAGNOSTICS

- PCR may be diagnostic if the test is specific for the adenovirus commonly isolated from the reptile species.
- Necropsy and histopathology: appropriate tissues need to be evaluated and, in some cases, additional tests such as TEM and/or PCR molecular diagnostics need to be performed.

PATHOLOGICAL FINDINGS

Sulawesi tortoises:

- Gross lesions: hepatosplenomegaly, thick fibrinonecrotic membranes in the lumen of the large intestine, segmental darkening of the serosal surfaces of the small and large intestine, oronasal fistulas, and tongue and oral mucosa ulceration.
- Histology: heterophilic and lymphoplasmacytic infiltration of intestinal enteritis and hepatic necrosis. The inclusions are basophilic or amphophilic.

TREATMENT

APPROPRIATE HEALTH CARE

N/A

NUTRITIONAL SUPPORT

- Nutritional support should be provided as needed only when the reptile is well hydrated and at an ideal environmental temperature for the species.
- An esophagostomy tube should be considered for long-term care.

CLIENT EDUCATION/HUSBANDRY RECOMMENDATIONS

- Quarantine: the current recommendation is for approximately 6 months isolation period for most reptiles, with PCR testing at various intervals.
- Post-outbreak: after diagnosis of an adenovirus infection in a collection, cages and hard surfaces should be thoroughly cleaned with a detergent, followed by disinfection with a 10% bleach solution. A minimum of 10-minute contact time with the bleach is recommended. All bleached supplies and cages should be thoroughly rinsed afterward and dried. Bleach can be corrosive and can cause respiratory irritation in enclosed spaces.
- Direct unfiltered sunlight or other intense ultraviolet sources may also aid disinfection. Proper contact time must be followed if using other disinfectants.
- All reptiles should be kept at appropriate temperature and humidity and offered food consistent with their dietary requirements.

MEDICATIONS

DRUG(S) OF CHOICE

N/A

PRECAUTIONS/INTERACTIONS

N/A

FOLLOW UP

PATIENT MONITORING

- Reptiles showing clinical signs should be isolated and provided supportive care.
- Any co-infections should be treated, if possible.
- Monitoring weight, appetite, and fecal production will help assess response to therapy and progression of infection.
- Utensils and cage furniture should not be transferred from room to room or animal to animal.

EXPECTED COURSE AND PROGNOSIS

- There is no specific treatment.
- Disease progression is unknown as antemortem diagnosis is seldom determined.
- Cases have ranged from acute to chronic protracted presentation of clinical signs.
- Identifying adenovirus from a healthy animal is not diagnostic for a disease caused by the virus.
- Reptiles can be inapparent hosts for adenoviruses.

MISCELLANEOUS

COMMENTS

N/A

ZOONOTIC POTENTIAL

N/A

SYNONYMS

N/A

ABBREVIATIONS

• AdV = Adenovirus
• PCR = polymerase chain reaction
• PCV = packed cell volume
• TEM = transmission electron microscopy

INTERNET RESOURCES

• Kik, MJL. Adenoviris infection in reptiles. Transmissible Diseases Handbook. 4th ed. European Association of Zoo and Wildlife Veterinarians. https://www.eazwv.org/page/inf_handbook
• Jacobson E, Wellehan J, Stacy B. Reptile Adenovirus PCR and Sequencing at the University of Florida CVM. www.dachiu.com/beardeddragons/Adenovirus.pdf

Suggested Reading

Doszpoly A, Wellehan J.F.X. Jr., Childress AL, et al. Partial characterization of a new adenovirus lineage discovered in testudinoid turtles. *Infect Genet Evol* 2013;17:106–112.

Papp T, Fledelius B, Schmidt V, et al. PCR-sequence characterization of new adenoviruses found in reptiles and the first successful isolation of a lizard adenovirus. *Vet Microbiol* 2009;134(3–4):233–240.

Author Drury R. Reavill, DVM, DABVP (Avian and Reptile & Amphibian Practice), DACVP

ANEMIA

BASICS

DEFINITION/OVERVIEW

Anemia is a sign of disease and is characterized by a decreased number of erythrocytes, hemoglobin deficiency or both. It can occur due to one of four main categories: decreased erythropoietic activity, hemorrhage, destruction of red blood cells, or sequestration.

ETIOLOGY/PATHOPHYSIOLOGY

- Traumatic
- Hemorrhagic
- Maladaptation syndrome associated anemia: reported in stressed reptiles, associated with captivity or with capture of wild reptiles
- Blood parasites
- Virus associated anemia
- Autoimmune hemolytic anemia: rare in reptiles

SIGNALMENT/HISTORY

Wild-caught reptiles or those housed under poor husbandry conditions may be more predisposed.

CLINICAL PRESENTATION

- Nonspecific clinical signs including lethargy, anorexia, and behavioral changes.
- Pallor of skin and mucus membrane color may also be observed.

RISK FACTORS

Husbandry

- Inadequate husbandry, including diet, is often a predisposing factor for many diseases of captive reptiles.
- Any reptile maintained under poor husbandry conditions should be considered susceptible to disease.
- Wild-caught reptiles are more likely to have underlying diseases, especially endoparasites and hemoparasites, which may be the underlying cause of chronic anemia.

Others

Any reptile with a chronic illness may be predisposed to anemia.

DIAGNOSIS

DIFFERENTIAL DIAGNOSIS

- Trauma leading to external or internal hemorrhage.
- Maladaptation syndrome associated anemia—reported in stressed reptiles, associated with captivity or trapping of wild reptiles.
- Hemoparasites
- Malnutrition
- Toxicity
- Weakness and prostration due to metabolic bone disease, pregnancy, or infectious disease.

DIAGNOSTICS

- Blood sampling is essential for diagnosis and monitoring of anemic reptiles.
- Patient's size, condition, and venous access must all be considered.
- Venipuncture sites with minimal lymphatic contamination are preferred, to obtain a more representative sample of the peripheral blood.
- In chelonians, the jugular vein is the site with the least amount of lymphatic contamination.
- Alternatively, the brachial plexus and coccygeal veins can be sampled.
- The subcarapacial sinus tends to have the largest amount of lymphatic contamination.
- In critically ill, possibly anemic, reptiles, aim to collect a blood volume of no more than 0.5% of the body weight (0.5 ml/100 g body weight) so as to not exacerbate the anemic condition.
- EDTA can cause hemolysis and artifacts in most chelonian, so lithium heparin is the preferred anticoagulant.

Physical Exam

- Mucous membranes and general pallor—compared with mammals, reptiles' mucous membranes are lighter in color but should still appear pink.
- One exception is the family Chelydridae, which normally have rather pale mucous membranes.
- Examination of the ocular conjunctiva and even the iris color in American box turtles (*Terrapene* sp.) has also been reported, associating the pale iris with low hematocrit and possible anemia.

Hematology

Although there is limited ability to assess all the same hematologic parameters as in mammals, some basic guidelines can be found for certain values.

Hematocrit/PCV

- Normal values range from 20 to 45. Values below 20 suggest anemia in most cases.
- A blood transfusion should be considered in animals with values below 10, although there is little research in reptilian blood transfusions.
- Seasonal variations in this parameter should also be considered before making clinical decisions.
- A low hematocrit with an increased polychromasia index is a normal physiologic change during brumation, but pathologic during the active season.

Hemoglobin

- Normal values are 6–10 g/dl according to the species.
- Lower values should suggest anemia. MCHC is calculated according to the hematocrit and hemoglobin, like MCH; these parameters show variation in case of anemia.
- Individual variations should also be considered, as reptiles have different types of hemoglobin, which may influence the expression of clinical signs.

Polychromasia and Erythroblasts

- An increased polychromasia and erythroblasts in general suggests an increased need for erythrocytes in peripheral blood and can be interpreted as evidence of a regenerative anemia.
- Occasionally, a high number of erythroblasts may be found in the micro-hematocrit tube, forming an intermediate layer between the buffy coat and the red blood concentrate.
- This activity is usually accompanied by the presence of erythrocyte precursors in peripheral blood (erythroblasts, occasionally polychromatophils).
- Hemoparasites may also lead to increased numbers of erythroblasts and polychromasia.
- Polychromasia may also occur in the absence of anemia as has been reported in shedding reptiles.

Erythrocytic Mitoses

- When detected in peripheral blood as an anecdotal finding, it is not a manifestation of anemia.
- Anemia should only be considered when mitoses appear in erythrocytes together with the presence of abundant erythroblasts and other markers described, such as altered hematocrit and irregular erythrocytic nucleus.

Erythrocyte Counts

- Total erythrocyte counts are lower than in mammals and birds.
- Erythrocytes in chelonians are larger compared with other reptiles; they tend to have counts below 500,000/µl.

Fecal Occult3 Blood Test and Urinalysis

- May allow for the detection of small amounts of blood in an animal's urine or feces.
- Fecal occult test may return false positives in carnivorous species.

PATHOLOGICAL FINDINGS

Pathologic findings will be specific to the underlying cause of anemia.

TREATMENT

APPROPRIATE HEALTH CARE

- Anemia is often a chronic presentation in most reptiles.
- A slower metabolism and physiologic adaptation mechanisms allow reptiles to compensate better than birds or mammals.

- Treatment is often not needed on an emergency basis, but is rather focused on addressing the underlying diseases and providing supportive therapy.

NUTRITIONAL SUPPORT

- Proper nutrition is key for the prevention and treatment of anemia.
- The diet should be as varied as possible and adapted to each species.
- Diet should be balanced and contain natural sources of vitamin B12 and iron.
- Nutritional support via gavage feeding should be implemented in very ill and/or anorectic animals.

CLIENT EDUCATION/HUSBANDRY RECOMMENDATIONS

- It is recommended to perform annual health evaluations of the animals at risk.
- These evaluations should include blood tests and fecal exams.
- Any treatments must be performed based on the results of the exams and the historical data for the collection.
- These tests should also be done on newly acquired and quarantined animals.
- A proper nutritional plan is also essential for good health.

MEDICATIONS

DRUG(S) OF CHOICE

- Hemorrhagic anemia: control bleeding by applying pressure. Efficacy of blood replacers or transfusions has not been well studied.
- Use of hemostatic agents such as D-aminocaproic acid or ethamsylate has not been reported in reptiles; doses are empirical (0.1 ml/kg).
- Fluid therapy: isotonic fluids should be administered at a rate of 20–30 ml/kg IV, IO, or SC for maintenance.
- Fluid losses can be replaced but be careful not to overhydrate the patient.
- Colloids may also be used at a rate 10–20 ml/kg with a bolus of 3–5 ml/kg IV or IO as needed.
- Blood transfusion: homologous transfusions are preferred over heterologous. Blood volume of up to 1% body weight is extracted from the donor, by means of syringes and needles filled with anticoagulant at a ratio of 1:6 to 1:9 anticoagulant to blood. The blood is administered to the recipient by means of an infusion pump at 5 ml/hour flow rate. True efficacy is not well documented but clinical experience suggests some short-term benefits.
- Maladaptation syndrome: treatment consists of fluid therapy and stimulation of blood regeneration by means of iron dextran (12 mg/kg, IM every 7 days) and cyanocobalamin (vitamin B12; 0.5 mg/kg or 10–2000 iu according to the animal weight as single IM or SC dose).
- Availability of blood replacers varies across the world. If available, products like Oxyglobin® (bovine hemoglobin glutamer) 1 ml/100 g IV for 5 minutes by means of perfusion; repeat 4 hours later) may improve success in severe anemia.
- Epoietin alfa (EPOGEN®, Amgen Inc., Thousand Oaks, CA) erythropoeisis stimulating agent is reported as safe and effective in *Chelonia mydas* and *Caretta caretta* when used at 100 U/kg SC 3 times weekly over 2 weeks. Similar dosing has not been useful in *Testudo hermanni*.

PRECAUTIONS/INTERACTIONS

N/A

FOLLOW-UP

PATIENT MONITORING

- Because of the small size of some chelonians, monitoring should rely on assessment of the behavior and clinical signs of the affected animal, not just on blood sampling.
- If the treatment is appropriate, the lizard should become progressively more active and alert, with interest in hunting, seeking shelter or mating behaviors.
- Normal attitude and feeding behavior are two common aspects that can be monitored in chelonians after the start of treatment, because they are related to the overall health.
- In addition, signs of healing of the other diseases that have contributed to the animal's anemia should be observed.

EXPECTED COURSE AND PROGNOSIS

- Repeated blood samplings after 1 week and 1 month may show early signs of regeneration.
- Repeated blood sampling may be contraindicated, especially in cases of non-regenerative anemia, when working with small patients, or if the underlying etiology is not being treated.
- If the underlying cause of anemia is properly diagnosed and can be effectively treated, prognosis is good.

MISCELLANEOUS

COMMENTS

N/A

ZOONOTIC POTENTIAL

N/A

SYNONYMS

- Inadaptation syndrome
- Maladaptation syndrome

ABBREVIATIONS

- EDTA = ethylenediaminetetraacetic acid
- IM = intramuscular
- MCH = mean corpuscular hemoglobin
- MCHC = mean corpuscular hemoglobin concentration
- MCV = mean corpuscular volume
- PCV = packed cell volume
- SC = subcutaneous

INTERNET RESOURCES

- Cital S. Exotic animal blood transfusions: An overview. VetBloom http://blog.vetbloom.com/exotics/exotic-animal-blood-transfusions-an-overview
- Martínez-Silvestre A. How I treat anemia in reptiles. Southern European Veterinary Congress Annual Conference, Barcelona, October 19, 2013. www.ivis.org/library/sevc/sevc-annual-conference-barcelona-2013/how-i-treat-anemia-reptiles

Suggested Reading

Boyer TH. Autoimmune hemolytic anemia in a parson's chameleon, *Calumna parsonii parsonii*. *Proc ARAV* 2002;9:81–84.

Saggese MD. Clinical approach to the anemic reptile. *J Exot Pet Med* 2009;18(2):98–111.

Wu C, Chie CHH. Case study: successful treatment of acute anaemia with whole blood transfusion and supportive care in two turtles. *Proc UPAV/AAVAC/ARA* 2014:13–20.

Author Albert Martínez-Silvestre, DVM, MSc, PhD, DECZM (Herpetology), EBVS European Veterinary Specialist in Herpetological Medicine and Surgery, Acred. AVEPA (Exotic Animals)

ANOREXIA

BASICS

DEFINITION/OVERVIEW

Anorexia is the lack of appetite or intake of food, and does not define an underlying cause. Many pathological and even physiological conditions can result in decreased food intake. Anorexia is distinct from decreased appetite, which is also known as hypophagia.

ETIOLOGY/PATHOPHYSIOLOGY

- Anorexia may be a normal physiologic/behavioral occurrence during certain times of the year (e.g., brumation, estivation, reproductive season).
- Pathologic causes of anorexia may stem from either GI or extra-GI disease (e.g., any painful condition or systemic illness).
- Improper husbandry, and offering the wrong type and size of food, may also lead to anorexia.
- Prolonged anorexia may lead to hepatic lipidosis, which may result in nausea, leading to continued lack of food intake.
- Nutritional imbalances and metabolic derangements can occur with chronic anorexia and cachexia may ensue.
- Primarily, the gastrointestinal and musculoskeletal systems are affected with anorexia.
- Animals that are not consuming food for prolonged periods of time may not defecate significant amounts.
- As the body begins to break down adipose tissue stores and muscle, bony prominences become more obvious as body condition decreases.

SIGNALMENT/HISTORY

- Anorexia has no age or sex predilection.
- It is important to differentiate physiologic/behavioral anorexia from that caused by an underlying pathology or disease process.

CLINICAL PRESENTATION

- An isolated incident or occasional episodes of anorexia in otherwise healthy animals may be inconsequential, especially in animals presenting in good body condition.
- Decreased food intake over an extended period.
- Clients may report repeated attempts at feeding.
- Clinical signs of chronic anorexia include a decreased body condition score with prominent bony protuberances, dehydration, and muscle wasting.

RISK FACTORS

- Any disease process could result in anorexia.
- Different types of stress may also result in decreased food intake.

Husbandry

- Adjusting to captivity—often seen in newly acquired animals. A period of time for acclimation may be necessary before an animal feels secure enough to start eating on its own.
- Improper husbandry—inappropriate environmental temperature or humidity, inappropriate food items (type and/or size), malnutrition, inadequate exposure to UVB lighting, poor water quality, overcrowding, rapid change of diet, lack of provision of hiding areas.
- Stress—social or environmental.

Others

- Physiologic
- Cardiovascular disease: cardiomyopathy, congestive heart failure
- Reproductive activity: gravid females, breeding males
- Reproductive disease: pre- or postovulatory dystocia
- Respiratory infections: upper and lower respiratory tract infections; mycoplasmosis
- Viral infections: herpesviral infections in *Testudo* spp; ranaviral infections; iridoviral infections
- Fungal infections: fungal pneumonia
- Systemic illness: septicemia
- GI disease: stomatitis, foreign bodies, neoplasia, intussusception, gastroenteritis, constipation, prolapses
- Parasitic disease: ectoparasites and endoparasites
- Neurologic disease
- Toxic diseases
- Urogenital: cystoliths; prolapsed phallus; renal disease
- Metabolic: nutritional secondary hyperparathyroidism; hypovitaminosis A
- Any potentially painful condition: ophthalmic disease, orthopedic conditions (including shell fractures), cellulitis, trauma

DIAGNOSIS

DIFFERENTIAL DIAGNOSIS

- Conditions that result in failed food prehension (disorders of the tongue or oral cavity) or processing may result in animals that attempt to eat (have an appetite) but are unable to do so successfully.
- Hypophagia may be mistaken for anorexia in certain circumstances.

DIAGNOSTICS

Diagnostic procedures should be tailored towards identifying the underlying cause of the anorexia and identifying potential negative sequelae (e.g., hepatic lipidosis).

Baseline Blood Work

- CBC, PCV, TS, biochemistry
- Findings on complete blood count and biochemistry panels are usually non-specific but may be suggestive of an underlying disease process(es) resulting in the observed anorexia.
- Bile acids and liver leakage enzymes (AST) may be increased if hepatic lipidosis is present secondary to prolonged anorexia.

Imaging

Radiography can help identify abnormalities of the GI tract such as foreign bodies and masses. Ultrasound and CT can provide more detailed information about possible hepatic lipidosis, ileus, and coelomic masses.

Other Tests

- Additional diagnostics, including infectious or parasitic disease testing, may be warranted based on patient history and physical examination findings.
- The presumed underlying causes should be thoroughly investigated.

PATHOLOGICAL FINDINGS

- Findings depend on underlying cause of the anorexia.
- Hepatic lipidosis may be suspected based on the findings of advanced imaging or biochemistry evaluation.

TREATMENT

APPROPRIATE HEALTH CARE

N/A

NUTRITIONAL SUPPORT

- Nutritional support should be started in anorectic animals that have lost 10% of their body weight acutely (7 days or less) or 20% chronically (longer than 7 days).
- This weight loss must also be monitored together with an assessment of body condition (BCS).
- Anorectic animals with a BCS of 2/5 or lower may be immediate candidates for nutritional support.
- Animals should be housed in appropriate environments and maintained at their preferred optimum temperature zones, to facilitate proper utilization of the provided nourishment.
- Liquid diets may be provided via gavage in smaller animals.
- Placement of an esophagostomy tube should be considered for long-term support and to minimize stress of force feeding.
- Although poorly understood in veterinary medicine, the potential exists for refeeding syndrome in chronically anorectic patients, necessitating careful planning of nutritional support in these animals.

• Recommendations include feeding chronically anorectic animals half their calculated energy requirements initially, then slowly increasing up to the full energy requirement over 7–10 days.

CLIENT EDUCATION/HUSBANDRY RECOMMENDATIONS

• The clinician should perform a thorough review of the patient's current husbandry, including feeding.
• It is important to ensure that a proper diet of an appropriate size is being offered.
• The diet must be presented to the animal appropriately (e.g., feeding diurnal animals during daylight hours, offering prey on land vs. in the water or vice versa).
• Any husbandry or dietary deficiencies should be corrected.
• Clients should be notified that offering live food items to anorectic animals could result in rapid, serious injury to their pet secondary to prey attacks.
• For most cases, live prey should not be offered to chelonians without direct supervision.

MEDICATIONS

DRUG(S) OF CHOICE

• Commercial, high-calorie formulations designed for nutritional support are recommended when feeding anorectic chelonians.
• Alternatively, a slurry can be made with a commercial pelleted diet.

PRECAUTIONS/INTERACTIONS

• Exercise caution when force feeding, to prevent oral, esophageal, or gastric trauma.
• Be careful not to administer too large a volume of nutritional formula in small patients.
• Feed 1–3% of body weight initially to ensure the animal will tolerate the feeding.

FOLLOW-UP

PATIENT MONITORING

• Individuals should be monitored for resolution of anorexia following correction of any husbandry and dietary deficiencies.
• Serial imaging and blood chemistry evaluation may be considered to monitor for development or resolution of secondary liver diseases such as hepatic lipidosis.
• In patients with esophagostomy tubes, the tube should be monitored for clogging and the stoma regularly evaluated for signs of infection.

EXPECTED COURSE AND PROGNOSIS

• Anorexia may continue until the underlying reason is identified and treated, if applicable.
• Prognosis for resolution of anorexia depends on the severity of the underlying cause.

MISCELLANEOUS

COMMENTS

• Simply providing appropriate husbandry will help prevent many causes of anorexia in chelonians.
• Prompt diagnosis of true anorexia enables initiation of proper nutritional support and may prevent formation of hepatic lipidosis, which can perpetuate the lack of appetite.
• Supportive care should be continued while an underlying cause for the anorexia is identified and corrected.
• Gravid individuals may decrease their amount of food consumption from lack of coelomic space for GI distension.
• Animals that are anorectic from an underlying pathologic condition may cease or abort reproductive activity due to preferential allotment of energy for other physiologic functions.

ZOONOTIC POTENTIAL

N/A

SYNONYMS

• Anophagia
• Aphagia
• Inappetence

ABBREVIATIONS

• AST = aspartate aminotransferase
• BCS = body condition score
• CBC = complete blood count
• CT = computed tomography
• GI = gastrointestinal
• PCV = packed cell volume
• TS = total solids
• UVB = ultraviolet B

Suggested Reading

De Voe RS. Nutritional support of reptile patients. *Vet Clin North Am Exot Anim Pract* 2014;17: 249–261.
Divers SJ, Stahl S, eds. *Mader's Reptile and Amphibian Medicine and Surgery*. 3rd ed. St. Louis, MO: Elsevier; 2019.

Author Grayson Doss, DVM, DACZM

AURAL ABSCESSES

BASICS

DEFINITION/OVERVIEW

Aural abscesses are a common presentation of captive chelonians. They can be sterile but the majority are associated with bacteria, usually of digestive origin. May be observed in turtles suffering from subclinical hypovitaminosis A.

ETIOLOGY/PATHOPHYSIOLOGY

- Otitis in chelonians is often due to secondary infections as result of squamous metaplasia from hypovitaminosis A leading to blockage of the auditory ducts causing lack of drainage.
- Poor husbandry conditions and trauma may also be contributing factors.
- Otitis caused by nematodes (due to internal duct migration) has also been described in *Testudo graeca*.
- In box turtles, (*Terrapene carolina*), a possible correlation between the occurrence of otitis and environmental levels of organochlorine pesticides acting as immunosuppressive agents has been suggested, but the link is not definitively proven.

SIGNALMENT/HISTORY

- Aural abscesses are observed almost exclusively in chelonians, with more frequent occurrences in American species (*Trachemys* sp., *Graptemys* sp., *Pseudemys* sp., *Terrapene* sp.) followed by European species (*Testudo* sp.).
- There are some cases in saurians, but they are much less frequent.
- Primarily seen in captive animals or wild-caught animals that have been kept as pets and fed an inadequate diet.

CLINICAL PRESENTATION

- Animals present with unilateral or bilateral swellings of the tympanic membrane.
- These swellings can cause severe external and internal deformations of the ear canal.
- The swelling may start with a soft consistency but quickly becomes firm to hard as the material becomes caseous.
- In extreme cases, abscesses can progress towards the inside of the skull and affect internal structures (brain, mandibular base, etc.).
- Some animals may also present with conjunctivitis, blepharedema, nasal discharge, and overgrown beak and nails.
- Some of these signs may suggest a concurrent respiratory infection.

RISK FACTORS

Husbandry

Poor hygiene and inappropriate diet (low in vitamin A) are the main contributing factors.

Others

Exposure of animals to toxins such as organochlorines, which inhibit the synthesis of vitamin A, or have an immunosuppressive effect must also be considered.

DIAGNOSIS

DIFFERENTIAL DIAGNOSIS

- Nutritional secondary hyperparathyroidism
- Neoplasia
- Parasites
- Upper respiratory tract disease

DIAGNOSTICS

Cytology

A cytological imprint or aspiration of the abscess helps in determining whether bacteria and/or fungi are involved.

Microbiology

Culture and sensitivity of the abscess material is recommended for proper identification of the bacteria involved (usually *Staphylococcus*, *Streptococcus* or *Pseudomonas*) and to ensure a proper antibiotic was selected.

Imaging

In cases with perceived skull deformities or non-responsive to therapy, radiographs or CT are recommended to determine whether osteolytic changes are present.

Histology

If the material extracted from the site does not have the appearance of an abscess or is closely attached to the bone, it should be submitted for histopathological evaluation to rule out neoplasia.

PATHOLOGICAL FINDINGS

- Lesions of the tympanic epithelium include hyperplasia, squamous metaplasia, hyperemia, cellular sloughing, granulomatous inflammation, and bacterial infection.
- Histopathologic changes in turtles with aural abscesses are consistent with a syndrome involving hypovitaminosis A.

TREATMENT

APPROPRIATE HEALTH CARE

- Aural abscesses require a dual approach of surgical debridement and medical therapy.
- Ophthalmic antibiotic drops may be instilled in the canal for local therapy in addition to the use of systemic antibiotics.
- The use of ointments should be reserved for the period when all the material can be easily flushed out of the canal.
- Some may elect to administer vitamin A (5,000–10,000 iu IM as a single dose), but this should be reserved for the most severe cases, as hypervitaminosis A from parenteral administration is a concern.

NUTRITIONAL SUPPORT

Natural sources of vitamin A in the diet (herbivorous—parsley, carrot, tomato, spirulina; carnivorous—liver, fish, eggs).

CLIENT EDUCATION/HUSBANDRY RECOMMENDATIONS

- Ensure a proper balanced diet for the species and consider oral vitamin A supplementation at a rate of 2–8 iu/g of feed.
- Improve hygiene to decrease bacterial load in the water/enclosure.
- Avoid fights or scratches among animals housed together.

SURGICAL CONSIDERATIONS

- The debridement must be performed with the animal under sedation or anesthesia with proper analgesia (NSAIDs and opioids, local block, etc.).
- The tympanic membrane can then be incised either in a vertical or horizontal manner.
- A horizontal incision on the ventral aspect of the membrane may allow for better drainage postoperatively.
- The tympanic membrane is usually edematous and vascularized leading to appreciable bleeding upon incision.
- If excessive bleeding occurs, topical hemostatics (silver nitrate) may be used.
- Once an opening is made, the caseous material must be removed in its entirety via manual manipulation and flushing.
- Chelonian ears have an inverted L shape, which means that there is often a dorsocaudal pocket that harbors more material.
- A cotton-tip applicator can be placed on the dorsocaudal aspect of the head/ear followed by applying pressure in a cranioventral direction, to help expel the material.
- Forceps are also helpful to remove excess material.
- It is not uncommon to remove a volume of material two to three times the size of the external swelling.
- Once the material is removed, the ear canal can be flushed with a disinfectant solution (iodine, chlorhexidine, etc.) and saline.
- The membrane is left open to heal by secondary intention.
- The ear canal can continue to be flushed once to twice daily until it closes.

MEDICATIONS

DRUG(S) OF CHOICE

- Antibiotics: broad-spectrum antibiotics (fluoroquinolones, cephalosporins) until resolution of clinical signs.
- Preventive vitamin A is recommended at 1000–2000 iu/kg every 7 days, but is best done by dietary supplementation at 2–8 iu/g of feed) to avoid overdosing.

PRECAUTIONS/INTERACTIONS

- With preventive vitamin A it is advisable to use a minimum dose.
- Overdosage of oily vitamin A causes exostosis, hepatomegaly, and skin lesions.

FOLLOW-UP

PATIENT MONITORING

- A thorough physical examination will confirm the healing of the tympanic membrane.
- It usually takes between 2 and 4 weeks.
- If vitamin A has been provided, no further relapses are expected.

EXPECTED COURSE AND PROGNOSIS

- Generally carries a good prognosis.
- Balance is not usually affected, although cases may be observed depending on the degree of injury to the inner ear.

MISCELLANEOUS

COMMENTS

- Recent research suggests that 6 months of exposure to selected organochlorine compounds (chlordane, aroclor, lindane), or similar duration of reduced dietary vitamin A concentrations, did not influence the formation of squamous metaplasia and aural abscesses in red-eared sliders (*Trachemys scripta*).
- Although the etiopathogenesis of otitis is known, there are probably more factors involved in the onset of this disease.

ZOONOTIC POTENTIAL

N/A

SYNONYMS

- Otic abscess
- Otitis

ABBREVIATIONS

- IM = Intramuscular
- NSAIDs = nonsteroidal anti-inflammatory drugs

INTERNET RESOURCES

- Center for Avian and Exotic Medicine. Aural Abscesses in Aquatic Turtles. http://avianandexoticvets.com/aural-abscesses-in-aquatic-turtles
- Kik, M JL. Adenovirus infection in reptiles. EAZWV Transmissible Disease Fact Sheet, sheet no. 2, April 2009. https://www.eazwv.org/page/inf_handbook
- PetMD Editorial. Ear Infections in Turtles and Tortoises. PetMD July 24, 2008. http://www.petmd.com/reptile/conditions/ears/c_rp_ear_infections

Suggested Reading

Christiansen JL, Grzybowski JM, Rinner BP. Facial lesions in turtles, observations on prevalence, reoccurrence, and multiple origins. *J Herpetol* 2004;37:293–298.

De la Navarre BJS. Diagnosis and treatment of aural abscesses in turtles. *Proc ARAV* 2000;7:9–13.

Kroenlein KR, Sleeman JM, Holladay SD, et al. Inability to induce tympanic squamous metaplasia using organochlorine compounds in vitamin A-deficient red-eared sliders (*Trachemys scripta elegans*). *J Wildl Dis* 2010;44:664–669.

McKlveen TL, Jones CJ, Holladay SD. Radiographic diagnosis: aural abscesses in a box turtle. *Vet Radiol Ultrasound* 2000;41(5):419–421.

Author Albert Martínez-Silvestre, DVM, MSc, PhD, DECZM (Herpetology), EBVS European Veterinary Specialist in Herpetological Medicine and Surgery, Acred. AVEPA (Exotic Animals)

BALANTIDIUM

BASICS

DEFINITION/OVERVIEW

Balantidium is a large ciliated protozoal organism that resides within the gastrointestinal tract. The trophozoite is elliptical in shape and ranges in size from 30–300 × 25–120 µm. It is densely covered with cilia along its surface. At the tapered front end lies the cystostome (mouth). Cysts have a thick wall, spherical in shape, and have a kidney bean-shaped macronucleus. *Balantidium testudinis* is a species commonly reported in turtle species. They are typically found in herbivorous reptiles. It is debated whether these organisms are considered commensal within reptiles.

ETIOLOGY/PATHOPHYSIOLOGY

- Transmission is through the fecal–oral route.
- Cysts are ingested and then undergo excystation in the intestinal tract.
- Trophozoites inhabit the large colon and replicate by binary fission.
- Trophozoites undergo encystation in which infective cysts are formed and then excreted in feces.
- *Balantidium* sp. are facultative parasites and only become pathogenic when other virulence factors such as hyaluronidase are present.
- This then allows them to penetrate the intestinal mucosa and cause extensive hemorrhage and necrosis.
- Balantidium is generally limited to the large intestinal tract.
- In severe infections, the protozoal organisms migrate to the liver and cause abscessation.

SIGNALMENT/HISTORY

No age or sex predisposition

CLINICAL PRESENTATION

- Diarrhea
- Tenesmus
- Inappetence
- Weight loss

RISK FACTORS

Husbandry

Improper husbandry

Others

Immunocompromised animals with active parasitic/bacterial infections are more predisposed for the protozoan to become pathogenic.

DIAGNOSIS

DIFFERENTIAL DIAGNOSIS

Nyctotherus sp.

DIAGNOSTICS

- Microscopic evaluation of fresh fecal material to visualize trophozoites and cysts.
- SAF technique can be used for better visualization.
- The addition of iodine will stain the contents of the cysts, making them more visible.

PATHOLOGICAL FINDINGS

Hemorrhagic necrotizing colitis

TREATMENT

APPROPRIATE HEALTH CARE

N/A

NUTRITIONAL SUPPORT

N/A

CLIENT EDUCATION/HUSBANDRY RECOMMENDATIONS

- Practice proper hygiene
- Wash fruits and vegetables before being fed
- House infected animals separately

MEDICATIONS

DRUG(S) OF CHOICE

- Metronidazole 50 mg/kg PO q24h for 7 days
- Nimorazole 125 mg/kg PO q24h for 4 days
- Tetracyclines 5–10 mg/kg q24h for 5–8 days

PRECAUTIONS/INTERACTIONS

N/A

FOLLOW-UP

PATIENT MONITORING

Recheck feces on a routine basis

EXPECTED COURSE AND PROGNOSIS

Treatment should only be started if clinical disease is observed.

MISCELLANEOUS

COMMENTS

N/A

ZOONOTIC POTENTIAL

Balantidium coli is the only known species to infect humans.

SYNONYMS

N/A

ABBREVIATIONS

SAF = sodium acetate acetic acid formalin

INTERNET RESOURCES

- De Bosschere H, Roels S. Balantidium sp. and Nyctotherus sp.: Two common members of the digestive-tract flora in Mediterranean tortoises. Tortoise Trust. https://www.tortoisetrust.org/articles/balantidium.htm
- Divers SJ. Parasitic Diseases of Reptiles. MSD Manual Veterinary Manual, June 2020. http://www.merckvetmanual.com/exotic-and-laboratory-animals/reptiles/parasitic-diseases-of-reptiles

Suggested Reading

Hnizdo J, Pantchev N., eds. *Protozoa (digestive tract). In: Medical Care of Turtles and Tortoises: Diagnosis, Surgery, Pathology, Parasitology. Frankfurt*, Germany: Edition Chimaira; 2011:194–195

Jacobson ER. Parasites and parasitic diseases of reptiles. In: Jacobson ER, ed. *Infectious Diseases and Pathology of Reptiles: Color Atlas and Text.* Boca Raton, FL: CRC Press; 2007:571–666.

Rataj AV, Lindtner-Knific R, Vlahovic K, et al. Parasites in pet reptiles. *Acta Vet Scand* 2011;53(1):33.

Author Elsburgh O. Clarke III, DVM, DACZM

BUPHTHALMOS

BASICS

DEFINITION/OVERVIEW
Buphthalmos is an enlarged globe that is positioned normally in the socket.

ETIOLOGY/PATHOPHYSIOLOGY
An increase in IOP causing enlargement and distention of the globe secondary to chronic glaucoma.

SIGNALMENT/HISTORY
- There is no standard signalment for this disease.
- Common findings in the history may include tearing and squinting noted by the owners, as well as an asymmetry of the globes and loss of vision on the affected side(s).

CLINICAL PRESENTATION
- While buphthalmos can be bilateral, most cases in chelonians are unilateral.
- The corneal diameter of the affected eye is increased due to globe stretching.
- There may be blepharospasm and epiphora.
- Unlike exophthalmia, the conjunctiva and position of the nictitans is usually normal.
- There may be red ciliary flush (red ring around the cornea) and congested episcleral vessels.
- There may be lens luxation and/or cataracts in the affected eye(s).
- Retropulsion of the globe is normal but the globe itself may feel firmer than normal.

RISK FACTORS

Husbandry
- Diet and environmental factors are likely to have an effect on the development of cataracts.
- Cataract development in brumating tortoises has been associated with damage from freezing temperatures.

Others
- Trauma, especially if there is corneal penetration, can induce uveitis and cataract formation.
- The presence of a cataract may increase the chance of lens luxation and/or lens induced uveitis, both of which can lead to glaucoma.

DIAGNOSIS

DIFFERENTIAL DIAGNOSIS
- It is important to first differentiate between exophthalmia and buphthalmos.
- Glaucoma in chelonians is usually secondary to outflow obstruction of the aqueous humor, which is most often caused by uveitis, lens luxation, or intraocular neoplasia.

DIAGNOSTICS
- Physical examination findings should raise suspicion of buphthalmos, which is confirmed by finding elevated IOP.
- Normal IOP in three tortoise species has been reported to be 15.74 ± 0.2 mm Hg (*Testudo hermanni*), 14.2 ± 1.2 mm Hg (*Geochelone denticulata*), and 15.3 ± 8.81 mm Hg (*Geochelone carbonaria*) and in six turtle species at 5.42 ± 0.96 mm Hg (*Emys orbicularis*), 6.7 ± 1.4 mm Hg (*Terrapene* sp.), 8.3 ± 1.5 mm Hg (*Terrapene* sp.), 5.42 ± 1.7 mm Hg (*Trachemys scripta elegans*), 10.02 ± 0.66 mm Hg (*Trachemys scripta elegans*), 6.5 ± 1.0 mm Hg (*Lepidochelys kempii*), 3.8 ± 1.1 mm Hg (*Lepidochelys kempii*), and 4–9 mm Hg (*Caretta caretta*).
- Since most cases are unilateral, a significant difference in IOP between the eyes may be most indicative of a problem.
- Ocular examination and ultrasound are helpful in further evaluating the root cause, although the scleral ossicles can limit visualization.

PATHOLOGICAL FINDINGS
Chronically elevated IOP will lead to pain and blindness.

TREATMENT

APPROPRIATE HEALTH CARE
N/A

NUTRITIONAL SUPPORT
- Additional nutritional support is not necessary in most cases if the IOP can be brought down.
- If needed, tube feeding can be used to provide nutritional support.

CLIENT EDUCATION/HUSBANDRY RECOMMENDATIONS
- While buphthalmos can occur in any animal, those with husbandry deficiencies may be at increased risk.
- In addition to medical and surgical therapy, maximizing the husbandry of the animal will improve the chance for a successful outcome.

MEDICATIONS

DRUG(S) OF CHOICE
- As most of these cases present in a chronic state, vision is often already lost, and medications are used to control pain and slow the disease process during diagnostic evaluation, but enucleation as a salvage procedure is usually indicated.
- If acute glaucoma is suspected, it is important to start treatment immediately with topical β-adrenergic blockers (such as timolol) and CAIs (such as dorzolamide) BID to TID and mannitol (1–2 g/kg IV slowly over 20–30 minutes) to reduce IOP and preserve vision.
- If uveitis is suspected, systemic and topical antibiotics (such as ceftazadime 20 mg/kg IM or SC q48–72h) and steroids (prednisolone 0.25–0.5 mg/kg daily or dexamethasone SP 0.04–0.08 mg/kg daily) should also be instituted.

PRECAUTIONS/INTERACTIONS
N/A

FOLLOW-UP

PATIENT MONITORING
Serial IOP measurements are useful to determine response to therapy.

EXPECTED COURSE AND PROGNOSIS
- Prognosis is related to the underlying cause of the glaucoma, which is not always readily identifiable.
- Enucleation of the diseased globe will resolve the issue in most cases.

MISCELLANEOUS

COMMENTS
N/A

ZOONOTIC POTENTIAL
Depends on the cause of the buphthalmos, but low to most often no zoonotic potential.

SYNONYMS
N/A

ABBREVIATIONS
- CAI = carbonic anhydrase inhibitor
- IOP = intraocular pressure
- IV = intravenous
- SC = subcutaneous

Suggested Reading

Chittick B, Harms C. Intraocular pressure of juvenile loggerhead sea turtles (*Caretta caretta*) held in different positions. *Vet Rec* 2001;149(19):587–589.

Delgado C, Mans C, McLellan GJ, et al. Evaluation of rebound tonometry in red-eared slider turtles (*Trachemys scripta elegans*). *Vet Ophthalmol* 2014;17(4):261–267.

Espinheira Gomes F, Brandão J, Sumner J, et al. Survey of ophthalmic anterior segment findings and intraocular pressure in 95 North American box turtles (*Terrapene* spp.). *Vet Ophthalmol* 2016;19(2):93–101.

Gornik KR, Pirie CG, Marrion RM, et al. Ophthalmic variables in rehabilitated juvenile Kemp's ridley sea turtles (Lepidochelys kempii). *J Am Vet Med Assoc* 2016;248(6):673–680.

CHELONIANS

BUPHTHALMOS (CONTINUED)

Hochleithner C, Holland M. Ultrasonography. In: Mader, DR, Divers SJ, eds. *Current Therapy in Reptile Medicine and Surgery*. Saint Louis, MO: Elsevier Saunders; 2014:107–127.

Lawton, MPC. Reptilian Ophthalmology. In: Mader DR, ed. *Reptile Medicine and Surgery*. 2nd ed. St. Louis, MO: Elsevier Saunders; 2006:323–342.

Rajaei S, Ansari mood M, Sadjadi R, Azizi F. Measurement of intraocular pressure using Tonovet® in european pond turtle (*Emys orbicularis*). *J Zoo Wildl Med* 2015;46(2):421–422.

Selleri P, Di Girolamo N, Andreani V, et al. Evaluation of intraocular pressure in conscious Hermann's tortoises (*Testudo hermanni*) by means of rebound tonometry. *Am J Vet Res* 2012;73(11):1807–1812.

Selmi AL, Mendes GM, MacManus C, Arrais P. Intraocular pressure determination in clinically normal red-footed tortoise (*Geochelone carbonaria*). *J Zoo Wildl Med* 2002;33(1):58–61.

Selmi AL, Mendes GM, MacManus C. Tonometry in adult yellow-footed tortoises (*Geochelone denticulata*). *Vet Ophthalmol* 2003;6(4):305–307.

Somma AT, Lima L, Lange RR, et al. The eye of the red-eared slider turtle: morphologic observations and reference values for selected ophthalmic diagnostic tests. *Vet Ophthalmol* 2015;18(Suppl 1):61–70.

Author Christopher S. Hanley, DVM, DACZM

CARDIAC DISEASE

BASICS

DEFINITION/OVERVIEW

Cardiovascular disease encompasses a group of disorders of the heart and blood vessels including:

- Cardiomyopathy
- Septic endocarditis
- Valvular insufficiency (with no current evidence of primary degenerative endocardiosis)
- Myocarditis
- Pericardial effusion
- Infarct
- Atherosclerosis
- Aneurysm (rupture of aortic or carotid aneurysm)
- Gout
- Arterial calcification
- Thrombus
- Parasitic infestations
- Congenital heart defects
- Tumors

ETIOLOGY/PATHOPHYSIOLOGY

Infectious

- Often secondary to systemic infections in captive reptiles.
- Bacterial: aerobic Gram-negative bacteria: *Salmonella* spp., *Corynebacterium* spp., *Pseudomonas* spp. (endocarditis). *Flavobacterium* spp. and *Vibrio* spp. in a Barber's map turtle (*Graptemys barbouri*) (myocarditis).
- Parasitic: Trematodes (spirorchid flukes: *Spirorchis* spp., *Learedius* spp.) have been reported in the heart chambers and major vessels of sea and freshwater turtles (*Chelonia mydas*, *Trachemys scripta elegans*, *Chrysemys picta*), causing arteritis, endocarditis, granulomatous myocarditis, thrombosis and aneurysm.

Non-Infectious

- Neoplastic (primary neoplasia is uncommon in reptiles): hemangioma, hemangiosarcoma, cardiac rhabdomyosarcoma, fibrosarcoma; disseminated coelomic papillomas affecting various organs, including the heart, are frequently found in sea turtles with fibropapillomatosis.
- Metastasis to the heart: metastatic chondrosarcoma, metastasis of oviductal adenocarcinoma, disseminated mast cell tumor, multicentric lymphoblastic lymphoma and lymphoblastic malignant lymphoma.
- Metabolic: visceral gout can cause urate crystals deposition in the pericardium.
- Cardiomyopathy is of undetermined origin in reptiles. Myocardial degeneration can be the consequence of gout (of metabolic, nutritional or iatrogenic origin) and/or vitamin E and selenium deficiencies. The myocardium and the major arteries may also be subject to mineralization (calcification) with a diet of excessive levels of calcium and vitamin D3.
- Pericardial effusion is reported in many species but a small amount of fluid within the pericardial sac may also be normal. The etiology of pathologic pericardial effusion is unknown.

SIGNALMENT/HISTORY

- There are no known species, sex, or age predilections.
- Weakness and dyspnea
- Swelling in the area of the neck and/or peripheral edema.

CLINICAL PRESENTATION

- Presentation is similar to that seen in mammals.
- Some differences exist due to differing cardiovascular physiology and anatomy.
- Non-specific clinical signs such as lethargy, depression, anorexia, weight loss, weakness, dyspnea, bilateral exophthalmia, and sudden death.
- Cyanosis
- Peripheral edema (e.g., in gular region)
- Pulmonary edema, ascites
- Neurological signs such as ataxia and head tilt in case of brain anoxia.
- Peripheral thrombosis and necrosis in case of filarial infestation of the cardiovascular system.
- Coughing is not a feature of congestive heart failure as observed in mammals.

RISK FACTORS

Husbandry

Inadequate husbandry, resulting in chronic stress, immune suppression and malnutrition, is the most likely common predisposing factor for the development of cardiovascular conditions in captive reptiles.

Others

Atherosclerosis and viral diseases can also be predisposing factors.

DIAGNOSIS

DIFFERENTIAL DIAGNOSIS

All other diseases that induce lethargy and/or respiratory distress.

DIAGNOSTICS

Ambient temperature can influence cardiopulmonary parameters in reptiles so must be considered during examination.

Auscultation

- The use of a stethoscope is impossible because of the osteodermic shell.
- A continuous Doppler ultrasonic probe (8 MHz) can also be used for cardiac "auscultation". It allows determination of heart rate and rhythm but only indicates blood flow (not valve closure).

Ultrasound

- The most practical diagnostic tool for antemortem evaluation of reptilian heart diseases.
- Allows visualization of blood flow within the heart. In chelonians, the transducer is placed in the cervicobrachial area.

Hematology and Biochemistry

Blood pressure measurement and pulse oximetry are not reliable in reptiles.

Clinical Pathology

- CK and LDH may increase with conditions affecting the cardiac muscle in reptiles, such as myocarditis or infarct. However, these are non-specific measurements and may also increase with skeletal muscle damage from traumatic injuries, loss of body condition, and intramuscular injections.
- Currently, cardiac troponins have not been assessed in chelonians.
- Leukocytosis, lymphocytosis, and heterophilia may be present, and are suggestive of underlying infections or hematopoietic neoplasia with secondary cardiac effects.

Electrocardiography

- Low electric amplitudes (usually < 1.0 mV) and standard parameters not established for many species.
- Common findings in the normal reptilian ECG include P-wave pleomorphism, very small Q and S deflections and prolonged Q-T intervals compared with similar-sized mammals.
- Correct electrode placement (challenging in reptiles) is essential to avoid erroneous ECG readings.

Radiography

Challenging to produce images of high diagnostic value, especially in chelonians.

CT and MRI

- Apart from obvious cardiomyopathy, neither CT nor MRI (unless using a very high magnetic field strengths) are of use for visualizing intracardiac structures and large vessels.
- Evaluate for concurrent disease to determine whether cardiac issue is primary or secondary (neoplastic, infectious).

PATHOLOGICAL FINDINGS

Gross and histopathologic findings depend on the type of heart disease.

TREATMENT

APPROPRIATE HEALTH CARE

- Little information
- The pharmacology of cardiac drugs in reptiles is poorly understood and few data are available in the literature (pharmacokinetics, toxicity, etc.).

NUTRITIONAL SUPPORT

No specific nutritional support considerations or recommendations.

CLIENT EDUCATION/HUSBANDRY RECOMMENDATIONS

Reduce stress by minimizing handling, separating from cage mates, and maintaining the reptile at its preferred optimum temperature.

MEDICATIONS

DRUG(S) OF CHOICE

- Beta-blockers: of unknown effectiveness in reptile patients.
- Methylatropine: administration results in an increase in resting heart rate of iguanas (*Iguana iguana*). No data available for chelonians.
- Pimobendan and digoxin: unknown effects in reptiles.
- Enalapril: inhibited angiotensin I conversion in alligators at 0.5–0.7 mg/kg once every 24 hours (combined with spironolactone and furosemide). No data available for chelonians.
- Furosemide: possible diuretic effect in chelonians despite lacking the loop of Henle.
- Hydrochlorothiazide has been used as a diuretic in lizards with renal disease. No data available for chelonians.
- Methylated xanthines (aminophylline and theophylline) have successfully induced diuresis.
- Nothing is known about the potential use of spironolactone in reptiles.

PRECAUTIONS/INTERACTIONS

N/A

FOLLOW-UP

PATIENT MONITORING

Hemoculture, repeated echocardiographic examinations

EXPECTED COURSE AND PROGNOSIS

As no specific treatment is available, fast deterioration can be expected.

MISCELLANEOUS

COMMENTS

N/A

ZOONOTIC POTENTIAL

Can be zoonotic in case of salmonellosis and other Gram-negative bacteria.

SYNONYMS

- Cardiovascular disease
- Heart disease

ABBREVIATIONS

- CK = creatine kinase
- CT = computed tomography
- ECG = electrocardiogram
- LDH = lactate dehydrogenase
- MRI = magnetic resonance imaging

Suggested Reading

Beaufrère H, Schilliger L, Pariaut R. Cardiovascular system. In: Mitchell MA, Tully TN, eds. *Current Therapy of Exotic Animal Practice*. St. Louis, MO: Elsevier; 2016:151–220.

Mitchell MA. Reptile cardiology. *Vet Clin North Am Exot Anim Pract* 2009;12:65–79.

Schilliger L, Girling S. Cardiology. In: Divers S, Stahl S, eds. *Mader's Reptile and Amphibian Medicine and Surgery*. St. Louis, MO: Elsevier; 2019:669–698.

Author Lionel Schilliger, DVM, DECZM (Herpetology), DABVP (Reptile & Amphibian Practice)

CLOACAL PROLAPSE

BASICS

DEFINITION/OVERVIEW

A prolapse is the moving or slipping of a body part from its usual position or anatomic relation. In the reptile, a prolapse from the vent may originate in the cloaca, rectum, phallus, oviduct, or bladder.

ETIOLOGY/PATHOPHYSIOLOGY

- The underlying causes for prolapse is often unknown.
- See Differential Diagnosis for a list of possible etiologies.

SIGNALMENT/HISTORY

- There appear to be no specific signalments or predilections noted for the various reptilian prolapses.
- Female reptilians may be overrepresented due to occurrences of dystocia.

CLINICAL PRESENTATION

- A prolapse is easy to visualize as abnormal tissue protruding from the cloacal/vent region.
- In reptiles housed outdoors and in case of small prolapses, the owners may not notice a problem until days after it has occurred.
- A prolapse should be considered as an emergency and evaluated promptly.
- The tissue should be kept moist by gently washing the area with water and loosely wrapping in a damp cloth or paper towel until the animal can be evaluated by a veterinarian.
- The extruded tissue should be identified to the tissue(s) involved such as cloacal, with/without bladder, oviduct, proctodeum, colon, phallus, etc.
- Once the issues are identified, the clinician may be able to narrow the differential diagnoses (see below) to determine the course of diagnostics and therapeutics.

RISK FACTORS

- In cases of nutritional secondary hyperparathyroidism, the muscle tone around the cloacal opening is decreased, leading to potential tissue exposure.
- Any generalized physical straining of the patient can lead to tissue exposure through the cloaca, such as dyspnea, obstipation, parasites, infection, etc.
- Space-occupying lesions located in the coelomic cavity, such as uroliths, neoplasia, hepto/renomegaly, eggs, etc., may also cause increase straining and cloacal prolapse.

Husbandry

- Several factors of husbandry may lead to one of the clinical conditions listed in the Differential Diagnosis section.
- Corrections of the deficient aspects of the husbandry can lead to reversal of some of those listed conditions.

Others

- Some cloacal tissue may prolapse during normal oviposition.
- Iatrogenic prolapses may occur when owners attempt to manually manipulate ova in suspected cases of dystocia or feces in constipated animals.

DIAGNOSIS

DIFFERENTIAL DIAGNOSIS

- Parasites
- Hypocalcemia
- Dehydration
- Metabolic disease
- Neoplasia
- Impaction
- Obstruction
- Trauma
- Coelomic space occupying lesion
- Obesity
- Bacterial Infection
- Intoxication

DIAGNOSTICS

- Radiography and ultrasound may be useful in determining internal abnormalities (e.g., impactions, masses, obstructions).
- The small size of some reptiles may lead to reduced imaging detail, which makes interpretation challenging.
- Dental radiographs may be a better alternative in smaller species (< 100 g).
- A fecal examination should be performed in all cases. This can be directly from the feces, a saline cloacal wash, or direct impression smear of the prolapsed tissue may reveal the presence of parasites such as nematode larvae or eggs.
- A CBC and chemistry panel may assist in the determination of underlying physiologic abnormalities.

PATHOLOGICAL FINDINGS

- Protozoal infections affecting the gastrointestinal tract may be diagnosed on histopathology.
- Other findings will be consistent with the underlying cause but often no specific cause or pathology can be identified.

TREATMENT

APPROPRIATE HEALTH CARE

- Treatment often involves direct replacement of the tissue back into normal anatomic position either by manual or surgical means in combination with correction of the underlying etiology.
- The patient should be fully evaluated for general health status and treated accordingly.
- The prolapsed tissue should be evaluated for presence of devitalization, which must be surgically or medically addressed prior to prolapse reduction.
- In severe oviductal prolapses, discussion with the owner about desired reproductive status should take place with a potential for coeliotomy and ovariosalpingectomy.
- In some cases, the internal reproductive structures may be medically or surgically repaired; further reproductive events could result in dystocia.
- The prolapse may be reduced in size by coating with a hyperosmotic solution such as 2–5% ophthalmic saline or concentrated sugar solution.
- Direct application of dry salt or sugar may be attempted, but the extreme osmolar difference could lead to direct tissue damage and should be closely monitored.
- After several minutes of application, the prolapsed tissue should become less edematous and capable of reduction back into the body cavity.
- A moistened and lubricated (water soluble) cotton tip applicator or metal probe is used to gently push the tissue back inside the body cavity aligning the lumen.
- Surgical options such as resection of the diseased tissue and double-layer closure can be performed prior to tissue replacement.
- In more extensive cases, a coeliotomy/plastronotomy may be undertaken, with the tissue resection performed within the coelomic cavity where the tissue is in approximate "normal" anatomic position.
- Colonic prolapses may require a colopexy where sutures are placed to facilitate the "tacking" of the colon to the dorsolateral body wall.
- In cases of reproductive system prolapse (i.e., oviduct), the tissue may be replaced but damage to the suspensory ligaments and internal vasculature may be present.
- A purse-string suture around the cloaca or lateral sutures across the cloacal margin may be placed for 10–14 days to allow for the tissue swelling to resolve in place.

NUTRITIONAL SUPPORT

The reptilian patient may need weight and body condition monitoring to determine whether additional caloric supplementation is needed.

CLIENT EDUCATION/HUSBANDRY RECOMMENDATIONS

- If surgical correction of the prolapse was undertaken, the client should be directed on postoperative care of any surgical sites, suture, etc.

CLOACAL PROLAPSE (CONTINUED)

- A detailed log of activity, as well as food intake/defecations, should be maintained and related back to the veterinarian.
- If any changes to the husbandry are determined, the owner should correct those prior to the patient returning home, such as changes to temperature and/or humidity, exposure UVB lighting, etc.

MEDICATIONS

DRUG(S) OF CHOICE

- NSAIDs or opioids may be used in management of the inflammation and pain associated with the physical discomfort of the prolapse or surgery.
- Depending on the determined etiology, antibiotics or anti-parasiticides may be indicated.

PRECAUTIONS/INTERACTIONS

- When replacing the prolapse, extreme care must be taken not to tear or perforate the delicate, inflamed tissue.
- After the sutures are removed, the tissue may re-prolapse if swelling/inflammation are still present or the underlying etiology has not been corrected.
- Placement of additional sutures may be required. Hydration status of the patent must be considered before use of NSAIDs.

FOLLOW-UP

PATIENT MONITORING

- The patient should be followed up daily after clinical repair of the prolapse for reoccurrence.
- The owner should monitor and record all food intake and defecations during this time.
- Any abnormal changes should be related back to the veterinarian to determine any further changes to the therapy.

EXPECTED COURSE AND PROGNOSIS

- Prolapses of the oviduct and bladder tend to have a guarded to grave prognosis due to the degree of underlying physical damage to the affected tissues and cloaca.
- Rectal and cloacal prolapses tend to have a fair prognosis if treated promptly.
- Phallus prolapses have excellent to good prognosis, as these are purely copulatory organs.
- The length of time the prolapse presents has an inverse effect on the prognosis.
- When treated early in the disease process and the tissue appears viable, cloacal prolapse replacement may lead to clinical resolution if the underlying etiology is addressed.
- Once the tissue begins to desiccate and become devitalized, there is a guarded to grave prognosis.

MISCELLANEOUS

COMMENTS

N/A

ZOONOTIC POTENTIAL

N/A

SYNONYMS

N/A

ABBREVIATIONS

- CBC = complete blood count
- NSAIDs = nonsteroidal anti-inflammatory drugs
- UVB = ultraviolet B

Suggested Reading

Barten, SL. Penile prolapse. In: Mader DR, ed. *Reptile Medicine and Surgery*. 2nd ed. St. Louis, MO: Elsevier Saunders; 2006:862–864.

Bennett, RA. Cloacal prolapse. In: Mader DR, ed. *Reptile Medicine and Surgery*. 2nd ed. St. Louis, MO: Elsevier Saunders; 2006:751–755.

Author Rob L. Coke, DVM, DACZM, DABVP (Reptile & Amphibian), CVA

CONJUNCTIVITIS

BASICS

DEFINITION/OVERVIEW

Conjunctivitis is defined as inflammation of the conjunctiva. In reptiles, conjunctivitis often presents concurrently with blepharedema, which is edema and swelling of the eyelids. In many cases, the blepharedema is severe enough to impede proper evaluation of the eye and hence identification of conjunctivitis. Blepharoconjunctivitis is a common presentation.

ETIOLOGY/PATHOPHYSIOLOGY

- Conjunctivitis is most often caused by viral or bacterial infections.
- Other etiologies include fungal or parasitic infection, poor water quality, and environmental irritants or toxins.
- Trauma may also be a cause, especially in cases of unilateral conjunctivitis.

SIGNALMENT/HISTORY

- There is no specific signalment for the occurrence of conjunctivitis.
- The main focus should be on obtaining a thorough history of the husbandry.

CLINICAL PRESENTATION

- In addition to the conjunctivitis itself, chelonians often present with blepharedema, blepharospasm, and/or periocular swelling usually affecting both eyes and causing blepharoconjunctivitis.
- Animals may also present with anorexia, depression and lethargy due to either the systemic effects of the underlying etiology (e.g., herpes virus) or simply from their inability to see properly.

RISK FACTORS

Husbandry

- Poor cleanliness and hygiene of the enclosure can lead to increased environmental bacterial load, which can contribute to conjunctivitis.
- Poor water quality for aquatic chelonians causing high ammonia levels.

Others

N/A

DIAGNOSIS

DIFFERENTIAL DIAGNOSIS

- Herpes virus
- Ranavirus
- Mycoplasmosis
- Chlamydiosis
- Toxin exposure (ammonia, aromatic oils from cedar chips)
- Trauma
- Parasitic (leeches or trematodes)

DIAGNOSTICS

- A complete ophthalmic examination with the use of magnification by direct or indirect ophthalmoscopy including fluorescein test for corneal ulcers.
- Sampling of the conjunctiva for bacterial culture and sensitivity.
- PCR for herpes virus, ranavirus, *Mycoplasma* sp., or *Chlamydia* sp., according to other clinical signs and presentation.

PATHOLOGICAL FINDINGS

- Blepharoconjunctivitis is a common presentation.
- Plaques or caseous material may be observed within the fornix or even covering the corneal surface.
- Mucopurulent discharge

TREATMENT

APPROPRIATE HEALTH CARE

- Treatment will be based on the underlying etiology; anti-inflammatories and analgesics should be considered in most cases.
- Treatment of viral infections is often unrewarding.
- Concurrent systemic and ophthalmic therapy is recommended for best response.
- Flushing and cleaning of the eyes is also necessary to remove any adhered material or plaques that may be harboring organisms.
- A solution of 1 part povidone iodine to 50 parts saline can be used.
- When blepharedema is present, a pipette tip, tomcat catheter, or intravenous catheter can be inserted between the eyelids to flush the eyes.

NUTRITIONAL SUPPORT

- In cases of anorectic animals, force-feeding with easily digestible proteins should be initiated.
- Direct feeding by stomach tubing can be performed in some species; placement of an esophagostomy tube should be considered for chronic management.
- Supportive fluid therapy should be provided.

CLIENT EDUCATION/HUSBANDRY RECOMMENDATIONS

- Remove and isolate sick individuals and reduce stress by providing optimal living conditions and hygiene.
- Thorough cleaning of cage to reduce environmental load of infectious organisms.
- Ensure that quarantine protocols have been implemented for all new arrivals.
- Treatment compliance is key for response to therapy.

MEDICATIONS

DRUG(S) OF CHOICE

Systemic Therapy

- Meloxicam: 0.5 mg/kg IM, PO q24h
- Dexamethasone sodium phosphate —0.1–0.3 mg/kg IM, SC, IV q24h for 3 days
- Ceftazidime: 22 mg/kg IM q72h
- Ceftiofur crytasalline free acid: 30 mg/kg SC q5d
- Amikacin: 5 mg/kg IM q48h
- Enrofloxacin: 5–10 mg/kg IM, PO q24–48h
- Oxytetracycline: 5–10 mg/kg IM q24h; 10 mg/kg IM q5d for long-acting formulation

Ophthalmic Therapy

- Ophthalmic antibiotics applied 3–4 times daily
- Ophthalmic anti-inflammatory applied 3–4 times daily

PRECAUTIONS/INTERACTIONS

Vitamin A must be administered only in cases with clear indication of hypovitaminosis A, otherwise there is a risk of causing hypervitaminosis A.

FOLLOW-UP

PATIENT MONITORING

Weekly to every two-week re-evaluations are recommended to determine response to therapy.

EXPECTED COURSE AND PROGNOSIS

- Course and prognosis will vary according to the etiology.
- Prognosis for viral infections is grave as these animals typically become progressively worse over time.
- For other etiologies prognosis is good to excellent.

MISCELLANEOUS

COMMENTS

Figure 2—see web image supplementary content for Section II (Chelonians).

ZOONOTIC POTENTIAL

Low for the most common etiologies.

SYNONYMS

N/A

CONJUNCTIVITIS (CONTINUED)

ABBREVIATIONS

- IM = intramuscular
- IV = intravenous
- PCR = polymerase chain reaction
- PO = per os
- SC = subcutaneous

Suggested Reading

Di Ianni F, Dodi PL, Cabassi CS, et al. Conjunctival flora of clinically normal and diseased turtles and tortoises. *BMC Vet Res* 2015;11:91.

Lawton, MPC. Reptilian Ophthalmology. In: Mader DR, ed. *Reptile Medicine and Surgery*. 2nd ed. St. Louis, MO: Elsevier Saunders; 2006:323–342.

Author Javier G. Nevarez, DVM, PhD, DACZM, DECZM (Herpetology)

CRYPTOSPORIDIUM

BASICS

DEFINITION/OVERVIEW

Cryptosporidia are apicomplexan parasites typified by possessing an apical complex, and with four naked sporozites within each oocyte. Cryptosporidia can be distinguished from other coccidian parasites by the location that they occupy within the host cell membrane, their capacity for autoinfection, and their resistance to anti-parasitic medication. Possessing a durable oocyst wall consisting of a double layer of a protein–lipid–carbohydrate matrix, cryptosporidia are highly resistant to environmental degradation and chemical disinfection. Historically, oocyst morphology has been used for species identification, but this is considered unreliable and species assignment is now determined by molecular characteristics. Cryptosporidia are ubiquitous in the environment and are globally distributed.

ETIOLOGY/PATHOPHYSIOLOGY

- *Cryptosporidium pestis* has been recovered from captive tortoises, with an additional species in chelonians, *C. ducismarci*, yet to be ratified.
- *C. ducismarci* has been isolated from intestinal lesions in tortoises and additionally from asymptomatic ball pythons and chameleons.
- Cryptosporidium oocysts from chelonians can cause severe infections in snakes when experimentally transferred.
- Transmission is direct, with reptiles becoming infected after ingesting oocysts that have been shed in feces.
- Autoinfection may also occur with some oocysts releasing their sporozoites within the host's body.
- No pre-patent period has been determined.

SIGNALMENT/HISTORY

Infected animals usually have a history of chronic wasting accompanied by diarrhea and inappetence.

CLINICAL PRESENTATION

- Subclinical (carrier state): animals may appear healthy and are able to shed oocysts intermittently for years.
- Enteritis: a chronic debilitating enteritis without gastric involvement that may be accompanied by concurrent disease.

RISK FACTORS

The greatest risk factor for developing infection is poor quarantine of new animals entering a collection.

Husbandry

N/A

Others

N/A

DIAGNOSIS

DIFFERENTIAL DIAGNOSIS

Enteritis—bacterial or other protozoal disease.

DIAGNOSTICS

- Examination of feces: unstained smears are useful but sensitivity of detection increases with an acid-fast stain and is greatest with an IFA stain.
- Sensitivity may be increased if performed postprandially.
- An important limitation of these tests is their lack of specificity to differentiate *Cryptosporidium* spp.
- False positive results can occur in animals that have ingested food items (i.e., mice) infected with other *Cryptosporidium* spp. that are not pathogenic to reptiles.
- Serum antibody titers: can be assessed using an ELISA but antibodies take 6 weeks to develop. Best if combined with fecal or gastric lavage.
  - ELISA positive, fecal positive—animal infected and shedding.
  - ELISA negative, fecal negative—not infected.
  - ELISA negative, fecal positive—recent infection (<6 weeks) or passing non-reptilian *Cryptosporidium* spp.
  - ELISA positive, fecal negative—has been infected at some point but not shedding or shedding at undetectable levels.
- PCR: a highly sensitive test that can be used for either fecal or lavage samples. Can also differentiate between *Cryptosporidium* spp.

PATHOLOGICAL FINDINGS

- Gross: intestinal lesions may include mucosal thickening with mucus accumulation.
- Histopathology: intestinal lesions consist of a mixed inflammatory response with up to 80% of epithelial cells containing parasites.

TREATMENT

APPROPRIATE HEALTH CARE

Elimination of cryptosporidia from reptiles is difficult and rarely rewarding.

NUTRITIONAL SUPPORT

- Force-feeding with easily digestible proteins.
- Direct feeding by stomach tubing can be performed in some species; placement of an esophagostomy tube should be considered for chronic management.
- Supportive fluid therapy should be provided.

CLIENT EDUCATION/HUSBANDRY RECOMMENDATIONS

- Clients should be made aware of the insidious nature of infection, the unlikelihood of successful treatment, the risks that affected animals pose to the remaining collection, and the known zoonotic potential of some species of *Cryptosporidium*.
- Cryptosporidium oocysts are hardy and can persist in the environment for long periods, so thorough cleaning and disinfection is important.
- Methods for disinfection include:
  - ammonia (5%) or formal saline (10%) solution contact for 18 hours
  - exposure to moist heat (45–60 degrees C) for 5–9 minutes
  - freezing
  - thorough desiccation alone, or after any chemical application

MEDICATIONS

DRUG(S) OF CHOICE

- Trimethoprim sulfonamide 30 mg/kg PO SID for 14 days, then 1–3 times weekly for 3 months may reduce oocyst shedding but does not eliminate cryptosporidium organisms from the gastrointestinal mucosa.
- Paromomycin 100 mg/kg PO SID for 7 days; then twice weekly for 6 weeks; and 360 mg/kg q48h for 10 days resulted in complete resolution in experimentally infected bearded dragons (*Pogona vitticeps*).
- Hyperimmune bovine colostrum 1% body weight by volume PO once weekly for 6 weeks. Currently not available commercially.

PRECAUTIONS/INTERACTIONS

- Euthanasia should be strongly considered for affected animals to limit spread.
- If euthanasia is not an option, diseased reptiles should be separated from the remaining collection and strict barrier nursing protocols enacted to prevent spread.

FOLLOW-UP

Regular fecal examination and ELISA assays for suspected at risk animals.

PATIENT MONITORING

Monitor for signs of disease, i.e., wasting, diarrhea, persistent regurgitation.

EXPECTED COURSE AND PROGNOSIS

Grave prognosis, likely chronic wasting and death.

MISCELLANEOUS

COMMENTS

N/A

ZOONOTIC POTENTIAL

- *C. pestis* is a known zoonotic risk; *C. ducismarci* shows genetic similarities to other zoonotic *Cryptosporidium* spp.
- Caution should be used when working with suspected cases.

SYNONYMS

N/A

ABBREVIATIONS

- ELISA = enzyme-linked immunosorbent assay
- IFA = immunofluorescent antibody
- IM = intramuscular
- IV = intravenous
- PCR = polymerase chain reaction
- PO = per os
- SC = subcutaneous

Suggested Reading

Cranfield MR, Graczyk TK. Cryptosporidiosis. In: Mader DR, ed. *Reptile Medicine and Surgery*. 2nd ed. St. Louis, MO: Elsevier Saunders; 2006:756–762.

Fayer R. Taxonomy and species delimitation in Cryptosporidium. *Exp Parasitol Jan* 2010; 124(1): 90–-97.

Fayer R, Graczyk TK, Cranfield MR. Multiple heterogenous isolates of *Cryptosporidium serpentis* from captive snakes are not transmissible to neonatal BALB/c mice (*Mus musculus*). *J Parasitol* 1995;81(3):482–484.

Graczyk TK, Owens R, Cranfield MR. Diagnosis of subclinical cryptosporidiosis in captive snakes based on stomach lavage and cloacal sampling. *Vet Parasitol* 1996;67:143–151.

Grosset C, Villeneuve A, Brieger A, Lair S. Cryptosporidiosis in juvenile bearded dragons (*Pogona vitticeps*) effects of treatment with paromomycin. *J Herp Med Surg* 2011;21:10–15.

Pedraza-Diaz S, Ortega-Mora LM, Carrion BA, et al. Molecular characterisation of Cryptosporidium isolates from pet reptiles. *Vet Parasitol* 2009;160(3–4):204–210.

Plutzer J, Karanis P. Genetic polymorphism in Cryptosporidium species: An update. *Vet Parasitol* 2009;165(3–4):187–199.

Richter B, Rasim R, Vrhovec MG, et al. Cryptosporidiosis outbreak in captive chelonians (*Testudo hermanni*) with identification of two Cryptosporidium genotypes. *J Vet Diagn Invest* 2012;24(3):591–595.

Scullion FT, Scullion MG. Gastrointestinal protozoal diseases in reptiles. *J Exot Pet Med* 2009;18(4):266–278.

Shahiduzzaman M, Daugschies A. Therapy and prevention of cryptosporidiosis in animals. *Vet Parasitol* 2012;188(3–4):203–214.

Traversa D. Evidence for a new species of Cryptosporidium infecting tortoises: *Cryptosporidium ducismarci*. *Parasit Vectors* 2010;3(21):1–4.

Traversa D, Iorio R, Otranto D, et al. Cryptosporidium from tortoises: Genetic characterisation, phylogeny and zoonotic implications. *Mol Cell Probes* 2008;22(2):122–128.

Uhl EW, Jacobson E, Bartick TE, et al. Aural-pharyngeal polyps associated with *Cryptosporidium* infection in three iguanas (*Iguana iguana*). *Vet Path* 2001;38:239–242.

Author T. Franciscus Scheelings, BVSc, MVSc, PhD, MANCVSc (Wildlife Health) DECZM (Herpetology)

DIARRHEA

BASICS

DEFINITION/OVERVIEW

Diarrhea is the production of unformed or liquid fecal matter. It is often associated with increased fecal volume and frequency of defection.

ETIOLOGY/PATHOPHYSIOLOGY

- Diarrhea is usually associated with enteritis due to primary infectious (e.g., endoparasites) or non-infectious (e.g., dietary) causes.
- In tortoises with a natural diet high in dietary fiber (e.g., African and European tortoises) ingestion of diets high in fermentable carbohydrates (e.g., fruits) and/or insufficient fiber ingestion can result in dysbacteriosis, which can result in diarrhea.
- Environmental factors, such as low temperatures, lead to decreased gastrointestinal motility, dysbacteriosis and diarrhea due overgrowth of opportunistic pathogens.
- Diarrhea is common in tortoises, but uncommon in freshwater turtles, which normally have unformed liquid feces.
- Most commonly kept tortoise species require a high-fiber, low sugar, and low protein diet, and therefore feeding large amounts of fresh fruits and starch containing vegetables will frequently lead to unformed feces or diarrhea.
- The following endoparasites can be associated with diarrhea in tortoises:
  - nematodes: oxyurids are very common in tortoises; ascarids are reported in wild-caught *Testudo* spp. (European tortoises) in captivity; other nematodes such as Strongyloides and Capillaria are uncommon
  - coccidia: uncommon
  - ciliated protozoa: *Nyctotherus* spp., *Balantidium* spp., *Entamoeba* spp. (*E. invadens*)
  - flagellates: *Trichomonas* spp.
- Bacteria: *Proteus* and *Salmonella* spp. are often asymptomatic carriers, but can lead to diarrhea.

SIGNALMENT/HISTORY

- Diarrhea is more common in tortoises than in turtles.
- Inappropriate husbandry: low environmental temperatures and overcrowding (stress) can lead to enteritis and diarrhea.
- Inappropriate diet: tortoises fed a low-fiber diet, high in fermentable sugars and protein, are prone to develop diarrhea.
- Owners report liquid feces, frequently malodorous, with increased frequency of defecation.
- Straining to defecate, anorexia, and cloacal prolapse may also be reported.

CLINICAL PRESENTATION

- Depending on duration (acute vs. chronic), severity and etiology of diarrhea.
- Fecal staining around cloaca, and ventral aspects of proximal hind limbs and tail base.
- Presence of abnormally soft or liquid fecal matter in transport container.
- Tortoises with diarrhea caused by an inappropriate diet might show no other clinical signs or may show unspecific clinical signs, such as lethargy, reduced food intake, or dehydration.
- Chronic diarrhea can lead to weight loss and cachexia due to malabsorption of nutrients.
- Cloacal tissue prolapse, such as rectal/distal colon prolapse, or true cloacal prolapse.

RISK FACTORS

Husbandry

- In most tortoises (except red- and yellow-footed tortoises)—diet low in fiber and/or high in fermentable simple carbohydrates (e.g., fruits).
- Change in diet
- Poor sanitation can lead to high endoparasite load due to the direct lifecycle of many intestinal parasites of chelonians.
- Overcrowding results in stress
- Inappropriate (too low or too high) environmental temperatures.

Others

- Wild-caught animals often have a high endoparasite load and are often stressed during acclimatization to captivity.
- Lack of fecal parasitology screening after acquisition.

DIAGNOSIS

DIFFERENTIAL DIAGNOSIS

- Enteritis - bacterial, parasitic, dietary

DIAGNOSTICS

- Fecal direct wet mount to evaluate for motile protozoa.
- Fecal flotation to evaluate for helminths and protozoa (e.g., amoeba cysts).
- Fecal cytology to rule out fungal infections
- Diagnostic imaging (radiographs, CT, ultrasound) as needed.
- Fecal bacterial cultures are rarely useful in the diagnosis and treatment of chelonians with diarrhea.

PATHOLOGICAL FINDINGS

- Enteritis
- Malodorous and liquid intestinal content
- Emaciation

TREATMENT

APPROPRIATE HEALTH CARE

N/A

NUTRITIONAL SUPPORT

- Correct diet to ensure sufficient fiber intake in herbivorous tortoises.
- Provide nutritional support to emaciated and/or anorexic animals.
- Provide fluid therapy to dehydrated animals.

CLIENT EDUCATION/HUSBANDRY RECOMMENDATIONS

N/A

MEDICATIONS

DRUG(S) OF CHOICE

- Metronidazole: 40–100 mg/kg PO repeat 10–14 days or 25 mg/kg PO q24h for 5 days. Effective against motile protozoal organisms.
- Emodepside/praziquantel (Profender®, Bayer DVM, Pittsburgh, PA): 1 ml/kg topical on skin. Repeat after 14 days. Effective against nematodes, trematodes and cestodes. Recommended in particular in animals that cannot be dosed orally. Animals should not be soaked for 24 hours after topical administration. Apply to skin around forelimbs and neck.
- Fenbendazole: 20 mg/kg PO q24h for 3–5 days. Effective against nematodes and flagellates.
- Pyrantel pamoate: 25 mg/kg PO q24h for 5 days, repeat in 3 weeks. Effective against nematodes including pinworms and ascarids.
- Keep on newspaper until treatment is completed and recheck fecal samples.
- Immediate removal of feces to prevent ingestion, bathing the tortoises, and cleaning of the pericloacal region to remove feces and eggs or cysts are strongly recommended.
- Prevention of reinfection is critically important during and following treatment against parasites with a direct lifecycle.

PRECAUTIONS/INTERACTIONS

- Fenbendazole has been shown to result in heteropenia and biochemical abnormalities in *Testudo hermanni* following administration of two courses of 50 mg/kg q24h for 5 days.
- Fenbendazole has been shown in other reptiles to cause bone marrow suppression and temporary pancytopenia. Avoid doses > 20 mg/kg.
- Do not use ivermectin or other macrocyclic lactones (e.g., selamectin) in chelonians.

DIARRHEA (CONTINUED)

FOLLOW-UP

PATIENT MONITORING

- Return to normal fecal consistency.
- Weight gain and maintenance of hydration.
- Repeat fecal exams to ensure treatment effectiveness.

EXPECTED COURSE AND PROGNOSIS

- If dietary causes are responsible for the diarrhea, then prognosis is good to excellent.
- Animals in good body condition with no concurrent morbidities have a good to excellent prognosis.
- Animals in poor body condition with signs of systemic illness (dehydration, lethargy, etc.) have a guarded to poor prognosis.

MISCELLANEOUS

COMMENTS

- Diarrhea is a clinical sign associated with an underlying diseases, improper husbandry, or nutrition.
- Identification of the underlying cause is necessary to improve outcome and reduce the risk of reoccurrence.
- Correction of husbandry is always recommended to in help improve the outcome.

ZOONOTIC POTENTIAL

Salmonella spp. are commonly shed from chelonians with and without diarrhea.

SYNONYMS

N/A

ABBREVIATIONS

- CT = computed tomography
- PO = per os

Suggested Reading

Funk RS. Diarrhea. In: Mader DR, ed. *Reptile Medicine and Surgery*. 2nd ed. St. Louis, MO: Elsevier Saunders; 2006:772–773.

Greiner EC, Mader DR. Parasitology. In: Mader DR, ed. *Reptile Medicine and Surgery*. 2nd ed. St. Louis, MO: Elsevier Saunders; 2006:343–364.

Author Christoph Mans, Dr. med. vet., DACZM

BASICS

DEFINITION/OVERVIEW

Dystocia is difficulty laying eggs.

ETIOLOGY/PATHOPHYSIOLOGY

- The reproductive hormone mechanism in reptiles is not as well understood as that of mammals.
- It is suspected that a multitude of environmental and behavioral factors, as well as underlying diseases, contribute to an abnormal function of the endocrine system, which in turn leads to dystocia.
- It is also possible that a lack of breeding and exposure to males may be contributing factors.
- In addition to basic husbandry aspects, such as UVB light, temperature, humidity, and a proper diet, female reptiles also have a need for appropriate substrate and environment that is conductive for egg laying.

SIGNALMENT/HISTORY

- Dystocia occurs in female chelonians of reproductive age or size.
- Most animals have a history of inadequate nutrition and husbandry lacking an appropriate area for laying eggs.

CLINICAL PRESENTATION

- Signs of dystocia may include straining with or without vocalization, decreased fecal production, cloacal prolapse, hind limb weakness/paresis, lethargy, and anorexia.
- Some animals may also appear restless and may be observed attempting to dig.
- In some instances, the eggs may be palpable through the prefemoral fossa during physical exam.
- Physical exam should be done carefully to avoid rupturing the eggs.
- In most cases, the owners are not aware of the fact that their chelonian is in dystocia.
- Other abnormalities identified in physical exam may include dehydration, poor body condition score, and pliable bones.

RISK FACTORS

Husbandry

- Inappropriate husbandry is likely a significant contributing factor to the occurrence of dystocia.
- Beyond temperature and humidity, inadequate UVB light exposure and calcium supplementation is key in the development of NSHP, which in turn can have a significant impact in calcium availability, egg calcification, and contractions of the reproductive tract.
- Chelonians presenting for dystocia may also have concurrent NSHP.
- An often-forgotten aspect of the husbandry of reproductive female chelonians is the provision of an adequate substrate for nesting.
- Reptiles that may not perceive the environmental conditions are adequate for successful oviposition may not have the proper stimuli to lay their eggs.

Others

- A less-discussed topic is the effect that lack of exposure to males may have on the reproductive cycle of reptiles.
- Many reptiles display courtship and breeding behaviors that likely influence the proper hormonal stimulation of prospective females.
- Many female chelonians in captivity are kept alone without the benefit of behavioral cues from a male counterpart.
- This possibility of a behavioral effect must be considered, especially when animals are maintained in proper husbandry and are otherwise healthy.

DIAGNOSIS

DIFFERENTIAL DIAGNOSIS

- Follicular stasis
- Neoplasia
- Egg yolk coelomitis
- Ovarian cysts
- GI obstruction

DIAGNOSTICS

Radiography

The eggs of most species appear calcified, round to ovoid, but sea turtle eggs are minimally calcified.

Ultrasound

- Appearance of calcified eggs is a well-delineated hyperechogenic eggshell membrane to significant acoustic shadowing.
- In those with poorly calcified eggshell, ultrasound may be more sensitive than radiographs at diagnosing broken eggs, which may be associated with egg yolk coelomitis.

CT and MRI

Both these modalities are extremely sensitive at identifying eggs and can better assess their structure, integrity, and location.

Coelioscopy

Coelioscopic examination allows for confirmation of the presence of eggs and ruling out egg yolk coelomitis. However, the presence of eggs makes coelioscopy more difficult due to their space-occupying nature. Coelioscopy can also be used to assess the viability of the oviduct based on appearance and coloration.

Hematology and Biochemistry

- A chemistry panel is essential to help to identify other possible underlying disease processes such as dehydration and NSHP. In addition to Ca and P, Mg levels should be documented, as Mg also plays an important role in Ca homeostasis. Levels of Mg below 1 mg/dl and/or ionized Ca below 1 mmol/l should be considered deficient. Hypercalcemia and hyperphosphatemia are common findings in reproductively active females.
- CBC: a leukocytosis indicates a significant inflammatory response, which may suggest an additional underlying disease like egg yolk coelomitis.

PATHOLOGICAL FINDINGS

- Grossly, dystocia can be identified by the presence of eggs within the oviduct.
- Pathologic findings may include variation in eggs size, calcification, malformations, broken eggshells, and oviduct torsions.
- Healthy eggs should be smooth, uniform in shape and white in color.
- A deviation from this appearance (i.e., dark, shriveled) is indicative of pathology.

TREATMENT

APPROPRIATE HEALTH CARE

- The treatment approach to dystocia is based on the species of chelonian, clinical condition at presentation, amount, and appearance of the eggs based on imaging or coelioscopy, and the ability to provide a suitable environment for egg laying.
- All chelonians will benefit from medical treatment even if surgery is ultimately required.
- Medical therapy consists of correcting the husbandry, providing an appropriate nesting area, and supportive therapy with emphasis on correcting calcium deficiencies.
- Oxytocin or arginine vasotocin can be administered as long as an obstructive process is not suspected.
- Some recommend the use of beta-adrenergic blockers such as propranolol or atenolol before administration of oxytocin, as these drugs have been shown to potentiate the effects of oxytocin in humans due to their ability to increase uterine activity.
- It is critical to provide an appropriate nesting box. A plastic container with a mixture of equal parts sand and soil can be used.
- The depth of the nesting material should be at least equivalent to the length of the carapace.
- If the chelonian appears to be stable, medical therapy alone can be attempted and

the animal monitored for evidence of egg laying.
- There are no specific timelines as to how quickly egg laying should occur once medical therapy is initiated.
- The majority of cases in which there are broken or malformed eggs require surgical intervention.
- Surgery is best performed before dystocia progresses while the animal is metabolically stable.
- Surgery should be an immediate consideration for chelonians with documented chronic dystocia, metabolic derangements, and when egg yolk coelomitis is suspected.
- The goal of surgery is to remove the eggs and perform an ovariosalpingectomy in order to avoid reoccurrence.
- Extreme care must be taken to not rupture the eggs in the coelomic cavity, as the yolk is extremely antigenic and will cause a severe inflammatory response.
- If leakage occurs, the coelomic cavity should be thoroughly lavaged before closure.

NUTRITIONAL SUPPORT

Dietary deficiencies must be corrected with special emphasis on UVB light and oral Ca supplementation.

CLIENT EDUCATION/HUSBANDRY RECOMMENDATIONS

- Clients should be encouraged to seek veterinary care of chelonians early on to establish individual baseline values and to confirm the sex of the animal.
- Dystocia likely has a multifactorial cause, so all husbandry deficiencies must be corrected with emphasis on UVB light, calcium supplementation, nutrition, temperature, humidity, and provision of adequate nesting substrate.
- Chelonians should be weighed at least weekly to document any sudden weight increases that may be indicative of egg development.

MEDICATIONS

DRUG(S) OF CHOICE

- Propranolol 1 mg/kg PO once at least 3 hours prior to administration of oxytocin or arginine vasotocin.
- Atenolol 7 mg/kg PO once at least 3 hours prior to administration of oxytocin or arginine vasotocin.
- Arginine vasotocin 0.5–1 μg/kg IV, IO, IM, ICe q12–24 h; should be administered 30–60 minutes after IM or SC injection of calcium gluconate.
- Oxytocin 5–10 iu/kg IM, IV, IO q4–8h; IV administration may be more efficacious but must be administered slowly.
- Calcium: start with calcium gluconate (100 mg/kg IM, SC q12–24h) followed by calcium glubionate (10–100 mg/kg PO q4–24h) long term.
- Magnesium: magnesium sulfate 20 mg/kg IM, SC q24–72h or magnesium lactate (Rescue Cal+, Repashy Ventures, CA) 20 mg/kg PO q24h.
- Crystalloid fluids 20–30 ml/kg SC, IV, IO q24h.
- Meloxicam 0.5 mg/kg PO, IM, SC q24–48h.

PRECAUTIONS/INTERACTIONS

- There is scant information about the safety and efficacy of oxytocin and arginine vasotocin when used for prolonged periods over 2–3 days.
- Intravenous administration of both these drugs should be done slowly as they can cause life-threatening hypotension.
- Beta-adrenergic blockers also may cause bradycardia and hypotension.

FOLLOW-UP

PATIENT MONITORING

- If performing medical therapy alone, especially with oxytocin or arginine vasotocin, the animals should be monitored closely to identify any signs of distress, although this is a rare occurrence.
- If an underlying disease process was diagnosed, appropriate follow-up diagnostics should be performed to determine improvement of that condition or the need to alter therapy.
- For those undergoing surgery, a re-evaluation within 1–2 weeks is recommended to evaluate the surgical site and overall recovery.

EXPECTED COURSE AND PROGNOSIS

- Ultimately, the prognosis will depend on the underlying cause of dystocia and the response to therapy.
- Cases with underlying infectious or metabolic disease that respond to medical therapy have a good prognosis.
- Many cases requiring surgical therapy have a good to guarded prognosis.

MISCELLANEOUS

COMMENTS

- The ultimate diagnosis of dystocia is based on interpretation of clinical signs, history, and results of physical exam and diagnostics.
- In all cases, it is essential to have at least one confirmatory test that there are indeed eggs present in the coelomic cavity.
- It must be mentioned that the sex of the animals must be confirmed as female before surgery is performed.
- While this may seem obvious, in some chelonians, sex determination can be quite challenging and males may present with coelomic neoplasias or GI obstructions that clinically appear very similar to dystocia.

ZOONOTIC POTENTIAL

N/A

SYNONYMS

- Egg bound
- Postovulatory follicular stasis

ABBREVIATIONS

- Ca = calcium
- CBC = complete blood count
- CT scan = computed tomography
- GI = gastrointestinal
- ICe = intracoelomic
- IM = intramuscular
- IO = intraosseous
- IV = intravenous
- Mg = magnesium
- MRI = magnetic resonance imaging
- NSHP = nutritional secondary hyperparathyroidism
- P = phosphorus
- PO = per os
- SC = subcutaneous
- UVB = ultraviolet B

Suggested Reading

Chitty J, Raftery A. Egg retention/dystocia. In: Chitty J, Raftery A, eds. *Essentials of Tortoise Medicine and Surgery*. Oxford, UK: Wiley Blackwell; 2003:195–197.

Hochleithner C, Holland M. Ultrasonography. In: Mader DR, Divers SJ, eds. *Current Therapy in Reptile Medicine and Surgery*. St. Louis, MO: Elsevier Saunders; 2014:107–127.

Jacobson ER. Overview of reptile biology, anatomy, and histology. In: Jacobson ER, ed. *Infectious Diseases and Pathology of Reptiles: Color Atlas and Text*. Boca Raton, FL: CRC Press; 2007:14–17.

McArthur S. Problem-solving approach to common diseases of terrestrial and semi-aquatic chelonians. In: McArthur S, Wilkinson R, Meyer J, eds. *Medicine and Surgery of Turtles and Tortoises*. Ames, IA: Blackwell; 2004:309–378.

Author Javier G. Nevarez, DVM, PhD, DACZM, DECZM (Herpetology)

EGG YOLK COELOMITIS

BASICS

DEFINITION/OVERVIEW

Egg yolk coelomitis occurs when yolk material is released into the coelomic cavity as a result of a ruptured follicle or egg due to oophoritis, follicular stasis, dystocia, salpingitis, or aggressive palpation.

ETIOLOGY/PATHOPHYSIOLOGY

- In all cases, yolk coelomitis is a result of yolk material free within the coelomic cavity overwhelming the body's activity to resorb the material. This leads to an intense inflammatory response that is often sterile but can also be associated with secondary bacterial infection.
- It can progress to adhesions throughout the coelomic cavity, septicemia, and death.

SIGNALMENT/HISTORY

- Egg yolk coelomitis occurs in female chelonians of reproductive age or size, usually older than 1 year.
- Most animals have a history of inadequate husbandry, being housed alone without access to a male, and lacking an appropriate area for laying eggs or giving birth.
- The majority of cases occur in captive animals, but the author has diagnosed yolk coelomitis in free-ranging gopher tortoises (*Gopherus polyphemus*).

CLINICAL PRESENTATION

- Chelonians with yolk coelomitis often present with non-specific clinical signs such as anorexia and lethargy.
- Other abnormalities identified in physical exam may include hind-limb weakness/paresis, dehydration, poor body condition score, and pliable bones.
- Some animals may present obtunded due to rapid progression of the disease.

RISK FACTORS

Husbandry

- Any factors that may result in follicular stasis or dystocia are also contributing factors to yolk coelomitis.
- These include inadequate husbandry, nutrition, brumation, and nesting environment.

Others

- A less discussed topic is the effect that lack of exposure to males may have on the reproductive cycle of reptiles.
- Many reptiles display courtship and breeding behaviors that likely influence the proper hormonal stimulation of prospective females.
- Many female chelonians in captivity are kept alone without the benefit of behavioral cues from a male counterpart.
- This possibility of a behavioral effect must be considered, especially when animals are maintained in proper husbandry and are otherwise healthy.

DIAGNOSIS

DIFFERENTIAL DIAGNOSIS

- Follicular stasis
- Dystocia
- Neoplasia
- Ovarian cysts
- GI obstruction
- Septicemia

DIAGNOSTICS

Cytology

- Evaluation of free fluid in the coelomic cavity will be a confirmatory test of yolk coelomitis. In acute cases, fluid is yellow to white, with a high amount of proteinaceous material and inflammatory cells.
- In chronic cases the fluid may appear cloudier.
- Blood and bacteria may also be observed with either presentation.

Imaging

- Radiography: findings may include free fluid, follicles, or ruptured eggs.
- Ultrasound: aspiration of any free fluid can be used to diagnose egg yolk coelomitis.
- CT scan and MRI: both modalities are extremely sensitive for evaluation of the reproductive tract. They can also help to assess damage to other organs.

Coelioscopy

Coelioscopic examination allows for confirmation of yolk coelomitis but may be confounded by changes in anatomy due to adhesions.

Hematology and Biochemistry

- A chemistry panel is essential to help identify other possible underlying disease processes such as dehydration and NSHP.
- In addition to Ca and P, Mg levels should be documented as Mg also plays an important role in Ca homeostasis.
- Levels of Mg below 1 mg/dl and/or ionized Ca below 1 mmol/l should be considered deficient.
- Hypercalcemia and hyperphosphatemia are common findings in reproductively active female chelonians.
- Hyperproteinemia, anemia, and hypoglycemia may also be identified.
- CBC: leukocytosis may be observed but does not always occur, especially in chronic cases. Leukopenia may be present if sepsis has ensued.

PATHOLOGICAL FINDINGS

- During the acute stages, egg yolk coelomitis presents as yellow to white, viscous, free fluid within the cavity.
- Fragments of more solid yolk may also be free floating within the cavity.
- Chronically more adhesions develop and form a white fibrinous to fibrotic membrane on the serosal surfaces of the organs.
- The lesions are often severe enough that surgical repair is not possible.
- Many cases are diagnosed postmortem.

TREATMENT

APPROPRIATE HEALTH CARE

- Animals with yolk coelomitis must undergo surgery in an attempt to correct the condition, but it is often fatal.
- In most chelonians, yolk coelomitis is a chronic presentation.
- The goal of exploratory coeliotomy is to determine the severity of the diseases and whether successful lavage and cleaning of the cavity can be performed.
- Any free-floating material must be removed and the cavity lavaged copiously to remove the protein.
- If it can be accomplished, an ovariosalpingectomy is performed.
- Surgery can be performed either through the prefemoral fossa, aided by an endoscope or by plastronotomy.
- A plastronotomy will allow for better lavage and evaluation of the cavity, but it carries a higher risk of postoperative complications.
- Any underlying abnormalities (e.g., NSHP, dehydration, anemia) must be treated accordingly.
- These animals must also receive anti-inflammatories and analgesics, as the reaction to the yolk and subsequent adhesions are extremely painful.

NUTRITIONAL SUPPORT

Dietary deficiencies must be corrected with special emphasis on UVB light and oral Ca supplementation.

CLIENT EDUCATION/HUSBANDRY RECOMMENDATIONS

- Clients should be encouraged to seek veterinary care of chelonians early on to establish individual baseline values and confirm the sex of the animal.
- Egg yolk coelomitis occurs as a sequel to multifactorial causes, so all husbandry deficiencies must be corrected, with emphasis on UVB light, calcium supplementation, nutrition, temperature,

humidity, and provision of adequate nesting substrate.

- Chelonians should be weighed at least weekly to document any sudden weight increases that may be indicative of follicular development that may lead to yolk coelomitis.

MEDICATIONS

DRUG(S) OF CHOICE

- Meloxicam 0.5 mg/kg PO, IM, SC q24–48h
- Morphine 1–10 mg/kg IM, SC q24h
- Hydromorphone 0.2–0.5 mg/kg IM, SC q12–24h

PRECAUTIONS/INTERACTIONS

- Morphine and hydromorphone can cause sedation and respiratory depression.
- Dose and frequency of administration should be refined based on the patient's response.

FOLLOW-UP

PATIENT MONITORING

- If an underlying disease process is diagnosed, appropriate follow-up diagnostics should be performed to determine improvement of that condition or the need to alter therapy.
- A re-evaluation within 1–2 weeks of surgery is recommended to evaluate the surgical site and overall recovery.

EXPECTED COURSE AND PROGNOSIS

- The overall prognosis will depend on the speed with which the disease is recognized by the owners and diagnosed and treated by the veterinarian.
- Per-acute to acute cases have a fair prognosis.
- Chronic cases have a grave prognosis.

MISCELLANEOUS

COMMENTS

N/A

ZOONOTIC POTENTIAL

N/A

SYNONYMS

- Egg coelomitis/peritonitis
- Yolk coelomitis/peritonitis

ABBREVIATIONS

- Ca = calcium
- CBC = complete blood count
- CT scan = computed tomography
- GI = gastrointestinal
- IM = intramuscular
- Mg = magnesium
- MRI = magnetic resonance imaging
- NSHP = nutritional secondary hyperparathyroidism
- P = phosphorus
- PO = per os
- SC = subcutaneous

INTERNET RESOURCES

Pollock C. Reproductive disease in reptiles: twelve key facts. LafeberVet, September 23, 2012. https://lafeber.com/vet/reproductive-disease-in-reptiles-twelve-key-facts

Author Javier G. Nevarez, DVM, PhD, DACZM, DECZM (Herpetology)

EIMERIA

BASICS

DEFINITION/OVERVIEW

Eimeria are apicomplexan parasites characterized by oocytes having four sporocysts that each contain two sporozoites. Eimeria are typically intracytoplasmic parasites, although some have been described as having intranuclear development. They rarely cause disease and commonly form a normal component of the GI flora of reptiles.

ETIOLOGY/PATHOPHYSIOLOGY

- Over 200 species of *Eimeria* have been described in reptiles and, with the advent of molecular techniques, the rate of species discovery is increasing.
- *Eimeria* have a direct lifecycle, with infective stages passed in the feces of the host. *Eimeria* can be found in the gallbladder, bile ducts, and intestinal epithelium of snakes, lizards, and crocodilians.
- Most reports of illness associated with *Eimeria* infection are from captive animals that have been housed under suboptimal conditions.
- Virulence may be exacerbated by a range of intrinsic and extrinsic factors such as concurrent disease and infective dose.
- Disseminated visceral coccidiosis due to an unspecified *Eimeria* sp. was the cause of death of two of Indo-Gangetic flap-shelled turtles (*Lissemys punctata andersonii*).
- An unspecified intranuclear coccidia has been responsible for the deaths of a range of chelonian species but, to date, identification to genus level has not been possible.

SIGNALMENT/HISTORY

Disease usually occurs under circumstances of high stocking density, unsanitary conditions, and maladaptation of wild animals entering captive situations.

CLINICAL PRESENTATION

- Most animals are asymptomatic carriers but, when disease occurs, clinical signs are reflective of host-cell destruction and are dependent on site of infection.
- Typically, signs are related to GI disorder and may include anorexia, weight loss, dehydration, diarrhea, and, in severe cases, death.
- In cases of disseminated coccidiosis in chelonians, clinical signs may include pneumonia, inner ear infection, pancreatitis, and nephritis.

RISK FACTORS

Husbandry

New (captive or wild) animals entering a collection with poor hygiene and high stocking densities.

Others

Concurrent disease or excessive stress may cause immunosuppression, thus increasing the risks of disease expression.

DIAGNOSIS

DIFFERENTIAL DIAGNOSIS

Other GI disease such as bacterial or protozoal infections (i.e., *Isospora*).

DIAGNOSTICS

- Examination of feces for presence of oocysts using light microscopy is the most reliable test.
- Molecular techniques such as PCR may aid in species delineation but are unlikely to improve treatment efficacy or prognosis.
- Protozoa may also be seen in biopsy or necropsy samples.
- For preservation of coccidia for future diagnostics, fecal samples should be stored in 2–3% of aqueous (w/v) $K_2Cr_2O_7$.

PATHOLOGICAL FINDINGS

- Lesions may include proliferation of connective tissue and erosions of epithelial cells lining the intestines, gallbladder, and extra hepatic ducts.
- There may also be an accompanying catarrhal or diphtheroid inflammatory response in the small and large intestines of affected animals.

TREATMENT

APPROPRIATE HEALTH CARE

N/A

NUTRITIONAL SUPPORT

- Ensure that animals are well hydrated, especially if medicating with sulfa drugs.
- In cases of anorectic animals, force-feeding with easily digestible proteins should be initiated.
- Some species can have direct feeding by stomach tubing, but placement of an esophagostomy tube should be considered for chronic management.
- Supportive fluid therapy should be provided.

CLIENT EDUCATION/HUSBANDRY RECOMMENDATIONS

- Remove and isolate sick individuals and reduce stress by providing optimal living conditions and hygiene.
- Thoroughly clean the animal's cage to reduce environmental contamination of oocysts.
- Ensure that quarantine protocols have been adopted for all new arrivals; during quarantine, all animals should undergo repeated clinical and fecal examinations.

MEDICATIONS

DRUG(S) OF CHOICE

- Because *Eimeria* spp. are rarely pathogenic, prophylactic therapy or treatment should not be based on the identification of *Eimeria* spp. alone, to avoid development of resistance.
- Treatment should only be performed after an *Eimeria* sp. has been confirmed to be causing clinical disease.
- Ponazuril 30 mg/kg PO q48h for 2 treatments, or 30 mg/kg PO q24h for 4 treatments, then repeat for 2–4 treatments 2 weeks apart.
- Toltrazuril 15 mg/kg PO q48h for 30 days
- Sulfadimethoxine 50 mg/kg q24h for 21 days
- Trimethoprim-sulfa 30 mg/kg daily for 5 days then q48h until the coccidia are eliminated.

PRECAUTIONS/INTERACTIONS

Sulfa drugs are known to be nephrotoxic and care should be taken with their use, particularly in dehydrated or severely compromised individuals.

FOLLOW-UP

PATIENT MONITORING

Repeat fecal examination at monthly intervals.

EXPECTED COURSE AND PROGNOSIS

- Treatment may have variable efficacy as many protozoa are resistant to a range of anti-coccidial medication.
- Prognosis is good to guarded and is determined primarily by the state of the animal at initial presentation and the presence or absence of concurrent disease.

MISCELLANEOUS

COMMENTS

N/A

ZOONOTIC POTENTIAL

High host-specificity. No known zoonotic risk with any *Eimeria* species.

SYNONYMS

N/A

EIMERIA (CONTINUED)

ABBREVIATIONS

- GI = gastrointestinal
- $K_2Cr_2O_7$ = potassium dichromate
- PCR = polymerase chain reaction
- w/v = weight by volume

Suggested Reading

Gibbons PM. Advances in reptile clinical therapeutics. *J Exot Pet Med* 2014;23(1):21–38.

Helke KL, Cooper TK, Mankowski JL, Poynton SL. Disseminated visceral coccidiosis in Indo-gangetic flap-shelled turtles, *Lissemys punctata andersonii*. *J Wildl Dis* 2006;42(4):788–796.

Jacobson ER. Parasites and parasitic diseases of reptiles. In: Jacobson ER, ed. *Infectious Diseases and Pathology of Reptiles: Color Atlas and Text*. Boca Raton, FL: CRC Press; 2007:571–665.

Scullion FT, Scullion MG. Gastrointestinal protozoal diseases in reptiles. *J Exot Pet Med* 2009;18(4):266–278.

Vetterling JM, Widmer EA. *Eimeria cascabeli sp.* n. (*Eimeriidae, Sporozoa*) from rattlesnakes, with a review of the species of *Eimeria* from snakes. *J Parasitol* 1968;54(3):569–576.

Author T. Franciscus Scheelings, BVSc, MVSc, PhD, MANCVSc (Wildlife Health), DECZM (Herpetology)

ENTAMOEBA

BASICS

DEFINITION/OVERVIEW

Entamoeba are characterized into two groupings based on morphology. The two groupings are based on the number of nuclei present. *Entamoeba* spp. in the group containing four nuclei are considered to be pathogenic and the main concern for reptilian species. Entamoeba spp. in the group containing eight nuclei are considered to be noninvasive. *E. invadens* is the most common pathogenic species seen in reptiles and has been known to cause significant mortality. Virulence can differ between strains of *E. invadens*; infectious cysts are 11–20.2 µm with four nuclei and a small central karyosome. Trophozoites are 17.5–50 µm in length (average 36.18 µm), 10–25 µm (average 12 µm) in width and average diameter of 24.1 µm. Trophozoites also possess a single nuclei with a large central karysome that is 5–7.5 µm (average 5.65 µm) in diameter.

ETIOLOGY/PATHOPHYSIOLOGY

- *E. invadens* has a direct life cycle and transmission is through the fecal–oral route.
- Cysts are ingested and then undergo excystation in the intestinal tract.
- In chelonians, cyst production occurs by cell division and one metacystic form gives rise to eight amoebas.
- *E. invadens* mainly inhabits the small and large intestines but can affect other adjacent organs, including the liver, kidneys, pancreas, and lungs via systemic circulation.
- The motile feeding trophozoite can also encyst and then be passed through the host's GI tract and out in the feces.
- Trophozoites undergo encystation in which infective cysts are formed and then excreted in feces.
- Cysts can remain infective for 14+ days at temperatures of 8 degrees C and several days at 37 degrees C.
- It was first considered that chelonians were only carriers and *E. invadens* were commensal parasites, but there is sufficient evidence that the parasite can affect and cause mortality in all chelonians, including terrestrial chelonians, freshwater and sea turtles.
- The disease process causes severe necrotizing colitis, hepatic and pancreatic necrosis with associated granulomas.
- Clinical signs occur approximately 2–10 weeks prior to death.

SIGNALMENT/HISTORY

- All ages can be affected. Animals consistently kept in temperatures between 25–33 degrees C.
- Carnivorous chelonians appear to be more susceptible versus herbivorous chelonians.
- Herbivorous chelonians can be asymptomatic carriers.

CLINICAL PRESENTATION

- Anorexia
- Diarrhea
- Dehydration
- Weight loss
- Bloody and mucoid stools
- Hardening of the large intestinal tract that can be palpated.
- Intussusception
- Vomiting
- Sudden death

RISK FACTORS

Husbandry

- Improper husbandry and hygiene, diarrhea, housed with infected animals, decreased immune status, temperatures held between 25 and 33 degrees C.
- Invertebrates (i.e., roaches and flies) act as mechanical vectors.

Others

N/A

DIAGNOSIS

DIFFERENTIAL DIAGNOSIS

- Salmonellosis
- GI helminths

DIAGNOSTICS

- Microscopic evaluation of fresh fecal material to visualize trophozoites and cysts.
- Trophozoites may be seen in fresh fecal but die rapidly within 20–30 minutes once outside the host.
- SAF technique can be used for better visualization.
- Fecal/cysts can be placed within a petri dish with water and trophozoites will emerge from the dissolved envelope within several hours.
- Immunohistochemistry with *E. invadens* poly clonal antibody is developed for snakes.
- Polymerase chain reaction assays can be used to distinguish species of *Entamoeba.*

PATHOLOGICAL FINDINGS

- Gross changes include thickening, edema, erosions, ulcers, and diphtheritic membranes of the large intestine.
- Liver abscesses may also be seen.
- Histologically, the primary finding is fibrinonecrotic colitis.

TREATMENT

APPROPRIATE HEALTH CARE

N/A

NUTRITIONAL SUPPORT

Nutritional supplementation may be indicated if diarrhea, dehydration is severe.

CLIENT EDUCATION/HUSBANDRY RECOMMENDATIONS

- Practice proper hygiene
- Wash fruits and vegetables before being fed.
- Do not house infected individuals with non-infected chelonians.

MEDICATIONS

DRUG(S) OF CHOICE

Metronidazole 25 mg/kg PO q24h for 5–7 days

PRECAUTIONS/INTERACTIONS

N/A

FOLLOW-UP

PATIENT MONITORING

- Monitor for weight gain
- Take fecal samples

EXPECTED COURSE AND PROGNOSIS

Good

MISCELLANEOUS

COMMENTS

- *E. invadens* in culture, dies at 37 degrees C, so can raise the temperature to 37 degrees C if it is within the animal's preferred optimum temperature range.
- *E. histolytica* and *E. dispar*, which are found in humans GI tracts, are morphologically similar to *E. invadens* but are considered to be non-pathogenic.

ZOONOTIC POTENTIAL

Unknown

SYNONYMS

Amebiasis

ABBREVIATIONS

- GI = gastrointestinal
- SAF = Sodium acetate acetic acid formalin

ENTAMOEBA (CONTINUED)

INTERNET RESOURCES

- de Cardenas C. Amebiasis in Reptiles. PetMD, October 1, 2008. www.petmd.com/reptile/conditions/digestive/c_rp_amebiasis
- Amebiasis in Snakes. Wag! 2020. https://wagwalking.com/reptile/condition/amebiasis-in-snakes
- Divers SJ. Parasitic Diseases of Reptiles. MSD Manual Veterinary Manual, June 2020. www.merckvetmanual.com/exotic-and-laboratory-animals/reptiles/parasitic-diseases-of-reptiles

Suggested Reading

Denver MC. Reptile protozoa. In: Fowler M, Miller E, eds. *Zoo and Wildlife Medicine: Current Therapy 6*. St. Louis, MO: Elsevier Saunders ; 2008:154–159.

Hnizdo J, Pantchev N., eds. *Protozoa (digestive tract). In: Medical Care of Turtles and Tortoises. Diagnosis. Surgery. Pathology. Parasitology. Frankfurt*, Germany: Edition Chimaira; 2011:194–195.

Jacobson ER. Parasites and parasitic diseases of reptiles. In: Jacobson ER, ed. *Infectious Diseases and Pathology of Reptiles: Color Atlas and Text*. Boca Raton, FL: CRC Press; 2007:571–665.

Author Elsburgh O. Clarke III, DVM, DACZM

EXOPHTHALMIA

BASICS

DEFINITION/OVERVIEW

Exophthalmia is the anterior protrusion of a normal-sized globe.

ETIOLOGY/PATHOPHYSIOLOGY

Space-occupying swelling or mass in the orbit placing pressure on the globe, displacing it anteriorly.

SIGNALMENT/HISTORY

- There is no standard signalment for this disease.
- Gradual protrusion of the eye, possibly preventing blinking, and potentially anorexia are common findings in the history.

CLINICAL PRESENTATION

- While it can be bilateral, exophthalmia is more commonly unilateral.
- The displacement of the globe will often push the eyelids forward and cause protrusion of the nictitans, and excessive conjunctiva will be visible.
- Retropulsion of the globe is met with resistance due to the presence of retrobulbar swelling.

RISK FACTORS

Husbandry

- Inadequate husbandry, especially hypothermia, may predispose animals to this condition due to decreased immune function leading to retrobulbar cellulitis and/or abscessation.
- Hypovitaminosis A in chelonians causes squamous metaplasia of the orbital glands and ducts, as well as decreased immune function, and may present as bilateral exophthalmia.

Others

N/A

DIAGNOSIS

DIFFERENTIAL DIAGNOSIS

- It is important to first differentiate between exophthalmia and buphthalmos.
- The most common cause for exophthalmia in chelonians is retrobulbar abscessation.
- Other differentials include cellulitis, trauma, granulomas, neoplasia, mucoceles, and sialadenitis.
- In tortoises, vascular obstruction and generalized edema have been reported to cause bilateral exophthalmia as well.

DIAGNOSTICS

- Physical examination will confirm exophthalmia, but additional diagnostics are necessary to determine the cause.
- Ocular ultrasound is helpful in evaluating the problem, although the scleral ossicles can limit visualization.
- Advanced imaging, such as CT or MRI, is most helpful in determining the extent of the mass and if resection is possible.
- Surgical exploratory of the retrobulbar space to collect biopsies and resect any masses present in the most definitive way to achieve a diagnosis but in many cases requires enucleation to reach the retrobulbar space.
- A CBC may provide information on the severity of the infection/inflammation.

PATHOLOGICAL FINDINGS

Histology and culture are most useful to diagnose the cause of the exophthalmia and allow the clinician to form an appropriate treatment plan.

TREATMENT

APPROPRIATE HEALTH CARE

N/A

NUTRITIONAL SUPPORT

- Additional nutritional support is not necessary if the animal is eating, but it may be necessary to tube feed or place an esophagostomy tube if the animal is anorexic.
- Assessment of the diet for adequate vitamin A levels is important and should be done to rule out hypovitaminosis A as a potential cause or contributor to this condition in chelonians.

CLIENT EDUCATION/HUSBANDRY RECOMMENDATIONS

- While exophthalmia can occur in any animal, those with husbandry deficiencies may be at increased risk.
- In addition to medical and surgical therapy, maximizing the husbandry of the animal will improve the chances of a successful outcome.

MEDICATIONS

DRUG(S) OF CHOICE

- Treatment should be based on results of culture, histology, and/or FNA.
- Starting an appropriate broad-spectrum antibiotic with a good Gram-negative spectrum (e.g., ceftazadime 20 mg/kg IM or SQ q48–72h) and anti-inflammatory (e.g., meloxicam 0.2–0.3 mg/kg IM or SQ q24–48h) can be helpful while test results are pending.

PRECAUTIONS/INTERACTIONS

N/A

FOLLOW-UP

PATIENT MONITORING

Serial CBC, especially if the first one was abnormal, may provide an indication of response to treatment.

EXPECTED COURSE AND PROGNOSIS

- Prognosis is related to the underlying cause of the exophthalmia.
- Cellulitis and trauma have the most favorable outcomes.
- Retrobulbar abscesses can be extensive and therefore carry a more guarded prognosis.
- Retrobulbar neoplasia usually carries a poor prognosis because of location and inability to get clean margins.

MISCELLANEOUS

COMMENTS

N/A

ZOONOTIC POTENTIAL

Depends on the cause of the retrobulbar swelling but generally low to no zoonotic potential.

SYNONYMS

- Exophthalmos
- Proptosis—severe case of exophthalmia

ABBREVIATIONS

- CBC = complete blood count
- CT = computed tomography
- FNA = fine-needle aspiration
- MRI = magnetic resonance imaging

Suggested Reading

Boyer TH. Turtles, Tortoises, and Terrapins. In: Mader DR, ed. *Reptile Medicine and Surgery*. 2nd ed. St. Louis, MO: Elsevier Saunders; 2006:696–704.

Hochleithner C, Holland M. Ultrasonography. In: Mader, DR, Divers SJ, eds. *Current Therapy in Reptile Medicine and Surgery*. Saint Louis, MO: Elsevier Saunders; 2014:107–127.

Lawton MPC. Reptilian Ophthalmology. In: Mader DR, ed. *Reptile Medicine and Surgery*. 2nd ed. St. Louis, MO: Elsevier Saunders; 2006:323–342.

Author Christopher S. Hanley, DVM, DECZM

FOLLICULAR STASIS

BASICS

DEFINITION/OVERVIEW

Follicular stasis is the retention of ovarian follicles. Normally, follicles ovulate into the oviduct or undergo atresia. If neither happens, the reptile is considered to be in follicular stasis. Identifying whether the presence of follicles is pathologic or physiologic is difficult given the fact that, most of the time, the stage of the reproductive cycle in an individual animal is unknown. A diagnosis of follicular stasis is often made once the animal starts showing clinical signs of illness or follicles are present for a longer period than expected for the species.

ETIOLOGY/PATHOPHYSIOLOGY

- Follicles can fail to ovulate and undergo atresia for a number of reasons, but in most cases an abnormal hormonal status can be assumed.
- The reproductive hormone mechanism in reptiles is not as well understood as it is in mammals.
- It is suspected that a multitude of environmental and behavioral factors, as well as underlying diseases, contribute to an abnormal function of the endocrine system, which in turn leads to follicular stasis.
- It is also possible that a lack of breeding and exposure to males may have a negative impact on reptiles' ability to properly ovulate.
- Inappropriate or lack of brumation may also be a contributing factor.
- In addition to basic husbandry aspects such as UVB light, temperature, humidity, and a proper diet, female reptiles also have a need for appropriate substrate and environment that is conductive for egg laying.

SIGNALMENT/HISTORY

- Follicular stasis occurs in female chelonians of reproductive age or size.
- Most animals have a history of inadequate husbandry, being housed alone without access to a male, and lacking an appropriate area for laying eggs.

CLINICAL PRESENTATION

- Chelonians with follicular stasis often present with non-specific clinical signs such as anorexia and lethargy.
- Other signs that may cue in the possibility of follicular stasis include hind-limb weakness or paresis and constipation.
- Significant weight gain that does not match the growth of the animal may also be identified.
- These changes could be due to the pathologic effects of the retained follicles, an underlying disease, or both.
- In most cases, this is a chronic disease and the owners are not aware of the fact that their chelonian is in follicular stasis.
- Other abnormalities identified in physical exam may include dehydration, poor body condition score, and pliable shell.

RISK FACTORS

Husbandry

- Inappropriate husbandry is likely a significant contributing factor to the occurrence of follicular stasis.
- Beyond temperature and humidity, inadequate UVB light exposure and calcium supplementation is key in the development of NSHP, which in turn can have a significant impact in calcium availability and follicular development.
- Many chelonians presenting for follicular stasis also have concurrent NSHP.
- An often-forgotten aspect of the husbandry of reproductive female reptiles is the provision of an adequate substrate for nesting/oviposition.
- It is often accepted that reptiles that may not perceive the environmental conditions are adequate for successful reproduction will resorb the follicles through atresia.
- In captivity, there may be a combination of factors that do not allow for normal follicular atresia.

Others

- A less discussed topic is the effect that lack of exposure to males may have on the reproductive cycle of reptiles.
- Many reptiles display courtship and breeding behaviors that likely influence the proper hormonal stimulation of prospective females.
- Many female chelonians in captivity are kept alone without the benefit of behavioral cues from a male counterpart.
- This possibility of a behavioral effect must be considered, especially when animals are maintained in proper husbandry and are otherwise healthy.

DIAGNOSIS

DIFFERENTIAL DIAGNOSIS

- Dystocia
- Neoplasia
- Egg yolk coelomitis
- Ovarian cysts
- GI obstruction
- Constipation

DIAGNOSTICS

Imaging

- Radiography: follicles appear as non-calcified, round to ovoid, variably sized soft-tissue opacities in the mid to caudal coelom. At times, the follicles may either be large enough, or in large enough numbers, to encompass over 50% of the coelomic cavity.
- Ultrasound: early follicles appear as anechoic and progress to have more echogenicity as they mature or fail to ovulate. Follicles with a more heterogeneous distribution within the lumen should be highly suspicious of being retained follicles as the material within becomes firmer and inspissated. Ultrasound examination and aspiration of any free fluid can also be used to rule out egg yolk coelomitis.
- CT scan and MRI: both these modalities are extremely sensitive at identifying follicles and can better assess the differences in size, shape and content of the follicles.
- Coelioscopy: coelioscopic examination allows for confirmation of the presence of follicles and evaluation of their color and size to help make a determination of whether the presentation may be pathologic.

Hematology and Biochemistry

- Chemistry panel: a chemistry panel is essential to help identify other possible underlying disease processes such as dehydration and NSHP. In addition to Ca and P, Mg levels should be documented as it also plays an important role in Ca homeostasis. Levels of Mg below 1 mg/dl and/or ionized Ca below 1 mmol/l should be considered deficient. Hypercalcemia and hyperphosphatemia are common findings in reproductively active female chelonians.
- CBC: a leukocytosis indicates a significant inflammatory response that may suggest an additional underlying disease like egg yolk coelomitis.

PATHOLOGICAL FINDINGS

- Grossly, follicular stasis can be differentiated from dystocia by the presence of follicles outside of the oviduct.
- At times, the follicles may be large enough to appear to be in chains but are surrounded by the ovarian membrane rather than the oviduct.
- Healthy follicles should be smooth and white to yellow in color.
- A deviation from this appearance (i.e., dark, shriveled, or cystic follicles) is indicative of pathology.
- Hepatic lipidosis may also be a common finding due to the chronicity of these cases.

TREATMENT

APPROPRIATE HEALTH CARE

- The treatment approach to follicular stasis is based on diagnosis and treatment of contributing factors leading to the stasis and treatment of the stasis itself.
- The species of chelonian, clinical condition at presentation, amount and appearance of

the follicles based on imaging or coelioscopy, and ability to provide a suitable environment all contribute to the decision-making process.

- All chelonians will benefit from medical treatment even if surgery is ultimately required.
- Medical therapy consists of correcting the husbandry, providing an appropriate nesting area, and supportive therapy with emphasis on correcting calcium deficiencies.
- If the chelonian appears to be stable, medical therapy alone can be attempted and the animal monitored for evidence of follicular atresia.
- There are no timelines as to how quickly atresia can be expected.
- The use of proligestone has been reported to have unreliable results.
- Ultimately, many if not most cases require surgical intervention.

NUTRITIONAL SUPPORT

- Dietary deficiencies must be corrected with special emphasis on UVB light and oral Ca supplementation.
- Supplemental feeding should also be considered, since many of these animals may have hepatic lipidosis.

CLIENT EDUCATION/HUSBANDRY RECOMMENDATIONS

- Clients should be encouraged to seek veterinary care of chelonians early on to establish individual baseline values and confirm the sex of the animal.
- Follicular stasis likely has a multifactorial cause, so all husbandry deficiencies must be corrected with emphasis on UVB light, calcium supplementation, nutrition, temperature, humidity, and provision of adequate nesting substrate for oviparous species.
- Chelonians should be weighed at least weekly to document any sudden weight increases that may be indicative of follicular development.

SURGICAL CONSIDERATIONS

- Surgery is best performed before stasis progresses while the animal is metabolically stable.
- Surgery should be an immediate consideration for chelonians with documented chronic stasis, metabolic derangements, and when egg yolk coelomitis is suspected.
- The goal of surgery is to remove the follicles and perform an ovariectomy, to avoid reoccurrence.
- Follicular stasis is commonly associated with follicles on both ovaries but even if only one is affected, bilateral ovariectomy is recommended.
- Extreme care must be taken to not rupture the follicles in the coelomic cavity, as the yolk is extremely antigenic and will cause a severe inflammatory response.
- If leakage occurs, the coelomic cavity should be thoroughly lavaged before closure.

MEDICATIONS

DRUG(S) OF CHOICE

- Calcium: start with calcium gluconate (100 mg/kg IM, SC q12–24h) followed by calcium glubionate (10–100 mg/kg PO q4–24h) long term
- Magnesium: magnesium sulfate 20 mg/kg IM, SC q24–72h or magnesium lactate (Rescue Cal+, Repashy Ventures, CA) 20 mg/kg PO q24h
- Crystalloid fluids: 20–30 ml/kg SC, IV q24h
- Meloxicam: 0.5 mg/kg PO, IM, SC q24–48h
- Morphine: 1–10 mg/kg IM, SC q24h
- Hydromorphone: 0.2–0.5 mg/kg IM, SC q12–24h

PRECAUTIONS/INTERACTIONS

- Morphine and hydromorphone can cause sedation and respiratory depression.
- Dose and frequency of administration should be refined based on the patient's response.

FOLLOW-UP

PATIENT MONITORING

- If performing medical therapy alone, the weight of the chelonian should be recorded daily to every other day to provide an early indication that follicle atresia may be occurring.
- Any acute weight losses beyond 10% of the body weight should prompt re-evaluation by a veterinarian.
- If an underlying disease process was diagnosed, appropriate follow-up diagnostics should be performed to determine improvement of that condition or the need to alter therapy.
- For those undergoing surgery, a re-evaluation with 1–2 weeks is recommended to evaluate the surgical site and overall recovery.

EXPECTED COURSE AND PROGNOSIS

- Ultimately, the prognosis will depend on the underlying cause of follicular stasis and the required therapy.
- Cases with underlying infectious or metabolic disease that respond to medical therapy have a good prognosis.
- Many cases requiring surgical therapy have a good to guarded prognosis.

MISCELLANEOUS

COMMENTS

- The ultimate diagnosis of follicular stasis is based on interpretation of clinical signs, history, and results of physical exam and diagnostics.
- Before ovariectomy is performed, it is essential to have at least one confirmatory test that there are indeed follicles present in the coelomic cavity.
- It must be mentioned that the sex of the animals must be confirmed as female before surgery is performed.
- While this may seem obvious, in some chelonians species sex determination can be quite challenging, especially when of small size, and males may present with coelomic neoplasias or GI obstructions that clinically appear very similar to follicular stasis.

ZOONOTIC POTENTIAL

N/A

SYNONYMS

Preovulatory follicular stasis

ABBREVIATIONS

- Ca = calcium
- CBC = complete blood count
- CT scan = computed tomography
- GI = gastrointestinal
- IM = intramuscular
- Mg = magnesium
- MRI = magnetic resonance imaging
- NSHP = nutritional secondary hyperparathyroidism
- P = phosphorus
- PO = per os
- SC = subcutaneous
- UVB = ultraviolet B

Suggested Reading

Chitty J, Raftery A. Follicular stasis. In: Chitty J, Raftery A, eds. *Essentials of tortoise medicine and surgery*. Oxford, UK: Wiley Blackwell; 2003:200–204.

Jacobson ER. Overview of reptile biology, anatomy, and histology. In: Jacobson ER, ed. *Infectious Diseases and Pathology of Reptiles: Color Atlas and Text*. Boca Raton, FL: CRC Press; 2007:14–17.

McArthur S. Problem-solving approach to common diseases of terrestrial and semiaquatic chelonians. In: McArthur S, Wilkinson R, Meyer J, eds. *Medicine and Surgery of Tortoises and Turtles*. Ames, IA: Blackwell; 2004:309–378.

Author Javier G. Nevarez, DVM, PhD, DACZM, DECZM (Herpetology)

GOUT

BASICS

DEFINITION/OVERVIEW

Gout is a common disease seen in reptiles, which occurs due to the buildup of uric acid crystals deposited in or around the joints or throughout visceral organs.

ETIOLOGY/PATHOPHYSIOLOGY

- Increased production of uric acid may occur due to excessive levels of dietary proteins, or potentially due to an inherited enzyme defect as occurs in humans.
- Excretion may be compromised, for example by dehydration, starvation, nephrotoxic drugs, or renal pathology.
- Uric acid is a relatively insoluble substance so when levels are elevated in the blood or in other body fluids, crystallization will occur and deposits will form.
- Uric acid crystals may deposit in the joints (articular gout), around the joints (periarticular gout) or throughout other internal organs (visceral gout).
- Common sites for visceral gout include the kidneys, liver, spleen, pericardial sac, lungs, and subcutaneous tissue.

SIGNALMENT/HISTORY

- More common in terrestrial species with a history of husbandry or diet deficits.
- Sometimes may have been previously treated with potentially nephrotoxic drugs.

CLINICAL PRESENTATION

- Animals with articular or periarticular gout usually present with obvious joint swellings.
- One or more joints may be affected, and the animal may be lame.
- Animals with visceral gout may be asymptomatic or may have non-specific signs such as lethargy and reduced appetite.
- Sometimes white nodules may be visualized on examination of the oral cavity or subcutaneously.

RISK FACTORS

Husbandry

- Inappropriate environmental temperatures
- Inappropriate water provision (e.g., low humidity or fresh water not supplied in an easily accessible way)
- High-protein diets

Others

Administration of potentially nephrotoxic drugs (e.g., aminoglycosides), especially to dehydrated patients.

DIAGNOSIS

Gout may be suspected on history and clinical examination, but diagnostic testing will be necessary for definitive diagnosis.

DIFFERENTIAL DIAGNOSIS

For articular swellings, differentials include pseudogout, septic arthritis, trauma, and metabolic bone diseases.

DIAGNOSTICS

- Cytologic examination of aspirates from affected joints for articular or periarticular gout. For visceral gout, biopsies need to be taken for histopathology.
- Demonstration of uric acid (usually monosodium urate) crystals is necessary for definitive diagnosis.
- Blood uric acid levels may be elevated, but this is not always a consistent finding as this depends on the stage in the disease process.
- On radiography of affected limbs, lytic lesions may be seen in and around joints. Crystals are radiolucent so will not be detected.
- Ultrasound of the coelomic organs may reveal echodense areas of precipitates within internal organs in cases of visceral gout.

PATHOLOGICAL FINDINGS

- On gross postmortem examination, small white nodules (tophi) can be seen scattered throughout visceral organs, within or around joints.
- On histopathological examination, tophi are often surrounded by granulomatous inflammation.

TREATMENT

APPROPRIATE HEALTH CARE

- Treatment aims to lower blood uric acid levels and promote uric acid excretion.
- Supportive treatment should always include appropriate analgesia, as in other species this is known to be a painful condition.
- Euthanasia may be considered in severe cases.

NUTRITIONAL SUPPORT

- Some patients may be anorexic and severely dehydrated on presentation.
- Fluid deficits should always be corrected, and nutritional support provided.
- Care should be taken to provide an appropriate diet low in dietary purines to minimize further uric acid production.

CLIENT EDUCATION/HUSBANDRY RECOMMENDATIONS

- Husbandry should be reviewed to identify any predisposing factors, such as inappropriate temperatures or low humidity, and these should be corrected.
- Clean fresh water should always be available in a recognizable form for the species.
- Diet should be reviewed to ensure that it is appropriate for the species and not too high in protein.
- Clients should be advised that this is a condition that will require long-term management and can potentially be very painful if allowed to progress.

SURGICAL CONSIDERATIONS

Surgical removal of tophi may be considered if only one joint is affected, but permanent damage to the joint may already have occurred.

MEDICATIONS

DRUG(S) OF CHOICE

- Allopurinol is the most common choice for treating gout. It is a xanthine oxidase-inhibiting drug that works by inhibiting the conversion of hypoxanthine and xanthine to uric acid in the liver, consequently reducing blood uric acid levels.
- If blood uric acid levels remain consistently low, existing deposits may potentially dissolve.
- Doses of 10–20 mg/kg PO q24h are recommended for most species.
- Long-term medication will be necessary to prevent relapses.
- Other drugs to promote uric acid excretion such as probenecid can theoretically be used but are contraindicated in dehydrated patients.
- In cases of visceral gout, allopurinol should also be avoided as it increases uric acid excretion by the kidneys and could theoretically make the condition worse.

PRECAUTIONS/INTERACTIONS

Allopurinol and probenecid may potentially interact, although the clinical significance of this interaction in reptiles is unknown.

FOLLOW-UP

PATIENT MONITORING

- Response to therapy is usually monitored by physical examination findings (e.g., increase in activity levels or no progression in joint swellings).
- Repeat blood samples can also be taken to recheck uric acid levels which would be expected to start reducing within 7 days of allopurinol treatment.

EXPECTED COURSE AND PROGNOSIS

- The prognosis for patients with severe widespread disease is poor, but if diagnosed early the condition could be managed successfully.
- If left untreated, the disease will progress with widespread uric acid deposition ultimately resulting in organ failure and death.

MISCELLANEOUS

COMMENTS

N/A

ZOONOTIC POTENTIAL

N/A

SYNONYMS

N/A

INTERNET RESOURCES

Veterinary Information Network: www.vin.com

Suggested Reading

Casimire-Etzioni AL, Wellehan JF, Embury JE et al. Synovial fluid from an African spur-thighed tortoise (*Geochelone sulcata*). *Vet Clin Path* 2004;33(1):43–46.

Dallwig R. Allopurinol. *J Exot Pet Med* 2010;19(3):255–257.

Mader DR. Gout. In: Mader DR, ed. *Reptile Medicine and Surgery*. 2nd ed. St. Louis, MO: Elsevier Saunders; 2006:374–379.

Author Joanna Hedley, BVM&S, DZooMed (Reptilian), DECZM (Herpetology), MRCVS

HEPATIC LIPIDOSIS

BASICS

DEFINITION/OVERVIEW

Hepatic lipidosis is the excessive accumulation of triglycerides in the hepatocytes and can result in altered hepatic function. It is expected to be a reversible lesion if the underlying cause is corrected. It is a common lesion diagnosed in reptiles.

ETIOLOGY/PATHOPHYSIOLOGY

- Triglyceride accumulation in hepatocytes can occur due to disturbances of lipid metabolism from primary metabolic liver disease, toxins, protein malnutrition, diabetes mellitus, obesity, anorexia (increased fatty acid mobilization from peripheral stores), extrahepatic visceral inflammation, and anoxia (inhibits fatty acid oxidation).
- In female reptiles, the change can be associated with folliculogenesis.
- The common factor for each of these possible etiologies is a negative balance between the rates of deposition and dispersal of fat from the liver, resulting in an accumulation of triglycerides in the liver.
- In reptiles, obesity from rich diets can result in hepatic lipidosis and enlargement of the coelomic fat bodies.
- Reduced activity will also contribute to increased fat deposits and is not uncommonly reported condition in monitors and turtles.
- In tortoises, a lack of normal hibernation and reproductive activity can lead to hepatic lipidosis.

SIGNALMENT/HISTORY

- Hepatic lipidosis is reported to be more common in turtles. Data from one laboratory (D Reavill, unpublished) found the percentages of hepatic lipidosis in the reptile groups with the liver submitted for evaluation, as follows:
    - chelonians (turtles and tortoises) (97/676) 14%
    - lizards (304/1485) 20%
    - snakes (91/1672) 5.4%
- There is a reported difference in tolerance to the condition, with turtles being more resistant to metabolic derangements.

CLINICAL PRESENTATION

- The clinical signs are generally non-specific.
- Signs include weakness, depression, pale oral mucous membranes, and non-specific neurologic signs.
- Green to blue urates are reported, and clay-like, tan, or watery feces may also be noted.

RISK FACTORS

Husbandry

- Inappropriate diet and overfeeding, such as chelonians fed only canned dog food.
- Chronic stress: inappropriate captive husbandry conditions (POTZ, cage size, feeding strategies).
- Inactivity: restricted physical activity due to space or adequate stimulation.
- Inappropriate support for reproduction
- Inappropriate hibernation conditions
- Anorexia/hyporexia: desert and sulcata tortoises that have failed to eat for more than 1 week.

Others

N/A

DIAGNOSIS

Although the presumptive diagnosis is based on history, clinical signs, laboratory data, and imaging, the definitive diagnosis is made by microscopic evaluation of a liver biopsy or necropsy examination.

DIFFERENTIAL DIAGNOSIS

- Hepatic lipidosis needs to be distinguished from other causes of hepatomegaly.
- Vascular congestion: underlying cardiovascular disease.
- Toxins: mycotoxins, pesticides, heavy metals
- Infectious diseases: herpesvirus, adenovirus, *Salmonella* spp., mycobacteria, Gram-negative bacterial infections, abscesses/granulomas, protozoa.
- Tumor: lymphoma, hepatoma

DIAGNOSTICS

Imaging

- Radiographs ± contrast, ultrasound, CT, and MRI.
- There may an enlarged hepatic silhouette on radiography.
- Ultrasound may reveal a brightly reflective, enlarged, rounded liver.
- CT provides measurements of radiodensity of the liver.
- CT values lower than 20 HU are compatible with hepatic lipidosis in red-footed tortoises (*Chelonoidis carbonaria*).

Hematology and Biochemistry

- Serum biochemistry: lack of species-specific reference ranges make interpretation challenging.
- In general, decreased plasma proteins; increased triglycerides, cholesterol, AST, and LDH; glucose and bile acid levels vary; blood is often noticeably lipemic.

PATHOLOGICAL FINDINGS

- The gross appearance is of an enlarged, friable liver, pale tan to yellow, and typically has a greasy feel.
- Biopsy and/or necropsy histopathology: the hepatocytes will be variably enlarged, and supporting cytoplasmic vacuolization with HE stain.
- Additional stains will demonstrate the prominent oil red O-positive lipid droplets in all the hepatocytes.

TREATMENT

APPROPRIATE HEALTH CARE

Administration of oral medications is recommended.

NUTRITIONAL SUPPORT

- Placement of an esophagostomy tube for feeding is recommended.
- Maintain at appropriate temperature and humidity; exercise.
- Caloric reduction with a nutritionally complete, low-fat, high-quality protein, liquid diet (Lafeber's Emeraid®, EmerAid, LLC, Cornell, IL; Oxbow Critical Care®, Oxbow Animal Health, Omaha, NE; or Oxbow Carnivore Care®, Oxbow Animal Health, Omaha, NE).
- Hydration

CLIENT EDUCATION/HUSBANDRY RECOMMENDATIONS

N/A

MEDICATIONS

DRUG(S) OF CHOICE

- Antibiotic of choice in reptiles if needed: ceftazidime.
- Nutriceuticals such as silymarin and milk thistle are reported to be an anti-inflammatory and antioxidant; however, there are no studies to support claims for hepatic benefits.

PRECAUTIONS/INTERACTIONS

Avoid hepatotoxic agents in reptiles:

- antibiotics: doxycycline, clindamycin, erythromycin
- antivirals: acyclovir
- antifungals: itraconazole, ketoconazole
- antiparasitic: metronidazole, dichlorvos, tiabendazole, ivermectin

FOLLOW-UP

PATIENT MONITORING

Regular checkups to assess body weight, change in serum biochemistries, and possibly rebiopsy.

EXPECTED COURSE AND PROGNOSIS

After support through any acute crisis, the long-term prognosis depends on associated conditions and whether these can be changed.

MISCELLANEOUS

COMMENTS

N/A

ZOONOTIC POTENTIAL

N/A

SYNONYMS

- Fatty liver
- Vacuolar hepatopathy

ABBREVIATIONS

- AST = aspartate aminotransferase
- CT = computed tomography
- HE = hematoxylin and eosin
- LDH = lactate dehydrogenase
- MRI = magnetic resonance imaging
- POTZ = preferred optimal temperature zone

Suggested Reading

Divers SJ, Cooper JE. Reptile hepatic lipidosis. *Semin Avian Exot Pet* 2000;9(3):153–164.

Knotková Z, Dorrestein GM, Jekl V, et al. Fasting and postprandial serum bile acid concentrations in 10 healthy female red-eared terrapins (*Trachemys scripta elegans*). *Vet Rec* 2008;163(17):510–514.

Marchiori A, da Silva ICC, de Albuquerque Bonelli M, et al. Use of computed tomography for investigation of hepatic lipidosis in captive *Chelonoidis carbonaria* (spix, 1824). *J Zoo Wildl Med* 2015;46(2):320–324.

Martínez-Silvestre, A. *Hepatic lipidosis in reptiles.* Proc SEVC, October 2013, Barcelona, Spain.

West G. Endoscopic hepatic biopsy in Coahuilan box turtles, *Terrapene coahuila. J Herpetol Med Surg* 2001;11(2):28–29.

Author Drury R. Reavill, DVM, DABVP (Avian and Reptile & Amphibian Practice), DACVP

HERPESVIRUSES

BASICS

DEFINITION/OVERVIEW

HV are double-stranded, enveloped DNA viruses. They can cause latent infections and infected animals can shed virus, in some cases without any clinical signs of disease. Infections are associated with various disease syndromes and clinical signs and severity of disease may depend on both the virus strain and the host species. Specific disease processes have been described in sea turtles and tortoises.

ETIOLOGY/PATHOPHYSIOLOGY

- HV in the genus *Scutavirus* have been described in sea turtles, tortoises, and aquatic turtles.
- HV infecting sea turtles include various strains of FPTHV, including chelonian chHV5, the type species of the genus *Scutavirus*, LEDV, and others.
- Four different HV have been described in tortoises: testudinid HV 1–4. Transmission is most likely via direct contact.
- In sea turtles, virus may survive for some time in sea water, and transmission via the environment may be possible.
- Environmental stressors lead to more severe disease, and other infectious agents likely also contribute to the development of severe disease (e.g., mycoplasma infections in tortoises).
- Animals that survive initial infection become carriers, and any animal that has been infected should be considered a lifelong carrier.

SIGNALMENT/HISTORY

- Can affect all age classes
- In sea turtles, fibropapillomatosis has been described in green (*Chelonia mydas*), loggerhead (*Caretta caretta*), hawksbill (*Eretmochelys imbricata*), and olive ridley (*Lepidochelys olivacea*) turtles around the world.
- TeHV has been described in various tortoise species:
  - TeHV1 most commonly in Russian tortoises (*Testudo horsfieldii*) in Asia and Europe.
  - TeHV2 in California desert tortoises (*Gopherus agassizii*) in the USA.
  - TeHV3 has been reported from a wide range of species, most commonly Mediterranean tortoise species (*Testudo* spp.). Hermann's (*T. hermanni*) and Russian tortoises appear to be highly susceptible to disease, while spur-thighed (*T. graeca*) and marginated (*T. marginata*) tortoises survive disease more often and are more likely to become clinically inapparent carriers.
  - TeHV4 has been described in a bowsprit tortoise (*Chersina angluata*) and a leopard tortoise (*Stignochelys pardalis*) in the USA and Europe (although both species are African in origin).
- In aquatic turtles, HV have been described in various emydid species, including pond, painted, map, and box turtles as well as in other taxonomic groups of turtles.
- Disease can occur year round, although tortoises may be particularly susceptible in the spring and fall.

CLINICAL PRESENTATION

Sea turtles

- Fibropapillomatosis: can develop externally on all parts of the body, including the eyes and around the cloaca, leading to difficulties in finding food and/or in defecating. Internal tumors can also occur. Affected animals may be cachectic.
- Other HV-associated diseases described in sea turtles: gray patch disease (skin lesions in young green sea turtles); LETD (respiratory disease in green sea turtles); LGRV, and LOCV in wild-caught loggerhead sea turtles.

Tortoises

- Acute: lethargy, anorexia, caseous plaques on the tongue and palate, dyspnea, hepatitis. Severe disease with high morbidity and mortality associated with TeHV3 infection in various tortoise species. Infection may be clinically inapparent in some cases, although disease can develop in any species. TeHV1 and TeHV4 may be associated with less severe disease or inapparent infections.
- Chronic: surviving tortoises may develop CNS signs, including paralysis or incoordination. Clinically healthy carriers are also possible.

Turtles

- Sudden death, weakness, nasal discharge, stomatitis, papillomatosis, and hepatitis.
- Herpesviruses have also been detected in apparently clinically healthy animals.

RISK FACTORS

Husbandry

- Mixing of different tortoise species leads to an increase in the probability of inapparent carriers transmitting virus to highly susceptible species.
- In sea turtles, sudden changes in temperature and exposure to environmental pollutants have both been shown to increase susceptibility to HV disease.

Others

N/A

DIAGNOSIS

DIFFERENTIAL DIAGNOSIS

- In tortoises: depending on the presentation, mycoplasma infections (esp. in cases with upper respiratory disease), ranavirus (family *Iridoviridae*) infections, topivirus (family *Picornaviridae*) infections, bacterial and/or fungal stomatitis.

DIAGNOSTICS

Virus detection

- Most commonly done using PCR detection of viral DNA.
- A pan-HV PCR can be used to detect all reptilian HV described so far.
- PCRs for specific chelonian HV have also been described.
- In sea turtles, material from fibropapillomas should be used for testing; in tortoises oral swabs, tongue, liver and brain can be tested.
- Material from any lesions observed should be included in any testing scheme.

Serology

- Virus neutralization tests have been used for the detection of antibodies against TeHV1 and 3 in tortoises.
- An ELISA has also been described for the detection of antibodies against these two viruses and against TeHV2, but may not be commercially available.

PATHOLOGICAL FINDINGS

- Ballooning degeneration and necrosis may be noted in infected epithelial cells, necrosis and inflammation in affected tissues.
- Fibropapillomas consist of a hyperplastic epidermis and a thickened hypercellular dermis.
- Infected cells may contain eosinophilic to amphophilic intranuclear inclusions.

TREATMENT

APPROPRIATE HEALTH CARE

- There are no standardized protocols for treating HV-infected reptiles.
- Strict quarantine, biosecurity, and hygiene are essential for the prevention of HV infections.
- Autovaccination with inactivated material from surgically removed fibropapillomas has been suggested.
- Keeping animals at the high end of their POTZ may help in recovery, as well as treatment of secondary bacterial infections.

NUTRITIONAL SUPPORT

- Herpesvirus infected reptiles may be anorexic and nutritional support may be necessary.
- In animals with oral lesions, esophagostomy tubes may be necessary.

CLIENT EDUCATION/HUSBANDRY RECOMMENDATIONS

- Testing for both virus and antibodies (in tortoises) should be in place.
- An effective quarantine regimen should be in place.
- Mixing of tortoise species should be avoided.
- Infected animals must be isolated

SURGICAL CONSIDERATIONS

For fibropapillomas—surgical removal of lesions.

MEDICATIONS

DRUG(S) OF CHOICE

• Acyclovir 80 mg/kg PO q24h (famciclovir has been shown to be safer in mammals and may be an alternative choice for treatment).
• Acyclovir topically on lesions or topical disinfection (e.g., with 0.5% chlorhexidine solution) have also been suggested.
• The use of immunomodulators (e.g., Zylexis (Pfizer AG, Zurich, Switzerland)) has been suggested in HV infected tortoises, but its efficacy is unproven.

PRECAUTIONS/INTERACTIONS

Affected animals should be barrier nursed and in-contact animals should be placed in quarantine.

FOLLOW-UP

PATIENT MONITORING

• Development of disease in contact animals may take several weeks, so monitoring of a collection (and barrier nursing of contact animals) should remain active for at least one season.
• There is some indication that brumation may provoke disease outbreaks, and intensified health monitoring should be carried out in the spring and again before the next brumation.

EXPECTED COURSE AND PROGNOSIS

• Morbidity and mortality can be high, depending on the virus strain and host species involved, although it can take an extended period of time for the disease to run its course within a collection.
• Surviving animals remain carriers

MISCELLANEOUS

COMMENTS

N/A

ZOONOTIC POTENTIAL

Herpesviruses of reptiles have not been shown to be zoonotic.

SYNONYMS

Fibropapillomatosis (FP) in sea turtles

ABBREVIATIONS

• chHV5 = chelonid alphaherpesvirus 5
• CNS = central nervous system
• ELISA = enzyme-linked immunosorbent assay
• FPTHV = fibropapillomatosis-associated turtle herpesvirus
• HV = herpesvirus
• LETD = lung = eye = and trachea disease
• LEDV = lung = eye = and trachea disease virus
• LGRV = loggerhead genital–respiratory herpesvirus
• LOCV = loggerhead orocutaneous herpesvirus
• PCR = polymerase chain reaction
• POTZ = preferred optimal temperature zone
• TeHV = testudinid herpesvirus

Suggested Reading

Gandar F, Wilkie GS, Gatherer D, et al. The genome of a tortoise herpesvirus (testudinid herpesvirus 3) has a novel structure and contains a large region that is not required for replication in vitro or virulence in vivo. *J Virol* 2015;89(22):11438–11456.
Marschang RE. Virology. In: Divers SJ, Stahl SJ, eds. *Mader's Reptile and Amphibian Medicine and Surgery*. St. Louis, MO: Elsevier; 2019:247–269.
Marschang RE. Viruses infecting reptiles. *Viruses* 2011;3:2087–2126.

Author Rachel E. Marschang, PD, Dr. med. vet., DECZM (Herpetology), FTÄ Mikrobiologie

HEXAMITA

BASICS

DEFINITION/OVERVIEW

Hexamita is a small flagellate parasite which can be found in the intestinal tract of chelonians and snakes. *Hexamita parva* is the usual cause of disease in chelonians. Disease has not been reported in other reptiles.

ETIOLOGY/PATHOPHYSIOLOGY

- Infection is thought to occur by ingestion of an infective cyst, which passes into the gastrointestinal tract.
- Reproduction is by simple binary fission. Subsequently, the parasite may ascend via the bile ducts to the gall bladder or via the ureters to the kidneys, where it encysts, resulting in inflammation.
- Alternatively, *Hexamita* may pass through the gastrointestinal tract without resulting in disease.
- Transmission can occur via urine or feces.

SIGNALMENT/HISTORY

Disease has been described in a wide variety of chelonian species with no "typical" signalment.

CLINICAL PRESENTATION

- Animals with *Hexamita* infection may be asymptomatic or have non-specific signs such as lethargy and reduced appetite.
- If significant renal pathology is present, weight loss and polydipsia may be seen.

RISK FACTORS

Husbandry

Poor hygiene will increase the risk of disease transmission.

Others

Pre-existing renal or biliary disease or concurrent parasite infection have been suggested to be potential risk factors.

DIAGNOSIS

- Identification of the parasite in a sample of urine ± feces may lead to suspicion of disease, but flagellates are not always associated with pathology.
- Definitive diagnosis requires detection of the parasite on renal biopsy in a live animal.

DIFFERENTIAL DIAGNOSIS

Parasites should be distinguished from commensal intestinal flagellates, especially trichomonads, which may commonly be seen in fecal samples or urine samples contaminated with feces.

DIAGNOSTICS

- Analysis of a fresh urine sample may reveal small fast-moving flagellates (< 8 microns) characterized by six anterior flagella.
- In small samples the parasite will rapidly desiccate and die.
- Renal biopsies should be submitted for histopathology.
- Biochemistry may be helpful to indicate degree of renal damage.

PATHOLOGICAL FINDINGS

- Characteristic postmortem findings include pale enlarged kidneys with dilated collecting tubules. Bile ducts appear thickened with a dilated lumen.
- On histopathological examination, flagellates may be visualized within the renal tubules and bile ducts with associated inflammatory changes.

TREATMENT

APPROPRIATE HEALTH CARE

- Treatment involves both eliminating the parasite and supportive care of the renal disease.
- Euthanasia may be considered in severe cases of renal failure.

NUTRITIONAL SUPPORT

- Some patients may be anorexic and severely dehydrated on presentation.
- Fluid deficits should always be corrected and nutritional support provided as needed.

CLIENT EDUCATION/HUSBANDRY RECOMMENDATIONS

Hygiene measures should be reviewed to minimize the risk of disease transmission.

MEDICATIONS

DRUG(S) OF CHOICE

- Metronidazole is the most common choice for treating *Hexamita*.
- Various treatment regimens have been recommended ranging from 100–125 mg/kg PO once, then repeated after 14 days to 50 mg/kg PO q24h for 3–5 days for severe infections.

PRECAUTIONS/INTERACTIONS

Hepatotoxicity and CNS toxicity have occasionally been reported in other species following metronidazole use, so care should be taken if pre-existing hepatic dysfunction is suspected.

FOLLOW-UP

PATIENT MONITORING

- Response to therapy is usually monitored by a reduction in clinical signs (e.g., improved appetite).
- Repeat blood samples can also be taken to recheck renal parameters.

EXPECTED COURSE AND PROGNOSIS

- The prognosis for patients with extensive biliary or renal damage is poor, but if diagnosed early the condition can be managed successfully.
- If left untreated, the disease will slowly progress to renal failure and death.

MISCELLANEOUS

COMMENTS

N/A

ZOONOTIC POTENTIAL

N/A

SYNONYMS

N/A

ABBREVIATIONS

- CNS = central nervous system
- PO = per oram

INTERNET RESOURCES

Veterinary Information Network: www.vin.com

Suggested Reading

Johns JD. Urogenital system. In: Girling SJ, Raiti P, eds. *BSAVA Manual of Reptiles*, 2nd ed. Quedgeley, UK: BSAVA; 2004:261–272.

Zwart P, Truyens EHA. Hexamitiasis in tortoises. *Vet Parasitol* 1975;1(2):175–183.

Author Joanna Hedley, BVM&S, DZooMed (Reptilian), DECZM (Herpetology), MRCVS

HYPERGLYCEMIA

BASICS

DEFINITION/OVERVIEW

Hyperglycemia is abnormally high blood glucose concentration. In most species, glucose concentrations fluctuate. Normal glucose concentration ranges from 60 mg/dl to 200 mg/dl (3.3–11 mmol/l).

ETIOLOGY/PATHOPHYSIOLOGY

- The etiology is largely unknown
- Transient hyperglycemia may be postprandial or stress induced.
- Elevated glucose may be seen during ovulation, and in certain neoplastic conditions.
- Iatrogenic from prior glucose or glucocorticosteroid administration.
- Hyperglycemia has been documented in parasitic pancreatitis (*Serpinema microcephalus*).
- It is speculated that endocrine pancreas disease may lead to insulin deficiency resulting in a diabetes mellitus-like syndrome, but this has not been documented.

SIGNALMENT/HISTORY

N/A

CLINICAL PRESENTATION

- Unspecific
- Possibly increased water consumption, increased urine (urate) production, and weight loss.

RISK FACTORS

Husbandry

- Largely unknown
- Stress from handling or improper housing may predispose.

Others

N/A

DIAGNOSIS

Blood glucose levels above 200 mg/dl (11 mmol/l) indicate hyperglycemia.

DIFFERENTIAL DIAGNOSIS

N/A

DIAGNOSTICS

- Blood glucose measurements should be repeated, as a single elevated value is likely insignificant.
- Persistent hyperglycemia is a more relevant finding.
- Glucosuria should be evaluated to identify chronic hyperglycemia.
- Underlying causes should be investigated: ovarian activity, neoplasia (particularly stomach and pancreas), metabolic disease.

PATHOLOGICAL FINDINGS

- The etiology for persistent hyperglycemia is unknown, but endocrine pancreas should be thoroughly evaluated.

TREATMENT

APPROPRIATE HEALTH CARE

N/A

NUTRITIONAL SUPPORT

N/A

CLIENT EDUCATION/HUSBANDRY RECOMMENDATIONS

N/A

MEDICATIONS

DRUG(S) OF CHOICE

- In cases with persistent hyperglycemia, where systemic disease has been ruled out, experimental insulin treatment may be attempted.
- Suggested starting dose: 1–5 iu q24–48h.

PRECAUTIONS/INTERACTIONS

N/A

FOLLOW-UP

PATIENT MONITORING

Follow up with repeated glucose measurements, and monitor general health of patient.

EXPECTED COURSE AND PROGNOSIS

Transient hyperglycemia is likely insignificant, while chronically elevated levels carry a poor prognosis.

MISCELLANEOUS

COMMENTS

N/A

ZOONOTIC POTENTIAL

N/A

SYNONYMS

N/A

INTERNET RESOURCES

Melissa Kaplan's Herp Care Collection. Hypoglycemia and Hyperglycemia in Reptiles. http://www.anapsid.org/diabetes.html

Suggested Reading

Campbell TW. Clinical pathology. In: Mader DR, Divers SJ, eds. *Current Therapy in Reptile Medicine and Surgery*. St. Louis, MO: Elsevier Saunders; 2014:70–92.

Stahl SJ. Hyperglycemia in reptiles. In: Mader DR, ed. *Reptile Medicine and Surgery*. 2nd ed. St. Louis, MO: Elsevier Saunders; 2006:822–830.

Author Mads F. Bertelsen, DVM, DVSc, DACZM, DECZM (Zoo Health Management)

HYPERVITAMINOSIS A

BASICS

DEFINITION/OVERVIEW

Hypervitaminosis A is well recognized health concern in chelonians. It can be caused by OTC supplements provided by well-meaning owners, parenteral overdosing by veterinarians, or diets with high animal vs. plant-based (beta carotene) vitamin A levels.

ETIOLOGY/PATHOPHYSIOLOGY

- In vertebrates, the vitamin A forms are trans-retinyl esters, trans-retinol, -retinal and -retinoic acid (99% of all vitamin A present in the body), while the major dietary provitamin A carotenoid is beta carotene.
- The all-trans-vitamin A isomers are the only forms used physiologically.
- The liver absorbs and stores preformed vitamin A; at a certain point, storage capacity is reached and toxicity occurs. Other storage sites include adipose tissue, lung, and kidney.
- In humans, the retinoid delivery pathway to tissues involves primarily retinol bound to retinol-binding protein; chylomicrons, very low density lipoprotein, low density lipoprotein, and albumin also provide transport.
- Adverse effects in humans include increased bone turnover by suppressing osteoblast activity and stimulating osteoclast formation. This can lead to hypercalcemia, osteoporosis, pathologic fractures, altered skeletal development in children, and skeletal pain.
- Vitamin A is fat soluble and high levels can affect metabolism of other fat-soluble vitamins (D, E, K); with the effects on vitamin D contributing to the aforementioned bone pathology, although stimulation of bone resorption by vitamin A is reported independent of effects on vitamin D.
- Vitamin A can have a toxic effect on mitochondrial function and is reported to cause hypothyroidism in mice.

SIGNALMENT/HISTORY

- First time owner of reptiles/species and young animals.
- Owner using OTC vitamin A drops, OTC multivitamin with vitamin A in formulation other than beta carotene, using cod liver oil or feeding liver to a carnivorous/omnivorous animal.
- Occasional issues with extruded diets with inadvertent toxic levels of non-beta carotene vitamin A.

CLINICAL PRESENTATION

- Patients present with vague signs such as anorexia, dehydration, lethargy.
- Usually has a dermatological component including: dysecdysis, epidermal flakiness, ulceration, and sloughing.
- Bilateral epiphora and periorbital edema may be noted.
- Ulcerative stomatitis can be seen.
- Secondary bacterial and fungal infections can occur.
- Based on pathophysiology, suspect that metabolic bone disease may have interplay with hypervitaminosis A.

RISK FACTORS

- Juvenile animal
- Reproductively active female
- Liver disease

Husbandry

N/A

Others

Iatrogenic dietary or parenteral over supplementation of non-beta carotene vitamin A.

DIAGNOSIS

DIFFERENTIAL DIAGNOSIS

- Hypovitaminosis A
- Infection
- Hepatic or renal disease
- UVB or thermal burns
- Poor overall husbandry or diet
- Improper conspecific arrangement
- Metabolic bone disease

DIAGNOSTICS

- Liver biopsy for histopathology and testing vitamin A levels (need normal values for the species).
- Presumptive diagnosis based upon history and clinical presentation.

PATHOLOGICAL FINDINGS

- Hepatic fibrosis
- Osteoporosis
- Decreased or abnormal bony growth in juvenile animals.
- Epidermal ulceration

TREATMENT

APPROPRIATE HEALTH CARE

N/A

NUTRITIONAL SUPPORT

- Often need assisted feeding
- Esophageal feeding tube is often recommended, especially in chelonians with skin sloughing, which makes it difficult to manipulate the head and neck.

CLIENT EDUCATION/HUSBANDRY RECOMMENDATIONS

- Proper education about the correct diet and formulation of vitamin A for the species.
- Education about differences between water soluble and fat-soluble vitamins.

MEDICATIONS

DRUG(S) OF CHOICE

- Discontinuing supplementation of non-beta carotene vitamin A.
- Other treatment focuses on supportive therapy and managing secondary infections.
- Systemic fluid therapy may be needed but with the goal of transitioning to oral fluids or passive soaking.
- Pain management can be important.
- Judicious topical use of silver sulfadiazine cream for epidermal ulcers can help.
- Vitamins E and K and taurine administration have all been shown to help mitigate hypervitaminosis A in rat studies, but no studies are available in reptiles.

PRECAUTIONS/INTERACTIONS

Oversupplementation of vitamin A can have negative interactions with other fat-soluble vitamins (D, E, K) leading to either decreased absorption or excess accumulation.

FOLLOW-UP

PATIENT MONITORING

- Reassessment of clinical manifestation
- Review of current diet plan
- Repeat liver biopsy if feasible

EXPECTED COURSE AND PROGNOSIS

- In the acute form, hypervitaminosis A generally resolves quickly and clinical manifestation is uncommon (except in very high overdosing).
- The chronic form is most common. Clinical resolution can take many months, with most dermatological manifestations resolving, although skeletal and hepatic damage may be permanent.

MISCELLANEOUS

COMMENTS

N/A

ZOONOTIC POTENTIAL

N/A

SYNONYMS

N/A

ABBREVIATIONS

- OTC = over the counter
- UVB = ultraviolet B

Suggested Reading

Chen LP, Huang CH. Effects of dietary β-carotene levels on growth and liver vitamin A concentrations of the soft-shelled turtle, *Pelodiscus sinensis* (Wiegmann). *Aquacult Res* 2011;42:1848–1854.

Chen LP, Huang CH. Estimation of dietary vitamin A requirement of juvenile soft-shelled turtle, Pelodiscus sinensis. *Aquacult Nutr* 2015;21:457–463.

Mans C, Braun J. Update on common nutritional disorders of captive reptiles. *Vet Clin North Am Exot Anim Pract* 2014;17(3):369–395.

Author Eric Klaphake, DVM, DACZM

HYPOGLYCEMIA

BASICS

DEFINITION/OVERVIEW

Abnormally low blood glucose concentration. In most species, glucose concentrations fluctuate; normal concentrations range from 60 mg/dl to 200 mg/dl (3.3–11 mmol/l), but lower values could be normal.

ETIOLOGY/PATHOPHYSIOLOGY

- Exhaustion, starvation, malnutrition
- Septicemia
- Hepatobiliary disease
- Pancreatic disease

SIGNALMENT/HISTORY

- Animals with severe systemic disease may be predisposed.
- Long-lasting anorexia

CLINICAL PRESENTATION

- Weakness
- Tremors
- Loss of righting reflex
- Torpor
- Unresponsiveness

RISK FACTORS

Husbandry

Poor nutritional status

Others

Systemic disease

DIAGNOSIS

Blood glucose levels below 20 mg/dl (1.1 mmol/l) indicate hypoglycemia.

DIFFERENTIAL DIAGNOSIS

N/A

DIAGNOSTICS

- Detection of hypoglycemia in a clinically healthy animal should not cause concern.
- In animals with clinical signs and hypoglycemia, attempts should be made to rule out septicemia, hepatobiliary disease, and pancreatic neoplasia.
- Glucose may be artificially low in blood samples stored for a prolonged period prior to separation of plasma/serum.

PATHOLOGICAL FINDINGS

- Depends on underlying etiology
- The pancreas should be thoroughly evaluated.

TREATMENT

APPROPRIATE HEALTH CARE

N/A

NUTRITIONAL SUPPORT

Consider energy-rich nutritional support by stomach tube in cases of anorexia.

CLIENT EDUCATION/HUSBANDRY RECOMMENDATIONS

If related to poor nutrition and management, educate clients on appropriate feeding practices.

MEDICATIONS

DRUG(S) OF CHOICE

- Treat underlying disease
- Supportive administration of glucose or dextrose parenterally (e.g., 2.5% in 0.45% saline, 20–40 mL/kg SC) or orally (3 g/kg PO) may be indicated.

PRECAUTIONS/INTERACTIONS

N/A

FOLLOW-UP

PATIENT MONITORING

Monitor glucose levels and clinical signs.

EXPECTED COURSE AND PROGNOSIS

- If related to nutritional status prognosis is good.
- If secondary to severe systemic disease prognosis is poor.

MISCELLANEOUS

COMMENTS

N/A

ZOONOTIC POTENTIAL

N/A

SYNONYMS

N/A

ABBREVIATIONS

PO = per os
SC = subcutaneous

INTERNET RESOURCES

Kaplan M. Hypoglycemia and Hyperglycemia in Reptiles. Melissa Kaplan's Herp Care Collection, January 1, 2014. www.anapsid.org/diabetes.html .

Suggested Reading

Campbell TW. Clinical pathology. In: Mader DR, Divers SJ, eds. *Current Therapy in Reptile Medicine and Surgery*. St. Louis, MO: Elsevier; 2014:70–92.

Stahl SJ. Hyperglycemia in reptiles. In: Mader DR, ed. *Reptile Medicine and Surgery*. 2nd ed. St. Louis, MO: Elsevier Saunders; 2006:822–830.

Author Mads F. Bertelsen, DVM, DVSc, DACZM, DECZM (Zoo Health Management)

HYPOVITAMINOSIS A

BASICS

DEFINITION/OVERVIEW

Hypovitaminosis A is a well-recognized health concern in pet carnivorous, insectivorous, and omnivorous chelonians. The primary cause is feeding food items deficient in the correct form of vitamin A for the species or in under/incorrectly supplementing vitamin A.

ETIOLOGY/PATHOPHYSIOLOGY

- In vertebrates, vitamin A forms are trans-retinyl esters, trans-retinol, -retinal and -retinoic acid (99% of all vitamin A present in body), while the major dietary provitamin A carotenoid is beta carotene.
- The all-trans-vitamin A isomers are the only forms used physiologically.
- Carnivores, insectivores, and possibly omnivores need these forms in their diet.
- While reptile herbivores can convert carotenoids lutein and canthaxanthin into trans-retinyl esters, beta carotene does not convert as well.
- Hypovitaminosis A in herbivores is extremely unlikely, excepting after long periods of anorexia.
- The liver absorbs and stores preformed vitamin A. Other storage sites include adipose, lung, and kidney.
- In humans, retinoid delivery pathway to tissues involves primarily retinol bound to retinol-binding protein; chylomicrons, very low density lipoprotein, low density lipoprotein, and albumin also provide transport.
- Adverse effects in humans include night blindness, impaired immune function, cancer, and birth defects.

SIGNALMENT/HISTORY

- First-time owner of reptiles/species.
- Supplementing with beta carotene-based vitamin A or no supplementation.
- Box turtles (*Terrapene carolina* sp.) and sliders (*Trachemys scripta* sp.) may present more commonly.

CLINICAL PRESENTATION

- Most present with non-specific signs such as anorexia, dehydration, and lethargy.
- Upper respiratory signs include bilateral nasal–ocular discharge, blepharedema, conjunctivitis, "pus" in conjunctival sacs (actually desquamated debris), swelling and closure of palpebral fissures due to squamous metaplasia and glandular hypertrophy, and secondary bacterial infections.
- Ulcerative stomatitis, glossal plaques, and glossitis may also be observed.
- Chelonian aural abscesses do not appear to be directly associated with hypovitaminosis A based on current findings, but squamous metaplasia may lead to secondary aural infections.

RISK FACTORS

Husbandry

Insectivore, carnivore not receiving vertebrate prey with liver.

Others

N/A

DIAGNOSIS

DIFFERENTIAL DIAGNOSIS

- Bacterial infection
- Hepatic/renal disease
- UVB/thermal burns
- Ocular trauma
- Water-based toxins
- Poor overall husbandry/diet
- Improper conspecific arrangement
- Metabolic bone disease

DIAGNOSTICS

- Presumptive diagnosis is based upon history, clinical presentation, and response to correct supplementation.
- Liver biopsy for histopathology and testing vitamin A levels can be performed, but there is a lack of normal values.
- Hepatic vitamin A levels are normally extremely high in carnivores, much lower in herbivores, and intermediate in insectivores and omnivores.
- Sex of animal, testing methodology, and reported units can affect results.

PATHOLOGICAL FINDINGS

- Squamous metaplasia
- Epidermal ulceration

TREATMENT

APPROPRIATE HEALTH CARE

N/A

NUTRITIONAL SUPPORT

- Omnivores and carnivores can be fed whole prey still containing liver, or for semiaquatic turtles, can offer extruded diet with correct form of vitamin A.
- Supportive feeding, including esophageal feeding tubes may be needed until the reptile feels better and can actually see the food.
- For herbivores, feed plenty of leafy greens and red/orange/yellow vegetables.
- Treatment for insectivores is more complex.
- Invertebrates store retinols in the retina only, so invertebrates (or juvenile forms) without eyes have no vitamin A.
- Dusting invertebrates must be done immediately before feeding, as the vitamin powder is usually often self-groomed off the invertebrate before the reptile has ingested it.
- Gut-loading guidelines are still controversial but seem to still be the best option—especially consider the Li diet (see Suggested Reading).
- Consider feeding non-toxic, wild-caught invertebrates, as they generally have much higher levels of vitamin A than captive-raised invertebrates.

CLIENT EDUCATION/HUSBANDRY RECOMMENDATIONS

- Proper education about correct diet for the species.
- Discuss correct formulation of vitamin A for the species.
- Correct invertebrates to offer and how to supplement them.
- Clear explanation of differences between water-soluble and fat-soluble vitamins.

MEDICATIONS

DRUG(S) OF CHOICE

- Parenteral treatment or oral supplementation of retinol forms to herbivores should be avoided.
- Use dietary carotenoids (non-beta carotene) instead.
- For omnivorous, carnivorous, and insectivorous reptiles, parenteral vitamin A (usually has vitamin D3 as well): 500–5,000 iu/kg IM q7–14d for up to 4 treatments.
- Dosing must be done carefully to avoid over supplementation with vitamin A in the retinol form.
- Other treatment focuses on managing with systemic antibiotics/antifungals for secondary infections.
- Judicious topical use of silver sulfadiazine cream for epidermal ulcers can help.
- Removal of conjunctiva plugs or flushing nasolacrimal ducts (when present) can be beneficial symptomatic treatment.

PRECAUTIONS/INTERACTIONS

Vitamin A interacts with other fat-soluble vitamins (D, E, K).

FOLLOW-UP

PATIENT MONITORING

- Re-evaluate for improvement of clinical signs.
- Review owner's diet plan
- Repeat liver biopsy if feasible

HYPOVITAMINOSIS A (CONTINUED)

EXPECTED COURSE AND PROGNOSIS

Usually chronic, clinical resolution can take several months with most manifestations resolving, though renal damage may be permanent.

MISCELLANEOUS

COMMENTS

N/A

ZOONOTIC POTENTIAL

N/A

SYNONYMS

N/A

ABBREVIATIONS

- IM = intramuscular
- UVB = ultraviolet B

Suggested Reading

Chen LP, Huang CH. Estimation of dietary vitamin A requirement of juvenile soft-shelled turtle, *Pelodiscus sinensis*. *Aquacult Nutr* 2015;21:457–463.

Li H, Vaughan MJ, Browne RK. A complex enrichment diet improves growth and health in the endangered Wyoming toad (*Bufo baxteri*). *Zoo Biol* 2009;28:197–213.

Mans C, Braun J. Update on common nutritional disorders of captive reptiles. *Vet Clin North Am Exot Anim Pract* 2014;17(3):369–395.

Miller EA, Green SL, Otto GM, Bouley DM. Suspected hypovitaminosis A in a colony of captive green anoles (Anolis carolinensis). *Contemp Top Lab Anim Sci* 2001;40:18–20.

Author Eric Klaphake, DVM, DACZM

HYPOVITAMINOSIS B

BASICS

DEFINITION/OVERVIEW

Hypovitaminosis B generally refers to hypothiaminosis and is a health concern in reptiles that are fed fish—whether live or frozen thawed. Other cases have been reported in herbivorous reptiles and reptiles fed vitamin supplements lacking in thiamine.

ETIOLOGY/PATHOPHYSIOLOGY

- In humans, thiamine deficiency can occur rapidly and advance to metabolic coma and death; causes being malnutrition, a diet high in thiaminase-rich foods (raw freshwater fish, raw shellfish, ferns), chronic gastrointestinal diseases, and diabetes mellitus.
- Thiamine derivatives and thiamine-dependent enzymes are present in all cells, but the nervous system is very sensitive, leading to nerve fiber myelin sheath degeneration causing necrotizing encephalopathy and peripheral neuritis.
- Bilateral vision loss due to optic neuropathy can occur.
- Thiamine is a water-soluble vitamin synthesized by bacteria, fungi, and plants.
- Captive fish-eating garter snakes and semi-aquatic turtles, and captive and free-ranging crocodilians are most commonly affected.
- Feeding fish high in thiaminase—goldfish and fathead minnow, improperly thawed fish (thawing too slowly), or fish that has been frozen a long time can all be factors.
- Some frozen thawed vegetables containing phytothiaminases lead to thiamine deficiency in green iguanas.
- Insectivorous anoles developed thiamine deficiency due to lack of any thiamine in the multivitamin supplement because of extensive storage before use.
- Thiamine is a rapidly deteriorating vitamin so it is important to ensure that supplements are stored and used properly.

SIGNALMENT/HISTORY

- Fish as primary diet
- Thawed frozen vegetables
- Using same container of vitamin supplement/powder beyond expiration date or past 6 months after opening.

CLINICAL PRESENTATION

Can present with non-specific signs such as anorexia, dehydration, and lethargy, but suspicions of thiamine deficiency are greater with torticollis, opisthotonus, muscle tremors, incoordination, blindness, jaw gaping, and sudden death.

RISK FACTORS

Husbandry

N/A

Others

- Piscivores
- Thawed frozen vegetables

DIAGNOSIS

DIFFERENTIAL DIAGNOSIS

- Trauma
- Infectious encephalitis
- Toxins
- Metabolic bone disease
- Hepatoencephalopathy
- Neoplasia
- Cardiac disease
- Renal disease
- Ruptured aneurysm

DIAGNOSTICS

Usually based upon history, clinical signs, and response to parenteral thiamine (B-complex vitamins).

PATHOLOGICAL FINDINGS

- Cerebral cortical necrosis
- Peripheral neuritis

TREATMENT

APPROPRIATE HEALTH CARE

N/A

NUTRITIONAL SUPPORT

- Avoid feeding fish known to have high thiaminase levels, such as goldfish and fathead minnows.
- Proper storage of frozen fish by not keeping beyond 6 months of death/freezing.
- Rapid thawing for five minutes in 80 degrees C (175 degrees F) water denatures thiaminase or thawing in refrigerator also avoids thiaminase activation.
- An added level of protection would be to add thiamine 25 mg/kg fish.
- Do not use vitamin supplements beyond expiration date or 6 months after opened.

CLIENT EDUCATION/HUSBANDRY RECOMMENDATIONS

- Proper education about expiration dates/opening dates of vitamin supplements, avoiding certain live fish species and carrying out proper thawing techniques for frozen fish.
- Avoidance of too many thawed frozen vegetables.

MEDICATIONS

DRUG(S) OF CHOICE

- Thiamine administered at 50–100 mg/kg IM, SC, or PO q24h until resolution of clinical signs.
- A vitamin B complex formulation is less ideal but can be used if a thiamine-only supplement is not available.

PRECAUTIONS/INTERACTIONS

N/A

FOLLOW-UP

PATIENT MONITORING

- Reassess diet
- Diet processing/handling
- Supplementation at every visit

EXPECTED COURSE AND PROGNOSIS

- If thiamine deficiency without concurrent issues, should have immediate response to therapy, although repeated treatments may be needed.
- In non-piscivores, often not considered and diagnosed postmortem on histopathology.

MISCELLANEOUS

COMMENTS

N/A

ZOONOTIC POTENTIAL

N/A

SYNONYMS

Thiamine deficiency

ABBREVIATIONS

- IM = intramuscular
- PO = per os
- SC = subcutaneous

Suggested Reading

Mans C, Braun J. Update on common nutritional disorders of captive reptiles. *Vet Clin North Am Exot Anim Pract* 2014;17(3):369–395.

Author Eric Klaphake, DVM, DACZM

IRIDOVIRUSES

BASICS

DEFINITION/OVERVIEW

Viruses in the family *Iridoviridae* are large, double-stranded DNA viruses that contain a lipid component and can be enveloped. Viruses in the genus *Ranavirus* are the most common iridoviruses described in chelonians and have the greatest clinical importance. They can infect a wide range of ectothermic vertebrates including reptiles, amphibians, and bony fish.

ETIOLOGY/PATHOPHYSIOLOGY

- Ranaviruses have been described in wild and pet chelonians, pet lizards, and occasionally in snakes.
- Numerous ranavirus strains can be transmitted between different animal classes. In North America, the ranaviruses described in reptiles have all been closely related to FV3, the type species of the genus, while ranaviruses found in reptiles in other parts of the world (particularly Europe) have been more genetically diverse.
- In infected reptiles, ranaviruses can cause severe disease, often associated with lesions in the mouth, liver, and blood vessels.

SIGNALMENT/HISTORY

- Ranaviruses have been found in terrestrial and aquatic species.
- Most chelonians appear to be highly susceptible to infection, and infection in these animals has been associated with large outbreaks.
- Virus has been detected in free-ranging box turtles in multiple states in the United States, while descriptions in Europe have mostly been in captive reptiles.
- Various age groups have been shown to be susceptible to ranavirus infection, although there may be some indication that juveniles are more susceptible to disease.
- Outbreaks are often associated with translocations, mixing of animals with unknown health status, or transport in the pet trade.
- The majority of viral strains detected in reptiles have been closely related to amphibian ranaviruses, and multiple studies have indicated that many of these viruses can switch between a wide range of ectothermic hosts.

CLINICAL PRESENTATION

- In chelonians, signs include ulcerative stomatitis, conjunctivitis, and nasal discharge.
- Subcutaneous cervical edema and erythema may also occur.
- Infected animals become lethargic and anorexic and may die acutely.
- Infection can cause hepatitis, enteritis, and pneumonia.
- Dermatitis has been described in some cases.

RISK FACTORS

Husbandry

- Close contact with infected amphibians, many of which can be inapparent carriers, can lead to virus transmission.
- Contaminated water can also lead to transmission.
- Ranaviruses do not replicate at high temperatures, so keeping animals at low temperatures may increase the risk of infection.

Others

N/A

DIAGNOSIS

DIFFERENTIAL DIAGNOSIS

- Herpesvirus infections
- Bacterial and/or fungal infections

DIAGNOSTICS

Virus detection

- In the United States, all the ranaviruses described in reptiles to date have been genetically closely related, and a highly sensitive real-time PCR is available for their detection.
- In other parts of the world, ranaviruses found in reptiles have been more genetically diverse, and PCRs capable of detecting these should be used.
- These viruses can also be relatively easily isolated in cell culture.
- Oral and cloacal swabs have been used to detect ranaviruses, as has blood, more invasive samples (tail clips, tissue biopsies) may be more sensitive.
- The liver and kidneys should also be tested if possible.

Serology

- An ELISA has been described for the detection of antibodies against ranaviruses in chelonians, although this is not widely commercially available.

PATHOLOGICAL FINDINGS

- Chelonians with ranavirus infections have been described with hepatitis, enteritis, and pneumonia.
- Vasculitis and formation of thrombi in various organs has also been described.
- In some, but not all, cases, infection may be associated with basophilic intracytoplasmic inclusions in in affected cells, especially hepatocytes and epithelial cells of the upper gastrointestinal tract.

TREATMENT

APPROPRIATE HEALTH CARE

- There is no specific treatment available for iridovirus infections in reptiles.
- All viruses in this family replicate at temperatures below 32 degrees C (89.6 degrees F), and environmental temperature has been shown to influence the pathogenicity of ranaviruses in turtles.
- It is, however, important to keep the POTZ of the affected species in mind when adjusting environmental temperature.

NUTRITIONAL SUPPORT

N/A

CLIENT EDUCATION/HUSBANDRY RECOMMENDATIONS

- Ranaviruses can be transmitted between various ectothermic vertebrate classes, and care should be taken not to mix species.
- Quarantine procedures for all ectothermic vertebrates in a collection should include testing for ranaviruses.
- Since wild reptiles and amphibians can be infected, and ranaviruses may survive for some time in the environment, especially under cold conditions, introduction of virus into a collection via the environment (e.g., water, soil) should be avoided.
- Conversely, in the case of an outbreak, special care should be taken to avoid contamination of the environment. All water and substrate that comes into contact with infected animals should be disinfected before it is disposed of, as should all husbandry items.
- Carcasses from dead animals should be disposed of appropriately, ensuring that they do not come in contact with other animals.
- Since ectoparasites may play a role in the transmission of various iridoviruses, effective measures for parasite control should be implemented.

MEDICATIONS

DRUG(S) OF CHOICE

N/A

PRECAUTIONS/INTERACTIONS

- Ranaviruses appear to be very infectious in chelonians, and affected animals should be barrier nursed.
- Viruses can cross species and class barriers, so contact with any other ectothermic vertebrates should be avoided.
- In has been suggested that ranaviruses may be transmitted by hematophagous invertebrates, so control of mosquito populations may be helpful.

FOLLOW-UP

PATIENT MONITORING

- The time to development of disease in contact animals can vary depending on the route of infection, amount of infectious material, virus strain and host species, so monitoring should be continued for several weeks to months in an affected collection.
- Surviving infected animals can become carriers.

EXPECTED COURSE AND PROGNOSIS

- Morbidity is usually very high, although recovery from infection has been described.
- Surviving animals may remain carriers and should be kept separate from susceptible animals including reptiles, amphibians, and fish.

MISCELLANEOUS

COMMENTS

N/A

ZOONOTIC POTENTIAL

Viruses in the family *Iridoviridae* are generally temperature restricted and can only replicate at temperatures below 32 degrees C (89.6 degrees F). They are therefore unable to infect mammals or birds.

SYNONYMS

Ranavirus

ABBREVIATIONS

- ELISA = enzyme-linked immunosorbent assay
- FV3 = Frog virus 3
- PCR = polymerase chain reaction
- POTZ = preferred optimal temperature zone

Suggested Reading

Allender MC, Mitchell MA, Torres T, Sekowska J, Driskell EA. Pathogenicity of frog virus 3-like virus in red-eared slider turtles (Trachemys scripta elegans) at two environmental temperatures. *J Comp Pathol* 2013;149:356–367.

Gray MJ, Chinchar VG, eds. *Ranaviruses: Lethal Pathogens of Ectothermic Vertebrates.* Heidelberg: Springer Nature; 2015.

Marschang RE. Virology. In: Divers SJ, Stahl SJ, eds. *Mader's Reptile and Amphibian Medicine and Surgery.* St. Louis, MO: Elsevier; 2019:247–269.

Author Rachel E. Marschang, PD, Dr. med. vet., DECZM (Herpetology), FTÄ Mikrobiologie

ISOSPORA

BASICS

DEFINITION/OVERVIEW

Isospora is a genus of apicomplexan parasites with two sporocysts containing four sporozoites. Isospora is typically an intracytoplasmic parasite, but some species may have intranuclear development.

ETIOLOGY/PATHOPHYSIOLOGY

- *Isospora* spp. have a direct life cycle, with infective stages passed in the feces of the host. Infections are confined to the intestines.
- Most reports of illness associated with *Isospora* infection are from captive animals that have been housed under suboptimal conditions with infection often further complicated by concurrent disease.
- *Isospora* infections are not commonly reported in chelonians.

SIGNALMENT/HISTORY

- High stocking density
- Unsanitary conditions
- Maladaptation of wild animals entering captivity.

CLINICAL PRESENTATION

None reported, but may be related to gastrointestinal upset.

RISK FACTORS

Husbandry

- Breeding colonies at high stocking density are at greatest risk.
- Poor hygiene and stress are likely to predispose to infection and disease.

Others

Concurrent disease or excessive stress may cause immunosuppression, thus increasing risks of disease expression.

DIAGNOSIS

DIFFERENTIAL DIAGNOSIS

Other gastrointestinal disease such as bacterial or protozoal infections (i.e., *Eimeria*).

DIAGNOSTICS

- Examination of feces for presence of oocysts using light microscopy.
- Molecular techniques such as PCR may aid in species delineation but are unlikely to improve treatment efficacy or prognosis.
- Protozoa may also be seen in biopsy or necropsy samples.
- Fecal samples should be stored in 2–3% of aqueous (w/v) $K_2Cr_2O_7$.

PATHOLOGICAL FINDINGS

- Gross lesions may be mild and unapparent in many cases.
- Histologically, there may be small intestinal villous atrophy with intracytoplasmic coccidia within enterocytes.

TREATMENT

APPROPRIATE HEALTH CARE

N/A

NUTRITIONAL SUPPORT

- Ensure that animals are well hydrated, especially if medicating with sulfa drugs.
- In cases of anorectic animals, force-feeding with easily digestible proteins should be initiated.
- Direct feeding by stomach tubing can be performed in some species.
- Placement of an esophagostomy tube should be considered for chronic management.
- Supportive fluid therapy should be provided.

CLIENT EDUCATION/HUSBANDRY RECOMMENDATIONS

- Remove and isolate sick individuals and reduce stress by providing optimal living conditions and hygiene.
- Thorough cleaning of cage to reduce environmental contamination of oocysts.
- Ensure that quarantine protocols have been adopted for all new arrivals.
- During quarantine, all animals should be subjected to repeated clinical and fecal examinations.
- Keep stocking densities as low as possible, especially in stressful conditions such as breeding colonies.

MEDICATIONS

DRUG(S) OF CHOICE

- Ponazuril 30 mg/kg PO q48h for 2 treatments, or 30 mg/kg PO q24h for 4 treatments, then repeat for 2–4 treatments 2 weeks apart.
- Toltrazuril 15 mg/kg PO q48h for 30 days.
- Sulfadimethoxine 50 mg/kg q24h for 21 days.
- Trimethoprim-sulfa 30 mg/kg daily for 5 days, then q48h until the coccidia are eliminated.
- Prophylactic therapy or treatment based on the identification of *Eimeria* spp. alone should not be performed, to avoid development of resistance. Treatment should only be performed after an *Isospora* sp. has been confirmed to be causing clinical disease.

PRECAUTIONS/INTERACTIONS

Sulfa drugs are known to be nephrotoxic.

FOLLOW-UP

PATIENT MONITORING

Repeat fecal examination at monthly intervals.

EXPECTED COURSE AND PROGNOSIS

- Treatment may have variable efficacy as many protozoa are resistant to a range of anti-coccidial medication.
- Prognosis is good to guarded and is determined primarily by the state of the animal at initial presentation and the presence or absence of concurrent disease.

MISCELLANEOUS

COMMENTS

N/A

ZOONOTIC POTENTIAL

N/A

SYNONYMS

N/A

ABBREVIATIONS

- $K_2Cr_2O_7$ = potassium dichromate
- PCR = polymerase chain reaction
- PO = per os

Suggested Reading

Gibbons PM. Advances in reptile clinical therapeutics. *J Exot Pet Med* 2014;23(1):21–38.

Jacobson ER. Parasites and Parasitic Diseases of Reptiles. In: Jacobson ER, ed. *Infectious Diseases and Pathology of Reptiles: Color Atlas and Text.* Boca Raton, FL: CRC Press; 2007:571–665.

Kim DY, Mitchell MA, Bauer RW, et al. An outbreak of adenoviral infection in inland bearded dragons (*Pogona vitticeps*) coinfected with *Dependovirus* and coccidial protozoa (*Isospora* sp.). *J Vet Diagn Invest* 2002;14:332–334.

Scullion FT, Scullion MG. Gastrointestinal protozoal diseases in reptiles. *J Exot Pet Med* 2009;18(4):266–278.

Walden M, Mitchell MA. Evaluation of three treatment modalities against *Isospora amphiboluri* in inland bearded dragons (*Pogona vitticeps*). *J Exot Pet Med* 2012;21(3):213–218.

Wolf D, Vrhovec MG, Failing K, et al. Diagnosis of gastrointestinal parasites in reptiles: comparison of two coprological methods. *Acta Vet Scand* 2014;56:1–13.

Author T. Franciscus Scheelings, BVSc, MVSc, PhD, MANCVSc (Wildlife Health), DECZM (Herpetology)

LEUKEMIA

BASICS

DEFINITION/OVERVIEW

Leukemia is a neoplasia of the white blood cells, which starts in the bone marrow.

ETIOLOGY/PATHOPHYSIOLOGY

- No confirmed etiology has been proved for any of the leukemia cases described in chelonians, including viral etiology.
- Leukemias are classified as myeloid or lymphoid, depending upon the neoplastic blood cell.
- It is generally accepted, based on previously reported cytochemical staining characteristics, that reptilian granulocytes, monocytes, and azurophils are from the myeloid cell lineage, whereas reptilian lymphocytes are from the lymphoid cell lineage.
- Leukemias are commonly graded as acute or chronic depending on the number of blast cells in peripheral circulation.
- Blast cells predominate in acute leukemia, whereas mature forms predominate in chronic onset leukemia, with less than 30% of the peripheral leukocytes being blast cells.
- Acute leukemias are rapidly fatal in untreated patients.

SIGNALMENT/HISTORY

Leukemia in chelonians has been reported in both adult and immature turtles.

CLINICAL PRESENTATION

- Anorexia and lethargy are frequently reported.
- Weight loss is common in chronic leukemia.

RISK FACTORS

Husbandry

N/A

Others

N/A

DIAGNOSIS

DIFFERENTIAL DIAGNOSIS

- Multiple myeloma or plasma cell myeloma.
- Monoclonal gammopathy

DIAGNOSTICS

- Hemogram: a marked leukocytosis characterized by lymphocytosis/monocytosis (depending upon the type of leukemia) can be observed.
- Cytological evaluation of blood smears and/or bone marrow biopsy (because of the extensive bony trabecular network, conventional bone marrow aspirates in chelonians have low cell yield; bone marrow may be collected from the gular projection of the plastron or the bridge of the plastron and carapace) (Silverstone et al, 2007).
- Necropsy and subsequent histopathology
- Cytochemical and immunocytochemical stains to confirm cell lineage.
- Cytochemical staining can include α-naphthyl butyrate esterase, chloroacetate esterase, Sudan black B, and alkaline phosphatase to distinguish myeloid or lymphoid origin; it is important to study comparison samples from both clinically healthy and affected animals of the same species because of the paucity of cytochemical characterization of blood cells for most reptiles. CD3 antibody identifies T-cell lymphocytes and Pax-5 and BLA36 antibodies identify B-cell lymphocytes (Silverstone et al, 2007; Bezjian et al, 2013). L1-calprotectin antibody has been used to identify myeloid cells in lizards.
- Transmission electron microscopy can be attempted to determine histogenesis and to identify viral particles.

PATHOLOGICAL FINDINGS

- Cytological evaluation of blood smears and/or bone marrow aspirates can reveal abnormal cell morphology of the neoplastic cells, abnormal nuclear to cytoplasm ratio, and anisokaryosis; mitotic figures are frequently detected.
- Histopathologic examination of tissue samples can reveal infiltration of neoplastic cells in several organs and occasional mitotic figures.

TREATMENT

APPROPRIATE HEALTH CARE

N/A

NUTRITIONAL SUPPORT

An esophagostomy tube should be considered in anorexic animals or for long-term administration of medications.

CLIENT EDUCATION/HUSBANDRY RECOMMENDATIONS

An early diagnosis can maximize the success of therapy.

MEDICATIONS

DRUG(S) OF CHOICE

- Silverstone et al (2007) treated a diamondback terrapin (*Malaclemys terrapin*) suffering from lymphoblastic leukemia with prednisone 0.6 mg/kg PO q48h, cytosine arabinoside 6 mg/kg SQ q7d for two treatments, and chlorambucil 1 mg/kg PO q7d for two treatments; at 24 days post-treatment, the WBC count and the turtle's activity had improved, but it died 46 days after the beginning of treatment.
- Cytosine arabinoside is the most frequently used treatment for small mammals with chronic monocytic leukemia, whereas prednisone therapy is widely used and accepted for small mammals with lymphoid leukemia and lymphoma; it is not effective for myeloid leukemias.

PRECAUTIONS/INTERACTIONS

Suspected cytosine arabinoside toxicity characterized by renal failure has been reported in a rhinoceros viper.

FOLLOW-UP

PATIENT MONITORING

Complete blood count must be done for monitoring the overall WBC count and different leukocyte counts to gauge response to the drugs.

EXPECTED COURSE AND PROGNOSIS

The prognosis of the disease, especially in acute leukemia, is poor.

MISCELLANEOUS

COMMENTS

N/A

ZOONOTIC POTENTIAL

N/A

SYNONYMS

N/A

ABBREVIATIONS

- PO = per os
- SC = subcutaneous
- WBC = white blood cells

Suggested Reading

Bezjian M, Diep AN, de Matos R, Schaefer D. Chinese box turtle (*Cuora flavomarginata*) with lymphoid leukemia characterized by immunohistochemical and cytochemical phenotyping. *Vet Clin Path* 2013;42:368–376.

Mauldin GN, Done LB2. Oncology. In: Mader DR, ed. *Reptile Medicine and Surgery*. 2nd ed. St. Louis, MO: Elsevier Saunders; 2006:299–322.

Silverstone AM, Garner MM, Wojcieszyn JW, et al. Acute lymphoblastic leukemia in a diamondback terrapin. *J Herp Med Surg* 2007;17:92–99.

Author Jorge Orós, DVM, PhD, DECZM

LOWER RESPIRATORY TRACT DISEASES

BASICS

DEFINITION/OVERVIEW

- Diseases of the respiratory tract are common and are often responsible for considerable morbidity and mortality in chelonians.
- Turtles and tortoises can be equally affected but possible etiologies and pathogens vary significantly.
- Tracheitis, glossitis, laryngitis and various types of pneumonia can have different causes in freshwater turtles, sea turtles, and tortoises.
- LRTD often occur concurrently with disease of the upper respiratory tract.
- In chelonians, the LRT consists of the glottis, larynx, trachea, paired bronchi, and paired, multichambered lungs.
- The trachea, bronchi, and lungs are covered by a ciliated glandular epithelium. In tortoises, the trachea divides relatively cranially into paired bronchi.
- The left and right lungs of chelonians are located in the dorsal coelom, and adhere dorsally to the dorsal peritoneum. Ventrally, they are attached to the septum horizontale or "pseudodiaphragm," which separates them from the coelomic viscera.
- In principle, expansion of the lung is almost equal on the left and right side, but is strongly correlated to the dimensions of the coelomic organs.
- Symptoms of LRTD in chelonians include obstructed external nares, nasal and ocular discharge or conjunctivitis, stridor or wheezing and dyspnea, mouth-breathing and increased front limb-motion (to assist breathing) as well as forced or open-mouth breathing in cases of major disease.
- Symptoms of lower respiratory tract diseases in turtles include additional symptoms such as bubbling noises especially when surfacing, increased time spent on land as well as buoyancy disorders in severe cases.

ETIOLOGY/PATHOPHYSIOLOGY

There is a wide range of etiologies associated with LRTD but infectious causes are some of the most common. LRTD may also be secondary to other diseases such as stomatitis.

Infectious

- Bacteria: mycobacteria; chlamydia; Gram-negatives such as *Pseudomonas* spp., *Morganella morganii*, *Acinetobacter* spp., *Serratia marcescens*, *Pasteurella* spp. In tortoises, *Mycoplasma agassizii* and *Mycoplasma testudineum* occasionally cause pneumonia in addition to URTD.
- Fungi: (*Sporotrichium* spp., *Cladosporium* spp., and *Paecilomyces* spp. in sea turtles; *Candida* spp. in tortoises).
- Parasites: (e.g., *Pentastomida* spp. and trematodes in turtles, *Spirorchida* spp. in sea turtles).
- Viral infection: (herpesvirus, ranavirus, reovirus, ferlavirus) sometimes in combination of mycoplasma.

Non-Infectious

- Tumors (pulmonary fibromas in sea turtles)
- Foreign bodies within the oral cavity, trachea, bronchus or lung.
- Drowning of tortoises (poorly secured pools or garden ponds)
- Inhalation of smoke, aerosols or other toxic compounds.
- Physical trauma/injuries
- Improper husbandry

SIGNALMENT/HISTORY

No age, sex or species predisposition.

CLINICAL PRESENTATION

- Depending on the underlying cause and chelonian species. Signs of LRTD in chelonians can include:
  - Nonspecific signs such as anorexia, lethargy, inactivity.
  - Dyspnea and/or tachypnea
  - Marked respiratory distress
  - Stridor, forced or open-mouth breathing, and increased front limb-motion (in association with breathing) in severe disease.
  - Sometimes nasal and ocular discharge and obstructed external nares.
  - Sneezing
  - Salivation
  - Stridor or wheezing
  - Cyanotic mucous membranes (especially in the oral cavity) in severe cases.
- In turtles:
  - Bubbling noises especially when surfacing.
  - Increased time spent on land.
  - Buoyancy disorders (including asymmetrical swimming in cases of unilateral pneumonia of the affected side and inability to dive).

RISK FACTORS

Husbandry

- Inadequate husbandry
- Stressors, such as overcrowding
- Poor hygiene
- Exposure to ill animals
- In some cases, brumation may predispose to recurrence of clinical signs due to immunosuppressed state.
- Inappropriate temperatures and humidity; sudden changes in temperature or humidity.
- Stagnant water
- Improper diet (including starvation) and endoparasitism.
- Substrate with irritating compounds (e.g., cedar shavings)
- Poor ventilation

Others

- Immunosuppression, which may be caused by stress.
- Relocation
- Concurrent disease

DIAGNOSIS

DIFFERENTIAL DIAGNOSIS

- Infectious diseases (bacterial, viral, fungal, parasitic)
- Trauma
- Neoplasia
- Foreign bodies
- Inhalation of irritating substances
- In cases with unilateral disease, noninfectious causes are more likely.
- When bilateral disease occurs, infectious diseases, smoke toxicity, and drowning are more likely.

DIAGNOSTICS

- Physical examination, including thorough exam of the oral cavity and choana. The use of magnification may aid in identifying subtle lesions.
- Bacterial culture and sensitivity (aerobic and anaerobic) and/or fungal culture. Tracheal or lung lavage are more difficult to perform in chelonians due to lung anatomy. Yield of fluid is not as large as with other reptiles and there is a higher risk of fluid retention in the lungs; extreme caution must be used.
- In mycoplasma is suspected: PCR of nasal flush and tracheal or lung lavage and mycoplasma-specific ELISA for detection of antibodies in plasma samples (serology).
- Cytology of oral mucus and tracheal or lung lavage.
- Diagnostic imaging (radiography, CT, MRI).
- Endoscopy, including nasal lavage and biopsy for further diagnostics such as cytology, histopathology, virology, and electron microscopy.
- Biopsy, cytology, and histopathology of the affected lung(s) may be beneficial in refractory cases.
- In cases of virus infections: virus isolation and/or PCR using tracheal or lung lavage, nasal flush or nasal swab, choanal, oral, esophageal swabs, or lung tissue; detection of antibodies in blood samples (serology).
- In case of suspected mycobacteria: immunohistochemistry and PCR.
- Fecal exam

PATHOLOGICAL FINDINGS

- Pathologic findings will vary according to the underlying cause and may range from mild to severe.
- In cases of mycoplasmosis in tortoises, the URT, especially the nasal cavity, is typically affected, but involvement of the LRT, including severe tracheitis and pneumonia, is possible in some cases.
- In cases of chronic bacterial pneumonia in box turtles, chronic, active inflammation with pseudomembrane formation in nasal sinuses and lungs and granuloma-like structures may be observed.
- Lungs may be expanded and turgid and can contain yellow mucoid exudate.
- Severe tracheitis and multifocal necrotizing pneumonia has been reported in ranavirus infection in a gopher tortoise.
- A smear from a lung lavage demonstrated numerous spherical yeast bodies and inflammatory cells in a Greek tortoise with pulmonary candidiasis.

TREATMENT

APPROPRIATE HEALTH CARE

N/A

NUTRITIONAL SUPPORT

- Force-feeding with easily digestible proteins.
- Direct feeding by stomach tubing can be performed in some species, however placement of an esophagostomy tube should be considered for chronic management.
- Fluid therapy at a fluid rate of 10–30 ml/kg/day as supportive care.

CLIENT EDUCATION/HUSBANDRY RECOMMENDATIONS

- Correct any husbandry deficiencies with special attention to temperature, humidity, and ventilation.
- Isolate animal from others in collection, especially when viral etiology is suspected.
- It is important to ensure a full course of treatment to avoid recurrence of disease.

MEDICATIONS

DRUG(S) OF CHOICE

Depending on the underlying cause and the affected chelonian species:

- Bacteria: systemic or nebulized antibiotics (enrofloxacin, cephalosporin, oxytetracycline, amikacin, doxycycline, ceftazidime, tylosin, trimethoprim/sulfadiazine), preferably according to sensitivity panel for at least 4–6 weeks. Local instillation of antibiotics (injectable or ophthalmic solutions) in the nasal passage may also be effective.
- Fungi: systemic, local, nebulized antifungals (e.g., terbinafine, voriconazole, amphotericin B).
- Nebulization with acetylcysteine for the elimination of exudates in severe cases.
- Confirmed mycobacterial infection: no treatment—euthanasia.
- Mycoplasmosis in tortoises:
  - In wild tortoises: isolation, no release because persistent risk of infection and deadly threat to wild populations.
  - In captive tortoises: fluoroquinolones and tetracycline are most effective; combining parenteral and nebulization of these two class of drugs may be beneficial.
  - Nasal flushing with physiologic saline solution (first once daily, then every third day).
- If secondary invading bacteria (e.g., *Pasteurella testudinis* and *Bortedella bronchiseptica*) antibiotics according to sensitivity panel.
- Herpes, ranavirus, reovirus, or ferlavirus (sometimes coinfection with *Mycoplasma* sp.): intensive symptomatic and supportive therapy; antiviral therapy effectiveness is not well documented. Euthanasia is often required, depending on the state of the animal.
- In cases of drowning of tortoises: diuretics and antibiotics (preferably according to resistogram).
- Oxygen cage therapy in severe cases.
- In cases of neoplasia, surgical removal, if feasible, followed by radiation or chemotherapy.
- Systemic use of itraconazole may cause severe adverse effects in some chelonians.
- Fluid therapy at a fluid rate of 10–30 ml/kg/day as supportive care.

PRECAUTIONS/INTERACTIONS

- Enrofloxacin is a fluoroquinolone with primary renal excretion; thus, adequate rehydration and regular monitoring of renal values are recommended if this antibiotic is chosen for treatment.

FOLLOW-UP

PATIENT MONITORING

- Improvement of clinical signs should be expected within 1–2 weeks for bacterial and fungal infections when definitive diagnosis and treatment are employed.
- It is critical to continue treatment until clinical signs are fully resolved and repeating cultures to confirm resolution of infection if unsure.
- In cases that do not show any improvement or worsen during the first 1–2 weeks of treatment, it should be considered that the etiology and/or treatment are not accurate.
- Viral infections should also be considered in cases that do not respond to therapy or have chronic, intermittent recurrence of disease.
- Repeat diagnostics may be needed to assess resolution or progression of disease.
- Treatment for mycoplasmosis may be longer than for other bacteria and animals may become subclinical carriers.
- Continued monitoring by PCR and serology may help to determine shedding and antibody status of the animal over time to may help in making management decisions.

EXPECTED COURSE AND PROGNOSIS

- Course and prognosis depend on the causative agent (see above).
- Bacterial: good prognosis depending on response to antibiotics.
- In case of mycoplasmosis:
  - No current standard therapy available to eliminate the pathogen.
  - Subclinically and clinically affected tortoises stay potentially infectious (all tortoise species should be considered as potentially susceptible).
  - In wild tortoises: no release due to persistent risk of infection and deadly threat to wild populations.
  - In captive tortoises: isolate. URTD may be triggered by certain factors and can lead to a fresh outbreak of the disease with possible fatal outcome at any time.
- Fungal: guarded to poor prognosis
- Viral (sometimes coinfection with mycoplasma): guarded to grave prognosis depending on the virus and host species.
- Neoplastic: poor to grave prognosis
- Drowning of tortoises: prognosis highly case dependent.
- Smoke toxicity: usually poor prognosis
- Others: depend on severity and involvement of other tissues.

MISCELLANEOUS

COMMENTS

N/A

ZOONOTIC POTENTIAL

Depending on the causative agent, mycobacteria, salmonella, pentastomids (rare), and other etiologies have zoonotic potential.

SYNONYMS

Pneumonia

LOWER RESPIRATORY TRACT DISEASES (CONTINUED)

ABBREVIATIONS

- CT = computed tomography
- ELISA = enzyme-linked immunosorbent assay
- LRT = lower respiratory tract
- LRTD = lower respiratory tract diseases
- MRI = magnetic resonance imaging
- PCR = polymerase chain reaction
- URT = upper respiratory tract diseases

Suggested Reading

Evans RH. Chronic bacterial pneumonia in free-ranging Eastern box turtles (*Terrapene carolina carolina*). *J Wildl Dis* 1983;19(4):349–352.

Fowler MF. Respiratory disease in reptiles. In: Kirk RW, ed. *Current Veterinary Therapy VII. Small Animal Practice*. 7th ed. Philadelphia, PA: WB Saunders; 1980:633–637.

Hernandez-Divers SJ. Pulmonary candidiasis caused by *Candida albicans* in a Greek tortoise (*Testudo graeca*) and treatment with intrapulmonary amphotericin B. *J Zoo Wildl Med* 2001;32(3):352–359.

Jacobson E. Diseases of the respiratory system in reptiles. *Vet Med Small Anim Clin* 1978;73(9):1169–1175.

Jacobson ER, Brown MB, Wendland LD, et al. Mycoplasmosis and upper respiratory tract disease of tortoises: A review and update. *Vet J* 2014;201(3):257–264.

Jacobson ER, Gaskin JM, Roelke M, et al. Conjunctivitis, tracheitis, and pneumonia associated with herpesvirus infection in green sea turtles. *J Am Vet Med Assoc* 1986;189(9):1020–1023.

Jacobson ER, Gaskin JM, Shields RP, White FH. Mycotic pneumonia in mariculture-reared green sea turtles. *J Am Vet Med Assoc* 1979;175(9):929–933.

Junge RE, Miller RE. Reptile respiratory diseases. In: Kirk RW, Bonagura JD, eds. *Kirk's Current Veterinary Therapy XI. Small Animal Practice*. 11th ed. Philadelphia, PA: WB Saunders; 1992:1204–1210.

Origgi FC, Jacobson ER. Diseases of the respiratory tract of chelonians. *Vet Clin North Am Exot Anim Pract* 2000;3(2):537–549.

Vanrompay D, De Meurichy W, Ducatelle R, Haesebrouck F. Pneumonia in Moorish tortoises (*Testudo graeca*) associated with avian serovar A *Chlamydia psittaci*. *Vet Rec* 1994;135(12):284–285.

Author Karina A. Mathes, DVM, Dr. med. vet., DECZM (Herpetology), European Veterinary Specialist in Zoological Medicine (Herpetology), Certified Specialist in Reptiles (Fachtieraerztin fuer Reptilien), Certified Specialist in Reptiles and Amphibians (ZB Reptilien und Amphibien)

LYMPHOMA

BASICS

DEFINITION/OVERVIEW

Lymphoma is a lymphoid neoplasia which originates in the lymphocyte cells.

ETIOLOGY/PATHOPHYSIOLOGY

- No viral etiology has been identified in most cases of lymphoid neoplasia in reptiles, including the scarce cases reported in chelonians. Most cases reported in chelonians have a multicentric distribution.
- There is insufficient information about lymphoma in reptiles to be able to meaningfully stage this entity.
- In some of the reptile lymphomas, immunohistochemistry has been attempted to determine the cellular origin, but no correlation to the biological behavior of the tumor has been made.

SIGNALMENT/HISTORY

Cases of lymphoma/lymphosarcoma have been reported in several tortoise (*Testudo hermanni*, *Chelonoidis nigra*, *Geochelone platynota*), and turtle species (*Trionyx ferox*, *Caretta caretta*).

CLINICAL PRESENTATION

- Anorexia and lethargy are frequently reported.
- CBC can reveal marked lymphocytosis.
- Physical examination can reveal single or multiple tumor nodules.

RISK FACTORS

Husbandry

Unknown

Others

Unknown

DIAGNOSIS

DIFFERENTIAL DIAGNOSIS

- Other tumors
- Inflammatory reactions (abscesses, granulomas, etc.)

DIAGNOSTICS

- Hemogram: a marked leukocytosis characterized by lymphocytosis can be observed.
- In advanced stages of the disease, it is unclear whether the neoplasia originated within the bone marrow or whether leukemia is a feature of disseminated, end-stage lymphoma.
- Histological examination of direct smears from a fine-needle aspirate of the nodular masses and/or of the biopsy specimen can reveal the presence of neoplastic lymphoid cells.
- Necropsy and subsequent histopathology
- Transmission electron microscopy can be attempted to identify viral particles.

PATHOLOGICAL FINDINGS

- Gross lesions include white and firm nodules in several organs, not limited to lymphoid organs.
- Splenomegaly is also frequently observed.
- Histologically, monotonous sheets composed of hyperchromatic neoplastic lymphoid cells are observed.
- Mitotic figures are variable

TREATMENT

APPROPRIATE HEALTH CARE

N/A

NUTRITIONAL SUPPORT

Esophagostomy tube should be considered in anorexic animals or for long-term administration of medications.

CLIENT EDUCATION/HUSBANDRY RECOMMENDATIONS

N/A

MEDICATIONS

DRUG(S) OF CHOICE

- No specific treatment protocol has been reported in chelonians.
- See Lymphoma in Section III Lizards for treatment protocol that can be used as a reference point.

PRECAUTIONS/INTERACTIONS

As in lizards, a heterophil count threshold can be used as an indicator of drug toxicity.

FOLLOW-UP

PATIENT MONITORING

As in lizards, it can be adequate to monitor the overall WBC count and lymphocyte count to gauge response to the drugs, together with reduction in tumor size, weight gain, and quality-of-life assessment.

EXPECTED COURSE AND PROGNOSIS

- Because little is known about most chemotherapeutic agents in chelonians, the prognosis of the disease is poor.
- Most cases are diagnosed postmortem.

MISCELLANEOUS

COMMENTS

N/A

ZOONOTIC POTENTIAL

N/A

SYNONYMS

- Lymphoid neoplasm
- Lymphosarcoma

ABBREVIATIONS

- CBC = complete blood count
- WBC = white blood cell

Suggested Reading

Frye FL. Diagnosis and surgical treatment of reptilian neoplasms with a compilation of cases 1966–1993. *In Vivo* 1994;8:885–892.

Harshbarger JC. *Activities Report Registry of Tumors in Lower Animals, 1965–1973.* Washington DC: Smithsonian Institution Press; 1974.

Machotka SV. Neoplasia in reptiles. In: Hoff CL, Frye FL, Jacobson ER, eds. *Diseases of Amphibians and Reptiles.* New York, NY: Plenum Press; 1984:519–580.

Mauldin GN, Done LB. Oncology. In: Mader DR, ed. *Reptile Medicine and Surgery.* 2nd ed. St. Louis, MO: Elsevier Saunders; 2006:299–322.

Orós J, Torrent A, Espinosa de los Monteros A, et al. Multicentric lymphoblastic lymphoma in a loggerhead sea turtle (*Caretta caretta*). *Vet Path* 2001;38:464–467.

Rideout BA, Worley MB, Anderson MP, Jacobson ER. Alimentary tract lymphomas in Galapagos tortoises. *Proc Am Assoc Zoo Vet* 1993;222–223.

Author Jorge Orós, DVM, PhD, DECZM

MYCOBACTERIOSIS

BASICS

DEFINITION/OVERVIEW

Mycobacteriosis is a cosmopolitan disease that affects all classes of vertebrates. Atypical or non-tuberculosis *Mycobacterium* spp. are most common. *Mycobacterium* spp. are more fastidious in ectothermic animals, and thus can appear as latent or chronic infections. While the apparent prevalence of mycobacteriosis in reptiles is low, it is likely underdiagnosed. Systemic and localized infections of *Mycobacterium* spp. have been documented in chelonians. Infections are more commonly reported in aquatic reptiles.

ETIOLOGY/PATHOPHYSIOLOGY

- Aerobic, acid-fast positive, Gram-positive rod bacteria.
- *Mycobacterium chelonae, M. szulgai, M. marinum, M. fortuitum, M. ulcerans, M. leprae, M. haemophilum, M. avium, M. leparemurium, M kansasii, M. terrae, M. intracellulare, M. genavense, M. kumamotonerse, M. fuscus, M. nonchromogenium, M. smegmatis, M. confluentis, M. hiberniae.*
- The epidemiology of mycobacteriosis in reptiles is not well documented.
- Transmission of *Mycobacterium* spp. in reptiles is most likely through direct and indirect contact with infected animals and materials in the captive environment.
- Infected animals can shed the organisms through various body excretions (e.g., respiratory, skin, gastrointestinal), contaminating the environment and directly exposing conspecifics.
- Non-tuberculosis mycobacterial species are ubiquitous within the environment; thus water, soil, dust, and plants can all serve as sources of exposure.
- Stress likely plays a role in the dissemination of this disease, as animals with compromised immune systems are more susceptible to infection.

SIGNALMENT/HISTORY

- No species, age, or sex predilection.
- Aquatic species more commonly affected than terrestrial species.
- Animals are typically housed under poor husbandry conditions: inappropriate environmental temperature, high organic loads, and poor water quality.

CLINICAL PRESENTATION

- Affected animals may be clinically inapparent carriers or show clinical signs that include emaciation and weight loss with or without anorexia.
- Skin lesions may be present that are draining or nodular.
- Animals with systemic mycobacteriosis may be dyspneic; aquatic chelonians with pneumonia may not be able to submerge (i.e., float at surface).
- Fecal production and consistency may vary in animals with lesions in their gastrointestinal tract.

RISK FACTORS

Husbandry

- Inappropriate husbandry, such as a low environmental temperature, can lead to immunosuppression, making individuals more susceptible to infection.
- An absence of a quarantine program can lead to the introduction of an infected animal to a collection.
- High stocking densities in a production system may lead to an increased risk of exposure in a closed system.
- Mycobacterial infections are more common in aquatic species.
- High organic load and poor water quality likely contribute to the buildup and dissemination of the bacteria in these systems.

Others

- Inappropriate nutrition
- Stress
- Chronic disease
- Captive wild animals—wild caught or imported animals.

DIAGNOSIS

DIFFERENTIAL DIAGNOSIS

- Any chronic disease process
- Sepsis
- Osteomyelitis—long bones/carapace and plastron.
- Cold stunning/stranded sea turtles.
- Osteoarthritis
- Organ dysfunction—liver failure (hepatomegaly, nodular hepatopathy), renal failure, splenomegaly.
- Pulmonary disease—fungal and bacterial pneumonia.
- Infectious—parasitism, viral disease, other bacterial disease.
- Neoplasia
- Malabsorptive gastrointestinal disease
- Disseminated intravascular coagulopathy

DIAGNOSTICS

Polymerase Chain Reaction

- PCR testing for *Mycobacterium* spp. does exist and is a more sensitive test than historical methodologies.
- The most common PCR primer used to diagnose *Mycobacterium* spp. in most laboratories is the 16s ribosomal RNA primer; however, a nested PCR assay targeting a 65 kDA heat shock protein (hsp65) has also been used as a diagnostic tool.
- Sensitives and specificities for these diagnostics have yet to be evaluated in reptiles. Sequencing is important to confirm the species of *Mycobacterium.*

Cytology

- Cytologic examination of skin lesions can be a useful first line diagnostic tool for diagnosing a *Mycobacterium* sp. infection. Cytology can be used to provide direct evidence of chronic inflammation in the lesions and demonstrate the presence of bacteria. Gram stain and acid-fast staining can be used to further characterize the presence of the bacteria, directing the clinician to other more sensitive diagnostics such as PCR and histopathology.
- Tissue biopsy and histopathology are considered the gold standard for diagnosing a *Mycobacterium* sp. infection. In addition to granulomatous lesions being present in the microscopic tissue architecture, acid-fast stains, including Ziehl–Neelsen and Fite's methods, can be used to confirm the presence of acid-fast bacteria within the lesions. The sensitivity of these stains is considered low for *Mycobacterium* spp.

Microbiological Culture

- Microbiological culture has fallen out of favor for clinical samples because of the special media required to culture *Mycobacterium* spp. and the long culture times associated with growing these organisms.
- Speciation can be performed on cultured samples.
- Antibacterial sensitivities can also be performed on cultured *Mycobacterium* spp. if therapy is elected.

Hematology and Biochemistry

- Hematology and biochemistry testing can be used to characterize the physiologic status of the reptile patient.
- A chronic inflammatory leukogram characterized by a heterophilia and monocytosis may be observed.
- Anemia of chronic disease is also common.
- Biochemistry testing typically reveals dehydration (hyperproteinemia, hyperuricemia, hypernatremia, hyperchloremia).
- If the liver is involved, elevated bile acids may be identified.

PATHOLOGICAL FINDINGS

- Gross necropsy findings can range from a single white to gray focal lesion/nodule to multifocal to coalescing white lesions/nodules within any organ system.
- Granulomatous inflammation is the most common histopathological finding in reptile mycobacteriosis cases.
- Granulomas can range from compact nests of macrophages containing intracellular acid-fast bacilli to complex granulomas containing caseated centers.

• Acute mycobacteriosis can have extracellular proliferation of acid-fast organisms with associated caseous necrosis and infiltrative heterophils and macrophages.

TREATMENT

APPROPRIATE HEALTH CARE

N/A

NUTRITIONAL SUPPORT

• If treatment is pursued, nutritional support should be considered.
• Mycobacteriosis in reptiles often leads to weight loss because of the negative energy balance that develops in these patients.
• Placement of an esophagostomy tube is indicated to provide critical care diets and medications.

CLIENT EDUCATION/HUSBANDRY RECOMMENDATIONS

• Disease exposure and dissemination can be limited by quarantine and testing (PCR) new arrivals.
• Implementing husbandry practices that reduce organic loads in both aquatic and terrestrial vivariums is highly recommended.
• Regular water changes can minimize pathogen build up in a closed system.
• Husbandry recommendations should be species specific to minimize stress and the potential for compromising the immune system of a reptile.
• Clients and veterinary staff should follow standard hygiene practices to minimize zoonotic potential.

MEDICATIONS

DRUG(S) OF CHOICE

• No proven or approved treatments exist for mycobacteriosis in reptiles.
• Treatment is controversial because of the lack of clinical data on appropriate therapy, poor response to therapy, and the implications that treating reptiles may have in the increase of multidrug-resistant *Mycobacterium* spp., which may have implications for human health.
• Euthanasia should be considered to mitigate zoonotic potential and further dissemination of the organism within a collection.
• In human medicine, *Mycobacterium* infections are treated based on culture and sensitivity results, with a multidrug treatment protocol including macrolides, aminoglycosides, ethambutol, and/or rifamycins.
• Treatment is long term until there is no evidence of disease for at least 12 months.

PRECAUTIONS/INTERACTIONS

If treatment is elected, owner compliance is critical to minimize the development of multidrug resistance.

FOLLOW-UP

PATIENT MONITORING

• Humane euthanasia is recommended
• If treatment is pursued, regular examinations and blood work (hematology and biochemistry testing) should be done to evaluate the patient's quality of life and physiologic status.

EXPECTED COURSE AND PROGNOSIS

• Reptiles diagnosed with *Mycobacterium* spp. have a grave prognosis.
• The likelihood for mycobacterial transmission to other reptiles and the zoonotic potential of these organisms present a challenge.
• Therapeutic options, if pursued, are long term and are not commonly reported to be successful in reptiles.
• Animals that do not undergo therapy often develop disseminated mycobacteriosis, which includes chronic weight loss, cachexia, and emaciation. Because of these challenges, euthanasia is recommended.

MISCELLANEOUS

COMMENTS

N/A

ZOONOTIC POTENTIAL

• *Mycobacterium* spp. can be zoonotic
• Atypical mycobacteria are most commonly isolated from reptiles and, while not the most common forms found in humans, they are known to infect humans.
• Atypical *Mycobacterium* spp. are classified as Runyon group IV and are characterized as antibiotic resistant.
• Preventive measures that should be followed to reduce the zoonotic potential of these organisms include minimizing direct contact with infected animals, wearing appropriate personal protective equipment (e.g., gloves, face mask) when handling infected animals, and following strict personal hygiene practices such as hand washing and not using human washbasins to clean these animals or materials from their environment.
• Immunocompromised individuals and children should avoid contact with infected animals and their environment.

SYNONYMS

• Atypical mycobacterium
• Granulomatous disease
• Vivarium granuloma

ABBREVIATIONS

PCR = polymerase chain reaction

Suggested Reading

Ebani VV, Fratini F, Bertelloni F, et al. Isolation and identification of mycobacteria from captive reptiles. *Res Vet Sci* 2012;93:1136–1138.

Jacobson ER. Bacterial diseases of reptiles. In: Jacobson ER, ed. *Infectious Diseases and Pathology of Reptiles: Color Atlas and Text.* Boca Raton, FL: CRC Press; 2007:461–526.

Mitchell MA. Mycobacterial infections in reptiles. *Vet Clin North Am Exot Anim Pract* 2012;15(1):101–111.

Author Sean M. Perry, DVM, PhD, and Mark A. Mitchell, DVM, MS, PhD, DECZM (Herpetology)

MYCOPLASMOSIS

BASICS

DEFINITION/OVERVIEW

Mycoplasma is the smallest bacterium identified to date. It lacks a cell wall, which makes it resistant to antibiotics targeting the cell wall (e.g., beta-lactams). Mycoplasmosis is most commonly reported in chelonians, causing primarily URTD that rarely progresses into pneumonia. In wild populations, initial mortality is high, and morbidity remains high in surviving animals. Mycoplasmosis is widespread in *Gopherus agassizii* and *G. polyphemus*. It can cause widespread mortality, but is not found in wild *G. berlanderi*. In captivity, mycoplasmosis has a low mortality with high morbidity. The severity of the clinical signs leads to appetite suppression, which causes a slow chronic progressive decline in overall health.

ETIOLOGY/PATHOPHYSIOLOGY

- Several *Mycoplasma* species are implicated, including *Mycoplasma agassizii*, *M. testudineum* and unidentified *Mycoplasma*, but not *M. testudinis*.
- *Mycoplasma* is spread directly via nasal exudates, horizontally, by nose to nose contacts, through courtship, mating or male agnostic behavior.
- Vertical transmission has not been documented.
- *Mycoplasma* spp. do not survive well in the environment, as they lack cell walls.
- *Mycoplasma* attaches to the surface of epithelial cells in the nasal sinus and choana, which causes an overexuberant host immune response.
- The nasal mucosa suffers from loss of ciliated epithelium, mucosal hyperplasia, and infiltration of lymphocytes and histiocytes.
- Normal olfactory mucosa becomes replaced with proliferating mucosal epithelial cells and proliferating basal cells, heterophils, and histiocytes.
- Infected areas slough large amounts of epithelial and inflammatory cells, which create the nasal discharge and, can over time, form caseous material filling and occluding the nasal sinus.
- Clinical impression is that most tortoises do not eat well because they use olfaction to find and select food and mycoplasmosis decreases olfaction.

SIGNALMENT/HISTORY

- More commonly diagnosed in tortoises of the genus *Gopherus* or other species housed with *Gopherus* spp., all tortoise species thought to be susceptible.
- Clinical signs may appear within 1–2 weeks of exposure, or may break out under adverse environmental conditions.

CLINICAL PRESENTATION

- Clinical signs include clear serous to tenacious mucoid bubbling to mucopurulent nasal discharge, sometimes also from the eyes, with mild conjunctivitis and palpebral edema.
- Infected tortoises are often inappetent, lethargic, with clear nasal discharge, bubbling from the nares or have clogged nares, and have lost weight or feel light.
- Chronic cases can have erosion of the nares and rhamphotheca.
- Hatchlings can have enlargement and distortion of the snout (reminiscent of atrophic rhinitis in swine).
- If nasal discharge is not apparent during clinical examination, pushing the tortoise's head straight back into its shell will often produce nasal discharge.
- Nasal discharge is always abnormal.
- Slight conjunctivitis can be difficult to appreciate clinically.

RISK FACTORS

Husbandry

- Exposure to other tortoises with mycoplasmosis.
- Lack of quarantine
- In the wild, disease incidence is higher in sexually mature adults, especially males, compared with juveniles.
- Adverse environmental conditions, such as brumation, or below normal environmental temperature, may cause latent infections to become clinical.

Others

N/A

DIAGNOSIS

DIFFERENTIAL DIAGNOSIS

- Most symptomatic tortoises the author has tested are positive. Clients often balk at the cost of testing, in which case the author proceeds to treatment without confirmation, provided there are no oral lesions or recent deaths in the collection.
- Other differentials for URTD and nasal discharge include herpes virus, ranavirus, adenovirus, intranuclear coccidiosis, chlamydiosis, reovirus, and paramyxovirus.
- A key difference between mycoplasmosis and these diseases is that tortoises often die quickly after the owner noticing something amiss, which is atypical for mycoplasmosis.
- Colonic foreign-body obstruction, with resulting gastric reflux, oronasal fistulas, and oronasal foreign bodies can also cause nasal discharge.

DIAGNOSTICS

Serology

- Serology is the test of choice for *Mycoplasma* infections.
- There is a statistically significant positive correlation between severity of clinical signs and serum antibody ELISA status.
- An ELISA test has been validated for desert and gopher tortoises by the Mycoplasma Testing Lab, University of Florida.
- The disadvantage of ELISA is that it only detects antibodies, which documents exposure, but not necessarily infection. Nonetheless, this is an important screening test when importing chelonians to a closed collection.

PCR

- Samples obtained by nasal flushing are more sensitive than nasal swabbing.
- A good nasal flush sample is best obtained in sedated or anesthetized animals.
- *Mycoplasma* numbers fall over time due to host response therefore a negative PCR does not necessarily mean that the tortoise is *Mycoplasma* negative, as bacteria may not have been in that sample.

Culture

- Culture is not recommended because it is extremely difficult due to slow growth (4–6 weeks for *M. agassizii*), small colony size (colonies not visible without dissecting microscope), and fastidious culture requirements (lower temperature, special expensive culture media, with serum added).
- Jacobson et al (1994) found that less than one-quarter of infected tortoises cultured positive.

PATHOLOGICAL FINDINGS

- Chronic nasal sinusitis
- Emaciation

TREATMENT

APPROPRIATE HEALTH CARE

- Four major classes of drugs are used to treat *Mycoplasma* including fluoroquinolones, macrolides, tetracyclines, and chloramphenicol. Aminoglycosides are not indicated.
- Antibiotics alone, even long term, do not seem to clear *Mycoplasma*, perhaps because *Mycoplasma* spp. live on the nasal epithelial surface and do not penetrate into tissue.
- The lack of pharmacokinetic data makes proper dosing more challenging.
- A retrospective preliminary study of 10 symptomatic desert tortoises showed promising results in eliminating clinical signs. Jarchow (2004) combined nasal flushing with systemic enrofloxacin and found 8 of 10 desert tortoises remained

asymptomatic while still being monitored, for 11–78 months, and 2 of 10 became symptomatic again, at 12 and 30 months post-treatment.
• Treatment consisted of 5 mg/kg enrofloxacin (100 mg/ml) IM in the brachial muscle q72h (range 48–96 hours) for a total of 3–5 treatments and, in addition, flushing the nasal sinus with a solution of 3.0 mg enrofloxacin (2.27%), 0.12 mg dexamethasone (not DexNaP), and 0.8 ml 0.9% sodium chloride, q72h (range 48–96 hours), also for 3–5 treatments.
• Nasal flushes were applied by placing the unsedated tortoise in dorsal recumbency, opening the mouth and flooding the choanae with the flush solution.
• The mouth was then closed and the solution forced through the nares by applying digital pressure on the intermandibular tissue, pushing the tongue into the choanae.
• The process was then repeated and the tortoise returned to sternal recumbency before again applying pressure to the intermandibular tissue.
• The nasal cavity was flushed repeatedly in this manner until only the flushing solution, with no obvious mucus, was expelled from the nares.
• Treatment was usually one time past resolution of clinical signs; five treatments were typically needed.
• The author has slightly modified the above technique as follows. Tortoises are first sedated, with 20 mg/kg Telazol® (Zoetis Services LLC, Parsippany, NJ) IM, unless small, or cooperative enough, that sedation is not needed. After 15–30 minutes, the sedated tortoise is placed in dorsal recumbency with the head extended downwards, the mouth opened and the glottis packed off with several cotton balls clamped to a hemostat, to prevent aspiration. Each nare is then flushed with 12 cc saline through small gavage needle to force thick mucus, solid cellular debris or foreign bodies out of the choanae and mouth, opening up the nasal sinuses, before slowly instilling the enrofloxacin/steroid/saline solution as above. Nasal sinus flush can be used for PCR testing. After treatment, most patients have improved appetite, activity and no further nasal discharge.

NUTRITIONAL SUPPORT

Esophagostomy tube should be considered in anorexic animals or for long-term administration of medications, most do not need this.

CLIENT EDUCATION/HUSBANDRY RECOMMENDATIONS

• Keep patients between 73 degrees F (low at night) to 86 degrees F (high during day), and improve the diet.
• *Mycoplasma*-positive chelonians, or chelonians with nasal discharge, should be isolated from negative tortoises as the disease is extremely contagious.
• Cages can be rinsed and disinfected with 0.15% sodium hypochlorite and substrates should be replaced.

MEDICATIONS

DRUG(S) OF CHOICE

Parenteral, or nasal topical antibiotics, alone or in combination, are not recommended without nasal flushing because they generally fail to clear infection (see previous section).

PRECAUTIONS/INTERACTIONS

N/A

FOLLOW-UP

PATIENT MONITORING

• Check for nasal discharge after last treatment and continue nasal flushing past resolution of clinical signs.
• Watch for recurrence of clinical signs, especially after the winter or periods of stress.

EXPECTED COURSE AND PROGNOSIS

• Prognosis is grave for wild tortoises. For captive tortoises the prognosis is good if treated as described in treatment. Without treatment captive tortoises typically survive with chronic nasal sinusitis and necrosis, but gradually decline.
• Prognosis may improve for animals that can be treated with both nasal flushing and systemic antibiotic therapy.

MISCELLANEOUS

COMMENTS

Figure 3 – see web image supplementary content for Section II (Chelonians).

ZOONOTIC POTENTIAL

Not thought to be zoonotic

SYNONYMS

• Nasal sinusitis
• Upper respiratory tract disease of tortoises (term used before the discovery of *Mycoplasma* spp. as causative agents; no longer current)

ABBREVIATIONS

• ELISA = enzyme-linked immunosorbent assay
• IM = intramuscular
• PCR = polymerase chain reaction
• PO = per os
• SC = subcutaneous
• URTD = upper respiratory tract disease

Suggested Reading

Brown MA, Schumacher IM, Klein PA, et al. *Mycoplasma agassizii* causes upper respiratory tract disease in the desert tortoise. *Infect Immun* 1994; 62(10):4580–4586.
Jacobson ER, Brown MB, Wendland LD, et al. Mycoplasmosis and upper respiratory tract disease of tortoises: A review and update. *Vet J* 2014;201(3):257–264.
Jacobson ER, Gaskin JM, Brown MB, et al. Chronic upper respiratory tract disease of free-ranging desert tortoises (*Xerobates agassizii*). *J Wildl Dis* 1991;27(3):296–316.
Jarchow J. *Treatment Protocol for Upper Respiratory Tract Disease of Desert Tortoises. Proceedings of the 7th International Symposium Pathology and Medicine of Reptiles and Amphibians*, Berlin, Germany, 2014.
Rettenmund CL, Boyer DM, Orrico WJ, et al. Long-term oral clarithromycin administration in chelonians with subclinical Mycoplasma spp. infection. *J Herpetol Med Surgery* 2017; 27 (1/2): 58–61.

Author Thomas H. Boyer, DVM, DABVP (Reptile and Amphibian Practice)

MYIASIS

BASICS

DEFINITION/OVERVIEW

Myiasis is infection with fly larva (i.e., maggots) from the order Diptera. It primarily affects animals housed in tropical and subtropical areas during warm climates. The fly either deposits the eggs directly into the skin/wound or onto mosquitoes, which then transmit the eggs upon inflicting their bites.

ETIOLOGY/PATHOPHYSIOLOGY

- The cycle of dipterous larva varies with the fly species, environmental temperature and tissues in which it occurs.
- A general cycle consists of the eggs deposited in the skin or wound of an animal. The eggs will hatch within 24 hours and begin burrowing. High temperatures stimulate hatching. Once the first stage larva hatch, it begins burrowing in the skin as a feeding larva that undergoes various molts for approximately 7 days until it develops into a pupa. The pupa emerges as an adult approximately 5 days. The whole cycle takes approximately 10–15 days to complete within the tissues of an animal, but under the right conditions it could take less than a week.

SIGNALMENT/HISTORY

- No sex or age predilection but more commonly diagnosed in terrestrial chelonians housed in warm climates.
- Animas usually present with a history of subcutaneous swellings.
- Common presentation in box turtles (*Terrapene carolina* sp.) in the United States.

CLINICAL PRESENTATION

- Chelonians present with subcutaneous swelling primarily along the neck and skin folds on the proximal aspect of the limbs.
- A 1–3 mm hole can sometimes be observed near the swellings.

RISK FACTORS

Husbandry

- Being housed outdoors in tropical and subtropical climates.
- Poor hygiene with high organic load in the enclosures may attract more flies.

Others

N/A

DIAGNOSIS

- Diagnosis is based on observation of subcutaneous swelling and breathing hole if present.
- Exploration of the swellings will reveal the larva or pupa.

DIFFERENTIAL DIAGNOSIS

Abscess

DIAGNOSTICS

Diagnosis is made based on finding fly larvae or pupa under the skin.

PATHOLOGICAL FINDINGS

- Fly larvae or pupa can be grossly identified upon exploration of the subcutaneous swellings.
- The surrounding tissues are usually healthy and not associated with necrosis.

TREATMENT

APPROPRIATE HEALTH CARE

- The animal must be maintained indoors to prevent additional infestation.
- Treatment relies on manual removal of the maggots and flushing the wound.
- It is critical to remember that usually there will be a large number of maggots and not just a few. The author has removed in excess of 300 from a single animal.

NUTRITIONAL SUPPORT

Usually not required, as mots animals are stable.

CLIENT EDUCATION/HUSBANDRY RECOMMENDATIONS

- It is important to maintain animals in a clean environment, especially during the warmer months of the year.
- Food remnants must be cleaned daily to prevent attracting flies to the enclosure.

SURGICAL CONSIDERATIONS

- The breathing hole can be incised to access the maggots.
- Forceps can be used for mechanical removal.
- Magnification or an endoscope can be used to explore the pocket and ensure that no more remain.
- It may take a few days to remove all maggots as buried larvae continue to molt from deep within the tissues.
- The wound should be cleaned and flushed with povidone iodine solution daily until no more maggots are present.
- Once clean, the wound can be left to heal by secondary intention.
- Antibiotic ointments can be placed within the subcutaneous space if there are concerns about bacterial infection.

MEDICATIONS

DRUG(S) OF CHOICE

- Povidone iodine 1 : 40 dilution. Flush the wound daily until all maggots are removed.
- Nitenpyram: mix a crushed 11.4-mg tablet with 10 ml sterile water. Flush the wound with this solution to kill the maggots or give 1 ml/kg PO once.

PRECAUTIONS/INTERACTIONS

Use of nitenpyram is empirical and in a small number of species so there is no safety data, especially for oral administration. Use with caution.

FOLLOW-UP

PATIENT MONITORING

Re-evaluate within 1–2 weeks to ensure that the skin is healing properly.

EXPECTED COURSE AND PROGNOSIS

- Prognosis is excellent to good.
- Cases of myiasis causing severe disease are rare and likely associated with underlying disease in those animals.

MISCELLANEOUS

COMMENTS

N/A

ZOONOTIC POTENTIAL

Myiasis can also occur in humans but there is low risk of becoming infected directly from working with myiasis in animals since it requires the first instar larva to burrow through the skin.

SYNONYMS

- Blowfly strike
- Fly strike
- Maggots

ABBREVIATIONS

PO = per os

Author Javier G. Nevarez, DVM, PhD, DACZM, DECZM (Herpetology)

NANNIZZIOPSIS MYCOSES

BASICS

DEFINITION/OVERVIEW

A newly recognized, often severe and deep, carapacial dermatomycosis of captive and free-ranging chelonians, which affects almost exclusively semi-aquatic or aquatic species.

ETIOLOGY/PATHOPHYSIOLOGY

A newly identified onygenalean fungus in a novel genus, *Emydomyces testavorans*, related to *Nannizziopsis*.

SIGNALMENT/HISTORY

- Usually adult turtles; up to 10 species are known to be affected.
- The disease can probably infect any aquatic or semi-aquatic chelonian.

CLINICAL PRESENTATION

- Ulcerative and granulomatous dermatitis of the plastron and/or carapace, with malacia and osteomyelitis of underlying bone, and with dermal inclusion cysts.
- May present as flakiness and discoloration of the shell in some species, and may cause dermatitis over the limbs, with swelling and paronychia, in other species.

RISK FACTORS

Husbandry

Poor husbandry and stress are likely contributors but has been reported from animals in zoological collections where husbandry should be optimal.

Others

Unknown

DIAGNOSIS

DIFFERENTIAL DIAGNOSIS

Viral dermatitis and/or bacterial dermatitis and osteomyelitis.

DIAGNOSTICS

- Both histopathology and culture of skin/shell biopsies are essential for definitive diagnosis.
- *Emydomyces testavorans* requires special growth media for culture.
- Correct identification requires molecular tools.

PATHOLOGICAL FINDINGS

- Ulcerative dermatitis, osteomyelitis, and often dermal inclusion cysts that will contain non-pigmented fungal elements.
- Inclusion cysts are highly suggestive of infection with this fungus.

TREATMENT

APPROPRIATE HEALTH CARE

- Topical antifungal lacquers may help with aquatic patients.
- Largely unknown
- Aggressive debridement of lesions and use of broad-spectrum antifungals, systemic and topical is warranted.

NUTRITIONAL SUPPORT

Assist-feeding if needed

CLIENT EDUCATION/HUSBANDRY RECOMMENDATIONS

Quarantine of incoming animals and thorough examination of any shell lesions.

MEDICATIONS

DRUG(S) OF CHOICE

- Unknown
- Based on what is known of other fungi in *Nannizziopsis* spp., triazoles and terbinafine might be effective.

PRECAUTIONS/INTERACTIONS

- Triazole antifungal and terbinafine possibly synergistic.
- Interactions with other drugs possible.

FOLLOW-UP

PATIENT MONITORING

- Monitor appetite and behavior
- Monitor for progression or regression of lesions.
- Bloodwork to monitor liver enzymes while on antifungals.

EXPECTED COURSE AND PROGNOSIS

Typically slowly progresses to fatal disease.

MISCELLANEOUS

COMMENTS

N/A

ZOONOTIC POTENTIAL

Unknown

SYNONYMS

N/A

Suggested Reading

Woodburn DB, Miller AN, Allender MC, et al. Emydomyces testavorans, a new genus and species of onygenalean fungus isolated from shell lesions of freshwater aquatic turtles. *J Clin Microbiol* 2019;57:1–11.

Woodburn D, Naples L, Poll C, et al. *Nannizziopsiacae* spp. infection in aquatic chelonians. *Proc Assoc Rept Amphib Vet* 2014:13.

Author Jean A. Paré, DMV, DVSc, DACZM, DECZM (Zoo Health Management)

NUTRITIONAL SECONDARY HYPERPARATHYROIDISM

BASICS

DEFINITION/OVERVIEW

NSHP is one of the most common disorders in captive reptiles. The disease is characterized by hypocalcemia caused by deficiency of calcium and/or vitamin D in the diet or a lack of UVB light exposure. This results in increased PTH production leading to increased calcium resorption from the bones. Affected reptiles typically present with functional and morphological bone changes, including pathological fractures and/or with tetany, seizure-like activity and muscle tremors.

ETIOLOGY/PATHOPHYSIOLOGY

- The etiology of NSHP is considered multifactorial.
- In herbivorous/omnivorous reptiles, a diet poor in calcium and high in phosphorus is a common cause.
- Low calcium intake in the diet results in low blood calcium concentrations.
- A blood calcium concentration below 2.3 mmol/l triggers the parathyroid glands to produce PTH to raise calcium concentrations.
- PTH stimulates the osteoclastic activity, resulting in different degrees of bone depletion. It also stimulates calcium reabsorption in the kidneys.
- The lack of UVB light exposure from the sun or UVB bulbs is another critical factor in the development of NSHP.
- The active form of vitamin D3 is 1,25-dihydroxycholecalciferol, which is mediated in most species by exposure to UVB light in the range of 280–315 nm.
- 1,25-dihydroxycholecalciferol increases intestinal calcium absorption and renal calcium reabsorption.
- In hibernating chelonians, lack of provision of correct temperatures for hibernation typically leads to excessive growth rates, that associated with inadequate calcium content in the diet triggers the development of NSHP.

SIGNALMENT/HISTORY

- NSHP is the most common nutritional disorder of captive reptiles, especially chelonians.
- It is most commonly observed in herbivorous and omnivorous species.
- Those in life stages experiencing intensive growth are most affected from the chronic form of the disease (i.e., skeletal deformities) due to the increased demand for calcium during this period.
- Those in life stages experiencing high demands of calcium for a short period (e.g., reproductive females), are usually presented with the acute form of the disease (i.e., hypocalcemia and tetany).

CLINICAL PRESENTATION

- Clinical signs vary depending on the severity of the disease.
- In tortoises, initial clinical signs of NSHP include beak overgrowth, scute pyramiding, and softening of the plastron and/or carapace.
- In more advanced cases, signs may include difficulty walking, non-weight bearing, anorexia and lethargy.
- Blood effusions under plastral scutes may also be observed.

RISK FACTORS

Husbandry

Diets that lead to NSHP generally present a combination of the following:

- Insufficient calcium intake
- Excessive phosphorus intake
- Insufficient vitamin D intake
- Excessive vitamin A intake

Husbandry errors that lead to NSHP include

- Insufficient exposure to UVB radiation in the range of 280–315 nm.
- Lack of hibernation in hibernating species, which results in excessive growth rates.

Others

Concurrent parasitism may exacerbate NSHP.

DIAGNOSIS

DIFFERENTIAL DIAGNOSIS

- Renal secondary hyperparathyroidism
- Primary hyperparathyroidism

DIAGNOSTICS

- In most cases, NSHP is diagnosed based on clinical presentation and history of inappropriate diet and/or management.
- Radiographs, blood work and fecal exams are indicated to confirm the clinical suspicion, determine the severity of the disease, and formulate a prognosis.
- These diagnostic tests are also useful to rule out concomitant conditions like urinary bladder overdistension, egg dystocia, endoparasitism, and constipation.

Radiography

- Decreased bony cortices and pathologic fractures may be observed.
- Depending on the duration of the disease, long-bone deformities may be observed.
- Animals with multiple fractures and decreased cortices across the majority of the long bones tend to have a worse prognosis for recovery.

Biochemistry

- Hypocalcemia is usually observed in the early and late stages of the disease; it is common for animals with NSHP to be normocalcemic or even hypercalcemic owing to the active resorption of calcium from the bones.
- Hyperphosphatemia may be observed concurrently, especially when hypocalcemia is present.
- A chemistry panel is particularly indicated in reptiles presenting with seizure-like activity or muscle tremors. It is also useful for monitoring response to therapy.
- Analysis should include measurement of ionized calcium. In general, values of ionized calcium lower than 1.0–1.2 mmol/l are abnormal.
- The calcium to phosphorus ratio is expected to be 1 : 5 to 2 : 1, and a decrease is suggestive of calcium depletion (e.g., NSHP, renal secondary hyperparathyroidism or renal disease).

Fecal Exams

Endoparasites may be a confounding factor in the development of this disease as they can contribute to depletion of nutrients.

PATHOLOGICAL FINDINGS

- Gross pathological findings include deformity and softening of bone tissue, including carapace and the plastron.
- Alterations of parathyroid glands may be present in form of generalized or focal enlargements.
- Histopathological lesions may range from increased osteoclastic resorption of otherwise well-formed and mineralized bone laminae to thinning of laminae and widening of medullary cavities, with scalloped endosteal surfaces due to massive resorptive activity.
- The cortices may be thinned and layers of osteoblasts and unmineralized osteoid on the periosteal surface may be present.

TREATMENT

APPROPRIATE HEALTH CARE

N/A

NUTRITIONAL SUPPORT

- Reptiles with chronic NSHP are often anorectic.
- The anorexia is usually transient and improves once the management is corrected.
- Reptiles with severe NSHP may not be able to ingest food due to the changes in the mandibular bones or concurrent diseases. In such cases, placement of an esophagostomy tube is indicated.

CLIENT EDUCATION/HUSBANDRY RECOMMENDATIONS

- NSHP is caused by improper husbandry and diet.
- Despite the efforts made to educate owners on adequate husbandry practices, NSHP is still one of the most common disorders of captive reptiles.
- Husbandry issues to consider in order to prevent NSHP are: provision of unfiltered sunlight (or as an alternative UVB through a UVB-emitting lamp), and provision of an environment adequate for brumation in brumating species.
- Dietary issues to consider to prevent NSHP are: provision of a diet that is naturally high in calcium and is low in phosphorus, and has the proper quantity of vitamins, especially vitamins A and D.

MEDICATIONS

DRUG(S) OF CHOICE

- In reptiles presented with acute hypocalcemic crisis, calcium should be administered intravenously, or intramuscularly when an intravenous line is not available.
- There is no dosage of calcium that has been evaluated for effectiveness and safety in reptiles.
- In reptiles presented with chronic NSHP, the mainstay of the therapy is an improvement in husbandry and diet.
- Fluid administration is also required, as reptiles presenting with this condition are usually severely dehydrated.
- Exposure to unfiltered sunlight is preferred over artificial UVB lights.
- When sunlight exposure is not possible or ideal (e.g., wintertime), proper selection and use of UVB lights is necessary.
- This can then be followed by oral supplementation once the animal is stabilized.
- Monitoring of calcium, heart activity through an ECG and other electrolytes is highly suggested during seizure-like crisis.
- A gradual change to a diet that contains the appropriate levels of calcium, vitamin D, and fibers, with low level of phosphorus is also required.
- Administration of oral calcium may assist in the recovery, but it must not be used as a standalone therapy.
- Calcium supplements containing vitamin D should be carefully dosed to avoid hypervitaminosis D.
- Calcium gluconate 50–100 mg/kg SC, IM, IV q6–24h
- Calcium glubionate 50–360 mg/kg PO q12–24h

PRECAUTIONS/INTERACTIONS

- It is presumed that, as in other vertebrates, parenteral calcium administration may provoke cardiac arrhythmias.
- Administration of exogenous vitamin D3 may result in excessive concentrations, resulting in intoxication and metastatic calcification of tissues.
- The only cases where exogenous vitamin D3 should be administered is when renal and/or hepatic functions are impaired, and endogenous vitamin D3 cannot be produced. In all the other cases, the exposure to unfiltered sunlight or UVB-emitting lamps is considered a safer approach.
- The absorption of dietary vitamin D3 can be variable across species of reptiles.

FOLLOW-UP

PATIENT MONITORING

- In cases of acute hypocalcemic crisis, the reptile requires intensive care and monitoring of ionized calcium levels and ECG activity.
- In cases of chronic NSHP, if the reptile is eating on its own, a physical exam once every 7–14 days, accompanied by radiography and blood work, is usually adequate to assess response to therapy.

EXPECTED COURSE AND PROGNOSIS

- The prognosis of the disease is strictly dependent on the chronicity of the improper husbandry and on the severity of clinical signs and pathology upon presentation.
- Older animals that present with chronic bone tissue depletion may have a worse prognosis.
- Different species have also different prognoses.
- Terrestrial chelonians in general are very sensitive to calcium deficiencies and have a poor prognosis once NSHP has developed.

MISCELLANEOUS

- Currently, there is a lack of information as to the proper amounts of calcium, vitamin D and other nutrients required for proper health of reptiles.
- The source of these nutrients may also influence their ability to be properly absorbed through the intestinal tract.
- It is possible that supplementation of these nutrients is not as effective as the natural ingestion via proper foods.

COMMENTS

N/A

ZOONOTIC POTENTIAL

N/A

SYNONYMS

- Fibrous osteodystrophy
- Metabolic bone disease
- Nutrition-related metabolic bone disease

ABBREVIATIONS

- ECG = electrocardiogram
- IM = intramuscular
- IV = intravenous
- NSHP = nutritional secondary hyperparathyroidism
- PTH = Parathyroid hormone
- SC = subcutaneous
- UVB = ultraviolet B

INTERNET RESOURCES

- Additional information on reptile endocrinology from Carl Gans Collections: BiologyoftheReptilia. http://carlgans.org/bor-view/?borv=3&borp=7
- Information on secondary hyperparathyroidism in humans: Kim L. Hyperparathyroidism. Medscape, August 18, 2020. http://emedicine.medscape.com/article/127351-overview?pa=mcKd1JF66kULHOzxxIxn2fK%2Bx5xE5kE6dUeU7dvJSrcnjyhACchqCtq5rNZR2UhkQPQxex%2Bo7mr5pATtx84gCBXKySxof3ndUJD5aivxmIc%3D#a4

Suggested Reading

Fledelius B, Jorgensen GW, Jensen HE, Brimer L. Influence of the calcium content of the diet offered to leopard tortoises (*Geochelone pardalis*). *Vet Rec* 2005;156(26):831–835.

Hoby S, Wenker C, Robert N, et al. Nutritional metabolic bone disease in juvenile veiled chameleons (Chamaeleo calyptratus) and its prevention. *J Nutr* 2010;140:1923–1931.

Mans C, Braun J. Update on common nutritional disorders of captive reptiles. *Vet Clin North Am Exot Anim Pract* 2014;17(3):369–395.

Author Paolo Selleri, DMV, PhD, SpecPACS, DECZM (Herpetology & Small Mammals), and Nicola Di Girolamo, DMV, MSc (EBHC), PhD, DECZM (Herpetology)

NYCTOTHERUS

BASICS

DEFINITION/OVERVIEW

Nyctotherus is a large ciliated protozoal organism that resides within the gastrointestinal tract. The trophozoite is dorsoventrally flattened like a bean and ranges in size from 60–200 µm. It has peristomal cilia that is characteristic for the organism. The cytostome (mouth) is long and curved. Cysts are brown, have a thick wall, ovoid in shape and have a polar cap. The polar cap is located more laterally in chelonians.

ETIOLOGY/PATHOPHYSIOLOGY

- Transmission is through the fecal–oral route.
- Cysts are ingested and then undergo excystation in the intestinal tract.
- Trophozoites hatch and emerge in the small intestine. They then migrate and manifest in the large colon and replicate by cell division.
- They feed on the chyme, bacteria, fiber, and other ingesta within the intestinal tract.
- Trophozoites undergo encystation in which infective cysts are formed and then excreted in feces.
- If in a moist environment, cysts remain infective for several weeks.
- *Nyctotherus* spp. are generally not considered to be pathogens of chelonians.
- Animals with diarrhea have been observed to have large amounts of trophozoites within fecals, but this is believed to be secondary due to the more liquid environment within the large intestine.

SIGNALMENT/HISTORY

All ages can be affected

CLINICAL PRESENTATION

- Diarrhea
- Dehydration
- Weight loss

RISK FACTORS

Husbandry

Improper husbandry

Others

Diarrhea

DIAGNOSIS

DIFFERENTIAL DIAGNOSIS

- Oxyurid nematodiasis
- Trematodes

DIAGNOSTICS

- Microscopic evaluation of fresh fecal material to visualize trophozoites and cysts.
- SAF technique can be used for better visualization.
- Fecal matter/cysts can be placed within a petri dish with water and trophozoites will emerge from the dissolved envelope within several hours.

PATHOLOGICAL FINDINGS

- Diarrhea, dehydration, weight loss
- Clinical signs are only likely to occur in severely immunocompromised individuals.

TREATMENT

APPROPRIATE HEALTH CARE

Treatment is rarely required because *Nyctotherus* are mostly non-pathogenic.

NUTRITIONAL SUPPORT

Nutritional supplementation may be indicated if diarrhea and dehydration is severe.

CLIENT EDUCATION/HUSBANDRY RECOMMENDATIONS

- Practice proper hygiene
- Wash fruits and vegetables before being fed.

MEDICATIONS

DRUG(S) OF CHOICE

Metronidazole 25 mg/kg PO q24h for 5–7 days

PRECAUTIONS/INTERACTIONS

N/A

FOLLOW-UP

PATIENT MONITORING

- Monitor for weight gain
- Take fecal samples

EXPECTED COURSE AND PROGNOSIS

Good

MISCELLANEOUS

COMMENTS

N/A

ZOONOTIC POTENTIAL

Unknown

SYNONYMS

N/A

ABBREVIATIONS

- PO = per os
- SAF = sodium acetate acetic acid formalin

INTERNET RESOURCES

- De Bosschere H, Roels S. *Balantidium* sp. and *Nyctotherus* sp: two common members of the digestive-tract flora in Mediterranean tortoises. Tortoise Trust. https://www.tortoisetrust.org/articles/balantidium.htm
- Divers SJ. Parasitic diseases of reptiles. MSD Manual Veterinary Manual, June 2020. http://www.merckvetmanual.com/exotic-and-laboratory-animals/reptiles/parasitic-diseases-of-reptiles

Suggested Reading

Hnizdo J, Pantchev N., eds. *Protozoa (digestive tract). In: Medical Care of Turtles and Tortoises. Diagnosis. Surgery. Pathology. Parasitology. Frankfurt*, Germany: Edition Chimaira; 2011:194–195.

Jacobson ER. Parasites and parasitic diseases of reptiles. In: Jacobson ER, ed. *Infectious Diseases and Pathology of Reptiles: Color Atlas and Text.* Boca Raton, FL: CRC Press; 2007:571–665.

Author Elsburgh O. Clarke III, DVM, DACZM

OTHER HYALOHYPHOMYCOSES

BASICS

DEFINITION/OVERVIEW

Refers to any infection with non-pigmented (hyaline) filamentous fungi such as *Aspergillus*, *Purpureocillium lilacinum* (formerly *Paecilomyces lilacinum*), *Fusarium*, *Metarhizium*, and many others fungi in genera other than *Chamaeleomyces*, *Nannizziopsis*, *Paranannizziopsis*, and *Ophidiomyces*.

ETIOLOGY/PATHOPHYSIOLOGY

- Ubiquitous environmental fungi that act as opportunistic pathogens in stressed/immunocompromised, or otherwise sick or debilitated animals.
- Some, like *Fusarium incarnatum* (formerly *F. semitectum*) in Texas tortoises or *Schizangiella serpentis* in snakes, may act as true pathogens, while others, like *P. lilacinum* or *F. solani*, seem to need little help in causing infection.
- Some are known insect pathogens, like *M. anisopliae* or *Beauveria bassiana*.

SIGNALMENT/HISTORY

- Any reptile, any age, any sex.
- History usually discloses substandard to outright deficient husbandry, poor hygiene, concurrent disease or infection, climactic extreme conditions (e.g., cold stunning in sea turtles) or life support system failure in captive animals (e.g., loss of heat from power failure), which result in immune suppression.

CLINICAL PRESENTATION

- Reflects the organ system affected.
- Dermatomycoses with epidermal necrosis, respiratory signs common in chelonians and crocodilians subject to hypothermia.
- Systemic, disseminated disease also often a consequence of prior hypothermia.

RISK FACTORS

Husbandry

- Climactic events in wild reptiles.
- Poor or deficient husbandry is probably the single most important predisposing factor.

Others

Chronic debilitating disease process, concurrent bacterial or other infections, prolonged antibiotic therapy.

DIAGNOSIS

DIFFERENTIAL DIAGNOSIS

- Depends on presentation and targeted organ system.
- Bacterial/mycobaterial, viral, and parasitic diseases
- Neoplasia when disseminated granulomas

DIAGNOSTICS

- Culture and cytology of material/clinical samples.
- Biopsy of lesions and histopathology to confirm causation.
- Blood work and imaging to determine extent of disease/lesions.

PATHOLOGICAL FINDINGS

Hyaline hyphae or other fungal elements within inflamed and/or necrotic tissue or within granulomas, consistent in morphology (e.g., diameter, septation, branching) to those of hyaline fungus isolated from the lesion.

TREATMENT

APPROPRIATE HEALTH CARE

- Fluids, antibiotic coverage, thermal and nutritional support.
- Correct perceived husbandry deficiencies
- Broad-spectrum antifungal drugs

NUTRITIONAL SUPPORT

Assist-feeding if needed

CLIENT EDUCATION/HUSBANDRY RECOMMENDATIONS

- Quarantine of incoming animals
- Thorough and meticulous captive husbandry.

SURGICAL CONSIDERATIONS

Debulking of lesions, when possible.

MEDICATIONS

DRUG(S) OF CHOICE

- Ideally based on fungal identification and known susceptibility of the causative fungus to the various antifungal drugs.
- In vitro assays might be available.
- Broad-spectrum antifungals that are efficacious against molds (itraconazole, voriconazole, terbinafine) are probably indicated pending culture and sensitivity results.

PRECAUTIONS/INTERACTIONS

- Triazole antifungal and terbinafine are possibly synergistic.
- Interactions with other drugs possible.

FOLLOW-UP

PATIENT MONITORING

- Monitor appetite, demeanor, and skin improvement with treatment.
- Blood work to monitor liver enzymes and other parameters while on antifungals and/or to assess immune status indicated.

EXPECTED COURSE AND PROGNOSIS

- Often diagnosed late in the course of disease.
- Early infection often subclinical in reptiles, which tend to be stoic, and fungal etiology often unsuspected by clinicians.
- Prognosis is therefore usually guarded to very poor, but may vary depending on duration, severity, and extent of lesions, and on the sensitivity pattern of the offending fungus.

MISCELLANEOUS

COMMENTS

S. serpentis causes a rare but serious and usually fatal disseminated granulomatous infection of snakes.

ZOONOTIC POTENTIAL

- Many fusaria and aspergilli carry some mild zoonotic impact.
- Dermatomycosis with *Trichophyton mentagrophytes var. interdigitale* has been reported in green iguanas in Iran.

SYNONYMS

Necrotizing scute disease refers to *F. incarnatum* infection of the shell in Texas tortoises.

Suggested Reading

Paré JA, Jacobson ER. Mycotic diseases of reptiles. In: Jacobson ER, ed. *Infectious Disease and Pathology of Reptiles, Color Atlas and Text.* Boca Raton, FL: CRC Press; 2007:527–570.

Author Jean A. Paré, DMV, DVSc, DACZM, DECZM (Zoo Health Management)

OXYURIDS

BASICS

DEFINITION/OVERVIEW

Oxyurids (pinworms) have a direct life cycle and are host specific. They are common in many chelonian species, particularly in herbivorous animals. Oxyurids are considered non-pathogenic in animals without clinical signs.

ETIOLOGY/PATHOPHYSIOLOGY

- Animals are usually asymptomatic
- Parasites inhabit the lower intestinal tract.
- Severe infestations may cause secondary problems, especially in debilitated and dehydrated animals.

SIGNALMENT/HISTORY

Oxyurids are most commonly found in herbivorous tortoises as commensal organisms of the lower intestinal tract.

CLINICAL PRESENTATION

- Disease caused by oxyurids is usually a secondary complication due to an underlying disease.
- Anorexia
- Lethargy
- Diarrhea
- Dehydration

RISK FACTORS

Husbandry

- Inadequate husbandry may lead to stress, immunosuppression, and a myriad of secondary conditions.
- Poor hygiene, high fecal loads, and overcrowding may contribute to higher infection rates.

Others

N/A

DIAGNOSIS

DIFFERENTIAL DIAGNOSIS

- In omnivorous chelonians, rule out prey items as the source of oxyurid ova.
- Commensals of the rodent cecum.
- Insects have species-specific pinworms in their gut flora.

DIAGNOSTICS

- Eggs vary in shape, can be ovoid, elongate, or D-shaped, and lack the thick wall of ascarid eggs.
- The eggs measure approximately 130 µm by 40 µm.
- Some eggs can be larvated.
- Adult worms are visible in fecal material.
- Oxyurid eggs are commonly seen in feces of herbivorous reptiles.

PATHOLOGICAL FINDINGS

Impaction of the intestinal tract may be observed in sick animals with severe pinworm infection.

TREATMENT

APPROPRIATE HEALTH CARE

Excessive numbers of these organisms in sick chelonians may require medical treatment.

NUTRITIONAL SUPPORT

- In ill animals, nutritional support after rehydration is needed to maintain positive nitrogen balance.
- Feed small amounts more frequently.
- Use high protein and fat diets for carnivores and complex carbohydrate diets for herbivores.

CLIENT EDUCATION/HUSBANDRY RECOMMENDATIONS

- Follow proper husbandry guidelines for the species.
- Environmental temperature, proper housing, and feeding regimen all play a crucial role in the wellbeing of reptilian species kept in captivity.

MEDICATIONS

DRUG(S) OF CHOICE

- Fenbendazole 25–50 mg/kg PO q24h for 5 days; 50–100 mg/kg PO q14d
- Oxfendazole 66 mg/kg PO once, may repeat in 14 days as needed
- Pyrantel pamoate 25 mg/kg PO q24h for 3 days; repeat in 3 weeks

PRECAUTIONS/INTERACTIONS

- Avoid fenbendazole and oxfendazole in severely debilitated and dehydrated animals to minimize the risk of the potential adverse effects (bone marrow suppression, intestinal cell damage) associated with these drugs.
- Lower doses of these drugs should also be considered in species of critical conservation status if previous safe use of these drugs is unknown.

FOLLOW-UP

PATIENT MONITORING

- Evaluate hydration frequently after starting treatment.
- Make husbandry changes to provide proper environment and nutrition.

EXPECTED COURSE AND PROGNOSIS

- Oxyurids are non-pathogenic in healthy, immunocompetent animals.
- In sick animals, treatment is aimed at decreasing the parasitic load in the gut to minimize the chance of impaction.
- Prognosis is excellent to good, as long as the underlying source of illness is identified and treated effectively (husbandry mismanagement, primary disease process).

MISCELLANEOUS

COMMENTS

N/A

ZOONOTIC POTENTIAL

N/A

SYNONYMS

N/A

ABBREVIATIONS

PO = per os

Suggested Reading

Mader DR, ed. *Reptile Medicine and Surgery*, 2nd ed. St Louis, MO: Elsevier Saunders; 2006.

McArthur S, Wilkinson R, Meyer J, eds. *Medicine and Surgery of Turtles and Tortoises*. Ames, IA: Blackwell; 2004.

Rataj AV, Lindtner-Knific R, Vlahović K, et al. Parasites in pet reptiles. *Acta Vet Scand* 2011;53(1):33.

Author Sam Rivera, DVM, MS, DABVP (Avian), DACZM, DECZM (Zoo Health Management)

PAPILLOMAVIRUS

BASICS

DEFINITION/OVERVIEW

Papillomaviruses cause mucocutaneous and cutaneous epithelial proliferative lesions in several vertebrate hosts, including reptiles.

ETIOLOGY/PATHOPHYSIOLOGY

- The members of the family *Papillomaviridae* are non-enveloped, icosahedral viral particles with a diameter of 50–55 nm and a small (7–8 kb), circular, double-stranded DNA.
- Papillomavirus-like particles were identified on electron microscopy in twist-necked turtles (*Platemys platycephala*) with skin lesions, and in a lung washing of a Russian tortoise (*Agrionemys horsfieldii*).
- Genomic characterization of two novel reptilian papillomaviruses, *Chelonia mydas* papillomavirus 1 and *Caretta caretta* papillomavirus 1, associated with proliferative dermatitis in a juvenile green turtle and a subadult loggerhead turtle, respectively, has also been reported; these chelonian papillomaviruses form a distinct clade most closely related to the avian papillomaviruses.

SIGNALMENT/HISTORY

Although papillomavirus-like particles and/or papillomavirus infection have been reported in several species of turtles (*P. platycephala*, *C. mydas*, *C. caretta*) and tortoises (*A. horsfieldii*), only turtle species had skin lesions.

CLINICAL PRESENTATION

- The first cases of papilloma-like virus infection in twist-necked turtles had multifocal, small, round to confluent, white skin lesions distributed over the head.
- The first documented cases of papillomavirus in marine turtles showed generalized proliferative dermatitis in the loggerhead turtle and localized proliferative dermatitis in the green turtle.

RISK FACTORS

Husbandry

Because transmission is likely by direct contact, absence of quarantine for newly admitted chelonians can contribute to widespread the disease.

Others

In mammals, the presence of papillomaviral lesions may be an indication of immunosuppression.

DIAGNOSIS

DIFFERENTIAL DIAGNOSIS

- Herpesvirus infection
- Gray patch disease of green turtles is caused by a herpesvirus and the lesions are similar.
- Fibropapillomatosis in sea turtles (associated with α-herpesviruses infection) is characterized by fibroblastic proliferation of the papillary dermis, degeneration of basilar epidermis, and orthokeratosis (lesions not found in papillomavirus infections).

DIAGNOSTICS

Although transmission electron microscopy can be used for detecting intranuclear aggregates of virions consistent in morphology with papillomavirus, a definitive diagnosis of papillomavirus in suspected samples must be made by PCR.

PATHOLOGICAL FINDINGS

- Gross lesions resemble very early papillomavirus lesions in mammals.
- In most cases, the lesions are circumscribed epidermal proliferations without progressing into the lobulated, pedunculated growths often observed in the mature papillomas.
- Histologically, the lesions are benign in appearance and consist of epidermal hyperplasia with prominent anisocytosis and anisokaryosis of keratinocytes and severe parakeratotic hyperkeratosis.

TREATMENT

APPROPRIATE HEALTH CARE

N/A

NUTRITIONAL SUPPORT

N/A

CLIENT EDUCATION/HUSBANDRY RECOMMENDATIONS

Affected turtles should be isolated, and their tanks should be cleaned and disinfected to minimize virus transmission and secondary infections.

MEDICATIONS

DRUG(S) OF CHOICE

- Surgical removal may be performed when lesions affect quality of life or normal function of the animal.
- No drug therapy has been reported in reptiles.
- Several antiviral drugs (cidofovir and imiquimod) have been effective in mammalian papillomavirus infections.

PRECAUTIONS/INTERACTIONS

N/A

FOLLOW-UP

PATIENT MONITORING

N/A

EXPECTED COURSE AND PROGNOSIS

- In most cases the lesions are benign, and regression of lesions is observed within 3–6 months.
- Secondary bacterial infections can be observed.

MISCELLANEOUS

COMMENTS

N/A

ZOONOTIC POTENTIAL

- Papillomaviruses are highly species-specific pathogens.
- There is no evidence for zoonosis from papillomaviruses affecting reptiles.

SYNONYMS

N/A

ABBREVIATIONS

PCR = polymerase chain reaction

Suggested Reading

Drury SEN, Gough RE, McArthur S, Jessop M. Detection of herpesvirus-like and papillomavirus-like particles associated with diseases of tortoises. *Vet Rec* 1998;143:639.

Herbst LH, Lenz J, Van Doorslaer K, et al. Genomic characterization of two novel reptilian papillomaviruses, *Chelonia mydas* papillomavirus 1 and papillomavirus 1. *Virology* 2009;383:131–135.

Jacobson ER, Gaskin JM, Clubb S, Calderwood MB. Papilloma-like virus infection in Bolivian side-neck turtles. *J Am Vet Med Assoc* 1982;181:1325–1328.

Manire CA, Stacy BA, Kinsel MJ, et al. Proliferative dermatitis in a loggerhead turtle, *Caretta caretta*, and a green turtle, *Chelonia mydas*, associated with novel papillomaviruses. *Vet Microbiol* 2008;130:227–237.

Author Jorge Orós, DVM, PhD, DECZM

PENTASTOMES

BASICS

DEFINITION/OVERVIEW

Pentastomids are crustacean endoparasites of the respiratory system of chelonians. Approximately 90% of pentastomids use carnivorous reptiles as their definitive hosts, with 70% being found in snakes. Turtles are often secondary hosts of pentastomes, but are not typically definitive hosts. Pentastomiasis occurs on all continents except Antarctica.

ETIOLOGY/PATHOPHYSIOLOGY

- Adult pentastomids live in the lungs of aquatic carnivorous turtles, where they breed and feed.
- Eggs are coughed up from the lungs or ingested and passed in feces.
- Intermediate hosts, such as insects, fish, anurans, reptiles, birds, or mammals ingest pentastomid eggs, which hatch, and go through two instars (growth periods between molts), before becoming encysted somewhere in the intermediate host's body.
- When the intermediate host is eaten by the definitive host, third-stage larvae emerge from the cyst and migrate to the host's lungs, where they feed on blood through the lung wall (hematophagous).
- Pentastomids damage the lungs, which may lead to secondary bacterial or fungal colonization, pneumonia, septicemia, or death.
- Heavy infestations can occlude the lungs or trachea.
- To date, the two monospecific genera, *Pelonia*, from the serrated hinged terrapin (*Pelusios sinuatus*) and African helmeted turtle (*Pelomedusa subrufa*), and *Diesingia* from Geoffroy's side-necked turtle (*Phrynops geoffroyana*) and Argentine snake-necked turtle (*Hydromedusa tectifera*) are the only adult chelonian pentastomes recovered worldwide.
- A possible exception is the crocodilian pentastome *Sebekia mississippiensis*, which can reach maturity in experimentally infected snapping turtles (*Chelydra serpentina*) and has also been described in softshell turtles (*Apalone* and *Chitra* spp.).

SIGNALMENT/HISTORY

Wild-caught turtles, including African and South American side neck turtles, soft shells and snapping turtles.

CLINICAL PRESENTATION

Can be subclinical or have respiratory tract disease, pneumonia, dyspnea, weight loss, or poor growth.

RISK FACTORS

Wild-caught aforementioned species

Husbandry

Yet another compelling reason for quarantine and fecal examinations.

Others

Feeding fresh wild caught fish that have not been frozen for three days.

DIAGNOSIS

- Detection of pentastomid eggs on fecal flotation, lung or cloacal washes, or tracheal discharge.
- Adult pentastomids are sometimes visible on radiography, or by pulmonoscopy or ultrasound.
- Adults may also be found during exploratory surgery, necropsy, or histopathology.

DIFFERENTIAL DIAGNOSIS

Respiratory signs may also be caused by other parasites, viruses, bacterial, fungi, neoplasia, trauma, or foreign bodies.

DIAGNOSTICS

- Fecal examination revealing thin-walled, large (up to 130 μm in diameter), distinct ova, containing larvae with four claw-like hooklets.
- A complete blood count might reveal anemia or eosinophilia.

PATHOLOGICAL FINDINGS

- Poorly described in chelonians
- Pentastomids are medium to large (0.25–15 cm), superficially segmented, wormlike parasites, with two compound pairs of hooks surrounding the mouth.
- Adults may be recovered from the lungs; encysted instars may be found throughout the body.
- In tissues, pentastomids are identified histologically by the presence of acidophilic glands adjacent to the intestine, and black sclerotized openings in the body wall.
- Inflammatory response in the lung may be mild with pentastomids because all life stages secrete surfactant very similar to host surfactant, which is thought to help them to evade the host's immune system.
- Degrading moulted pentastomid cuticles shed into the lung lumen may induce putrid pneumonia.
- Feed attachment sites on the lung surface can cause multiple crateriform ulcers.
- Pentastomids can be identified by morphological and molecular techniques.

TREATMENT

APPROPRIATE HEALTH CARE

Stabilize patient first with antibiotics, fluids and nutritional support, if indicated.

NUTRITIONAL SUPPORT

Feeding of Emeraid™ Carnivore (LaFeber Co., Cornell, IL), or Oxbow Carnivore Care® (Oxbow Animal Health, Murdock, NE) via esophagostomy tube in anorexic animals or those in poor body condition.

CLIENT EDUCATION/HUSBANDRY RECOMMENDATIONS

- Do not feed raw fish to turtles unless frozen first for at least 3 days.
- Wash hands after handling turtles or wear gloves.

SURGICAL CONSIDERATIONS

In otherwise stable patients, consider benign neglect or removal through transcarapacial pulmonary laparoscopy.

MEDICATIONS

DRUG(S) OF CHOICE

Ivermectin and other avermectins, macrocyclic lactones, are the treatment of choice for pentastomids; however, these are contraindicated in chelonians due to reports of paralysis and death.

PRECAUTIONS/INTERACTIONS

Living pentastomids secrete surfactant that helps them evade the host's immune system but, upon their death in tissue or lungs, a severe antigenic release, or putrefaction, with serious and potential lethal complications can occur.

FOLLOW-UP

PATIENT MONITORING

Perform serial fecal examinations post-treatment to gauge effectiveness.

EXPECTED COURSE AND PROGNOSIS

- Highly variable, dependent on parasitic burden, chronicity, condition of patient, and response to therapy.
- Given the inability to treat with macrocyclic lactones, long-term prognosis is guarded, as the parasites will continue to thrive within the host.

MISCELLANEOUS

COMMENTS

Figure 4 – see web image supplementary content for Section II (Chelonians).

ZOONOTIC POTENTIAL

- Species infecting humans belong to the families Linguatulidae, Armilliferidae, Porocephalidae, and Raillietiellidae, which have not been reported in chelonians.
- Nonetheless, all pentastomids should be considered potentially zoonotic.
- In the intermediate hosts, pentastome larvae often hatch and bore through the stomach wall and encyst in nearby mesentery, serosa or viscera.
- *Sebekia* spp. can cause a parasitic dermatitis in humans.

SYNONYMS

- Pentastomiasis
- Tongue worms

Suggested Reading

Jacobson ER. Parasites and parasitic diseases of reptiles. In: Jacobson ER, ed. *Infectious Disease and Pathology of Reptiles*. Boca Raton, FL: CRC Press; 2007:571–665.

Junker K, Boomker J. A check-list of the pentastomid parasites of crocodilians and freshwater chelonians. *Onderstepoort J Vet Res* 2006;73:27–36.

Paré JA. An overview of pentastomiasis in reptiles and other vertebrates. *J Exot Pet Med* 2008;17:285–294.

Author Thomas H. Boyer, DVM, DABVP (Reptile and Amphibian Practice)

PHAEOHYPHOMYCOSES

BASICS

DEFINITION/OVERVIEW

Phaeohyphomycoses refers to any infection with dematiaceous (pigmented) fungi, such as *Exophiala*, *Cladosporium*, *Ochroconis*, *Ulocladium*, *Trichoderma*. The cell wall of these fungi contains variable amounts of melanin, and hyphae are therefore easily seen on routine H&E histological sections. These are relatively uncommon in reptiles.

ETIOLOGY/PATHOPHYSIOLOGY

- Dematiaceous fungi are environmental fungi often found in soil and/or water.
- They usually infect cutaneous wounds or, less often, infect sick or debilitated animals.
- These opportunistic pathogens typically cause deep granulomatous infections of the feet, especially in tortoises, and rarely disseminate.
- *Exophiala* species in particular have been isolated with some regularity from reptiles with phaeohyphomycosis.

SIGNALMENT/HISTORY

- Any reptile, any age or sex.
- Tortoises and box turtles (*Terrapene* spp.) seem overrepresented.

CLINICAL PRESENTATION

- Swellings, nodules, wounds, often on the feet or ventrum (body parts in contact with soil).
- Slow progression
- Tends to not disseminate

RISK FACTORS

Husbandry

- Substandard or otherwise deficient husbandry.
- Soil substrate
- Poor water quality

Others

Open wounds or other cutaneous breaches may facilitate invasion by these opportunistic fungi.

DIAGNOSIS

DIFFERENTIAL DIAGNOSIS

- Other fungal infections
- Mycobacteriosis
- Abscesses
- Even neoplasia

DIAGNOSTICS

- Biopsy and histopathology
- Culture of biopsy tissue or PCR.
- Pigmented fungi associated with inflammation/necrosis in histological section, and morphology of fungi in tissues consistent with morphology of putative isolate cultured from biopsy.

PATHOLOGICAL FINDINGS

Pigmented hyphae or other fungal elements within inflamed and/or necrotic tissue or within granulomas, consistent in morphology (e.g., pigmentation, diameter, septation, branching) with those of fungal isolate from the lesion.

TREATMENT

APPROPRIATE HEALTH CARE

- Fluids, antibiotic coverage, thermal and nutritional support.
- Correct perceived husbandry deficiencies

NUTRITIONAL SUPPORT

Assist-feeding if needed

CLIENT EDUCATION/HUSBANDRY RECOMMENDATIONS

- Quarantine of incoming animals
- Thorough and meticulous captive husbandry.

SURGICAL CONSIDERATIONS

- Debulking of lesions, when possible.
- Amputation may be indicated when deep lesion located on/in feet.

MEDICATIONS

DRUG(S) OF CHOICE

- Ideally based on fungal identification and known susceptibility of the causative fungus to the various antifungal drugs.
- In vitro assays might be available.
- Many if not most pigmented fungi display resistance to triazoles and allylamines.

PRECAUTIONS/INTERACTIONS

N/A

FOLLOW-UP

PATIENT MONITORING

- Monitor appetite, demeanor, and skin improvement with treatment.
- Blood work to monitor liver enzymes and other parameters while on antifungals and/or assess immune status indicated.

EXPECTED COURSE AND PROGNOSIS

- Often diagnosed late in the course of disease when lesions chronic and/or extensive.
- Prognosis usually guarded, but may vary depending on duration, severity, and extent of lesions, and on the sensitivity pattern of the offending fungus.

MISCELLANEOUS

COMMENTS

N/A

ZOONOTIC POTENTIAL

- Minimal
- Some pigmented fungi can cause local infections and onychomycosis in humans and, rarely, fungemia and disseminated disease.

SYNONYMS

N/A

ABBREVIATIONS

- H&E = hematoxylin and eosin
- PCR = polymerase chain reaction

Suggested Reading

Paré JA, Jacobson ER. Mycotic diseases of reptiles. In: Jacobson ER, ed. *Infectious Disease and Pathology of Reptiles, Color Atlas and Text.* Boca Raton, FL: CRC Press; 2007:527–570.

Author Jean A. Paré, DMV, DVSc, DACZM, DECZM (Zoo Health Management)

PHALLUS PROLAPSE

BASICS

DEFINITION/OVERVIEW

A prolapse is the moving or slipping of a body part from its usual position or anatomic relation. A prolapse of the single penis or phallus happens in chelonians.

ETIOLOGY/PATHOPHYSIOLOGY

- The underlying causes for prolapse is often unknown.
- See Differential Diagnosis for a list of possible etiologies.

SIGNALMENT/HISTORY

There appears to be no specific signalment or predilections noted for the various reptilian prolapses.

CLINICAL PRESENTATION

- A prolapse is easy to visualize as abnormal tissue protruding from the cloacal/vent region.
- With any prolapse of tissue it should be communicated to the owner that this is an emergency and should be evaluated immediately.
- The tissue should be kept moist either through gentle washing the area with water and loosely wrapped in a damp cloth or paper towel.
- The phallus may revert inside the cloaca when examined.
- The extruded tissue should be identified to the tissue(s) involved.
- In the case of the phallus, the tissue may be pink to purple, though some species have black pigmentation normally.
- The phallus may have a spade-shaped end.
- Exposure of the prolapsed tissue may result in further damage due to desiccation and trauma.
- The act of crawling and walking exposes the prolapsed organ to mechanical damage from the ground, branches, etc.

RISK FACTORS

- In cases of NSHP, the muscle tone around the cloacal opening is decreased, leading to potential tissue exposure.
- Any generalized physical straining of the patient can lead to tissue exposure through the cloaca, such as dyspnea, obstipation, parasites, infection.
- Space-occupying lesions located in the coelomic cavity such as uroliths, neoplasia, hepato/renomegaly may also cause increased straining and phallus prolapse.
- The act of copulation may result in trauma to the phallus, resulting in swelling and the inability to invert tissue.
- Any eversion of the organ may result in direct trauma with the environment (e.g., ground, dirt, etc.) or bite wounds from a cage mate.
- Even animals housed singly may attempt copulation.

Husbandry

- Several factors of husbandry may lead to one of the clinical conditions listed in the Differential Diagnosis section.
- Corrections of the deficient aspects of the husbandry can lead to reversal of some of those listed conditions.

Others

N/A

DIAGNOSIS

DIFFERENTIAL DIAGNOSIS

- Trauma
- Sexual activity
- Constipation
- Cloacal impaction (urates, cystic calculi, cage substrate)
- Neurological deficits
- Parasites
- Hypocalcemia
- Bacterial infection
- Metabolic disease
- Neoplasia

DIAGNOSTICS

- Radiography and ultrasound may be useful in determining internal abnormalities (e.g., impactions, masses, obstructions).
- The small size of some reptiles may lead to reduced imaging detail, which makes interpretation challenging.
- Dental radiography may be a better alternative in smaller species (< 100 g).
- A fecal examination should be performed in all cases.
- This can be directly from the feces, from a saline cloacal wash, or direct impression smear of the prolapsed tissue may reveal the presence of parasites such as nematode larvae or eggs.
- CBC and chemistry panel may assist in the determination of underlying physiologic abnormalities.

PATHOLOGICAL FINDINGS

- The length of time the prolapse presents inversely affects the prognosis.
- The longer an internal mucosal tissue is exposed to the outside environment, the higher the risk for the tissue to desiccate and potentially devitalize.
- Any devitalized tissue must be removed, and the greater the amount of tissue devitalized the lower the prognosis to save the organ.

TREATMENT

APPROPRIATE HEALTH CARE

- Treatment often involves direct replacement of the tissue back into normal anatomic position either by manual or surgical means, in combination with correction of the underlying etiology.
- The patient should be fully evaluated for general health status and treated accordingly.
- The prolapsed tissue should be evaluated for presence of devitalization, which must be surgically or medically addressed prior to prolapse reduction.
- The phallus prolapse may be reduced in size by coating with a hyperosmotic solution such as 2–5% ophthalmic saline or concentrated sugar solution.
- Direct application of dry salt or sugar may be attempted, but the extreme osmolar difference could lead to direct tissue damage and should be closely monitored.
- After several minutes of application, the prolapsed tissue should become less edematous and capable of reduction back into the body cavity.
- A moistened and lubricated (water-soluble) cotton tip applicator or metal probe is used to gently push the tissue by inversion back inside the body cavity aligning the lumen.

NUTRITIONAL SUPPORT

The reptilian patient may need weight and body condition monitoring to determine whether additional caloric supplementation is needed.

CLIENT EDUCATION/HUSBANDRY RECOMMENDATIONS

- If surgical correction of the prolapse is undertaken, the client should be directed on postoperative care of any surgical sites, suture, etc.
- A detailed log of activity as well as food intake/defecations should be maintained and related back to the veterinarian.
- If any changes to the husbandry were determined, the owner should correct those prior to the patient returning home, such as changes to temperature and/or humidity, exposure to UVB lighting.

SURGICAL CONSIDERATIONS

- Lateral sutures across the cloacal margin may be placed for 10–14 days to allow for the tissue swelling to resolve in place.
- If the tissue is devitalized or traumatized, the best option may be amputation.
- To perform amputation, the exteriorized tissue should be further removed to identify and isolate the base of the organ.
- The base should be ligated with a transfixation and/or mattress suture.
- A double ligation is warranted due to the well-developed vascular system, and the vascular stimulation secondary to the prolapse.
- The remaining surgical stump should be replaced back into the cloaca.

PHALLUS PROLAPSE (CONTINUED)

MEDICATIONS

DRUG(S) OF CHOICE

- NSAIDs or opioids may be used to manage the pain and inflammation associated with the physical discomfort of the prolapse or surgery.
- Depending on the underlying etiology, antibiotics or anti-parasiticides may be indicated.

PRECAUTIONS/INTERACTIONS

- When replacing the prolapse, extreme care must be taken not to tear or perforate the delicate, inflamed tissue.
- After the sutures are removed, the tissue may re-prolapse if swelling/inflammation are still present or the underlying etiology has not been corrected.
- Placement of additional sutures may be required.
- Hydration status of the patent must be considered before use of NSAIDs.

FOLLOW-UP

PATIENT MONITORING

- The patient should be followed up daily after clinical repair of the prolapse for reoccurrence.
- The owner should monitor and record all food intake and defecations during this time.
- Any abnormal changes from the routine should be related back to the veterinarian to determine any further changes to the therapy.

EXPECTED COURSE AND PROGNOSIS

- Phallus prolapses have excellent to good prognosis, as it is a purely copulatory organ, so even in amputation is required, there are rarely any ill effects on the patient.
- The phallus does possess a long groove along its length that allows for sperm to travel to the end during copulation.
- Amputation of a phallus would render the patient unable to copulate, although sperm could theoretically be collected for artificial placement.

MISCELLANEOUS

COMMENTS

N/A

ZOONOTIC POTENTIAL

N/A

SYNONYMS

N/A

ABBREVIATIONS

- CBC = complete blood count
- NSAIDs = nonsteroidal anti-inflammatory drugs
- NSHP = nutritional secondary hyperparathyroidism
- UVB = ultraviolet B

Suggested Reading

Barten, SL. Penile prolapse. In: Mader DR, ed. *Reptile Medicine and Surgery*. 2nd ed. St. Louis, MO: Elsevier Saunders; 2006:862–864.

Bennett, RA. Cloacal prolapse. In: Mader DR, ed. *Reptile Medicine and Surgery*. 2nd ed. St. Louis, MO: Elsevier Saunders; 2006:751–755.

Author Rob L. Coke, DVM, DACZM, DABVP (Reptile & Amphibian), CVA

PSEUDOGOUT

BASICS

DEFINITION/OVERVIEW

Pseudogout is a condition that occurs due to the deposition of crystals, other than uric acid, in or around the joints.

ETIOLOGY/PATHOPHYSIOLOGY

- Crystals may be deposited for a variety of reasons.
- In humans, these include previous joint damage, hyperparathyroidism or sometimes hereditary factors.
- In reptiles, the exact etiology is unclear but deposition of calcium crystals in and around joints may be seen, especially CPPD.
- This can result in an acute inflammatory response in the affected joint.

SIGNALMENT/HISTORY

- Pseudogout may be seen in chelonians with a history of inappropriate husbandry or diet.
- Signs may also be seen in combination with gout.

CLINICAL PRESENTATION

- Animals with pseudogout usually present with obvious joint swellings.
- One or more joints may be affected, and the animal may be lame.

RISK FACTORS

Husbandry

Excessive calcium and vitamin D supplementation may be a predisposing factor.

Others

Previous joint damage, previous metabolic bone disease, or renal disease are all thought to predispose to the development of pseudogout.

DIAGNOSIS

DIFFERENTIAL DIAGNOSIS

- Gout
- Septic arthritis
- Trauma
- Metabolic bone diseases

DIAGNOSTICS

- Pseudogout may be suspected based on history and clinical examination, but diagnostic testing will be necessary for definitive diagnosis.
- On radiography of affected limbs, calcified lesions may be seen in and around joints.
- Metastatic calcification on whole body radiography may also be seen concurrently affecting internal organs, but is not always a feature.
- Demonstration of calcium crystals in joints or within diseased tissue is necessary for definitive diagnosis.
- Aspirates may be taken from affected joints and examined microscopically for the presence of crystals or the whole joint may be submitted for histopathology if amputation is performed.
- Von Kossa or Alizarin red S stain may help aid in the identification of calcium crystals.

PATHOLOGICAL FINDINGS

- On gross postmortem examination, pale nodules can be seen within or around joints.
- On histopathological examination, nodules are often surrounded by granulomatous inflammation.

TREATMENT

APPROPRIATE HEALTH CARE

- Amputation of the affected digit or limb may be considered if signs are localized.
- If signs are mild, NSAIDs can be given to reduce inflammation and pain.
- Euthanasia may be considered in severe cases.

NUTRITIONAL SUPPORT

N/A

CLIENT EDUCATION/HUSBANDRY RECOMMENDATIONS

- Diet should be reviewed to ensure that it is appropriate for the species and not does not contain excessive levels of calcium or vitamin D3.
- Clients should be advised that this is a condition that will require long-term management and can potentially be very painful if allowed to progress.

MEDICATIONS

DRUG(S) OF CHOICE

N/A

PRECAUTIONS/INTERACTIONS

N/A

FOLLOW-UP

PATIENT MONITORING

Response to therapy is usually monitored by physical examination findings (e.g., increase in activity levels or no progression in joint swellings).

EXPECTED COURSE AND PROGNOSIS

- The prognosis for patients with severe widespread signs is poor, but if diagnosed early the condition can often be managed successfully.
- If the underlying cause is not addressed, disease can progress to affect multiple joints.

MISCELLANEOUS

COMMENTS

N/A

ZOONOTIC POTENTIAL

N/A

SYNONYMS

- Chondrocalcinosis
- CPPD crystal deposition disease

ABBREVIATIONS

- CPPD = calcium pyrophosphate dihydrate
- NSAIDs = non-steroidal anti-inflammatories

INTERNET RESOURCES

Veterinary Information Network: www.vin.com

Suggested Reading

Chambers JK, Suzuki T, Une Y. Tophaceous pseudogout of the femorotibial joint in a painted turtle (*Chrysemys picta*). *J Vet Med Sci* 2009;71(5):693–695.

Jones YL, Fitzgerald SD. Articular gout and suspected pseudogout in a Basilisk lizard (*Basilicus plumifrons*). *J Zoo Wildl Med* 2009;40(3):576–578.

Mader DR. Gout. In: Mader DR ed. *Reptile Medicine and Surgery*. 2nd ed. Philadelphia, PA: Elsevier Saunders; 2006: 374–379.

Rosenthal AK, Ryan LM. Calcium pyrophosphate deposition disease. *N Engl J Med* 2016;374(26):2575–2584.

Author Joanna Hedle,y BVM&S, DZooMed (Reptilian), DipECZM (Herpetology), MRCVS

REGURGITATION

BASICS

DEFINITION/OVERVIEW

Regurgitation is the passive discharge through the mouth of undigested food or other contents within a short time after eating.

ETIOLOGY/PATHOPHYSIOLOGY

- Regurgitation usually originates as an esophageal or pharyngeal problem.
- May be gastric if the gastroesophageal sphincter is incompetent or the stomach is markedly diseased.

SIGNALMENT/HISTORY

- All species, ages, sexes may be affected.
- Owner may report observing regurgitation or only that regurgitated material was found.
- Other notable history may include lethargy, anorexia, weight loss, respiratory distress, or increased basking frequency; ingestion of foreign material.

CLINICAL PRESENTATION

- No clinical signs are specific to regurgitation, and physical exam may be normal.
- Presentation varies depending on the underlying cause and chronicity.
- Dehydration and/or emaciation/cachexia.
- Hard mass on palpation of the coelomic cavity due to an obstructive lesion or organomegaly.
- Skeletal abnormalities that may include pathological fractures or abnormal growth patterns.
- Lethargy and/or obtunded mentation.
- Ulceration and accumulation of caseous material in the oral cavity.
- Secondary respiratory disease (e.g., oral/nasal discharge, abnormal respiratory sounds) or enteritis (e.g., diarrhea).

RISK FACTORS

Husbandry

- Too much disturbance or lack of hiding places (increases stress/anxiety).
- Poor sanitation, overcrowding, hyper/hypothermia, lack of quarantine for new individuals (increases stress, possibility of secondary infections, and disease transmission).
- Toxin exposure (cleaning chemicals, pesticides, heavy metals).
- Excessive/inappropriate handling (especially soon after feeding).
- Inadequate diet (incorrect calcium/phosphorus ratio, improper prey items, excessive feeding).
- Inappropriate substrate (may be accidentally ingested).

Others

Concomitant infectious or parasitic disease.

DIAGNOSIS

DIFFERENTIAL DIAGNOSIS

- Stomatitis
- Esophagitis
- Esophageal stricture
- Gastritis
- Handling/stress (e.g., excessive pressure to coelom)
- Obstructive lesions (e.g., GI foreign body, intussusception, neoplasia, abscess, granuloma)
- Metabolic disease (e.g., nutritional secondary hyperparathyroidism, renal or hepatic dysfunction)
- Toxicoses (e.g., zinc)
- Iatrogenic (e.g., enrofloxacin, xylazine, levamisole)
- Trauma to esophagus or stomach.
- Parasites (e.g., *Cryptosporidium*, amoebiasis, ascaridiasis, cestodiasis)
- Viruses
- Bacteria/septicemia (e.g., *Chlamydophila*)
- Congenital GI defects

DIAGNOSTICS

- Husbandry review
- Physical examination
- Complete blood count and plasma biochemistries.
- Radiography with or without contrast.
- Ultrasound
- Fecal parasite exam
- Other diagnostics to consider: bacterial cultures from oral lesions; GI endoscopy or coeliotomy (direct tissue evaluation and biopsy).

Suspected Cryptosporidiosis

Acid-fast staining and/or indirect fluorescent antibody of feces, regurgitated material, or gastric wash (best collected 3 days after feeding); PCR of feces, regurgitated material, gastric wash, or biopsy from affected tissues (e.g., stomach).

PATHOLOGICAL FINDINGS

- Dependent on underlying cause
- Cryptosporidiosis in chelonians primarily affects the GI tract, but could also potentially affect the stomach.

TREATMENT

APPROPRIATE HEALTH CARE

The primary goal is to identify and address the underlying cause.

NUTRITIONAL SUPPORT

- Correct fluid deficits and maintain hydration. Intracoelomic, subcutaneous, or intravenous routes for administration of a reptile Ringer's solution are most effective. Maintenance rate is 10–30 ml/kg/day.
- Tube or assist-feeding liquid or gel diets (e.g., Oxbow Critical Care®, Oxbow Animal Health, Omaha, NE, formulas) may be beneficial during initial treatment/recovery. Gradually add normal diet items as the animal improves.

CLIENT EDUCATION/HUSBANDRY RECOMMENDATIONS

- Review husbandry and correct any problems.
- Institute quarantine procedures for new animals, including 30–60-day period, veterinary evaluation, and 1–3-weekly fecal exams for parasites.

MEDICATIONS

DRUG(S) OF CHOICE

- Cimetidine 4 mg/kg IM, PO q8–12h, or famotidine 0.25–0.5 mg/kg SC, PO q24–72h
- Metoclopramide 0.06 mg/kg PO q24h for 7 days or 1–10 mg/kg PO q24h, or cisapride 0.5–2 mg/kg PO q24h
- Sucralfate 500–1000 mg/kg PO q6–8h

PRECAUTIONS/INTERACTIONS

N/A

FOLLOW-UP

PATIENT MONITORING

Monitor for continued signs of regurgitation and possible complications.

EXPECTED COURSE AND PROGNOSIS

- The prognosis is dependent on the underlying cause.
- Regurgitation and vomiting are rare in chelonians, and their presence worsens the prognosis.
- The prognosis for subclinical cryptosporidiosis is fair to good.
- The prognosis for clinical disease is poor to grave, and euthanasia is often indicated.

MISCELLANEOUS

COMMENTS

N/A

ZOONOTIC POTENTIAL

N/A

SYNONYMS

Reflux

ABBREVIATIONS

- GI = gastrointestinal
- PCR = polymerase chain reaction
- IM = intramuscular
- PO = per os
- SC = subcutaneous

Suggested Reading

Funk RS. Vomiting and regurgitation. In: Mader DR, ed. *Reptile Medicine and Surgery*. 2nd ed. St. Louis, MO: Elsevier Saunders; 2006:939–940.

Gibbons PM, Klaphake E, Carpenter JW. Reptiles. In: Carpenter JW, Marion CJ, eds. *Exotic Animal Formulary*. 4th ed. St. Louis, MO: Elsevier Saunders; 2013:83–182.

Mitchell MA, Diaz-Figueroa O. Clinical reptile gastroenterology. *Vet Clin N Am Exot Anim Pract* 2005;8:277–298.

Authors Tamara Kruse, DVM, MS, and Trevor T. Zachariah, DVM, MS, DACZM

RENAL SECONDARY HYPERPARATHYROIDISM

BASICS

DEFINITION/OVERVIEW

RSHP can be a common occurrence in captive reptiles. It is a consequence of late-stage chronic renal failure, where calcium and vitamin D levels are depleted. The decrease in blood calcium triggers an overproduction of PTH, which stimulates resorption of bone tissue. Prognosis for this disease is poor to guarded, because even if calcium imbalances can be corrected, the renal function is rarely improved by means of current treatments.

ETIOLOGY/PATHOPHYSIOLOGY

- RSHP develops in reptiles suffering of chronic renal failure.
- Reduction in renal mass results in diminished elimination of phosphorus with a consequent increase in serum phosphate concentrations and decreased 1,25-dihydroxycholecalciferol (vitamin D3) formation.
- Both these perturbations lead to a decrease of blood calcium, which is followed by an uncontrolled, diffuse proliferation of parathyroid cells (polyclonal proliferation) in the initial stages of the disease, and subsequently in nodular proliferation (monoclonal proliferation) in patients with higher stages of chronic kidney disease.
- The consequent increase in PTH concentrations result in increased osteoclastic activity and severe bone resorption.
- In humans, the cardiovascular system is also affected as a consequence of increased PTH levels, with increased risk of congestive heart failure and coronary artery disease.
- Chronic renal failure may be triggered by degenerative disease, as caused by diets with excess in proteins, and infectious diseases, including picornavirus infection.

SIGNALMENT/HISTORY

- Compared with NSHP, RSHP is more commonly seen in older animals, where a chronic decline in kidney function leads to the aforementioned metabolic disturbances.
- Aquatic turtles that develop RSHP have a typical history of diet with excess in animal proteins, and lack of proper brumation.
- Less commonly, an entire group of young reptiles presents with clinical signs related with metabolic bone disease, without any history of poor diet or improper husbandry. An infectious agent affecting the kidneys should be considered in these cases.

CLINICAL PRESENTATION

- Compared with NSHP, reptiles with RSHP do not have significant bone resorption when presented for clinical examination.
- Most reptiles with RSHP are presented for clinical signs caused by renal failure, including celomic effusion, anorexia, and lethargy.
- Alternatively, they may present with the acute consequence of hypocalcemia, which includes seizures-like crisis, muscle tremors, depression, and collapse.
- Reptiles with RSHP and chronic renal failure may present with increase in kidney size.
- Abnormally enlarged kidneys may be palpated in chelonians through the prefemoral fossae.

RISK FACTORS

Husbandry

- Chelonians that develop RSHP during adulthood typically have a chronic history of poor husbandry and diet.
- Factors that may result in chronic renal failure and consequent RSHP include:
  - Excess in dietary protein intake.
  - Low fiber content in the diet.
  - Low environment humidity resulting in chronic dehydration.
  - Inappropriate environment temperatures resulting in inadequate metabolism.
  - Lack of brumation in brumating species resulting in excessive growth rates.

Others

- Toxic exposure
- Neoplasia
- Infectious disease
- Degenerative renal changes including fluid-filled and epidermoid cyst formation may all result in decreased kidney function and RSHP.

DIAGNOSIS

DIFFERENTIAL DIAGNOSIS

- Differential diagnoses for seizure-like activity and muscle tremors include other causes of hypocalcemia, particularly NSHP and primary hyperparathyroidism.
- Differential diagnoses for increased renal size include gout and neoplasia.
- Other forms of renal failure may mimic the clinical signs of RSHP.

DIAGNOSTICS

- In most cases, a clinical suspicion of chronic kidney disease is made based on history of long-term inappropriate diet and/or husbandry and clinical signs.
- Diagnosis of RSHP is supported by hyperphosphatemia with concurrent hypocalcemia.
- Increased uric acid and/or urea may also be observed.
- Alterations in phosphorus, calcium and uric acid/urea due to RSHP typically do not improve with fluid therapy.
- PTH levels may be measured but reference intervals are lacking for most reptile species.
- Radiography can be used to evaluate bone cortices.
- Ultrasound can be used to evaluate renal and parathyroid parenchyma.
- If coelomic effusion is present, perform standard cytological and microbiological analyses.

PATHOLOGICAL FINDINGS

- Grossly, kidneys may be enlarged and may present superficial and/or parenchymal alterations.
- Depending on the severity of the RSHP, bone softening or deformity may be observed, including the carapace and plastron.
- Alterations of parathyroid glands may be present as generalized or focal enlargements.
- Histopathology of kidneys may reveal different degrees and types of renal alterations.
- Histopathological bone lesions may range from increased osteoclastic resorption of otherwise well-formed and mineralized bones, to thinning of lamina and widening of medullary cavities, with scalloped endosteal surfaces due to increased resorptive activity.
- Long bones may show thinned cortices with layers of osteoblasts and unmineralized osteoid on the periosteal surface.

TREATMENT

APPROPRIATE HEALTH CARE

N/A

NUTRITIONAL SUPPORT

- Reptiles with RSHP are often anorectic.
- The anorexia is usually associated with the concurrent renal failure and may persist for long period.
- Chelonians with severe bone depletion may not be able to ingest food due to the changes in the mandibular bones.
- In either case, placement of an esophagostomy tube must be implemented to provide nutritional support.

CLIENT EDUCATION/HUSBANDRY RECOMMENDATIONS

- Chronic renal failure is more common in animals that had improper husbandry and diet during their life.
- Owners should be informed that at the very first signs of renal failure (e.g., limb/celomic swelling, anorexia, decreased activity), a thorough veterinary assessment is required for early diagnosis and to limit phosphorus increase, calcium depletion, and consequent PTH increase.
- Owners should be advised to feed diets low in proteins and high in fiber.
- For non-aquatic species, a low environmental humidity may result in chronic dehydration, which exacerbates renal failure.

- It is believed that either excessive or insufficient environmental temperatures may worsen renal disease.
- In brumating species, the procedure of systematic skipping brumation by artificial provision of heat during the winter can lead to physiologic strain on the organs.

MEDICATIONS

DRUG(S) OF CHOICE

- Give fluid therapy 20–30 ml/kg/day IV, IO, SC, ICe.
- In reptiles suffering of RSHP, both the hyperparathyroidism and the renal disease should be corrected.
- Treatment of RSHP includes therapy designed to minimize the clinical and pathophysiological consequences of reduced kidney function and at correcting the primary cause of the renal impairment, including bacterial, fungal and parasitic disease.
- The main goal of therapy is to correct calcium, phosphorus, and uric acid/urea levels.
- In cases where renal disease has been caused by improper husbandry, the mainstay of the therapy is an improvement in husbandry and diet.
- Expose animal to UVB light daily.
- Phosphate binders (lanthanum carbonate octahydrate) 120–200 mg/kg mixed with feed q24h.
- Calcium gluconate 50–100 mg/kg SC, IM, IV q6–24h followed by calcium glubionate at 50–360 mg/kg PO q12–24h.
- Allopurinol 100 mg/kg q24h if hyperuricemic
- Angiotensin-converting enzyme inhibitors and antihypertensive therapy may also be considered on a case-by-case basis.

PRECAUTIONS/INTERACTIONS

N/A

FOLLOW-UP

PATIENT MONITORING

- If reptiles are presented for acute hypocalcemic crisis, intensive care and frequent monitoring of phosphorus and calcium levels (ionized and total), as well as other electrolytes and ECG activity is essential.
- In young reptiles with RSHP as a consequence of bacterial or viral renal infection, intensive care should be provided until the infection is resolved.
- In cases of chronic RSHP, if the reptile is eating on its own, a physical exam once every 7–14 days, accompanied by blood work (hematocrit, uric acid/urea, calcium and phosphorus) is recommended to assess response to therapy.

EXPECTED COURSE AND PROGNOSIS

- The prognosis for animals suffering RSHP is poor.
- Even if calcium and phosphorus imbalances can be corrected via fluid therapy, exogenous supplementation, and phosphate binder administration, there is currently no effective treatment for renal failure in reptiles.

MISCELLANEOUS

There is a need of development of novel diets that may reduce the protein intake in carnivorous/omnivorous reptiles suffering of renal disease while at the same time providing the correct amount of nutrients.

COMMENTS

N/A

ZOONOTIC POTENTIAL

N/A

SYNONYMS

Renal-related metabolic bone disease

ABBREVIATIONS

- ECG = electrocardiogram
- ICe = Intracoelomic
- IO = Intraosseous
- IV = Intravenous
- NSHP = Nutritional secondary hyperparathyroidism
- PTH = parathormone
- RSHP = renal secondary hyperparathyroidism
- SC = Subcutaneous
- UVB = ultraviolet B

INTERNET RESOURCES

- Additional information on reptile renal physiology from Carl Gans Collections: Biology of the Reptilia. http://carlgans.org/bor-view/?borv=5&borpage=447&borp=459
- Information on secondary hyperparathyroidism in humans: Kim L. Hyperparathyroidism. Medscape, August 18, 2020. http://emedicine.medscape.com/article/127351-overview?pa=mcKd1JF66kULHOzxxIxn2fK%2Bx5xE5kE6dUeU7dvJSrcnjyhACchqCtq5rNZR2UhkQPQxex%2Bo7mr5pATtx84gCBXKySxof3ndUJD5aivxmIc%3D#a4

Suggested Reading

Hernandez-Divers SJ, Martínez-Jimenez D, Bush S, et al. Effects of allopurinol on plasma uric acid levels in normouricaemic and hyperuricaemic green iguanas (*Iguana iguana*). *Vet Rec* 2008;162(4):112–115.

Heuser W, Pendl H, Knowles NJ, et al. Soft plastron, soft carapace with skeletal abnormality in juvenile tortoises: Histopathology and isolation of a novel picornavirus from *Testudo graeca* and *Geochelone elegans*. *Tierarztl Prax Ausg K Kleintiere Heimtiere* 2014;42(5):310–320.

Selleri P, Hernandez-Divers SJ. Renal diseases of reptiles. *Vet Clin North Am Exot Anim Pract* 2006;9(1):161–174.

Author Paolo Selleri, DMV, PhD, SpecPACS, DECZM (Herpetology & Small Mammals), and Nicola Di Girolamo, DMV, MSc (EBHC), PhD, DECZM (Herpetology)

SALMONELLOSIS

BASICS

DEFINITION/OVERVIEW

- Salmonellosis is a cosmopolitan disease and an important reptile zoonosis. The current approach to reptile-associated salmonellosis in the United States is based on our experiences with chelonians. Identified in the 1960s, chelonian-associated salmonellosis led to inter- and intrastate restrictions on the sale of turtles. At that time, it was estimated that more than 200,000 children were being impacted by the disease.
- Currently, chelonians with a carapace length of less than 10.2 cm (4 inches) are not allowed to be sold in the United States. Vendors on the internet, flea markets, and elsewhere can be found selling these animals. Thus, veterinarians may see these animals in their practice and should be prepared to educate their clients about the zoonotic potential of *Salmonella* spp.
- There is no difference in the prevalence of *Salmonella* spp. between turtles larger or smaller than 10.2 cm. This size designation was based on the desire of children to have smaller animals, which would increase the likelihood of exposure to the pathogen.
- Chelonians rarely develop salmonellosis; however, when it does occur presentation appears similar to that in other reptiles, including enteritis, focal abscesses, and osteomyelitis.

ETIOLOGY/PATHOPHYSIOLOGY

- Anaerobic, Gram-negative, straight rods, flagellated.
- Species: *Salmonella enterica* and *S. bongori*
- Subspecies: *S. enterica* [1], *salamae* [II], *arizonae* [IIIa], *diarizonae* [IIIb], *houtenae* [IV], and *indica* [VI].
- Reptile patients often are infected with *S. arizonae* [IIIa] and *diarizonae* [IIIb].
- Serovars: 2,637 extant serovars, determined by phenotype of the O (somatic) and H (flagellar) antigens. Common serovars identified in chelonians include Newport, Poona, Saint-Paul, Typhimurium, Pomona, and Rubislaw. It is not uncommon to have multiple serotypes in the same chelonian.
- The prevalence of *Salmonella* spp. in wild and captive chelonians can vary between 0% and 100%.
- Captive-raised animals have a higher prevalence because of stocking densities leading to increased exposure, and hygiene practices.
- The low prevalence reported in wild chelonians may be associated with the sampling method; single samples are typically collected for prevalence studies and may misclassify animals due to intermittent shedding.
- The epidemiology of *Salmonella* infection in chelonians has been evaluated using the red-eared slider turtle (*Trachemys scripta elegans*) as a model. Red-eared sliders raised at breeding farms were found to be exposed through both horizontal and vertical routes of transmission.
- Horizontal transmission can occur via contaminated sources of food and water. This was one of the concerns with turtles housed in bowls during the 1960s and 1970s. Children would become exposed to *Salmonella* when they placed their hands into the aquatic habitat of their turtle.
- Vertical transmission is likely at the level of the follicle (*Salmonella* spp. has been isolated from the ovary of red-eared sliders) and during egg deposition; exposure during egg deposition is likely more common.
- The first eggs being oviposited are exposed through the cloaca, while the other eggs are exposed during incubation or after the hatchlings ingest the eggshells.
- Egg washing with non-antibiotic drugs (e.g., bleach, polyhexamethylene biguanide) can reduce the prevalence of *Salmonella* spp. to less than 1% in hatchling turtles.
- While research has primarily focused on aquatic turtles, tortoises should also be considered *Salmonella* spp. positive.
- Clients should not allow their pet chelonians to roam free in their house or place them on countertops or other surfaces that they can contaminate.
- It is important for clients to wash their hands after each exposure to their pet chelonian, as cases of reptile-associated salmonellosis in infants are typically associated with indirect contamination via parents or caretakers.

SIGNALMENT/HISTORY

Because many of the cases of chelonian-associated salmonellosis are from latent carriers, all animals should be considered *Salmonella* spp. positive.

CLINICAL PRESENTATION

- Chelonians that are carriers of *Salmonella* spp. typically appear healthy on physical examination or present for another illness.
- Those presenting with primary salmonellosis may show lethargy, anorexia or hyporexia, and diarrhea.
- Because *Salmonella* spp. can enter systemic circulation by ascending through the bile duct system, multisystemic disease, such as abscesses and shell lesions, can develop.

RISK FACTORS

Husbandry

- Inappropriate husbandry conditions can potentiate the likelihood of infection for conspecifics and the human caretakers of chelonians.
- Environmental temperatures should be appropriate for the species, as low or high temperatures can lead to stress and the potential for increased shedding of the organism.
- In aquatic habitats, water should be changed regularly as high organic loads can increase the potential growth of *Salmonella* spp.
- For tortoises, substrate should also be replaced regularly to minimize organic build-up.
- Animal density and mixing of chelonians can increase stress levels and *Salmonella* spp. shedding.
- Routine cleaning and disinfection of a chelonian's enclosure is necessary to prevent dissemination of *Salmonella* spp.

Others

- Confiscated or imported animals have an increased risk associated with clinical illness and zoonotic potential because of the increased likelihood of shedding *Salmonella* spp.
- Shipping, overcrowding and suboptimal husbandry conditions can lead to stress, infection or increased shedding of *Salmonella* spp.

DIAGNOSIS

DIFFERENTIAL DIAGNOSIS

- Enteritis (other species of *Enterobacteriaceae*)
- Renal disease
- Liver disease
- Primary and secondary bacterial infections.
- Fungal infections
- Neoplasia
- Osteomyelitis (shell lesions)

DIAGNOSTICS

- Microbiological culture of a gastrointestinal sample or abscess can be used to confirm the presence of *Salmonella* spp.
- Positive fecal cultures in clinically normal animals are not uncommon.
- These animals should not be treated for *Salmonella* spp., as this can lead to the development of antimicrobial resistance.
- Culture of *Salmonella* spp. requires special consideration, as the organism can be outcompeted by other *Enterobacteriaceae* under standard culture methods.
- It is important to specifically request a *Salmonella* culture from your diagnostic laboratory if the organism is suspected.
- Enrichment with selenite or tetrathionate is required. Samples are then plated onto specific agars such as XLD, SS Agar, or XLT-4 Agar. XLD and XLT-4 agars have a hydrogen sulfide indicator system to detect lactose fermenting *Salmonella* spp.

• Factors that influence the reliability of culture include the collection method, quantity and/or type of sample collected, temporal variation in shedding, and culture methods. Time to perform culture can delay appropriate antimicrobial therapy and control/mitigation procedures.
• PCR testing can be used to confirm the presence of *Salmonella* spp. in a sample. This test is considered more sensitive than culture and provides faster turnaround times. One limitation of PCR is that it cannot provide an antibiotic sensitivity profile to guide treatment.
• Parallel testing with PCR and culture is recommended to increase the sensitivity of the testing methods.
• Complete blood counts can be used to confirm an inflammatory leukogram or toxic changes that might occur with salmonellosis.
• Radiography can be used to examine the coelomic cavity for organomegaly and bony structures for osteomyelitis.
• Ultrasound can be used to improve visualization of the coelomic organs.
• Fine-needle aspiration of coelomic fluid and cytologic review of the sample can be used to confirm the presence of Gram-negative bacteria and inflammatory cells.

PATHOLOGICAL FINDINGS

• *Salmonella* spp. are commonly isolated from the gastrointestinal tract of chelonians on postmortem examinations as an incidental finding.
• Chelonian that have clinical salmonellosis will have typical inflammatory signs associated with the pathogen causing an enteritis, osteomyelitis, or systemic infection.

TREATMENT

APPROPRIATE HEALTH CARE

• Chelonians that are clinically normal and not showing signs of disease should never be treated for salmonellosis. Treating animals that are latent carriers could potentiate antimicrobial resistance.
• Animals that are clinically affected by *Salmonella* spp. should only be treated if an antibiotic sensitivity profile is available. This will help to minimize the likelihood of resistance.
• Some clinicians elect to not treat affected animals with antibiotics but instead provide supportive care and allow the infection to run its course.

NUTRITIONAL SUPPORT

• Nutritional support should be implemented in patients that have concurrent weight loss, hyporexia, or anorexia; however, fluid support should be provided first to ensure that the gastrointestinal tract is functioning properly.
• In animals with diarrhea, nutritional support can exacerbate the diarrhea.
• Assist-feeding can support the daily nutritional requirements of these patients with a highly digestible diet, which should be based on the species life history and nutritional requirements of the species.

CLIENT EDUCATION/HUSBANDRY RECOMMENDATIONS

• Clients should be educated on the risks of keeping chelonians and provided with information on the most appropriate husbandry and sanitation procedures.
• Owners should be made aware that it is not recommended to allow their pet to free roam in their household. This can serve as a source of indirect exposure for children.
• To minimize the zoonotic potential of chelonians, it is important to practice strict hygiene and biosecurity.
• Hand washing with soap and warm water is one of the simplest and most effective methods of eliminating exposure to *Salmonella* spp.
• Individuals handling these animals or any part of their captive habitat should wash their hands thoroughly after working with them.
• Clients should be made aware of the importance of making regular water changes for their pet turtles. The water removed from the enclosures should be discarded outside or down a toilet. It should never be discarded down a sink used for cooking or cleaning food or where water is obtained for drinking or a bathtub.
• The enclosure and its contents should be cleaned outside, if at all possible, and never in an area where food or drink is prepared.
• Separate washing receptacles, such as a plastic container, are recommended.
• Dilute bleach solution can be used to clean the environment and food and water bowls; it is important that the client rinse these thoroughly to minimize the potential for bleach toxicity.

MEDICATIONS

DRUG(S) OF CHOICE

• As with any bacterial disease, therapy should be driven by culture and sensitivity testing in addition to mean inhibitory concentration, target plasma concentration, and volume of distribution of the medication.
• *Salmonella* spp. isolated from chelonians are typically susceptible to the following antibiotics:
  ◦ Ceftazidime 22 mg/kg IM q72h
  ◦ Amikacin 5 mg/kg IM q48h
  ◦ Enrofloxacin 5–10 mg/kg IM, PO q24–48h
  ◦ Oxytetracycline 42 mg/kg IM q6d

PRECAUTIONS/INTERACTIONS

N/A

FOLLOW-UP

PATIENT MONITORING

• Serial culture and PCR testing can be done to monitor the *Salmonella* spp. status and antimicrobial sensitivity profile of a patient or captive population of chelonians.
• Serial complete blood counts to monitor responses to treatment.
• Repeat radiographs to monitor for progression or resolution of osseous lesions.

EXPECTED COURSE AND PROGNOSIS

• Chelonians diagnosed with salmonellosis from culture or PCR and without clinical signs may not require any intervention.
• Many chelonians test positive for *Salmonella* spp.; however, these are often latent carriers and do not show signs of disease.
• Additionally, animals that test negative for *Salmonella* spp. on a single test may still be positive because intermittent shedding is common.
• Overall prognosis for recovery from salmonellosis is good to fair according to severity of disease and level of supportive care.

MISCELLANEOUS

COMMENTS

N/A

ZOONOTIC POTENTIAL

• *S. enterica* zoonotic infections linked to aquatic turtles have been considered an important source of human illness since the 1960s.
• Federal regulations established in 1975 that restrict the sale of turtles less than 10.2 cm remain in place today.
• These restrictions have not limited their zoonotic potential. From 2006 to 2014, 15 multistate outbreaks of turtle-associated salmonellosis were reported within the United States. These outbreaks accounted for 921 illnesses, 156 hospitalizations, and the death of an infant.
• Chelonians continue to serve as a source of reptile-associated salmonellosis for humans.
• Because these animals serve as reservoirs and latent carriers of *Salmonella* spp., clients are often unaware as to the risks associated with maintaining these animals as pets.

SALMONELLOSIS (CONTINUED)

- It is important to recognize that these animals may also serve as a potential source of infection to the veterinary staff working with them or that the treatment used (e.g., antibiotics) could alter the pathogenicity of the *Salmonella* sp.

SYNONYMS

- Salmonella infection
- Typhoid fever

ABBREVIATIONS

- PCR = polymerase chain reaction
- SS = Salmonella–Shigella
- XLD = xylose lysine deoxycholate
- XLT-4 = xylose lysine Tergitol 4

INTERNET RESOURCES

- Center for Food Security and Public Health. Reptile Associated Salmonellosis. January 2013.http://www.cfsph.iastate.edu/DiseaseInfo/factsheets.php
- Association of Reptile and Amphibian Veterinarians: http://www.ARAV.org

Suggested Reading

Bosch S, Tauxe R, Behravesh C. Turtle-associated salmonellosis, United States, 2006–2014. *Emerg Infect Dis* 2016;22(7):1149–1155.

Clancy MM, Davis M, Valitutto MT, et al. Salmonella infection and carriage in reptiles in a zoological collection. *J Am Vet Med Assoc* 2016;248(9):1050–1059.

Gray TZ. Update: reptiles and salmonella. *J Exot Pet Med* 2011;20(1):14–17.

Author Sean M. Perry, DVM, PhD, and Mark A. Mitchell, DVM, MS, PhD, DECZM (Herpetology)

SAPROLEGNIASIS

BASICS

DEFINITION/OVERVIEW

Saprolegniasis refers to mycosis caused by several species of aquatic oomycetous fungi (water molds). The genus *Saprolegnia* is most often associated with this condition. Saprolegniasis can affect a wide range of freshwater chelonians.

ETIOLOGY/PATHOPHYSIOLOGY

- *Saprolegnia* species are typically opportunistic pathogens of traumatized or devitalized tissue.
- They are primitive fungi with a complex life cycle that includes flagellated zoospores.
- Infection is usually superficial.
- Primary or secondary bacterial infection may be present.

SIGNALMENT/HISTORY

- Most *Saprolegnia* species thrive in cold, stagnant water.
- Infections can be found in aquatic chelonians.

CLINICAL PRESENTATION

- A white, cottony film or fuzzy growth over open lesions or the shell is suggestive of saprolegniasis.
- The cottony film is the mycelium, which may become grayish or greenish as debris and algae become entrapped in the mycelial mat.
- Fungal growth usually collapses when removed from water.
- Rare systemic infection

RISK FACTORS

- Water molds are primarily opportunists; they often infect open wounds.
- Water temperature is an important factor in the development of saprolegniasis as its incidence rate decreases at water temperatures higher than 19 degrees C (68 degrees F).

Husbandry

- Environmental and husbandry co-factors can be very important in the development of saprolegniasis.
- Low environmental temperatures (< 20 degrees C) enhances the growth of fungus.
- High environmental organic loads may be a predisposing factor.
- Poor water quality (ammonia) can lead to stress and immunosuppression, facilitating infection.

Others

N/A

DIAGNOSIS

DIFFERENTIAL DIAGNOSIS

Other oomycetes

DIAGNOSTICS

- Characteristic appearance of white to tan cotton-like material that covers skin or shell ulcers.
- Microscopic examination of wet mounts from a skin scraping will confirm the diagnosis; may see branching non-septate hyphae and zoospores (flagellated oospore).

PATHOLOGICAL FINDINGS

- The characteristic gross appearance of white to tan cotton-like material covering skin ulcers is best appreciated when viewing the affected animal under water.
- Infections can occur anywhere; shell or skin may be affected.

TREATMENT

APPROPRIATE HEALTH CARE

- Underlying causes such as substandard water quality, inter- or intraspecies aggression, or bacterial disease should be corrected.
- Elevation of water temperatures may also be useful if the patient can tolerate the higher water temperature.
- Correction of predisposing factors is essential.

NUTRITIONAL SUPPORT

N/A

CLIENT EDUCATION/HUSBANDRY RECOMMENDATIONS

- Aquatic turtles kept under inappropriate husbandry (i.e., overcrowding and poor water quality) may be prone to saprolegniasis.
- Proper nutrition, sanitation, stock density, and water quality are essential for the prevention of saprolegniasis.
- Adequate basking areas where the turtle can get out of the water will minimize the risk of saprolegniasis.

MEDICATIONS

DRUG(S) OF CHOICE

- Chlorhexidine, 0.05% solution
- Povidone-iodine, 0.05% solution
- Scrub the affected area with disinfectant once or twice daily; keep the animal out of water for 20–30 minutes after treatment.
- Lesions usually resolve within a few days after starting topical treatment.
- Treat any underlying conditions (i.e., lacerations/abrasions) as necessary.

PRECAUTIONS/INTERACTIONS

N/A

FOLLOW-UP

PATIENT MONITORING

- Effective treatment will eliminate the "cottony" growth on the affected area which can be assessed visually.
- Return to normal behavior is expected after resolution of lesions.

EXPECTED COURSE AND PROGNOSIS

- Prognosis is good to excellent for localized infections.
- Prognosis is greatly enhanced by correcting any husbandry deficiencies that may be contributing to the disease.

MISCELLANEOUS

COMMENTS

N/A

ZOONOTIC POTENTIAL

N/A

SYNONYMS

- Cotton wool disease
- Water mold

INTERNET RESOURCES

Saprolegnia. Science Direct. https://www.sciencedirect.com/topics/veterinary-science-and-veterinary-medicine/saprolegnia

Suggested Reading

Mader DR, ed. *Reptile Medicine and Surgery*, 2nd ed. St Louis, MO: Elsevier Saunders; 2006.

Author Sam Rivera, DVM, MS, DABVP (Avian), DACZM, DECZM (Zoo Health Management)

SEPTICEMIC CUTANEOUS ULCERATIVE DISEASE (SCUD)

BASICS

DEFINITION/OVERVIEW

SCUD is a syndrome that primarily affects aquatic turtles. First described in 1957, this term is still in use today; however, a more accurate description would be carapacial/plastral osteomyelitis. Underlying factors associated with this disease are inappropriate husbandry practices such as poor water quality, overcrowding, temperature extremes, and trauma. Ultimately, immunosuppression permits overwhelming bacterial infection, including sepsis, culminating in high morbidity and mortality.

ETIOLOGY/PATHOPHYSIOLOGY

- Although over the years specific bacteria have been identified as etiologic agents (i.e., *Citrobacter freundii*, *Beneckea chitinovora*), this syndrome is now considered to be associated with a variety of bacteria that are classified as opportunistic pathogens (i.e., *Morganella morganii*, *Aeromonas hydrophila*, *Serratia* spp. and *Bacteroides* spp.).
- In the past, *B. chitinovora*, a common infectious agent of crustaceans, has been implicated as a primary pathogen in SCUD; hence, the feeding of crayfish to aquatic turtles is discouraged.
- Opportunistic pathogens are a component of normal environmental microbiota including the reptilian gastrointestinal tract.
- Under appropriate conditions mentioned above, these microorganisms become invasive and capable of causing disease in immunosuppressed animals.
- Commonly, there is a break in the integrity of the epidermis secondary to trauma.
- High bacterial concentrations that are present in fecal-contaminated water then gain entrance to the body.
- Anorexia, lethargy, and petechial hemorrhages of the shell and skin are seen.
- This is followed by circular lesions forming between the scutes and dermis.
- Scutes become ulcerated and may slough with an underlying purulent discharge.
- In advanced cases sepsis and organ failure (liver, kidneys) occur.

SIGNALMENT/HISTORY

- SCUD can be encountered in freshwater turtles of any age.
- Affected turtles commonly present with a history of anorexia and lethargy.
- Anamnesis includes poor husbandry practices such as improper temperatures, inadequate nutrition, poor water quality, lack of a dry basking area, overcrowding with other turtles, abrasive cage furniture and lack of UVB light.

CLINICAL PRESENTATION

- Skin and shell lesions are readily visualized.
- Initially, epidermal vesicles can be present eventually progressing to pustules and ulcerations.
- Heavily keratinized structures such as the rhamphothecae, scutes, and claws may loosen and slough exposing underlying muscle and bone.
- Commonly, the shell will be ulcerated and hemorrhagic.
- Deeper ulcerations can penetrate bone and expose the coelomic cavity.
- A foul odor may accompany the osteomyelitis.
- If sepsis has occurred, petechiae and ecchymoses may be visible on the shell and skin.

RISK FACTORS

- Environmental stressors secondary to inappropriate husbandry practices include poor water quality, suboptimal temperatures, overcrowding, lack of basking areas, abrasive cage furniture, conspecific aggression, and absence of UVB lighting.
- Immunosuppression of affected individuals plays a large role.

Husbandry

N/A

Others

N/A

DIAGNOSIS

DIFFERENTIAL DIAGNOSIS

- Severe dermal mineralization associated with RSHP.
- Shell deformities associated with NSHP.
- Thermal burns
- Dysecdysis
- Neoplasia

DIAGNOSTICS

- Diagnosis is based upon history and clinical signs.
- All bony lesions should be gently probed and checked for depth and osteolysis.
- Microbiological (bacterial and fungal) samples should be harvested from deeper sites after debridement of superficial lesions.
- Biopsy of affected areas is important for bacterial culture/sensitivities and confirmation of diagnosis.
- Radiography (three orthogonal views) and hematology/plasma biochemical analysis are recommended.
- Leukocytosis is common and renal status should be evaluated by assessment of calcium, phosphorus and urea/uric acid values.
- If sepsis is suspected, blood cultures may be indicated.

PATHOLOGICAL FINDINGS

- Grossly, hemorrhagic and ulcerative lesions are observed on the carapace and plastron.
- Histologically, lesions are characterized by bacterial colonization of the keratin, dermis and bone.
- There is accompanying infiltration with heterophils and inflammatory cells.
- Osteolysis secondary to increased osteoclast activity leads to fibrosis of bones.

TREATMENT

APPROPRIATE HEALTH CARE

- Quarantine of individual animals to be maintained in optimal conditions (daily water changes, dry docking on moistened paper towels for 4–6 hours/day to encourage desiccation and granulation formation of lesions, proper temperatures and exposure to UVB light.
- Debridement of deeper lesions while animals are under sedation/anesthesia and with analgesics.
- Weekly rechecks should be done with continued debridement as required.

NUTRITIONAL SUPPORT

- Nutrition is critical for convalescence.
- If the patient has been anorexic for several days to weeks, assist-tube feeding or an esophagostomy tube should be used for administration of critical care diets and/or medications.

CLIENT EDUCATION/HUSBANDRY RECOMMENDATIONS

- Adhere to strict guidelines regarding quarantine of new acquisitions.
- Use appropriate mechanical filtration systems, with complete water changes at appropriate intervals (every 2–4 weeks at a minimum).
- Feed individual animals outside of the community enclosure.
- Avoid sharp cage furniture (abrasive rocks) and examine all animals daily for abrasions, skin discoloration and shell lesions.

MEDICATIONS

DRUG(S) OF CHOICE

- Appropriate analgesics such as NSAIDS (meloxacam at 0.2–0.5 mg/kg IM/SC q24–48h).
- Narcotics (hydromorphone 0.5 mg/kg IM q24h, tramadol 5–10 mg/kg PO, SC q24h)
- Appropriate systemic antibiotics based upon culture and sensitivities.
- Topical antibacterials (chlorhexidine, silver sulfadiazine, betadine)

• Note that if empiric antimicrobial treatment is chosen, the use of "four quadrant" antibiotics is recommended (piperacillin at 100 mg/kg IM q24h, ceftazidime at 20 mg/kg IM q72h combined with enrofloxacin at 5 mg/kg IM, PO q48h, amikacin at 5 mg/kg loading dose followed by 2.5 mg/kg IM q72h or enrofloxacin combined with metronidazole at 20 mg/kg PO q24h).

PRECAUTIONS/INTERACTIONS

• Penicillins, aminoglycosides and fluoroquinolones should be used with caution in reptiles that have compromised renal and hepatic function.
• Antiseptic soaks such as betadine and chlorhexidine may be toxic if ingested.

FOLLOW-UP

PATIENT MONITORING

• Affected animals should be rechecked every 1–2 weeks preferably with a "hands on" examination.
• Debriding should be done as needed.
• If rechecking is not feasible, pictures can be sent by the owner to the veterinarian for appraisal until healing is progressing in a positive manner.

EXPECTED COURSE AND PROGNOSIS

• Prognosis depends on chronicity and severity of lesions and any underlying organ function.
• Treatment may take several weeks to months before healing is observed.
• Extensive scar formation associated with osteomyelitis should be expected.

MISCELLANEOUS

COMMENTS

• Two types of SCUD have been described: the "wet" form described above; and the "dry" form characterized by the presence of dry white patches on the carapace and plastron. In the author's opinion, the so-called "dry" form is not a variation of SCUD but rather dysecdysis associated with unshed scutes. The combination of desiccation from basking and rehydration from immersion causes contraction and expansion of the older superficial scutes, which consequently aids in ecdysis. Hence, turtles that are either continuously immersed in water or continuously basking are prone to this problem. Mineral oil or a similar emollient can be applied to the affected areas and 12–24 hours later the affected scutes can be gently lifted using a small spatula.
• Figures 5, 6 and 7 – see web image supplementary content for Section II (Chelonians).

ZOONOTIC POTENTIAL

• Potential zoonosis from opportunistic pathogens is a possibility particularly if the handler has breaks in the skin.
• Latex examination gloves should be worn when handling affected turtles.

SYNONYMS

• Carapacial/plastral osteomyelitis
• Shell rot

ABBREVIATIONS

• IM = intramuscular
• NSAIDs = nonsteroidal anti-inflammatory drugs
• NSHP = nutritional secondary hyperparathyroidism
• PO = per os
• RSHP = renal secondary hyperparathyroidism
• SC = subcutaneous
• SCUD = septicemic ulcerative cutaneous disease
• UVB = ultraviolet B

INTERNET RESOURCES

• Ma, V. Red-Eared Slider Care Sheet. *Reptiles Magazine*, November 7, 2013. www.reptilesmagazine.com/Red-Eared-Slider-Care-Sheet
• Divers SJ. Parasitic Diseases of Reptiles. MSD Manual Veterinary Manual, June 2020. https://www.msdvetmanual.com/en-gb/exotic-and-laboratory-animals/reptiles/parasitic-diseases-of-reptiles

Suggested Reading

McArthur S, Wilkinson R, Meyer J, eds. *Medicine and Surgery of Tortoises and Turtles*. Ames, IA: Blackwell; 2004.
Zych J, Hnizdo J, eds. *Medical Care of Turtles and Tortoises: Diagnosis, Surgery, Pathology, Parasitology*. Frankfurt, Germany: Edition Chimaira; 2011.

Author Paul Raiti, DVM, DABVP (Reptile and Amphibian Practice)

SHELL FRACTURES

BASICS

DEFINITION/OVERVIEW

Fractures of the shell are any fractures of the carapace, plastron, or bridge of chelonians. This is a common presentation in both captive and free-ranging animals.

ETIOLOGY/PATHOPHYSIOLOGY

- Shell fractures are almost always traumatic in origin, but pathologic fractures due to underlying NSHP may also occur.
- The anatomy of the shell consists of an exterior layer of beta keratin forming the scutes, which are attached to the bone itself through dermal connective tissue.

SIGNALMENT/HISTORY

- No sex, age, or species predilection.
- May be more common during reproductive season when wild chelonians are more prone to crossing roads or getting closer to shore.

CLINICAL PRESENTATION

- Animals present with complete or incomplete fractures of the shell and exposed body membranes or organs.
- Some may be missing bone fragments that cannot be reattached.
- Most animals present in a stable condition, despite severe injuries that may expose internal organs.
- In severe or chronic cases, the chelonian may present obtunded due to shock, anemia, dehydration, and/or septicemia.

RISK FACTORS

The primary risk factors for traumatic fractures are simply being dropped by a handler, exposure to vehicles on roads, exposure to boats and boat propellers, dog bites, and any situation that puts the animal in contact with machinery (e.g., lawn mowers) that can traumatize the shell.

Husbandry

Inadequate UVB light exposure, calcium supplementation, and nutrition are contributing factors to NSHP, which in turn can lead to pathologic fractures or can make it easier for traumatic fractures to occur.

Others

N/A

DIAGNOSIS

Diagnosis is based on gross observation of the fractures.

DIFFERENTIAL DIAGNOSIS

- NSHP
- RSHP
- Trauma

DIAGNOSTICS

- Radiography to evaluate all the bones in the body to determine the extent of the fractures, coelomic involvement and whether NSHP may be an underlying factor.
- Bacterial culture and sensitivity in cases when there is a large amount of organic matter within the fracture line, body tissues, or cavity.
- Baseline blood work (CBC, chemistry panel) to establish the current condition of the animal and to monitor response to therapy.

PATHOLOGICAL FINDINGS

- Fractured shell with compression or collapse of fragments.
- Hemorrhage, inflammation, and maggots may also be present.

TREATMENT

APPROPRIATE HEALTH CARE

- The goal of treatment is stabilization, pain control, and allowing time for healing.
- Infection is a common sequela, since the shell is exposed to the environment.
- If bone fragments are missing, most animals will develop a membrane that will seal the defect but this may leave the area more susceptible to future trauma such as attacks by predators.
- It is important to recognize that this membrane may take on a yellow to pigmented coloration which must not be confused with necrosis. If there is no foul-smelling odor from the wound, it is likely to be part of the normal healing process.
- Any bone defects with exposed membranes/tissues should be treated as an open wound (copiously lavaged and treated with bandaging) until it is clean and not infected before attempting to close over the defect.
- Shell fractures can be repaired with any material that allows reduction of the fracture fragments and/or stabilization of collapsed segments.
- Metal screws, wire, plates and plastic fasteners are among the most common materials used. Many can be purchased at a hardware store and sterilized at the veterinary clinic.
- The equipment and materials are really only limited by the veterinarian's imagination.

Wound Care

- Any open wounds with exposed tissues must be thoroughly cleaned to get rid of any infection.
- Wet-to-dry bandages are still very effective at removing organic debris from the area.
- Sugar, honey, and hypertonic saline are also effective in the acute stages of wound cleaning and healing. However, these products can quickly dry out the tissues and must not be left in place for more than 6–12 hours at a time.
- The author routinely places a wet-to-dry bandage with sugar or hypertonic saline in the morning that is the replaced with a wet bandage in the evening to prevent drying of tissues.
- Frequency and products used should be determined based on the tissue appearance and viability.
- Product selection is ultimately based on what is available and the veterinarian's experience in working with them.
- Another technique that works well is vacuum-assisted closure. This technique has been described in chelonians and can help to speed up the healing process. It must be noted that it can be painful/uncomfortable in humans and so proper analgesia should be considered when using this technique.
- Once a wound is healed, there is the option to either leave the healed membrane exposed or seal the area with an epoxy or similar material.
- Some do not advocate sealing these wounds due to the risks of developing infection under the material. However, in some instances, such as aquatic chelonians, this is the best option to ensure that the animal can be placed back in the water.
- For desert species living in high humidity environments, leaving the area exposed can create a nidus for infections.
- Using a clear epoxy or acrylic and performing routine health evaluations of captive animals can help to monitor the wound and ensure that no infection is occurring.
- For animals being released to the wild, each veterinarian must make a decision based on the type of wound and the species.
- In the author's experience, sealing a healed, clean wound is the best option to avoid contamination of the area. The caveat is that the edges must be sealed properly to ensure that they are watertight.

Fracture Repair

- A combination of screws and wire can be used to achieve the desired reduction of the fractures and replace bone fragments.
- The screws must be fully seeded within the bone but trying to not penetrate the coelomic cavity.
- Wire can be either passed around the head of the screws or through holes drilled through the shell.
- Sometimes full-thickness drilling is necessary to pass wire through the carapace or plastron, even if it penetrates the coelomic cavity.

• Drill-hole and wire entry points can be sealed as needed with bone wax, epoxy, dental acrylic or any other material that has lo exothermal reaction.

Plastic Fasteners/Cable Ties

• There is a wide array of plastic fasteners that can be glued onto the shell itself and used to reduce fractures.
• These are inexpensive and do not require drilling into the bone.
• The scute should be sanded before gluing to ensure a tight grip. Nonetheless, this technique may be prone to failure in high-tension areas.
• There are a wide variety of products such as epoxy, fiberglass, and dental acrylics that can be used as primary (fissures and incomplete fracture) or supportive material for fracture repair.
• These products must have low exothermic reaction during the curing process to avoid thermal damage to the keratin and dermal tissue.

NUTRITIONAL SUPPORT

• Dietary deficiencies must be corrected with special emphasis on UVB light and oral calcium supplementation.
• Placement of an esophagostomy tube in anorexic animals or those requiring long-term oral therapy is recommended.

CLIENT EDUCATION/HUSBANDRY RECOMMENDATIONS

• Correct any husbandry deficiencies with emphasis on UVB light and calcium supplementation. Owners and caretakers must be committed to comply with therapy and follow-up visits until healing has occurred.
• Before cutting grass, all animals must be accounted for and the yard surveyed to ensure that there are no buried animals that could be traumatized by the lawnmower.
• Outdoor enclosures must be predator proof.

MEDICATIONS

DRUG(S) OF CHOICE

• Meloxicam 0.5 mg/kg PO, IM, SC q24–48h
• Opioids (hydromorphone 0.2–0.5 mg/kg IM, SC q12–24h, morphine 1–10 mg/kg IM, SC q24h
• Lidocaine 1 : 1 to 1 : 5 dilution of lidocaine to sterile saline (can be used as a splash for analgesia over exposed membranes and on the edges of fractures).

PRECAUTIONS/INTERACTIONS

• Morphine and hydromorphone can cause sedation and respiratory depression.
• Dose and frequency of administration should be refined based on the patient's response.
• Bandages with hypertonic products must not be left in place for longer than 6–12 hours to avoid desiccation of tissues.

FOLLOW-UP

PATIENT MONITORING

• The chelonian must be monitored daily for development of any foul odors, which may be indicative of infection.
• Urination and defecation must be recorded to ensure that no neurologic damage has occurred affecting the animal's ability to urinate or defecate.

EXPECTED COURSE AND PROGNOSIS

• Most fractures have excellent to good prognosis as long as the integrity of the shell can be preserved.
• If the fractures are such that the shell's integrity is compromised to the point that it collapses into the cavity, or there is spinal trauma, then prognosis is guarded to grave.
• Chelonians are very resilient and can overcome even the most aggressive of shell fractures as long as they can be housed and cared for the required convalescent time which is a minimum of 6–9 months for fracture stabilization and up to 2 years for complete fracture healing.
• Exposed tissues with missing bone over the area will typically heal within 6-8 weeks.

MISCELLANEOUS

COMMENTS

N/A

ZOONOTIC POTENTIAL

N/A

SYNONYMS

N/A

ABBREVIATIONS

• CBC = complete blood count
• IM = intramuscular
• NSHP = nutritional secondary hyperparathyroidism
• PO = per os
• RSHP = renal secondary hyperparathyroidism
• SC = subcutaneous
• UVB = ultraviolet B

Suggested Reading

Chitty J, Raftery A. Fractures of the shell. In: Chitty J, Raftery A, eds. *Essentials of Tortoise Medicine and Surgery*. Oxford, UK: Wiley Blackwell; 2003:403–464.

Lafortune M, Wellehan JFX, Haerd DJ, et al. Vacuum-assisted closure (Turtle VAC) in the management of traumatic shell defects in chelonians. *J Herp Med Surg* 2005;15(4):4–8.

McArthur S, Hernandez-Divers S. Surgery; Shell trauma. In: Stuart McArthur, Roger Wilkinson, and Jean Meyer, eds. *Medicine and Surgery of Turtles and Tortoises*. Ames, IA: Blackwell; 2004:441–447.

Author Javier G. Nevarez, DVM, PhD, DACZM, DECZM (Herpetology)

SQUAMOUS CELL CARCINOMA

BASICS

DEFINITION/OVERVIEW

SCCs are malignant epithelial cell tumors, most commonly associated with cutaneous or mucocutaneous regions of the body. SCCs are most commonly found on the skin or associated with oropharyngeal tissues. They tend to be well differentiated, with some evidence of local infiltration of adjacent tissues and limited evidence of metastatic behavior. SCCs are not uncommon in reptile species, and have been identified in a variety of chelonians.

ETIOLOGY/PATHOPHYSIOLOGY

- An underlying cause of SCCs in reptiles is unknown.
- Published hypotheses with respect to risk factors and etiology include those based on mammalian or avian examples: overexposure to ultraviolet radiation, including exposure at higher altitudes, light skin color, chronic hypovitaminosis A, and possibly chronic viral infections.
- There is no evidence that any of these risk factors are associated with reptile SCCs.
- No viruses have been associated with SCCs in reptiles.
- Most reptile SCCs are locally invasive, but not associated with metastatic behavior.
- Two free-ranging, stranded, loggerhead sea turtles were found to have SCCs of the skin with metastasis in the lungs, liver, and myocardium of one sea turtle, and in the lungs, liver, and kidneys of the second turtle.

SIGNALMENT/HISTORY

- In the reptile neoplasia literature, there is no clear predisposition with respect to species or sex.
- There may be an association between the presence of SCCs and increasing age of the reptile, but this has not been evaluated systematically.
- Historically, reptiles diagnosed with SCC are observed to have a focal mass or masses anywhere on the skin, within the oral cavity or at other mucocutaneous junctions.
- The raised tissue may become hemorrhagic, ulcerative and/or necrotic.
- With chronicity, bacterial abscessation may develop within or in close association with the tumor.
- Most commonly, the neoplastic cells invade adjacent tissues.
- Depending on the site of the tumor, the animal may become hyporexic/anorexic, exhibit a depressed attitude, and/or favor a limb/eye or other anatomical sites that may be involved.
- If the eyes are involved, vision may become impaired and the animal may, uncharacteristically, fall from cage furniture or not be able to find food.

CLINICAL PRESENTATION

- The clinical signs may be somewhat variable depending on the anatomic locations of the mass.
- Discrete skin lesions tend to appear raised, with erythema, hemorrhage, and/or ulceration, or appear as chronic nonhealing wounds.
- If the lesions involve the digits, there may be more diffuse swelling and some degree of lameness.
- With SCCs of the oropharynx, hyporexia or anorexia may be present, in addition to masticatory dysfunction and mild oral hemorrhage.

RISK FACTORS

Husbandry

- Purely hypothetical risk factors in reptiles are based on mammalian or avian risk factors.
- In the case of husbandry, hypovitaminosis A or excessive ultraviolet light exposure could be predisposing risk factors but there is no evidence documenting a link between these factors and SCCs.

Others

N/A

DIAGNOSIS

DIFFERENTIAL DIAGNOSIS

- Bacterial abscesses
- Fungal granulomas (especially *Chrysosporium* species)
- Viral papillomatous lesions
- Chronic traumatic wounds with fibrosis.
- Cloacal prolapse
- Other neoplastic diseases (e.g., melanomas, fibrosarcomas, cutaneous papillomas, fibropapillomas, lipomas, spindle-cell sarcomas, and chromatophormas)

DIAGNOSTICS

- Histopathology of the lesion is the gold standard for diagnosis, through complete surgical excision or biopsy of the mass.
- A fine-needle aspirate with cytologic evaluation may or may not be diagnostic.
- Imaging modalities, such as radiography or CT may be helpful in detecting local soft tissue or bone involvement.
- Contrast CT may be useful when trying to evaluate for metastases.

PATHOLOGICAL FINDINGS

- In domestic mammals, histologic subtypes of SCCs are typically described as poorly differentiated, moderately differentiated, or well differentiated.
- In general, SCCs are histopathologically characterized as round to polygonal-shaped cells with varying amounts of basophilic cytoplasm, and keratinization.
- The nuclei tend to be round, with significant variation in size and chromatin pattern, from coarsely stippled to pyknotic, and commonly with perinuclear vacuoles.
- Frequently, there is marked variation in nucleus to cytoplasmic ratio because the cells vary in degree of differentiation.
- In reptiles, the histologic description of SCC is similar. Typically, there are anastomosing cords and nests of polygonal cells with abundant eosinophilic cytoplasm, distinct intercellular bridges, and round to oval nuclei with finely stippled chromatin and multiple nucleoli, with occasional mitotic figures.
- Neoplastic cells are described as having differing levels of anisokaryosis, and frequently form circular keratinized foci consistent with keratin pearls and usually invade and/or replace adjacent tissues.

TREATMENT

APPROPRIATE HEALTH CARE

N/A

NUTRITIONAL SUPPORT

- Nonspecific nutritional support may include regular force-feeding of an appropriate commercial diet and/or placement of an esophagostomy tube to facilitate administering nutritional supplements.
- The directions on the label of the commercial diet can be followed for appropriate volume per feeding and frequency.

CLIENT EDUCATION/HUSBANDRY RECOMMENDATIONS

N/A

MEDICATIONS

DRUG(S) OF CHOICE

- There are no data demonstrating adverse effects of NSAIDs such as renal impairment and/or gastrointestinal bleeding.
- Surgical excision with histopathologic evidence of clean margins is the treatment of choice.
- In birds and mammals, focal SCCs have been treated with surgical debulking and intralesional platinum-based chemotherapeutic agents (e.g., cisplatin or carboplatin-impregnated beads).
- There is one report of electrochemotherapy using intratumoral administration of bleomycin followed by electric pulses in a yellow-bellied slider turtle.

- Antimicrobial drugs may be used as needed for secondary bacterial infections.
- NSAIDs may help with any discomfort, but there are no systematically derived data with respect to efficacy of NSAIDS in any reptile species.
- Depending on the species, meloxicam may be administered orally or subcutaneously (0.2–0.5 mg/kg).

PRECAUTIONS/INTERACTIONS

- With surgical excision of a SCC, recurrence should be considered and discussed with the owner.
- Should the owner elect intralesional chemotherapy, the possible outcomes include lack of therapeutic response, systemic absorption of the chemotherapeutic agent causing hyporexia/anorexia, depressed attitude, anemia or other blood cell changes, and necrosis of surrounding healthy tissues.

FOLLOW-UP

PATIENT MONITORING

- SCCs are likely to recur with incomplete surgical excision, and may recur regardless of complete surgical excision.
- There are a few documented cases of local tissue invasion and/or metastasis.
- The patient should be monitored for recurrence of the tumor, and contrast CT may be of some use in monitoring for local invasion or metastatic disease.
- If treatment is recommended and accepted by the owner (partial excision and intralesional chemotherapy or electrochemotherapy), the treatment site should be monitored for secondary microbial infection or self-trauma.
- The owner should be instructed to report any signs of skin discoloration, discharge, or dysfunction of the anatomical region of the original tumor.
- Because of possible systemic absorption of locally administered chemotherapeutic agents, a complete blood count and biochemical profile should be evaluated prior to the start of chemotherapy, and serially evaluated during and after the course of chemotherapy.

EXPECTED COURSE AND PROGNOSIS

- With complete surgical excision and clean tissue margins as evidenced by histopathology, the prognosis is good to guarded, with the possibility of recurrence.
- With recent published cases documenting metastatic disease, a guarded prognosis is wise until we know more about the behavior of SCCs across multiple reptile species.
- There may be some promising new intralesional chemotherapeutic techniques or refined radiation therapy techniques applied to future cases of SCCs in reptiles, which may improve prognostic factors.

MISCELLANEOUS

COMMENTS

N/A

ZOONOTIC POTENTIAL

N/A

SYNONYMS

N/A

ABBREVIATIONS

- CT = computed tomography
- NSAID = nonsteroidal anti-inflammatory drug
- SCC = squamous cell carcinoma

Suggested Reading

Christman J, Devau M, Wilson-Robles H, et al. Oncology of reptiles: Diseases, diagnosis, and treatment. *Vet Clin North Am Exot Anim Pract* 2017;20(1):87–110.

Lanza A, Baldi A, Spugnini EP. Surgery and electrochemotherapy for the treatment of cutaneous squamous cell carcinoma in a yellow-bellied slider (*Trachemys scripta scripta*). *J Am Vet Med Assoc* 2015;246(4):455–457.

Orós J, Tucker S, Fernández L, Jacobson ER. Metastatic squamous cell carcinoma in two loggerhead sea turtles (*Caretta caretta*). *Dis Aquat Org* 2004;58(2–3):245–250.

Sykes JM, Trupkiewicz JG. Reptile neoplasia at the Philadelphia Zoological Garden, 1901–2002. *J Zoo Wildl Med* 2006;37(1):11–19.

Author Kurt K. Sladky, MS, DVM, DACZM, DECZM (Zoo Health Management & Herpetology)

STOMATITIS

BASICS

DEFINITION/OVERVIEW

Stomatisis is inflammation of the soft tissues of the oral cavity, which may be caused by a local or systemic process.

ETIOLOGY/PATHOPHYSIOLOGY

- Immunosuppression or trauma can lead to bacterial or fungal colonization of oral tissues.
- Normal bacterial flora secondarily infect damaged oral tissue, particularly Gram-negative rods.
- Fungi—particularly *Candida* spp., *Penicillium* spp., *Aspergillus* spp. and *Mucor* spp.
- Systemic infections
- Adenovirus, herpesvirus, iridovirus
- Foreign objects—splinters, food debris, cactus spines, bedding material.
- Electric burns—biting electric cord
- Lacerations
- Prey injuries—bite or claw wounds from live prey; Injuries from sharp teeth or claws from previously frozen prey.
- Rough handling and damage of teeth and oral mucosa during physical examination
- Trauma during tong-feeding.
- Improper assisted feeding resulting in oral, pharyngeal or esophageal injuries.
- Vomiting and regurgitation may create mucosal defects in esophagus, pharynx or oral mucosa.
- Neoplasia
- NSHP can lead to mandibular swelling and exposure of oral mucosa.
- Hypovitaminosis A

SIGNALMENT/HISTORY

- No specific age, breed, sex predisposition.
- Animals with a history of poor husbandry, specifically inappropriate temperatures and hygiene.

CLINICAL PRESENTATION

- Anorexia, dysphagia
- Periorbital swelling, exophthalmos
- Nasal discharge and secondary tracheitis or pneumonia.
- Diphtheritic plaques on oral cavity, nasal discharge, petechia or ecchymosis of gingiva, ulcerated oral and pharyngeal mucosa, and thick saliva often associated with *Herpesvirus*.
- White plaques on mucous membranes, particularly with oral candidiasis.
- Rostral abrasions or callus from persistent facial rubbing or scratching.
- Hemorrhage, edema, swelling of lips and gingiva, ulceration, plaques, ptyalism, tongue dysfunction, halitosis, anorexia, or dysphagia.
- Dyspnea in some animals with choanal or periglottal lesions.
- Electrocution—vesicular and/or charred tissue often associated with a flared pattern; lesions usually associated with tongue and oral cavity.
- Non-specific clinical signs associated with infiltrating bacteria causing lesions in liver, kidney, heart or CNS secondary to osteomyelitis.

RISK FACTORS

Husbandry

- Chronic suboptimal temperature is considered one of the most important risk factors.
- Poor hygiene
- Overcrowding
- Improper light cycles
- Poor air quality
- Excess or insufficient humidity
- Toxin exposure
- Improper brumation
- Malnutrition

Others

- Pathogen-contaminated food or water.
- Hay-based bedding subject to molding.
- Bite wounds and facial injuries from territorial disputes.
- Feeding live prey

DIAGNOSIS

DIFFERENTIAL DIAGNOSIS

- Rule out septicemia as cause of oral petechiation. Usually ulceration and caseous lesions with stomatitis.
- Ulcerated neoplasms are usually focal, whereas stomatitis more typically diffuse.
- Consider neoplasia in cases unresponsive to supportive therapy and correction of improper husbandry.
- Abnormal maxilla and/or mandibles with NSHP.
- Tongue dysfunction from infection, trauma, electrocution, inflammatory masses, neoplasia and NSHP.

DIAGNOSTICS

- Physical examination: pay particular attention to eyes, teeth, choana and oral tissues.
- Use of a small otoscope or endoscope may be necessary for complete examination and to facilitate collection of samples. Anesthesia or sedation may be necessary.
- Cytology and culture: must target the deeper layers of affected tissue to minimize superficial contamination. The surface of the lesions can also be cleaned /disinfected prior to collection of samples. Aerobic, anaerobic and fungal cultures should be considered.
- Biopsy: particularly in recurring or persistent lesions; pre-clean tissue to collect samples for culture. Histopathology is key to further understanding the results of cytology and culture. Herpesvirus is often associated with intranuclear inclusion bodies associated with necrotic epithelium.
- CBC and plasma biochemistry may be useful to detect systemic disease and severity of tissue damage. CBC may be normal or may see toxic changes within heterophils if bacterial or fungal infection.
- Imaging: radiography, CT or MRI to identify severity of bone or ocular involvement.

PATHOLOGICAL FINDINGS

Histopathologic findings will vary depending on the etiologic agent involved.

TREATMENT

APPROPRIATE HEALTH CARE

- Therapy will fail if the underlying cause is not identified and corrected.
- Maintain sick reptiles, and those receiving medications, at high end of POTZ for the species, (80–90 degrees F for most reptiles; 100 degrees F for desert species).
- Some pathogens may be less pathogenic at higher temperatures and the reptile immune system may be more efficient.
- A higher temperature increases the heart rate, improves circulation, improves fluid and antibiotic distribution, improves neural response, increases muscular activity, and stimulates enzyme activity.
- Oral lesions and rostral abrasions should be debrided, cleaned, and treated with an appropriate antimicrobial.
- Mild and acute lesions: debride and clean lesions followed by application of topical antimicrobial and/or antifungal.
- Deep and severe lesions: require topical treatment described above as well as broad-spectrum systemic antimicrobials for bacteria (aerobic or anaerobic) or fungi based on results of cytology. Adjust therapy as needed based on results of culture.

NUTRITIONAL SUPPORT

- Correct dehydration and maintain normal hydration level (15–25 ml/kg/24 hours, IV, IO, ICe in divided dose) during treatment; reptiles that are sufficiently ill to require antimicrobial therapy should be considered to be dehydrated.
- After rehydration, supportive nutrition is needed to maintain positive nitrogen balance.
- Feed small amounts more frequently.
- Use high protein and fat diets for carnivores and complex carbohydrate diets for herbivores.
- Esophagostomy tube may be needed in severe cases.

CLIENT EDUCATION/HUSBANDRY RECOMMENDATIONS

- Quarantining new arrivals will minimize the risk of introducing a new pathogen to an established collection and will allow the new arrival time to acclimatize to its new environment.
- Follow proper husbandry guidelines for the species at hand.
- Environmental temperature, proper housing, and feeding regimen all play a crucial role in the wellbeing of reptilian species kept in captivity.

MEDICATIONS

DRUG(S) OF CHOICE

- Antimicrobial therapy alone is unlikely to be successful if the infection is walled off. There is poor drug penetration into exudates. A combination of aggressive debridement, wound care, and antibiotic therapy is likely to yield better results.
- Antibiotic selection is largely empiric based initially on in-clinic cytology and Gram staining, owing to the delay in return of culture results; disease associated organisms may be noted on cytology that are not cultured.
- Bactericidal drugs are preferable to bacteriostatic drugs.
- Topical antimicrobials/antifungals: iodine, chlorhexidine, and silver-based products.
- Herpesvirus in tortoises: topical and systemic acyclovir (80 mg/kg PO q72h); there is often varied and poor response to therapy across species.
- Antimicrobials may be required for 4–8 weeks.

Antibiotics of Choice for Empirical Treatment

- Amikacin 5 mg/kg IM, then 2.5 mg/kg q72h
- Azithromycin 10 mg/kg PO q3–7d
- Carbenicillin 200 mg/kg IM q24h
- Ceftazidime 20 mg/kg IM q72h
- Enrofloxacin 5–10 mg/kg IM q48h
- Metronidazole 20 mg/kg PO q48h

PRECAUTIONS/INTERACTIONS

Enrofloxacin given parentally can cause tissue necrosis; use with caution.

FOLLOW-UP

PATIENT MONITORING

- Evaluate hydration frequently after starting treatment.
- Make husbandry changes to provide proper environment and nutrition.

EXPECTED COURSE AND PROGNOSIS

- Varies with underlying cause, chronicity and condition of the patient.
- Lesions can progress from petechial hemorrhage to overwhelming infection and septicemia within 2–3 days.
- Acute and uncomplicated lesions usually respond to appropriate therapy.
- Untreated infections frequently progress to osteomyelitis, septicemia and death.
- Prognosis is guarded to poor with osteomyelitis depending on chronicity and severity.
- Neoplasia has a poor prognosis unless completely resected and with no metastasis.

MISCELLANEOUS

COMMENTS

Associated Conditions

- Osteomyelitis, sinusitis, septicemia, pneumonia and/or gastroenteritis.
- Ocular or periocular disease
- Permanent tongue damage resulting in dysphagia or anorexia.
- Pharyngeal cellulitis

ZOONOTIC POTENTIAL

- Many bacteria and fungi that infect reptiles can also cause disease in humans.
- Any bites from reptiles should be treated as contaminated; immediately wash wounds with soap and water and seek medical attention; humans with open wounds on the hands should not handle reptiles or their secretions or excretions without gloves.

SYNONYMS

- Infectious stomatitis
- Mouth rot
- Ulcerative stomatitis

ABBREVIATIONS

- CBC = complete blood count
- CNS = central nervous system
- CT = computed tomography
- ICe = intracoelomic
- IM = intramuscular
- IO = intraosseous
- IV = intravenous
- MRI = magnetic resonance imaging
- NSHP = nutritional secondary hyperparathyroidism
- POTZ = preferred optimal temperature zone

INTERNET RESOURCES

- Suedemeyer K, Pollock C. Presenting problem: stomatitis in reptiles. LafeberVet, November 11, 2013. https://lafeber.com/vet/presenting-problem-stomatitis-in-reptiles
- Divers SJ. Bacterial diseases of reptiles. MSD Manual Veterinary Manual, June 2020. https://www.merckvetmanual.com/exotic-and-laboratory-animals/reptiles/bacterial-diseases-of-reptiles

Suggested Reading

Jacobson ER, ed. *Infectious Diseases and Pathology of Reptiles: Color Atlas and Text.* Boca Raton, FL: CRC Press; 2007.

Mader DR, Divers SJ, eds. *Current Therapy in Reptile Medicine and Surgery.* St. Louis MO: Elsevier Saunders; 2014.

Author Sam Rivera, DVM, MS, DABVP (Avian), DACZM, DECZM (Zoo Health Management)

THERMAL BURNS

BASICS

DEFINITION/OVERVIEW

Reptiles are classified as ectothermic, meaning that they actively seek appropriate environmental temperatures to satisfy their metabolic requirements. Periods of increased metabolic activity such as foraging and digestion are usually preceded and followed by actively raising core body temperature. Traditionally, heat production has been categorized into three types: radiant heat such as solar energy, convective heat such as currents of warm air, and conductive heat such as direct contact with a heat source. Reptiles usually use a combination of all three types of heat acquisition. Ventilation and humidity are also important components of thermodynamics. Most thermal burns are associated with excessive exposure to radiant and/or conductive heat.

ETIOLOGY/PATHOPHYSIOLOGY

- Thermal burns have assorted causes, most of which fall into the following categories: close/direct contact with an unprotected focal heat or light source, faulty electrical equipment, human error.
- Burns can occur when the heating elements are placed dangerously close to the reptile.
- Overhead lights should be entirely outside the tank, with a tank lid between the lamp and the reptile, or placed high enough in the enclosure that the reptile cannot reach it.
- Malfunctions of submersible thermostats can lead to hyperthermia, burns, and acute death of aquatic chelonians.
- Thermal burns can also occur when a reptile is weak or lethargic due to systemic disease and cannot move away from the heat source.
- A complete clinical examination should be performed to determine whether there is an underlying disease.

SIGNALMENT/HISTORY

- Thermal burns may affect reptiles of all ages and may be more prevalent during the cooler seasons when additional heating devices are used.
- History usually involves prolonged exposure to heating elements or bulbs.

CLINICAL PRESENTATION

- Clinical signs depend primarily on the severity of lesions.
- Traditionally, thermal burns have been classified according to the depth of damaged tissue.
- First-degree burns cause damage confined to the epidermis and present as erythema and sloughing of damaged scales.
- Second-degree burns involve the epidermis and dermis. These burns present as erythema plus vesicles. The vesicles may rupture, causing loss of tissue fluid and protein, with a higher risk of secondary bacterial infections.
- Third-degree burns involve destruction of epidermis, dermis, and underlying tissues.
- Secondary bacterial and/or fungal infections commonly occur.
- A more recent classification makes use of the terms "partial thickness" and "full thickness" when defining the severity of burns.

RISK FACTORS

Husbandry

- Exposure to inappropriate or malfunctioning heat sources is the most common cause of thermal burns.
- This may occur in both terrestrial and aquatic species.

Others

Debilitation secondary to internal disease can predispose a reptile to being too weak to move away from a heat source.

DIAGNOSIS

DIFFERENTIAL DIAGNOSIS

Other causes of dermatoses should be excluded such as chronic dysecdysis, bacterial/fungal infections, trauma and neoplasia.

DIAGNOSTICS

Diagnosis is based upon history, clinical signs and physical examination.

PATHOLOGICAL FINDINGS

- For a description of gross lesions see Clinical Presentation.
- Histopathologic findings of first-degree burns consist of dilatation of arterioles and venules, increased capillary permeability with filtration of plasma into tissue spaces, and migration of erythrocytes and leukocytes.
- Second-degree burns consist of vesicles filled with an acellular transudate in addition to changes associated with first-degree burns.
- Third-degree burns are characterized by destruction of the entire integument followed by sloughing of necrotic tissue.
- Surrounding this zone are areas of lesser-degree burns, as described above.

TREATMENT

APPROPRIATE HEALTH CARE

N/A

NUTRITIONAL SUPPORT

- Nutritional support and proper temperatures are important factors that influence tissue regeneration.
- A 2.7–5.5 degrees C (5–10 degrees F) increase in the basking area may help improve healing but care must be taken that this does not cause additional evaporative losses.
- If the affected reptile was in a positive energy balance prior to the thermal injury and the wounds are not severe, most reptiles resume feeding as healing commences aided with the judicious use of analgesics.
- A weight loss of 10% acutely or 20% chronically should prompt nutritional intervention.
- Tube feeding with the use of an appropriate enteral (i.e., Oxbow Critical Care Herbivore® (Oxbow Animal Health, Omaha, NE, or EmerAid Sustain Herbivore® (EmerAid, LLC, Cornell, IL) aid in promoting anabolism and healing).
- An esophagostomy tube should be considered for long-term feeding and medication in anorectic, difficult to handle, or stressed animals.

CLIENT EDUCATION/HUSBANDRY RECOMMENDATIONS

- The owner should check the affected reptile's condition daily, implement suggested husbandry modifications and administer medications as directed.
- Follow-up veterinary visits at prescribed intervals should be adhered to.

MEDICATIONS

DRUG(S) OF CHOICE

- If the affected reptile presents acutely after a burn (less than 30 minutes), cooling of skin is recommended with the application of cold compresses for 15–20 minutes to further reduce inflammation and limit tissue swelling.
- Where blisters form, an effort should be made to minimize trauma and resultant rupture, to limit tissue fluid loss and prevent secondary infection.
- Patients should be kept on non-adherent substrates to minimize further wound trauma and infection; an empty glass enclosure is the simplest to keep clean.

• Wet-to-dry sterile bandages infused with sterile saline, or even honey bandages, also work well and initially should be changed every 24 hours.
• Other products that have been used widely include the porcine xenograft dressing VetBioSISt® (Cook Veterinary Products, Bloomington, IN), a sterile non-allergenic dressing that may be sutured over extensive wounds to provide a semi-permeable membrane, protecting the granulation bed and encouraging rapid epithelialization.
• Aquatic chelonians can be dry-docked during the day and kept on damp towels. In the evenings they can be placed in their aquatic environment composed of bottled spring water.
• Treatment can last weeks to months depending on the severity and extent of the burns.
• Permanent scarring with abnormal pigmentation usually occurs in the burn area.
• A complete blood count and biochemical analysis should also be done, especially in reptiles with third-degree burns.
• Topical therapy, such as dilute chlorhexidine (0.05%) and silver sulfadiazine cream, together with the use of non-adherent sterile dressings, is advised to limit secondary infection.
• Silver sulfadiazine is particularly useful due to its broad-spectrum activity and its efficacy against *Pseudomonas*, common contaminants of burns, as well as its ability to reduce further fluid loss from evaporation.
• Ophthalmic ointments can also be used topically.
• IV, IO or ICe crystalloid fluid therapy is recommended for second- and third-degree burns.
• For extensive wounds in chelonians, a semi-permeable hydrophilic wound dressing (e.g., Granuflex®, ConvaTec Inc., Oklahoma City, OK), may be used to cover defects.
• Narcotic analgesics (hydromorphone 0.5–1 mg/kg IM q12–24h, tramadol 5–10 mg/kg PO, SC q24h), NSAIDs (meloxicam 0.2–0.5 mg/kg IM, SC q24–48h), parenteral fluids (lactated Ringer's solution 10–25 ml/kg IV, IO, ICe, SC q24h), and antibiotics, based upon microbiological culture and sensitivities, are recommended.
• Depending on the severity of lesions, the author prefers the use of antibacterials such as piperacillin 100 mg/kg IM q24h, ceftazidime 20 mg/kg IM q72h, or amikacin 5 mg/kg loading dose followed by 2.5 mg/kg q72h, combined with metronidazole 20 mg/kg q24h.

PRECAUTIONS/INTERACTIONS

• Adequate hydration should be addressed, particularly for those reptiles being treated with aminoglycosides.
• Soaking the animal in sterile saline or water for 2–4–hours on the days antibiotics are administered can help provide additional hydration.
• Care must be taken when soaking reptiles in antiseptic solutions (dilute betadine, dilute chlorhexidine) because of the risk of ingestion; rather, direct application of these solutions to the wounds is recommended.

FOLLOW-UP

PATIENT MONITORING

• Affected animals should be re-evaluated every 1–2 weeks by a veterinarian.
• If a visit is not feasible, the owner can send pictures for appraisal until healing is progressing in a positive manner.

EXPECTED COURSE AND PROGNOSIS

• First-degree burns: damaged tissue heals in approximately 2–4 weeks.
• Second-degree burns: healing usually takes 6–8 weeks; eschar may form.
• Third-degree burns: healing can take from months to years, with extensive scarring. The prognosis is guarded for third-degree burns due to the possibility of sepsis.

MISCELLANEOUS

COMMENTS

• It should be noted that exposure to high-intensity and/or inappropriate wavelengths of ultraviolet radiation can cause signs of phototoxicity such as photokeratoconjunctivitis and photodermatitis. Affected reptiles can present acutely with corneal and dermal opacities, excessive ecdysis, hyperkeratosis, and epidermal erosions.
• Chronic cases may present with cataracts and cutaneous neoplasia. These cases must be differentiated from thermal burns.
• Figures 8 and 9 – see web image supplementary content for Section II (Chelonians).

ZOONOTIC POTENTIAL

N/A

SYNONYMS

N/A

ABBREVIATIONS

• ICe = intracoelomic
• IM = intramuscular
• IO = intraosseous
• IV = intravenous
• NSAID = nonsteroidal anti-inflammatory drug
• PO = by mouth
• SC = subcutaneous

INTERNET RESOURCES

Divers SJ. Management and husbandry of reptiles. MSD Manual Veterinary Manual, June 2020. https://www.msdvetmanual.com/en-gb/exotic-and-laboratory-animals/reptiles/management-and-husbandry-of-reptiles

Suggested Reading

Girling SJ, Raiti P, eds. *BSAVA Manual of Reptiles*. 2nd ed. Gloucester, UK: BSAVA; 2004.
Mader DR, ed. *Reptile Medicine and Surgery*. 2nd ed. St. Louis, MO: Elsevier Saunders; 2006.
Zych J, Hnizdo J, eds. *Medical Care of Turtles and Tortoises: Diagnosis, Surgery, Pathology, Parasitology*. Frankfurt, Germany: Edition Chimaira; 2011.

Author Paul Raiti, DVM, DABVP (Reptile and Amphibian Practice)

TICKS

BASICS

DEFINITION/OVERVIEW

Ticks are ectoparasites that feed on blood and can potentially transmit disease through their bite, along with causing local irritation, secondary infection, or, rarely, anemia. They are mainly seen in wild-caught animals, so any known wild-caught animals should be closely examined for their presence. They may also be found on animals that are otherwise weak or debilitated. Rarely, they may be seen in captive specimens that spend time outdoors.

ETIOLOGY/PATHOPHYSIOLOGY

- Seven genera of ticks can parasitize reptiles. These include the hard ticks of the genera *Ixodes*, *Hyalomma*, *Haemaphysalis*, *Amblyomma*, and *Aponomma*, and the soft ticks *Argasidae* and *Ornithodoros*.
- Soft ticks live in nests and burrows while hard ticks live in fields or scrub areas and attach to a host as it passes by. Some are host specific.
- Ticks use their mouthparts to attach and feed on blood.
- Soft ticks become engorged and drop off within hours and may feed repeatedly, while hard ticks remain attached for several days.
- Females lay eggs after a blood meal.
- Eggs hatch as a larval stage, which feed on blood from the host as well.
- They progress through two or more nymph stages before becoming adults, feeding on blood between each stage.
- Larvae, nymphs, and adults can live for months without a blood meal.

SIGNALMENT/HISTORY

- No age or gender predisposition.
- Typically only seen in wild-caught animals, those that spend significant time outdoors, or are kept in unsanitary conditions with poor husbandry.

CLINICAL PRESENTATION

- Identification of tick attached to skin. Ticks often attach in skin folds, under scales, or around the ears, lips, or cloaca.
- There may be swelling, erythema, or discharge at the site of attachment from local irritation or secondary bacterial infection.
- In some cases, animals may be otherwise debilitated, weak, or have other underlying problems.
- Animals may also soak frequently in an attempt to dislodge the parasites.
- If the infestation is severe, there may be signs of dysecdysis, anemia, or disease possibly transmitted by the tick.

RISK FACTORS

Husbandry

- Ticks are typically only seen in wild-caught animals, and rarely in captive animals that spend significant time outdoors.
- There is no specific way to avoid ticks other than regular control measures such as mowing the lawn regularly, removing debris piles or refuse, avoid overwatering or standing water, limiting access by wildlife, and using tick-control pesticides in the enclosure.
- Infestations can also occur in severe cases of poor husbandry and sanitation, stress and other underlying medical conditions.

Others

N/A

DIAGNOSIS

DIFFERENTIAL DIAGNOSIS

- Diagnosis is pathognomonic
- Other ectoparasites such as mites, chiggers, etc. are significantly smaller and not confused for ticks.

DIAGNOSTICS

- Diagnosis of ticks is based on physical exam alone.
- Additional tests to evaluate the animal's overall condition may be necessary if the animal is otherwise weak or debilitated.
- This may include a fecal exam, complete blood count and chemistry panel, and/or radiography.

PATHOLOGICAL FINDINGS

- Ticks are obvious on physical exam.
- There may be evidence of inflammation or secondary bacterial colonization at the attachment site.
- Anemia is possible, although, because ticks are large, they are often removed before significant anemia can occur.
- Other pathologic findings could include those from a pathogen transmitted by the tick.

TREATMENT

APPROPRIATE HEALTH CARE

N/A

NUTRITIONAL SUPPORT

- Not needed for this condition unless animal is otherwise debilitated.
- Chelonians typically need to be force fed using a stainless-steel, ball-tipped feeding needle.
- An esophagostomy tube may need to be placed.
- Feed 1–2% of body weight once or twice daily.

MEDICATIONS

DRUG(S) OF CHOICE

- Physical removal is recommended
- The tick must be grasped under the head on the mouthparts for full extraction.
- Secondary infection of the attachment site can be treated with topical antibacterial ointment, such as silver sulfadiazine cream, and systemic antibiotics if needed.
- FRONTLINE® Plus (Boehringer Ingelheim International GmbH, Ingelheim am Rhein, Germany) spray is effective for prevention and may aid in removal. It should never be sprayed directly on the animal; spray on a towel and wipe the animal from head to tail.
- Provent-a-Mite™ (Pro Products, Mahopac, NY) is an OTC permethrin product that appears to be both safe and effective. It can be applied to the animal or sprayed in the environment.
- Additional treatments may be needed based on the animal's overall condition.
- If the animal is anemic due to blood loss, consider additional therapies, such as B vitamins, iron dextran, or even a blood transfusion.
- A product containing permethrin and 0.01% cyfluthrin (Tempo™, Bayer, Kansas City, MO) formulated for premise treatment can be used to control ticks in outdoor tortoise enclosures.

PRECAUTIONS/INTERACTIONS

- Do not use ivermectin in chelonians. It is toxic in this group of reptiles and will cause death.
- Use caution with any OTC remedies, particularly organophosphates or permethrins, as toxicity is possible.

FOLLOW-UP

PATIENT MONITORING

- None needed if ticks are physically removed.
- If secondary bacterial infection is present, resolution of clinical signs will indicate response to therapy.

EXPECTED COURSE AND PROGNOSIS

- The prognosis is excellent. Once the ticks are removed there should be no further complications.
- The prognosis for secondary infection of the skin is also good.
- The main concern is if the animal is weak or debilitated overall, or there is potential for disease transmission from the tick. Depending on the animal's overall condition, the prognosis may be fair to guarded.

MISCELLANEOUS

COMMENTS

- One concern with ticks on wild-caught animals is potential foreign-animal disease transmission.
- For example, before captive breeding of sulcata tortoises (*Geochelone sulcata*) and leopard tortoises (*G. pardalis*) was commonplace, wild-caught animals were brought in from Africa.
- These animals frequently were infected with ticks of the genus *Amblyomma*, which can carry and transmit the rickettsia *Ehrlichia ruminantium*, the causative agent of Heartwater disease.
- Heartwater disease can affect any ruminant, wild or domestic, and causes an accumulation of fluid in the chest and pericardium.
- Mortality approaches 100% and the disease is not treatable.
- Heartwater is not present in the United States, and could be devastating for the goat, sheep, and cattle industries if introduced.
- Any tick on a wild-caught animal from another country and the animal itself should be treated with suspicion.

ZOONOTIC POTENTIAL

- Ticks affecting reptiles can potentially attach to humans and cause irritation and pruritis at the site of a bite.
- Many of these can also carry and transmit disease to humans such as tularemia, Lyme disease, and other encephalitis-causing viruses.
- Use caution during removal and kill the tick immediately.

SYNONYMS

N/A

ABBREVIATIONS

OTC = over the counter

INTERNET RESOURCES

- Burridge, MJ. Controlling and Eradicating Tick Infestations on Reptiles. Veterinary Compendium, 2005. https://vetfoliovetstreet.s3.amazonaws.com/mmah/5d/12368b9df24fabb6fd86b1b65e51df/filePV_27_05_371.pdf
- PetCoach Editorial. Reptile Tick and Mite Infestation: Causes, Signs, Diagnosis, and Treatment. Petco Animal Supplies Stores, Inc. http://www.peteducation.com/article.cfm?c=17+1796&aid=2433
- Greek T. How to Recognize and Treat Reptile Ectoparasites. Reptiles, July 1, 2014. http://www.reptilesmagazine.com/Snake-Care/How-to-Recognize-and-Treat-Reptile-Ectoparasites

Suggested Reading

Burridge MJ, Simmons L. Control and eradication of exotic tick infestations on reptiles. *Proc ARAV* 2001:21–23.

Fitzgerald KT, Vera R. Acariasis. In: Mader DR, ed. *Reptile Medicine and Surgery*. 2nd ed. St. Louis, MO: Elsevier Saunders; 2006:720–738.

Jacobson ER. Parasites and parasitic disease of reptiles. In: Jacobson ER, ed. *Infectious Diseases and Pathology of Reptiles*. Boca Raton, FL: CRC Press; 2007:571–665.

Author Stacey Leonatti Wilkinson, DVM, DABVP (Reptile and Amphibian)

UPPER RESPIRATORY TRACT DISEASE

BASICS

DEFINITION/OVERVIEW

URTD in chelonians is a common syndrome, especially in tortoises. It can be seen in turtles as well, but most likely has a different etiology than in tortoises. In many cases, URTD in tortoises has a bacterial (*Mycoplasma* sp.) or viral (herpesvirus, ranavirus) etiology. Fungi, parasites, and environmental factors (such as drought and dust) can also cause URTD. In turtles, it is mainly caused by foreign bodies in the URT (e.g., the nasal cavity, choana, or oral cavity) or nasal discharge secondary to infection of the LRT. Signs of URTD in tortoises include nasal and/or ocular discharge, conjunctivitis, palpebral edema and stridor or wheezing, typically recurring after treatment or over seasons. Signs in turtles include nasal discharge, palpebral edema, and bubbling noises, especially when surfacing. Chelonians breathe with a closed mouth, with air entering the URT through the external nares. Tortoises have a short, keratinized vestibule extending from the external nares to the membrane-lined nasal cavities. Conchae are typically absent. A cartilaginous septum separates left and right nasal cavity. Each cavity is lined with multilayered olfactory epithelium, located dorsally, and with a mucous membrane ventrally, which has a ventral recess of its own and opens into the roof of the pharynx roof as the left and right choana.

ETIOLOGY/PATHOPHYSIOLOGY

- There is a wide range of etiologies associated with URTD but infectious causes are some of the most common.
- URTD may also be secondary to other diseases such as stomatitis.

Infectious

- Bacterial: in tortoises, *Mycoplasma agassizii* and *M. testudineum* are the most common pathogens. Others, such as *Pasteurella testudinis*, usually occur as secondary invaders after damage of the nasal mucosa.
- Fungal
- Viral: herpesvirus, picornavirus, reovirus, adenovirus, ranavirus. Often seen in conjunction with mycoplasmosis.
- TINC in tropical tortoises

Noninfectious

- Foreign bodies within the choana, nasal or oral cavity.
- Physical trauma/injuries affecting the nasal or oral cavity or the choana.
- Tumors
- Improper husbandry

SIGNALMENT/HISTORY

- No age or sex predisposition
- Some infectious diseases (e.g., *Mycoplasma* spp. and herpesvirus) are more commonly documented in tortoise species and box turtles.

CLINICAL PRESENTATION

- Depends on the underlying cause and chelonian species.
- Nasal discharge (clear to yellow)
- Ocular discharge
- Palpebral edema
- Sneezing
- Excess salivation or mucous secretion in the oral cavity.
- Dyspnea, open mouth-breathing
- Stridor or wheezing
- Lightening of tissue around the nares.
- May include epistaxis in severe cases.
- Unilateral or bilateral decreased nasal airflow.
- Dyspnea, open mouth-breathing and increased front limb-motion (in conjunction with breathing) in cases of severe bilateral obstruction.
- In turtles, bubbling noises, especially when surfacing; buoyancy disorders if LRT is affected as well.
- Nonspecific signs such as anorexia, lethargy, inactivity.

RISK FACTORS

Husbandry

- Improper husbandry, including inappropriate temperatures and humidity, stagnant water, substrate with irritating compounds (e.g., cedar shavings), poor ventilation.

Others

- Immunosuppression, which may be caused by stress, overcrowding, relocation, concurrent disease or inappropriate husbandry.
- Sudden changes in temperature or humidity.
- Improper diet (including starvation) and endoparasitism may also be predisposing factors.
- Exposure to heavy metals and other toxicants.

DIAGNOSIS

DIFFERENTIAL DIAGNOSIS

- Unilateral: most likely foreign body, injury, tumor, (infectious agents possible).
- Bilateral: most likely infectious agents or improper husbandry (injuries, foreign bodies, and tumors also possible).
- Unilateral or bilateral: retained slough or occluded nostrils (especially in tortoises) after severe infection.

DIAGNOSTICS

- Physical examination, including thorough exam of the oral cavity and choana. The use of magnification may aid in identifying subtle lesions.
- Bacterial culture and sensitivity (aerobic and anaerobic) and/or fungal culture of nasal discharge, nasal flush, or inflamed tissue.
- In cases of suspected mycoplasmosis: PCR of nasal flush, detection of antibodies by ELISA.
- In cases of suspected viral infections: PCR of nasal flush or nasal swab, oral swab, histopathology of oral or nasal mucosa, serology.
- PCR for TINC
- Diagnostic imaging (radiographs, CT, MRI) for detection of foreign bodies, osteolysis, osteomyelitis, or concurrent LRTD.
- Endoscopy of the URTD (and LRTD); possibly including nasal lavage and biopsy for further diagnostics, such as cytology, histopathology, virology, and electron microscopy.
- Histopathology of the URT and LRT (if available).

PATHOLOGICAL FINDINGS

- Depending on the underlying cause, signs of mild to severe inflammation and lesions of the nasal and oral mucosa may be found.
- Bacteria (including mycobacteriosis), fungal hyphae, virus-associated inclusion bodies, and cell and bone destruction (if aggressive bacteria or fungi or tumor are the underlying cause) may be seen.
- In cases of mycoplasmosis in tortoises, the URT, especially the nasal cavity, is typically affected, and involvement of the LRT (e.g., tracheitis and pneumonia) is possible.
- Mycoplasma-induced pathological findings of the nasal cavity include mucosal basal cell hyperplasia and submucosal infiltrates of heterophils and histiocytes, and lymphoid hyperplasia.
- Viral inclusions may be observed but are not always present.

TREATMENT

APPROPRIATE HEALTH CARE

N/A

NUTRITIONAL SUPPORT

- Force-feeding with easily digestible proteins.
- Direct feeding by stomach tubing can be performed in some species, but placement of an esophagostomy tube should be considered for chronic management.

CLIENT EDUCATION/HUSBANDRY RECOMMENDATIONS

- Correct any husbandry deficiencies, with special attention to temperature, humidity, and ventilation.
- Isolate the animal from others in collection, especially when viral etiology is suspected.
- It is important to ensure a full course of treatment to avoid recurrence of disease.

MEDICATIONS

DRUG(S) OF CHOICE

- Depends on the underlying cause and the affected chelonian species.
- Bacteria: systemic or nebulized antibiotics (e.g., amikacin, ceftazidime, ceftiofur, enrofloxacin, tylosin), preferably according to sensitivity panel, for at least 4–6 weeks. Local instillation of antibiotics (injectable or ophthalmic solutions) in the nasal passage may also be effective.
- In case of confirmed mycobacterial infection, there is no treatment; the animal should be euthanased.
- In cases of mycoplasmosis: in wild tortoises, isolation, no release because of the persistent risk of infection and deadly threat to wild populations; in captive tortoises, fluoroquinolones and tetracycline are most effective; combining parenteral and nebulization of these two class of drugs may be beneficial. Nasal flushing with physiologic saline solution (first once daily, then every third day) is also helpful.
- Fungi: systemic, local, nebulized, antifungals (e.g., terbinafine, voriconazole, amphotericin B).
- Systemic use of itraconazole may cause severe adverse effects in some chelonians.
- Herpes or ranavirus (sometimes co-infection with *Mycoplasma* spp.); intensive symptomatic and supportive therapy; effectiveness of antiviral therapy is not well documented.
- Individual housing and barrier nursing of affected animals; hygiene and strict quarantine.
- Foreign body within the choana, nasal/oral cavity: extraction
- Neoplasia: surgical removal if feasible.
- Supportive fluid therapy at a rate of 10–30 ml/kg/day as supportive care.

PRECAUTIONS/INTERACTIONS

- Exposure to heavy metals (such as mercury) and other toxicants may be a predisposing factor for outbreaks of the disease.
- Enrofloxacin is a fluoroquinolone with primary renal excretion; thus, adequate rehydration and regular monitoring of renal values are recommended if this antibiotic is chosen for treatment.

FOLLOW-UP

PATIENT MONITORING

- Improvement of clinical signs should be expected within 1–2 weeks for bacterial and fungal infections when definitive diagnosis and treatment are employed.
- It is critical to continue treatment until clinical signs are fully resolved and repeating cultures to confirm resolution of infection if unsure.
- In cases that do not show any improvement or worsen during the first 1–2 weeks of treatment, it should be considered that the etiology and/or treatment are not accurate.
- Viral infections should also be considered in cases that do not respond to therapy or have chronic, intermittent recurrence of disease.
- Repeat diagnostics may be needed to assess resolution or progression of disease.
- Treatment for mycoplasmosis may be longer than for other bacteria and animals may become subclinical carriers.
- Continued monitoring by PCR and serology may help to determine shedding and antibody status of the animal over time to help in making management decisions.

EXPECTED COURSE AND PROGNOSIS

- Depends on the causative agent (see above).
- Bacterial: good prognosis, depending on response to antibiotics.
- In case of mycoplasmosis, no current standard therapy is available to eliminate the pathogen. Subclinically and clinically affected tortoises stay potentially infectious (all tortoise species should be considered as potentially susceptible). In wild tortoises, no release due to persistent risk of infection and deadly threat to wild populations. In captive tortoises: isolation. URT disease may be triggered by certain factors and can lead to a fresh outbreak of the disease with possible fatal outcome at any time.
- Fungal: guarded to poor prognosis.
- Herpesvirus/ranavirus (sometimes co-infection with *Mycoplasma*): guarded to grave prognosis depending on the virus and host species.
- Neoplastic: poor to grave prognosis.
- Others: prognosis depends on severity and involvement of other tissues.

MISCELLANEOUS

COMMENTS

N/A

ZOONOTIC POTENTIAL

- Depending on the causative agent
- Mycobacteria and salmonella (rare causes) have zoonotic potential.

SYNONYMS

- Mycoplasmosis in tortoises and box turtles.
- Runny nose syndrome
- Tortoise mycoplasmosis
- Upper respiratory disease syndrome

ABBREVIATIONS

- CT = computed tomography
- ELISA = enzyme-linked immunosorbent assay
- LRT = lower respiratory tract
- MRI = magnetic resonance imaging
- PCR = polymerase chain reaction
- TINC = intranuclear coccidiosis of testudines
- URT = upper respiratory tract
- URTD = upper respiratory tract disease

Suggested Reading

Feldman SH, Wimsatt J, Marchang RE, et al. A novel mycoplasma detected in association with upper respiratory disease syndrome in free-ranging eastern box turtles (*Terrapene carolina carolina*) in Virginia. *J Wildl Dis* 2006;42(2):279–289.

Innis CJ, Garner MM, Johnson AJ, et al. Antemortem diagnosis and characterization of nasal intranuclear coccidiosis in Sulawesi tortoises (*Indotestudo forsteni*). *J Vet Diagn Invest* 2007;19(6):660–667.

Jackson OF, Needham JR. Rhinitis and virus antibody titres in chelonians. *J Small Anim Pract.* 1983;24:31–36.

Jacobson ER, Brown MB, Wendland LD, et al. Mycoplasmosis and upper respiratory tract disease of tortoises: A review and update. *Vet J* 2014;201(3):257–264.

Wendland LD, Brown DR, Klein PA, Brown MB. Upper respiratory tract disease (mycoplasmosis) in tortoises (Specific diseases and clinical conditions). In: Mader DR, ed. *Reptile Medicine and Surgery*. St. Louis, MO: Elsevier Saunders; 2006:931–938.

Author Karina A. Mathes, DVM, Dr. med. vet., DECZM (Herpetology), European Veterinary Specialist in Zoological Medicine (Herpetology), Certified Specialist in Reptiles (Fachtieraerztin fuer Reptilien), Certified Specialist in Reptiles and Amphibians (ZB Reptilien und Amphibien)

UROLITHIASIS

BASICS

DEFINITION/OVERVIEW

Urolithiasis is the formation of calculi within the urinary tract. While most reptiles are uricotelic, some can be ureotelic, ammoniotelic, or a combination of the two. Uric acid is actively secreted by the proximal tubules of the kidneys and excreted in the urine. It is the end product of nitrogen metabolism through a series of enzymatic reactions that involve xanthine oxidase. Endogenous uric acid production results from de novo purine synthesis and tissue catabolism. The form in which uric acid is excreted is dependent on urine pH. When urine pH is less than 5, uric acid is present in the urine, whereas when urine pH is greater than 6.5, most of the uric acid is excreted as urate salts. Tortoises, like other herbivores, tend to have alkaline urine, which favors the physiologic formation of urate salts. The majority of uroliths are composed of salts of uric acid and ammonium, sodium, potassium, or calcium. In reptiles, urinary calculi have been identified in the kidneys, ureters, urinary bladder, urodeum and distal cloaca. Urinary calculi have been reported most commonly in tortoises, with aquatic turtles being a distant second. Inciting factors for calculus formation are chronic dehydration, renal insufficiency, high-protein diets, and lack of exercise.

ETIOLOGY/PATHOPHYSIOLOGY

- The Sonoran Desert tortoise (*Gopherus agassizii*) is the best-studied tortoise with regard to physiology and urolithiasis.
- Urea is the main nitrogenous waste when the Sonoran Desert tortoise is well hydrated and has access to plenty of drinking water or moist food plants.
- Urea requires less energy to form than uric acid, but it is more toxic than uric acid and therefore requires more water to keep it dilute enough to avoid tissue damage.
- Uric acid requires an additional investment of energy but is relatively insoluble in water and significantly less toxic than urea.
- Uric acid will crystallize out of solution at low concentrations and can be voided from the body in a paste that allows the tortoise to retain much more water per unit of nitrogen excreted than for urea.
- There is an advantage for a tortoise to excrete urea when water is abundant because more energy is conserved and used for other purposes and the nitrogenous wastes are eliminated from the body without reaching harmful levels.
- Xeric-adapted tortoises such as the Sonoran Desert tortoise tend to produce uric acid preferentially as a nitrogenous waste product compared to rainforest tortoises such as red-footed tortoises (*Chelonoidis carbonaria*).
- Cilia lining the chelonian bladder aid in keeping microcrystals of urates in suspension.
- The formation of urinary calculi is initiated by the precipitation of excretory metabolites in supersaturated urine.
- Factors credited with stone nidation include dehydration, alterations in urinary pH, abnormalities of urinary tract structure and function, high levels of urolith mineral components in the diet, nutrient deficiencies such as hypovitaminosis A, atypical metabolism of calculus precursors, and the presence of bacteria and other foreign materials within the urinary tract.
- An additional characteristic of reptiles is that urine is not sterile, since the bladder communicates with the coprodeum (the opening of the gastrointestinal tract into the cloaca).
- Some organisms, such as the flagellated protozoa *Hexamita*, have been frequently found in the urine of tortoises with bladder stones; however, the role of this protozoan in the formation of urinary calculi is uncertain.
- Tortoise urine is influenced by diet and water consumption and likely has many complicated interactions between nitrogenous wastes, electrolytes, proteins, other waste products, and bladder microbial populations.
- Whatever the factors that promote uroliths in tortoises, once a nidus is formed that is too large to pass through the urethra, a bladder stone results.
- In a retrospective study involving the diagnosis and treatment of 40 cases of urolithiasis in captive chelonians, the majority of urolith cases were identified in desert tortoises (70.5%), African spurred tortoises (*Centrochelys sulcata*) (7.5%), red-eared sliders (*Trachemys scripta elegans*) (5%) and Hermann tortoises (*Testudo hermanni*) (2.5%). Uroliths have also been identified in leopard tortoises (*Stigmochelys pardalis*), Russian tortoises (*Agrionemys horsfieldii*) a wild western spiny softshell turtle (*Apalone [Trionyx] spiniferus hartwegi*, and yellow-bellied sliders (*T. scripta scripta*).

SIGNALMENT/HISTORY

- Urolithiasis is usually a problem of adult herbivorous reptiles.
- Deficiencies in husbandry, such as chronic dehydration, suboptimal ambient temperatures, and inappropriately high-protein diets (usually mammalian based) are commonly identified during anamnesis.

CLINICAL PRESENTATION

- Many chelonians with small uroliths show no clinical signs.
- Some tortoises may lose their appetites; others may simply be less active.
- Small uroliths are usually voided; however, larger calculi may pass from the urinary bladder into the cloaca and obstruct the vent.
- In tortoises, as calculi grow larger, hematuria, hindleg dysfunction, tenesmus, audible "grunting" noises, prolapse of the phallus/clitoris/ cloaca, dystocia, dysuria, or tenesmus may occur.
- More serious signs are straining or failure to defecate.
- Gravid females may repeatedly dig nests and strain to lay eggs without success.
- In chelonians, an egg may pass from the oviduct into the urinary bladder, particularly after severe trauma or oxytocin administration. These eggs often serve as a nidus where urates are deposited and eventually grow into larger calculi.
- Some tortoises appear paralyzed or paretic in their hind limbs or may walk with an exaggerated limp on one or both sides, a sign sometimes described as a "wheelbarrow gait."
- In severe cases left untreated, bladder necrosis and death may occur.
- It is also common that a tortoise is presented with another problem, such as an upper respiratory infection, and the bladder stone is detected incidentally in the course of examination and diagnostics.
- In one study, only 10 of 40 (25%) chelonians had a solid coelomic mass palpable in the prefemoral fossa and abnormalities associated with the urogenital system were recorded for only 5 (12.5%). Interestingly, the most common abnormality identified during physical examination of the 40 chelonians was a change in mentation (15), followed by nasal discharge (12), weakness (7), soft bones (5), wounds (5), edema (4), dehydration (3), hyperemic skin (3), evidence of previous plastronotomy (3), chemosis (3), pale mucous membranes (2), carapacial pyramiding (2), shell lesions (2), peeling skin (2), thickened skin (2), stomatitis (2), expiratory wheezes (2), ocular discharge (2), and cardiac arrhythmia, straining to defecate or urinate, yellow-colored urates, open-beak breathing, palpebral thickening, hyphema, and cataracts (1 each).

RISK FACTORS

Husbandry

- Urolith formation is commonly associated with chronic dehydration, high-protein diets and lack of exercise.
- Exogenous uric acid production is dependent on diet and is particularly high when the diet is rich in animal protein; hence, the inappropriateness of feeding dog or cat food to herbivorous reptiles.
- Fresh water should always be present in the enclosure and supplemented with daily misting.
- Weekly soakings for most reptiles are also recommended.

Others
Underlying renal insufficiency

DIAGNOSIS

DIFFERENTIAL DIAGNOSIS

Space-occupying lesions of the intestinal tract including cloaca, gastrointestinal foreign bodies, ileus, dystocia and constipation.

DIAGNOSTICS

• In chelonians (smaller individuals), palpation of the inguinal fossae is done as the animal is gently rocked from side to side while held in a vertical position.
• Radiography is considered the gold standard.
• Dorsoventral and horizontal lateral views are useful to identify the size and shape of the urolith and to provide surgical landmarks if a plastronotomy is required.
• If a radiolucent calculus or soft tissue mass is suspected, ultrasound should be done.
• Ultrasound is also useful to determine whether an ectopic egg is located in the urinary bladder.

PATHOLOGICAL FINDINGS

• Uroliths cause mucinosis, cystitis, and inflammatory hypertrophy of the bladder wall, while very large uroliths can cause pressure necrosis of the bladder wall with subsequent rupture and septic coelomitis.
• Necropsies have revealed concurrent renal gout, membranous glomerulopathy, renal interstitial fibrosis, glomerulonephritis and interstitial fibrosis, and renal interstitial fibrosis with mineralization.

TREATMENT

APPROPRIATE HEALTH CARE

N/A

NUTRITIONAL SUPPORT

• Reptiles that are anorexic benefit from tube feeding for several days prior to an invasive procedure.
• Tortoises that have undergone celiotomy commonly require an esophagostomy tube prior to awakening from anesthesia.
• The esophagostomy tube is used for administering oral medications and feeding up to several months postoperatively.
• Oxbow Critical Care for Herbivores® (Oxbow Animal Health, Omaha, NE) or EmerAid Sustain Herbivore® (EmerAid, LLC, Cornell, IL) are commonly used to provide proper nutrition during the recovery period.

CLIENT EDUCATION/HUSBANDRY RECOMMENDATIONS

• Husbandry parameters should be adhered to meticulously, with special emphasis on ambient temperature ranges, diet, hydration, and hygiene during the immediate and long-term convalescent period.
• Follow-up visits with the veterinarian are also important for successful recovery.

MEDICATIONS

DRUG(S) OF CHOICE

• Currently, there are no drugs that have been used to successfully dissolve uroliths in reptiles; however, allopurinol, a xanthine oxidase inhibitor, 10–20 mg/kg PO q24h is used to reduce uric acid levels in reptiles to discourage stone formation.
• Extraction of the urolith is required and can be done via an assortment of techniques.
• Sometimes, smaller calculi can be passed successfully by soaking of affected animals.
• Calculi present in the cloaca can usually be removed under sedation, using forceps to fragment them into smaller pieces.
• Visualization is dramatically enhanced with the use of endoscopic guidance (cloacoscopy).
• The use of a dental drill to fragment cloacoliths in tortoises has been described.
• Coeliotomy and cystotomy are the procedures most commonly used to remove calculi located in the urinary bladder.
• In chelonians, cystotomy via marsupialization of the bladder through the prefemoral fossa can be used to remove most, if not all, calculi.
• Large calculi that do not fit though the marsupialized bladder can usually be fragmented and removed in smaller pieces.
• A drill or Carmalt forceps can then be used to fragment the calculi.
• The fragmented calculi are then grasped with sponge forceps and extracted from the marsupialized bladder.
• In chelonians, plastron osteotomy (plastronotomy) may be required for access to remove larger stones that cannot be fragmented or if there is concern for bladder necrosis.
• Successful cystoscopic lithotripsy has been described in a yellow-bellied slider.
• It is generally recommended that celiotomy/plastronotomy patients be administered postsurgical broad-spectrum antibiotics.

PRECAUTIONS/INTERACTIONS

N/A

FOLLOW-UP

PATIENT MONITORING

• Any reptile recovering from an invasive surgical procedure should be isolated so it may be carefully monitored.
• It is essential to keep the cage warm. A basking light, typically a 60–100-watt spotlight, should be set-up at one end of the tank. The temperature underneath the spotlight should reach 35–37 degrees C (95–100 degrees F). The other end of the cage should be about 8–10 degrees C (15–20 degrees F) cooler.
• It is recommended that the owner uses an infrared (laser) thermometer to directly measure the temperature of the reptile. If the patient spends all its time on the heated side, the cage may be too cool. If it spends all its time at the cool end of the cage, the basking spot may be too hot.
• Some source of floor heat, such as heat tape, is useful for night-time heat.
• Ultraviolet B lighting should be provided for proper vitamin D synthesis and to stimulate proper healing. Lights should be set up to illuminate the area around the basking light.
• The reptile should have a shallow water bowl for drinking, but it should not be soaked until the incision has healed or the patch has been on long enough that there is good granulation tissue beneath.
• Appetite should be closely monitored.
• Esophagostomy tubes can be removed once the patient begins feeding.
• It is also important to monitor urine and fecal output throughout recovery.

EXPECTED COURSE AND PROGNOSIS

• In the author's experience, reptiles that have been diagnosed concurrently with urinary calculi and gout (articular/visceral) carry a significantly more guarded prognosis than those that are not hyperuricemic.
• Clinicians considering surgical removal of uroliths, particularly via plastronotomy, should be aware of potential postoperative complications such as infected or delayed healing time, particularly if the bone flap has been completely severed on four sides, in which case it may be years before new bone forms underneath.
• It is also important place a barrier (i.e., bone wax) between the edges of the flap and the plastron to prevent epoxy from leaking into the bone incisions.
• For chelonians where celiotomies are done using a soft-tissue approach, complications associated with bladder dehiscence have been reported, presumably due to mural necrosis that was missed due to limited visibility of the urinary bladder.

MISCELLANEOUS

COMMENTS

Figures 10, 11 and 12 – see web image supplementary content for Section II (Chelonians).

SYNONYMS

- Bladder stones
- Cystic calculi
- Cystoliths
- Urinary concretions
- Urolithiasis
- Uroliths

ABBREVIATIONS

PO = per os

INTERNET RESOURCES

Mader D. Tortoise Bladder Stones. Reptiles Magazine, December 1, 2011. https://www.reptilesmagazine.com/tortoise-bladder-stones

Suggested Reading

Keller KA, Hawkins MG, Scott Weber EP III, et al. Diagnosis and treatment of urolithiasis in client-owned chelonians: 40 cases (1987–2012). *J Am Vet Med Assoc* 2015;247(6):650–658.

Mader DR. Calculi: Urinary. In: Mader DR, ed. *Reptile Medicine and Surgery.* 2nd ed. St. Louis, MO: Elsevier Saunders; 2006:763–771.

Mans C, Sladky K. Endoscopically-guided removal of cloacal calculi in three African spurred tortoises (*Geochelone sulcata*). *J Am Vet Med Assoc* 2012;240(7):869–875.

Nardini G, Leopardi S, Di Girolamo N. Endoscopic laser lithotripsy in a freshwater turtle. *Proc ARAV* 2013:23.

Wright K. Clinical management of bladder stones in tortoises. *Proc NAVC Conference* 2008:1804–1806.

Author Paul Raiti, DVM, ABVP (Reptile and Amphibian Practice)

VOMITING

BASICS

DEFINITION/OVERVIEW

Vomiting is the forcible ejection of partially or wholly digested contents from the stomach and small intestine through the mouth.

ETIOLOGY/PATHOPHYSIOLOGY

- Vomiting in reptiles is under active neural control from the autonomic and somatic nervous systems.
- Details are not completely understood, but they are likely similar to those of mammals.
- The difference between vomiting and regurgitation may be difficult to discern.

SIGNALMENT/HISTORY

- All species, ages, sexes may be affected.
- Owner may report observing vomiting or only that vomited material was found.
- Other notable history may include lethargy, anorexia, weight loss, respiratory distress, or increased basking frequency, or ingestion of foreign material.

CLINICAL PRESENTATION

- No clinical signs are specific to vomiting, and physical exam may be normal.
- Presentation varies depending on the underlying cause and chronicity.
- Dehydration and/or emaciation/cachexia.
- Hard mass on palpation of the coelomic cavity due to an obstructive lesion or organomegaly.
- Skeletal abnormalities that may include pathological fractures or abnormal growth patterns.
- Lethargy and/or obtunded mentation.
- Ulceration and accumulation of caseous material in the oral cavity.
- Secondary respiratory disease (e.g., oral/nasal discharge, abnormal respiratory sounds) or enteritis (e.g., diarrhea).

RISK FACTORS

Husbandry

- Too much disturbance or lack of hiding places (increases stress/anxiety).
- Poor sanitation, overcrowding, hyper- or hypothermia, lack of quarantine for new individuals (increases stress, possibility of secondary infections, and disease transmission).
- Toxin exposure (cleaning chemicals, pesticides, heavy metals).
- Excessive/inappropriate handling (especially soon after feeding).
- Inadequate diet (incorrect calcium/phosphorus ratio, improper prey items, excessive feeding).
- Inappropriate substrate (may be accidentally ingested).

Others

Concomitant infectious or parasitic disease.

DIAGNOSIS

DIFFERENTIAL DIAGNOSIS

- Stomatitis
- Esophagitis
- Esophageal stricture
- Gastritis
- Handling/stress (e.g., excessive pressure to coelom)
- Obstructive lesions (e.g., GI foreign body, intussusception, neoplasia, abscess, granuloma)
- Metabolic disease (e.g., NSHP, renal or hepatic dysfunction)
- Toxicoses (e.g., zinc)
- Iatrogenic (e.g., enrofloxacin, xylazine, levamisole)
- Trauma to esophagus or stomach.
- Parasites (e.g., *Cryptosporidium*, amoebiasis, ascaridiasis, cestodiasis)
- Viruses
- Bacteria/septicemia (e.g., *Chlamydophila*)
- Congenital GI defects

DIAGNOSTICS

- Husbandry review
- Physical examination
- Complete blood count and plasma biochemistries.
- Radiography with or without contrast.
- Ultrasound
- Fecal parasite exam
- Other diagnostics to consider: bacterial cultures from oral lesions, GI endoscopy or coeliotomy (direct tissue evaluation and biopsy), and testing for cryptosporidiosis.

PATHOLOGICAL FINDINGS

- Dependent on underlying cause
- Cryptosporidiosis in chelonians primarily affects the intestinal tract, but could also potentially affect the stomach.

TREATMENT

APPROPRIATE HEALTH CARE

The primary goal is to identify and address the underlying cause.

NUTRITIONAL SUPPORT

- Correct fluid deficits and maintain hydration.
- Intracoelomic, subcutaneous, or intravenous routes for administration of a reptile Ringer's solution are most effective. Maintenance rate is 10–30 ml/kg/day.
- Tube or assist-feeding liquid or gel diets (e.g., Oxbow Critical Care® formulas, Oxbow Animal Health, Omaha, NE) may be beneficial during initial treatment/recovery.
- Gradually add normal diet items as animal improves.

CLIENT EDUCATION/HUSBANDRY RECOMMENDATIONS

- Review husbandry and correct any problems.
- Institute quarantine procedures for new animals, including 30–60 day period, veterinary evaluation, and 1–3-weekly fecal exams for parasites.

MEDICATIONS

DRUG(S) OF CHOICE

- Cimetidine 4 mg/kg IM, PO q8–12h, or famotidine 0.25–0.5 mg/kg SC, PO q24–72h
- Metoclopramide 0.06 mg/kg PO q24h for 7 days or 1–10 mg/kg PO q24h, or cisapride 0.5–2 mg/kg PO q24h
- Sucralfate 500–1000 mg/kg PO q6–8h

PRECAUTIONS/INTERACTIONS

N/A

FOLLOW-UP

PATIENT MONITORING

Monitor for continued signs of vomiting and possible complications.

EXPECTED COURSE AND PROGNOSIS

- Dependent on underlying cause
- Vomiting is rare in chelonians, and often carries a fair to poor prognosis.
- Prognosis for subclinical cryptosporidiosis is fair to good.
- Prognosis for clinical disease is poor to grave, and euthanasia is often indicated.

MISCELLANEOUS

COMMENTS

N/A

ZOONOTIC POTENTIAL

N/A

SYNONYMS

Emesis

ABBREVIATIONS

- GI = gastrointestinal
- IM = intramuscular
- NSHP = nutritional secondary hyperparathyroidism
- PO = per os
- SC = subcutaneous

VOMITING (CONTINUED)

Suggested Reading
Funk RS. Vomiting and regurgitation. In: Mader DR, ed. *Reptile Medicine and Surgery*. 2nd ed. St. Louis, MO: Elsevier Saunders; 2006:939–940.

Gibbons PM, Klaphake E, Carpenter JW. Reptiles. In: Carpenter JW, Marion CJ, eds. *Exotic Animal Formulary*. 4th ed. St. Louis, MO: Elsevier Saunders; 2013:83–182.

Mitchell MA, Diaz-Figueroa O. Clinical reptile gastroenterology. *Vet Clin N Am Exot Anim Pract* 2005;8:277–298.

Authors Tamara Kruse, DVM, MS, and Trevor T. Zachariah, DVM, MS, DACZM

WEIGHT LOSS

BASICS

DEFINITION/OVERVIEW

Weight loss can take the form of body mass loss (i.e., cachexia) or fluid loss. In mammals, it is generally accepted that weight loss becomes clinically significant when the loss exceeds 10% of normal body weight (and when it is not completely due to fluid loss). From a clinical perspective, weight loss of more than 10–20% of a healthy, species-specific body weight is significant and must be systematically evaluated, with rapid weight loss being considered most urgent. Weight loss in reptiles may be a normal physiologic process (e.g., brumation/estivation, reproductive activity, or behavior), and is not considered a primary disease, but, rather, a clinical manifestation of other disease processes.

ETIOLOGY/PATHOPHYSIOLOGY

- Normal weight loss (fluid and body mass loss) will occur during times of torpor or brumation/estivation.
- Once post-torpor normal behavior returns, the reptile will replenish lost fluids and body mass under normal circumstances, or given normal access to clean water and appropriate food and environmental conditions.
- Normal weight loss may be associated with reproductive behavior or gravidity as well.
- Pathologic weight loss may be associated with a variety of noninfectious and infectious disease processes.
- In pet reptiles, inappropriate husbandry is the most common underlying cause of pathologic weight loss.
- Poor husbandry may frequently lead to metabolic diseases of secondary infectious diseases due to immune system compromise of the animal.
- Infectious diseases and debilitating noninfectious diseases will commonly result in weight loss due to both body mass and fluid loss.
- In some cases, reptiles succumb to a nonspecific disease process referred to as "maladaptation or failure to thrive syndrome," which is characterized by the failure of a captive reptile to adapt to its current conditions, or a wild-caught reptile unable to adapt to the captive environment.
- Many of these animals will lose weight and die, and a specific disease process is not diagnosed.

SIGNALMENT/HISTORY

- Weight loss in reptiles has no specific signalment, and can affect males or females of any species and any age.
- A typical history suggests rapid weight loss of 10% or more acutely or 20% or more chronically.
- Weight loss in reptiles typically includes some degree of dehydration, in addition to loss of body mass and/or fat stores.
- If the individual or species normally brumates/estivates, weight loss can be expected as a normal physiologic process.
- With pathologic weight loss, the husbandry and environment must be evaluated thoroughly, and infectious and noninfectious diseases must be considered as underlying causes to the weight loss.

CLINICAL PRESENTATION

- Reptiles presenting for weight loss typically show observable loss of muscle mass.
- The vertebral column and pelvic bones become more readily apparent, and the hind limb muscles will decrease in mass.
- In some chelonians, the base of the neck and prefemoral fossa may appear more sunken in and lack skin tone.
- The musculature over the skull may also become atrophied.
- With dehydration, the eyes may sink into the bony orbits, and the severe tenting of the skin may become distinct, depending on the species.

RISK FACTORS

Husbandry

- Poor husbandry is the most common contributing factor to pathologic process in reptiles, including weight loss.
- Poor husbandry might include: inappropriate housing type or improper placement within a client's household or other facility; ambient temperature and humidity; lack of access to clean water or dechlorinated water in aquatic species; lack of presence and appropriate maintenance of an ultraviolet light source (position, distance from reptiles, appropriate duration between bulb changes); inappropriate type, quality and quantity of food offered for the species; intra- or inter-specific competition for food; type of substrate, cage furniture, and frequency of cleaning/replacing substrate; toxicity associated with environmental cleaning solutions.
- Common diseases associated with inappropriate husbandry include: foreign-body ingestion and GI impaction; thermal burns; NSHP (metabolic bone disease); dental disease; chronic renal disease; starvation due to competition for food by other individuals; and exposure to toxic chemicals (e.g., ammonia, nitrites, or chloramines in aquatic species; heavy metals; cleaning solutions; toxic food items, such as fireflies).
- In some cases, maladaptation syndrome or failure to thrive syndrome should also be considered as an underlying cause of weight loss.

Others

- It is critical to ensure that chelonians undergoing brumation have access to water on a scheduled basis to prevent dehydration, which leads to weight loss.
- An over 20% decrease in body weight during brumation is suggestive of dehydration.
- Brumation temperatures must also be low enough for the species to avoid the animal retaining an active metabolism that may lead to muscle wasting.

DIAGNOSIS

DIFFERENTIAL DIAGNOSIS

Normal Behavior

- Periods of torpor, brumation and estivation are normal for some species and may be associated with weight loss (loss of body mass and fluids).
- In some species, fluid loss during brumation/estivation can contribute to over 10% of total weight loss.
- Reproductive activity, behavior and gravidity may contribute to normal seasonal weight loss.

Non-Infectious Diseases

Exposure to toxic substances, especially in aquatic species, or developing disease processes secondary to poor husbandry or nutrition will commonly lead to weight loss.

Neoplasia

- A number of neoplastic diseases have been identified in reptile species, with many different organ systems affected.
- Most of these neoplastic diseases have an expected clinical sequela of hyporexia, dehydration, and weight loss.

Infectious Diseases

- Reptiles are susceptible to many infectious diseases, all of which can contribute to hyporexia, dehydration, and weight loss.
- Simply attempting to list all infectious diseases of reptiles that may contribute to weight loss is beyond the scope of this chapter. However, common reptile diseases observed in clinical practice, include endoparasites (GI protozoa, nematodes, amoebae, and hemoparasites); ectoparasites (mites, ticks); Gram-negative bacterial infections and septicemia; *Chrysosporium* species and other fungal infections; and viruses (e.g., adenoviruses, paramyxoviruses, herpesviruses, retroviruses).

DIAGNOSTICS

- Since weight loss is not a specific disease, a significant clinical diagnostic workup will be necessary.
- A thorough history will be useful, including housing, feeding practices, maintenance

temperature and humidity, presence of other animals, access to UVB light spectrum, ad libitum access to water and water quality.
• Comparison with conspecifics housed in the same environment may confirm individual versus group disease.
• A complete physical examination is critical to identify obvious lesions on the skin, within the oral cavity, on the extremities, or associated with the eyes.
• A fecal sample should be evaluated by direct smear and fecal float, if possible.
• A complete blood count and biochemical profile, together with imaging modalities (radiography, ultrasound, and/or CT), should be considered.
• Aerobic and anaerobic bacterial cultures of blood samples can be useful in debilitated reptiles due to the possibility of sepsis.
• Intracoelomic or gastrointestinal endoscopy, with or without biopsy and histopathology, may help with the diagnosis.
• In cases of obvious skin disease, a biopsy with histopathologic examination is important.

PATHOLOGICAL FINDINGS

• Pathologic findings are non-specific for weight loss, but the underlying cause may be associated with obvious gross pathologic or histopathologic lesions.
• Gross pathology of nonspecific weight loss might include loss of intracoelomic fat bodies, lack of intracoelomic organ-associated fat, and generalized muscle wasting.

TREATMENT

APPROPRIATE HEALTH CARE

N/A

NUTRITIONAL SUPPORT

• Nonspecific nutritional support may include regular force-feeding of an appropriate commercial diet and/or placement of a pharyngostomy tube to facilitate administering nutritional supplements.
• The directions on the label of the commercial diet can be followed for appropriate volume per feeding and frequency.

CLIENT EDUCATION/HUSBANDRY RECOMMENDATIONS

N/A

MEDICATIONS

DRUG(S) OF CHOICE

• Based on the diagnosis of the underlying cause of weight loss, treatment should be focused on the primary disease process.
• Over-supplementation of vitamins and minerals may need to be discontinued if this appears to be causing primary disease.
• Correct hydration status by soaking or administering appropriate fluid therapy due to fluid loss (typically an isotonic solution), as any debilitated reptile will likely be moderately to severely dehydrated.
• Based on the primary disease process underlying the weight loss, antimicrobial and anti-inflammatory drugs may be warranted.
• In cases of some infectious diseases, antimicrobials can be administered for bacterial or fungal diseases using topical, parenteral, or oral solutions.
• In addition, vitamin and mineral supplements (e.g., calcium in the form of parenteral calcium gluconate or oral calcium glubionate) may be beneficial if nutritional deficiencies underlie the weight loss.

PRECAUTIONS/INTERACTIONS

N/A

FOLLOW-UP

PATIENT MONITORING

• If appropriate, medical therapy can be initiated and the patient monitored for improving condition.
• Correction of inappropriate husbandry and/or feeding practices will significantly benefit the reptile patient.
• If medical treatment is necessary, the body weight can be measured and the body condition assessed daily.

EXPECTED COURSE AND PROGNOSIS

• Replenishing lost fluids from normal physiologic processes, such as brumation/estivation, may be warranted and should improve the reptiles' condition and provide a good prognosis.
• Depending on the primary underlying disease process and duration, the prognosis will range from poor to good for re-establishing normal body weight and condition.
• If husbandry problems can be corrected in a relatively short amount of time, the prognosis may be good.
• If the underlying disease process is progressive and debilitating, the prognosis will be poor.

MISCELLANEOUS

COMMENTS

N/A

ZOONOTIC POTENTIAL

N/A

SYNONYMS

• Cachexia
• Wasting

ABBREVIATIONS

• CT = computed tomography
• GI = gastrointestinal
• NSHP = nutritional secondary hyperparathyroidism
• UVB = ultraviolet B

Suggested Reading

Mader DR. *Reptile Medicine and Surgery, Reptile Medicine and Surgery*. 2nd ed. St. Louis, MO: Elsevier Saunders; 2006.

Author Kurt K. Sladky, MS, DVM, DACZM, DECZM (Zoo Health Management & Herpetology)

YEAST INFECTIONS

BASICS

DEFINITION/OVERVIEW
Infection with *Candida* spp., *Cryptococcus* spp., or, exceptionally other yeasts, is rare in reptiles, in comparison with mammals and birds.

ETIOLOGY/PATHOPHYSIOLOGY
- Many yeasts, especially *Candida* species, are normal constituents of reptile GI and even respiratory tracts.
- Typically, they occur secondary to concurrent condition or infection.

SIGNALMENT/HISTORY
Any reptile species, any sex, any age.

CLINICAL PRESENTATION
- Anorexia, diarrhea, weight loss, debilitation.
- Signs may be non-specific or depend on affected organ system.
- Cryptococcosis has manifested as a granulomatous pneumonia and meningoencephalitis in an anaconda, but as a cutaneous swelling in a skink.

RISK FACTORS

Husbandry
Poor husbandry is likely a factor with these often opportunistic pathogens.

Others
- Breaches in mucosal epithelia from concurrent issues/infections may allow deep tissue access to yeasts.
- Prolonged antibiotic treatment may also favor yeast proliferation.

DIAGNOSIS

DIFFERENTIAL DIAGNOSIS
- Viral and/or bacterial stomatitides and enteritides, or even protozoal GI infections.
- Viral/bacterial/parasitic or other respiratory infections.

DIAGNOSTICS
- Cytology of swabs or washes that demonstrate budding yeast, and ideally inflammatory cells.
- Culture of swabs, exudates, and biopsies are needed but the isolation of *Candida* is insufficient to confirm causality.
- Concurrent histopathological evidence of yeast infection in biopsy/tissue sections is essential to establish causality.

PATHOLOGICAL FINDINGS
Necrosis, inflammation, and budding yeast with pseudohyphae.

TREATMENT

APPROPRIATE HEALTH CARE
- Systemic antifungals, fluid therapy, thermal and nutritional support.
- Isolation of sick animals
- Review of captive husbandry

NUTRITIONAL SUPPORT
Assist-feeding if needed

CLIENT EDUCATION/HUSBANDRY RECOMMENDATIONS
- Isolation of sick animals and thorough hygiene.
- Critical review of husbandry

MEDICATIONS

DRUG(S) OF CHOICE
- Fluconazole may be efficient in treating yeast infections, but some *Candida* species are inherently fluconazole resistant.
- Superficial GI mucosal infections may respond to nystatin.
- Probably better to use wider-spectrum, systemically absorbed triazoles like itraconazole.

PRECAUTIONS/INTERACTIONS
N/A

FOLLOW-UP

PATIENT MONITORING
- Might require intensive care
- Monitor response to antifungal therapy and supportive measures.

EXPECTED COURSE AND PROGNOSIS
- Variable, depending on duration and severity of disease, affected organ systems, and extent of lesions.
- As these infections are often diagnosed late in the disease process, prognosis should be guarded.

MISCELLANEOUS

COMMENTS
- A presumptive diagnosis of candidiasis or other yeast infection may be possible cytologically from clinical samples.
- Every effort should be made to pursue identification of these yeast to species.
- Yeast identification may carry treatment implications, as sensitivity panels can be determined.
- Only with proper identification can we understand which yeasts carry pathogenic potential.

ZOONOTIC POTENTIAL
- Cryptococcosis, a zoonotic disease, has been documented in reptiles.
- Candidiasis is rare in reptiles, but also is a potential zoonosis.

SYNONYMS
N/A

ABBREVIATIONS
GI = gastrointestinal

Suggested Reading

Paré JA, Jacobson ER. Mycotic diseases of reptiles. In: Jacobson ER, ed. *Infectious Disease and Pathology of Reptiles, Color Atlas and Text.* Boca Raton, FL: CRC Press; 2007:527–570.

Author Jean A. Paré, DMV, DVSc, DACZM, DECZM (Zoo Health Management)

Section III

Lizards

ABSCESSES

BASICS

DEFINITION/OVERVIEW

Abscesses are non-fluctuating hard masses of variable size, formed by concentric layers of purulent material in which the outermost layer has the most liquid consistency. All purulent material is contained in a fibrous capsule. Coloration ranges from brown to yellow. Adhesions occasionally occur with adjacent tissues. There are no general symptoms if the abscesses do not result from a systemic infection (salmonellosis, pseudomoniasis, microsporidiosis, etc.). Dermal abscesses in reptiles evolve from external wounds, ectoparasites or contamination by direct contact with feces or water with a high bacterial population, all of which may be exacerbated by immunosuppression.

ETIOLOGY/PATHOPHYSIOLOGY

- Abscesses can be a result of local or systemic infections.
- Local infections are typically isolated to the skin and are caused by contamination of wounds with environmental, fecal, or normal flora leading to abscess formation.
- The existence of local infections in the skin is very frequent.
- Cultures show a high causative flora including bacteria, fungi, and viruses.
- Systemic infections may also lead to abscess formation, particularly in internal organs.
- Some local abscesses may spread and become systemic if environmental conditions are favorable.
- In some cases, abscesses may also be the manifestation of systemic diseases (e.g., *Microsporidium* in *Pogona*).

SIGNALMENT/HISTORY

- There is no specific signalment for the occurrence of abscesses.
- The main focus should be on obtaining a thorough history of the husbandry and social interactions of the reptiles.
- A history of aggression in a group of reptiles may contribute to the appearance of abscesses.
- Poor cleanliness and hygiene of the enclosure can lead to increase environmental bacterial load that can contribute to skin lesions and abscess formation.

CLINICAL PRESENTATION

- Reptiles may present with cutaneous abscesses ranging in size from a few millimeters to larger ones that are centimeters in diameter. They can either be freely moveable or firmly attached to the underlying tissues.
- Some of these abscesses become chronic and expel a malodorous, purulent discharge.
- The content of the abscess is mostly caseous in nature.
- Sometimes abscesses can affect nearby bones, and animals may present with lameness.
- Dysecdysis may also be observed in association with the abscess or through the animal's body.
- In iguanas, the most affected parts are the sides, the jaw, the ventral zone, and the tail.

RISK FACTORS

Husbandry

- Husbandry factors that can contribute to the appearance of abscesses are poor hygiene and overpopulation leading to increased bacterial load in the enclosure and possibly stress and immunosuppression.
- Rough substrate or surfaces in the terrarium can lead to cuts or abrasions that may become infected.
- Inappropriate diet and/or UVB exposure may also lead to a weakened immune status.

Others

N/A

DIAGNOSIS

DIFFERENTIAL DIAGNOSIS

- Chronic dysecdysis
- Blister disease
- Limb fractures may have symptoms similar to osteolytic abscesses at the same extremities (limb malposition, lameness, etc.)

DIAGNOSTICS

Cytology

- Cytology can be used as the first screening tool to identify whether a mass is an abscess, either via an aspirate or an impression smear of the material within.
- Abscesses usually reveal a large number of leukocytes, cellular detritus, tissue remnants, and desquamation of cells.
- Infectious organisms may also be observed, but their absence does not rule out an infection.

Microbiology

- Bacterial culture and sensitivity are essential for identification of the existing bacterial population and the best antibiotic treatment to follow.
- Obtaining bacterial growth from abscesses can be difficult. Samples must be obtained not only from the abscess material but also from the wall of the abscess to maximize the possibility of bacterial growth.
- It is also worth noting that anaerobic cultures must be considered, especially when there is no aerobic growth and in cases of malodorous discharge.
- 16sRNA PCR is another tool that is becoming more readily available for bacterial identification. Fungal cultures can also be considered, especially if hyphae are observed in the cytologic exam.

Hematology and Biochemistry

- Some changes that may be observed include leukocytosis, heterophilia, and eosinophilia. The heterophils may appear reactive (toxic granulation).
- Thrombocytes are also activated
- Mitosis may be observed in many leukocytes.
- Total protein values (gammaglobulins and alpha-globulins), and the enzymes AST, CPK, and ALP may be elevated.
- Most of these changes are not consistent and may vary according to the nature of the abscess and how well encapsulated it is.

Histology

Histopathologic exam of a suspected abscess can more definitively confirm the diagnosis and help to identify the presence of infectious organisms.

Imaging

- Radiography: in cases where an abscess is firmly attached to underlying bone, radiography can help determine whether there is bony involvement and osteomyelitis.
- Ultrasound: abscesses (regardless of their location) have a hyperechogenic capsule that creates intense acoustic shadowing with a hypoechogenic interior, especially when they still have a liquid content (the first stage of internal caseum formation). In advanced stages, there is a thin layer of fibrin that surrounds the abscess and under it the inflammatory liquid that forms the internal caseum.

PATHOLOGICAL FINDINGS

- Histologically, necrotic cell layers and a thin layer of phagocytic mononuclear cells in palisade are observed delimiting the core of the abscess.
- Organisms may be visible on numerous sections.
- A correct differential diagnosis of diseases such as mycosis, neoplasias or myiasis must be carried out.

TREATMENT

APPROPRIATE HEALTH CARE

- As with most abscesses, treatment often requires a combination of medical and surgical therapy for best results.
- Any suspected or confirmed bacteria should be treated with appropriate systemic antibiotics until results of sensitivity panel confirm its effectiveness.
- For suspected fungal infections, systemic therapy may not be necessary if the infection is restricted to the abscess.
- Topical antibiotic ointments can also be applied within the abscess cavity.
- An additional treatment is the placement of antibiotic-impregnated beads or dental antibiotic gels, especially in non-responsive cases, fractious animals, or those that cannot be easily treated on a daily basis.

- Most abscesses will take between two weeks and a month to heal.
- In some cases, once the caseous material has been completely removed and there is certainty that only healthy tissue remains, the wound can be sutured.
- In conjunction with medical therapy, surgery to either remove or debride the abscess must be performed.
- Complete removal of the whole abscess and capsule is preferred but is often not possible owing to size limitations for skin closure or involvement of underlying tissues. A debridement is more commonly performed.
- The abscess should be opened to extract the purulent material and as much of the capsule as possible. It can then be irrigated with a disinfectant solution (iodine, chlorhexidine, etc.) and left open to heal by secondary intention.
- Daily flushing and cleaning should be performed until no more purulent material is observed.

NUTRITIONAL SUPPORT

- Proper nutrition is key for response to therapy.
- The diet should be as varied as possible and adapted to each species.
- Nutritional support via gavage feeding should be implemented in very ill and/or anorectic animals.

CLIENT EDUCATION/HUSBANDRY RECOMMENDATIONS

- Correct any husbandry deficiencies, with special attention to hygiene, temperature, humidity, and ventilation.
- Isolate animal from others in collection during treatment.
- It is important to ensure a full course of treatment to avoid recurrence.

MEDICATIONS

DRUG(S) OF CHOICE

- The most commonly used antibiotics are broad-spectrum antibiotics, such as fluoroquinolones, aminoglycosides, sulfamides, or some penicillins, such as carbenicillin or ampicillin.
- Antibiotic (amikacin, cephalosporins) impregnated beads or dental antibiotic gels, such as doxycycline hyclate (DOXIROBE® gel, Zoetis Services, LLC, Parsippany, NJ; or clindamycin hydrochloride 1% (ClinzGard®, TriLogic Pharma, LLC, Tallassee, AL).

PRECAUTIONS/INTERACTIONS

- Fluid therapy should be considered when administering systemic antimicrobials, especially aminoglycoside antibiotics (gentamicin, streptomycin, amikacin, kanamycin) because of their nephrotoxic potential.
- Systemic antifungals should also be used and monitored cautiously.

FOLLOW-UP

PATIENT MONITORING

- Abscesses should not grow out again one month after treatment.
- If there is a recurrence, a more aggressive approach is needed.
- Scarring and pigmentation changes may be observed at the site of the healed abscess.

EXPECTED COURSE AND PROGNOSIS

- Generally, abscesses heal well, are not complicated, and have a good prognosis.
- If allowed to become chronic they can become systemic, affect the internal viscera, and compromise the life of the reptile. At this point, the prognosis would be guarded to grave.

MISCELLANEOUS

COMMENTS

N/A

ZOONOTIC POTENTIAL

- The zoonotic potential will depend on the type of bacteria associated with the abscess.
- Appropriate precautions must be taken when working with reptile abscesses to minimize exposure to zoonotic organisms.

SYNONYMS

- Purulent dermatitis
- Subcutaneous abscesses
- Superficial pyoderma

ABBREVIATIONS

- ALP = alkaline phosphatase
- AST = aspartate aminotransferase
- CPK = creatine phosphokinase
- PCR = polymerase chain reaction
- UVB = ultraviolet B

INTERNET RESOURCES

- Kaplan M. Treating Abscesses in Reptiles. 1996. Melissa Kaplan's Herp Care Collection. Last updated January 1, 2014. http://www.anapsid.org/abscess.html
- Negron V. 4 Diseases Your Pet Reptile Can Give You. PetMD, May 1, 2015. http://www.petmd.com/reptile/care/diseases-your-pet-reptile-can-give-you
- PetMD Editorial. Internal Abscesses in Reptiles. PetMD, July 28, 2008. http://www.petmd.com/reptile/conditions/skin/c_rp_internal_abscesses

Suggested Reading

Huchzermeyer FW, Cooper JE. Fibriscess, not abscess, resulting from a localized inflammatory response to infection in reptiles and birds. *Vet Rec* 2000;147:515–517.

Mayer J, Pizzirani S, DeSena R. Bilateral exophthalmos in an adult iguana (*Iguana iguana*) caused by an orbital abscess. *J Herp Med Surg* 2010;20:5–10.

Williams SR, Sims M, Roth-Jonson L, Wickes B. Surgical removal of an abscess associated with Fusarium solani from a Kemp's ridley sea turtle (*Lepidochelys kempii*). *J Zoo Wildl Med* 2012;43:402–406.

Author Albert Martínez-Silvestre, DVM, MSc, PhD, DECZM (Herpetology), EBVS European Veterinary Specialist in Herpetological Medicine and Surgery, Acred. AVEPA (Exotic Animals)

ADENOVIRUS

BASICS

DEFINITION/OVERVIEW

AdVs have been found to infect all classes of bony vertebrates and most appear to have co-evolved with their hosts. Adenoviral infections in reptiles have ranged from clinically inapparent to enteritis, necrotizing hepatitis, esophagitis, splenitis, and encephalopathy.

ETIOLOGY/PATHOPHYSIOLOGY

- AdVs are double-stranded, non-enveloped DNA viruses.
- They fall in the family *Adenoviridae*, which is further classified into five currently accepted genera: *Mastadenovirus* isolated from mammals; *Aviadenovirus* in birds; *Atadenovirus* isolated from squamates; *Siadenovirus* found in some chelonians, amphibians, and birds; and *Ichtadenovirus* isolated from a sturgeon.
- A sixth genus, *Testadenovirus*, isolated from tortoises, has been proposed.
- AdV infections have been identified in wild-caught and captive lizards, snakes, chelonians, and crocodiles.
- Disease is often a combination of other disease agents and/or stress and the viral infection.

SIGNALMENT/HISTORY

- The species reported with an adenovirus isolate are: bearded dragons, Gila monsters, beaded lizards, Savannah monitor, central netted dragon, leopard geckos, fat-tailed geckos, tokay gecko, mountain chameleon, green tree monitors, emerald monitor.
- With molecular diagnostics, more affected species are expected to be identified.
- There is no sex predilection
- Juvenile and/or stressed animals are more frequently reported with disease.

CLINICAL PRESENTATION

- The clinical presentation is non-specific and often the animal is found dead.
- Clinical signs in lizards include weight loss, anorexia, diarrhea, and some neurologic clinical signs such as head tilt and circling.

RISK FACTORS

Husbandry

- AdVs are very stable in the environment and are commonly spread through fecal–oral transmission.
- Poor biosecurity can help disseminate the virus throughout a collection.

Others

- Stressors such as capture, substandard housing, nutritional inadequacies, or underlying disease play a role in the development of clinical infection.
- Concurrent disease and/or immunosuppression increases the likelihood of severe systemic disease.
- Bearded dragons have been co-infected with *Dependovirus* and *Isospora* spp.

DIAGNOSIS

DIFFERENTIAL DIAGNOSIS

- Septicemia, gastroenteritis from any cause
- Bearded dragons: coccidia, microsporidia

DIAGNOSTICS

- PCR may be diagnostic if the test is specific for the adenovirus commonly isolated from the reptile species.
- Necropsy and histopathology: the appropriate tissues need to be evaluated and, in some cases, additional tests such as TEM and/or PCR molecular diagnostics need to be performed.

PATHOLOGICAL FINDINGS

Bearded dragons

- Gross lesions: coelomic effusion
- Histology: basophilic intranuclear viral inclusions and severe coagulative necrosis of the liver, intestine, lymphohistiocytic interstitial nephritis, and bile duct.

TREATMENT

APPROPRIATE HEALTH CARE

N/A

NUTRITIONAL SUPPORT

- Nutritional support should be provided as needed, only when the reptile is well hydrated and at an ideal environmental temperature for the species.
- An esophagostomy tube should be considered for long-term care.

CLIENT EDUCATION/HUSBANDRY RECOMMENDATIONS

- Quarantine: the current recommendation is for an approximately six months isolation period for most reptiles, with PCR testing at various intervals.
- Post-Outbreak: after diagnosis of an AdV infection in a collection, cages and hard surfaces should be thoroughly cleaned with a detergent, followed by disinfection with a 10% bleach solution.
- A minimum of 10-minutes contact time with the bleach is recommended. All bleached supplies and cages should be thoroughly rinsed afterward and dried. Bleach can be corrosive and can cause respiratory irritation in enclosed spaces.
- Direct unfiltered sunlight or other intense ultraviolet sources may also aid disinfection.
- Proper contact time must be followed if using other disinfectants.
- All reptiles should be kept at appropriate temperature and humidity, and offered food consistent with their dietary requirements.

MEDICATIONS

DRUG(S) OF CHOICE

N/A

PRECAUTIONS/INTERACTIONS

N/A

FOLLOW-UP

PATIENT MONITORING

- Reptiles showing clinical signs should be isolated and provided with supportive care.
- Any co-infections should be treated, if possible.
- Monitoring weight, appetite, and fecal production will help to assess response to therapy and progression of infection.
- Utensils and cage furniture should not be transferred from room to room or animal to animal.

EXPECTED COURSE AND PROGNOSIS

- There is no specific treatment
- Cases have ranged from acute to chronic protracted presentation of clinical signs.
- Identifying AdV from a healthy animal is not diagnostic for a disease caused by the virus.
- Reptiles can be inapparent hosts for AdVs.
- The disease progression is unknown as antemortem diagnosis is seldom determined.

MISCELLANEOUS

COMMENTS

N/A

ZOONOTIC POTENTIAL

N/A

SYNONYMS

N/A

ABBREVIATIONS

- AdV = Adenovirus
- PCR = polymerase chain reaction
- TEM = transmission electron microscopy

INTERNET RESOURCES

- Kik MJL. Adenovirus Infection in Reptiles. EAZWV Transmissible Disease Fact Sheet No. 2, April 2009. http:www.eazwv.org/resource/resmgr/Files/Transmissible_Diseases_Handbook/Fact_Sheets/002_Adenovirus_Infection_In_.pdf
- Jacobson E, Wellehan J, Stacy B. Reptile Adenovirus PCR an Sequencing at the University of Florida CVM. http://www.dachiu.com/beardeddragons/Adenovirus.pdf

Suggested Reading

Ball I, Ofner S, Funk RS, et al. Prevalence of neutralising antibodies against adenoviruses in lizards and snakes. *Vet J* 2014;202(1):176–181.

Papp T, Fledelius B, Schmidt V, et al. PCR-sequence characterization of new adenoviruses found in reptiles and the first successful isolation of a lizard adenovirus. *Vet Microbiol* 2009;134(3–4):233–240.

Author Drury R. Reavill, DVM, DABVP (Avian and Reptile & Amphibian Practice), DACVP

ANEMIA

BASICS

DEFINITION/OVERVIEW

Anemia is a sign of disease and is characterized by a decreased number of erythrocytes, hemoglobin deficiency, or both. Anemia can occur due to one of four main categories: decreased erythropoietic activity, hemorrhage, destruction of red blood cells, or sequestration.

ETIOLOGY/PATHOPHYSIOLOGY

- Traumatic
- Hemorrhagic
- Maladaptation syndrome-associated anemia is reported in stressed reptiles, associated with captivity or with capture of wild reptiles.
- Blood parasites
- Virus-associated anemia
- Autoimmune hemolytic anemia is rare in reptiles.

SIGNALMENT/HISTORY

Wild-caught reptiles or those housed under poor husbandry conditions may be more predisposed.

CLINICAL PRESENTATION

- Anemic reptiles often present with nonspecific clinical signs including lethargy, anorexia and behavioral changes.
- Pallor of skin and mucus membrane color may also be observed.

RISK FACTORS

Wild-caught reptiles are more likely to have underlying diseases, especially endoparasites and hemoparasites, which may be the underlying cause of chronic anemia.

Husbandry

- Inadequate husbandry including diet, is often a predisposing factor for many diseases of captive reptiles.
- Any reptile maintained under poor husbandry conditions should be considered to be susceptible to disease.

Others

Any reptile with a chronic illness may be predisposed to anemia.

DIAGNOSIS

DIFFERENTIAL DIAGNOSIS

- Trauma leading to external or internal hemorrhage.
- Maladaptation syndrome associated anemia is reported in stressed reptiles, associated with captivity or trapping of wild reptiles.
- Hemoparasites
- Malnutrition
- Toxicity
- Weakness and prostration due to metabolic bone disease, pregnancy, or infectious disease.

DIAGNOSTICS

- Blood sampling is essential for diagnosis and monitoring of anemic reptiles.
- Patient's size, condition, and venous access all must be considered.
- Venipuncture sites with minimal lymphatic contamination are preferred, to obtain a more representative sample of the peripheral blood. In lizards, the jugular, ventral coccygeal, and ventral abdominal vein are all options.
- The level of contamination at each site is highly variable across species.
- In critically ill, possibly anemic reptiles, one should aim to collect a blood volume of no more than 0.5% of the body weight (0.5 ml/100 g body weight) so as to not exacerbate the anemic condition.
- The use of EDTA vs. lithium heparin is widely debated in reptile medicine, and is largely based on experience and a few scientific studies.
- In general, EDTA is recommended unless artifacts are documented for a particular species.

Physical Exam

- Examination of mucous membranes and general pallor.
- Compared with mammals, reptiles' mucous membranes are lighter in color but should still appear pink.
- In some lizards, such as bearded dragons, the mucous membranes normally have a yellow pigmentation, which can make it more difficult to assess pallor.

Hematology

- Although there is limited ability to assess all the same hematologic parameters as in mammals, some basic guidelines can be found for certain values.

Hematocrit/PCV

- The normal values range from 20% to 45%. Values below 20% suggest anemia in most cases. A blood transfusion should be considered in animals with values below 10%, although there is little research in reptilian blood transfusions. Seasonal variations in this parameter should also be considered before making clinical decisions. A low hematocrit with an increased polychromasia index is a normal physiologic change during brumation, but pathologic during the active season.

Hemoglobin

- The normal values are 6–10 g/dl according to the species. Lower values suggest anemia. The MCHC is calculated according to the hematocrit and hemoglobin, so these parameters show variation in cases of anemia. However, individual variations should also be considered, as reptiles have different types of hemoglobin, which may influence the expression of clinical signs.

Polychromasia and Erythroblasts

- Increased polychromasia and erythroblasts in general suggest an increased need for erythrocytes in peripheral blood and can be interpreted as evidence of a regenerative anemia.
- Occasionally, a high number of erythroblasts can be found in the microhematocrit tube, forming an intermediate layer between the buffy coat and the red blood concentrate.
- This activity is usually accompanied by the presence of erythrocyte precursors in peripheral blood (erythroblasts, occasionally polychromatophils).
- Hemoparasites may also lead to increased erythroblast and polychromasia.
- Polychromasia may also occur in the absence of anemia, as has been reported in shedding reptiles.

Erythrocytic Mitoses

- Erythrocytic mitoses, when detected in peripheral blood as an anecdotal finding, are not a manifestation of anemia.
- Anemia should only be considered when mitoses appear in erythrocytes together with the presence of abundant erythroblasts and other markers described, such as altered hematocrit and irregular erythrocytic nucleus.

Erythrocyte Counts

- Total erythrocyte counts are lower than in mammals and birds.
- Erythrocytes in lizards are smaller compared with other reptiles; they tend to have higher erythrocyte counts between 1 and 1.5 million erythrocytes/microliter.

Fecal Occult Blood Test and Urinalysis

- Fecal occult blood test and urinalysis may allow for the detection of small amounts of blood in an animal's urine or feces.
- Fecal occult tests may give false positives in carnivorous species.

PATHOLOGICAL FINDINGS

Pathologic findings will be specific to the underlying cause of anemia.

TREATMENT

APPROPRIATE HEALTH CARE

- Anemia is often a chronic presentation for most reptiles.
- A slower metabolism and physiologic adaptation mechanisms allow reptiles to compensate better than birds or mammals.
- Treatment is often not needed on an emergency basis, but is rather focused on addressing the underlying diseases and providing supportive therapy.

NUTRITIONAL SUPPORT

- Proper nutrition is key for the prevention and treatment of anemia.
- The diet should be as varied as possible and adapted to each species.
- Diet should be balanced and contain natural sources of vitamin B12 and iron.
- Nutritional support via gavage feeding should be implemented in very ill and/or anorectic animals.
- Isotonic fluids should be administered at a rate of 20–30 ml/kg IV, IO, or SC for maintenance. Fluid losses can be replaced but be careful not to overhydrate the patient. Close monitoring is needed when treating hypoproteinemic patients to avoid overhydration.

CLIENT EDUCATION/HUSBANDRY RECOMMENDATIONS

- It is recommended to perform annual health evaluations of animals at risk. These evaluations should include blood tests and fecal exams.
- Any treatments must be performed based on the results of the exams and the historical data for the collection.
- These tests should also be done on newly acquired and quarantined animals.
- A proper nutritional plan is also essential for good health.

MEDICATIONS

DRUG(S) OF CHOICE

- Hemorrhagic anemia: control bleeding by applying pressure. The use of hemostatic agents such as D-aminocaproic acid or ethamsylate has not been reported in reptiles; doses are empirical (0.1 ml/kg). The efficacy of blood replacers or transfusions has not been well studied.
- Colloids may also be used, at a rate of 10–20 ml/kg with a bolus of 3–5 ml/kg IV or IO as needed.
- Blood replacers: availability varies across the world. If available, products like bovine hemoglobin glutamer (Oxyglobin®, Biopure Corporation, Cambridge, MA) 1 ml/100 g IV for 5 minutes by means of perfusion; repeat 4 hours later) may improve the urgency success of such cases of severe anemia.
- Blood transfusion: homologous transfusions are preferred over heterologous. A blood volume of up to 1% body weight is extracted from the donor by means of syringes and needles filled with anticoagulant at a ratio of 1 : 6 to 1 : 9 anticoagulant to blood. The blood is administered to the recipient by means of an infusion pump at 5 ml/hour flow rate. True efficacy is not well documented but clinical experience suggests some short-term benefits.
- Treatment for maladaptation syndrome consists of fluid therapy and stimulation of blood regeneration by means of iron dextran (12 mg/kg, IM q7d) and cyanocobalamin (vitamin B12) (0.5 mg/kg or 10–2000 IU according to the animal's weight as single IM or SC dose).

PRECAUTIONS/INTERACTIONS

N/A

FOLLOW-UP

PATIENT MONITORING

- Because of the small size of some lizards, monitoring should rely on assessment of the behavior and clinical signs of the affected animal, not just on blood sampling.
- If the treatment is appropriate, the lizard should become progressively more active and alert, with interest in hunting, seeking shelter, or mating behaviors.
- Normal attitude and shedding are two common aspects that can be monitored in reptiles after the start of treatment, because they are related to the overall health of the animal.
- In addition, signs of healing of the other diseases that have contributed to the animal's anemia should be observed.

EXPECTED COURSE AND PROGNOSIS

- Repeated blood samplings after 1 week and 1 month should show a compensated status and corrected anemia.
- Repeated blood sampling may be contraindicated, especially in cases of non-regenerative anemia, when working with small patients, or if the underlying etiology is not being treated.
- If the underlying cause of anemia is properly diagnosed and can be effectively treated, the prognosis is good.

MISCELLANEOUS

COMMENTS

N/A

ZOONOTIC POTENTIAL

N/A

SYNONYMS

- Inadaptation syndrome
- Maladaptation syndrome

ABBREVIATIONS

- EDTA = ethylenediaminetetraacetic acid
- IM = intramuscular
- IO = intraosseous
- IU = international units
- IV = intravenous
- MCHC = mean corpuscular hemoglobin concentration
- SC = subcutaneous

INTERNET RESOURCES

Cital S. Exotic Animal Blood Transfusions: An overview. VetBloom. http://blog.vetbloom.com/exotics/exotic-animal-blood-transfusions-an-overview

Suggested Reading

Boyer TH. Autoimmune hemolytic anemia in a parson's chameleon, *Calumna parsonii parsonii*. *Proc ARAV* 2002;9:81–84.

Martínez-Silvestre A. How do I treat anemia in reptiles. *Proc SEVC- AVEPA* 2013;48:1–5.

Saggese MD. Clinical approach to the anemic reptile. *J Exot Pet Med* 2009;18(2):98–111.

Wu C, Chie CHH. Case study: successful treatment of acute anaemia with whole blood transfusion and supportive care in two turtles. *Proc UPAV/AAVAC/ARAV* 2014:13–20.

Author Albert Martínez-Silvestre, DVM, MSc, PhD, DECZM (Herpetology), EBVS European Veterinary Specialist in Herpetological Medicine and Surgery, Acred. AVEPA (Exotic Animals)

ANOREXIA

BASICS

DEFINITION/OVERVIEW

Anorexia is the lack of appetite or intake of food, and does not define an underlying cause. Many pathologic and even physiologic conditions can result in decreased food intake. Anorexia is distinct from decreased appetite, which is also known as hypophagia.

ETIOLOGY/PATHOPHYSIOLOGY

- Anorexia may be a normal physiologic/behavioral occurrence during certain times of the year (e.g., brumation, estivation, reproductive season).
- Pathologic causes of anorexia may stem from either GI or extra-GI disease (e.g., any painful condition or systemic illness).
- Decreased to absent food intake often results in dehydration as well, as many lizards derive hydration through food items.
- Prolonged anorexia may lead to hepatic lipidosis, which may result in nausea, leading to continued lack of food intake.
- Nutritional imbalances and metabolic derangements can occur with chronic anorexia, and cachexia may ensue.
- Primarily, the GI and musculoskeletal systems are affected with anorexia.
- Lizards that are not consuming food for prolonged periods of time may not defecate significant amounts.
- As the body begins to break down adipose tissue stores and muscle, bony prominences become more obvious as body condition decreases.

SIGNALMENT/HISTORY

- Anorexia has no age or sex predilection.
- It is important to differentiate physiologic/behavioral anorexia from that caused by an underlying pathology or disease process.

CLINICAL PRESENTATION

- An isolated incident or occasional episodes of anorexia in an otherwise healthy animal may be inconsequential, especially in an animal presented in good body condition.
- Decreased food intake over an extended period.
- Clients may report repeated attempts at feeding.
- Clinical signs of chronic anorexia include a decreased body condition score with prominent bony protuberances, dehydration, and muscle wasting.

RISK FACTORS

Stress, social or environmental factors, may result in anorexia.

Husbandry

- Adjusting to captivity: often seen in newly acquired animals. A period of time for acclimation may be necessary prior to an animal feeling secure enough to start eating on its own.
- Improper husbandry: inappropriate environmental temperature or humidity, inappropriate food items (type and/or size), malnutrition, inadequate exposure to UVB lighting, poor water quality, overcrowding, rapid change of diet, lack of provision of hiding areas.

Others

- Physiologic
- Cardiovascular disease: cardiomyopathy, congestive heart failure
- Any disease process can result in anorexia
- Reproductive activity: gravid females, breeding males
- Reproductive disease: pre- or postovulatory dystocia; yolk coelomitis
- Respiratory infections
- Viral infections
- Fungal infections: *Nannizziopsis* spp. infections
- Systemic illness: septicemia
- Gastrointestinal disease: stomatitis, foreign bodies, neoplasia, intussusception, gastroenteritis, constipation, prolapses
- Parasitic disease: ectoparasites and endoparasites
- Neurologic disease
- Toxic diseases
- Urogenital: renal disease
- Metabolic: nutritional secondary hyperparathyroidism; hypovitaminosis A
- Any potentially painful condition: ophthalmic disease, orthopedic conditions, cellulitis, trauma

DIAGNOSIS

DIFFERENTIAL DIAGNOSIS

- Conditions that result in failed food prehension (disorders of the tongue or oral cavity) or processing may result in animals that attempt to eat (have an appetite) but are unable to do so successfully.
- Hypophagia may be mistaken for anorexia in certain circumstances.

DIAGNOSTICS

- Diagnostic procedures should be tailored towards identifying the underlying cause of the anorexia and identifying potential negative sequelae (e.g., hepatic lipidosis).

Baseline Blood Work

- CBC, PCV, TS, biochemistry
- Findings on CBC and biochemistry panels are usually non-specific but may be suggestive of underlying disease process(es) resulting in the observed anorexia.
- Bile acids and liver leakage enzymes (AST) may be increased if hepatic lipidosis is present secondary to prolonged anorexia.

Imaging

Radiography can help to identify abnormalities of the GI tract such as foreign bodies and masses. Ultrasound and CT can provide more detailed information about possible hepatic lipidosis, ileus, and coelomic masses.

Other Tests

- Additional diagnostics, including infectious or parasitic disease testing, may be warranted based on patient history and physical examination findings.
- The presumed underlying causes should be thoroughly investigated.

PATHOLOGICAL FINDINGS

- Findings depend on underlying cause of the anorexia.
- Hepatic lipidosis may be suspected based on the findings of advanced imaging or biochemistry evaluation.

TREATMENT

APPROPRIATE HEALTH CARE

N/A

NUTRITIONAL SUPPORT

- Nutritional support should be started in anorectic animals that have lost 10% of their body weight acutely (7 days or less) or 20% chronically (> 7 days).
- Weight loss must be monitored together with an assessment of BCS. Anorectic animals with a BCS of 2/5 or lower may be immediate candidates for nutritional support.
- Animals should be housed in appropriate environments and maintained at their preferred optimum temperature zones to facilitate proper use of the provided nourishment.
- Liquid diets may be provided via gavage in smaller animals.
- Placement of an esophagostomy tube should be considered for long-term support and to minimize stress of force-feeding.
- Although poorly understood in veterinary medicine, the potential exists for refeeding syndrome in chronically anorectic patients, necessitating careful planning of nutritional support in these animals.
- Recommendations include feeding chronically anorectic animals half of their calculated energy requirements initially, then slowly increasing up to the full energy requirement over 7–10 days.

CLIENT EDUCATION/HUSBANDRY RECOMMENDATIONS

- The clinician should perform a thorough review of the patient's current husbandry including feeding.
- Any husbandry or dietary deficiencies should be corrected.

- It is important to ensure that a proper diet of an appropriate size is being offered.
- The diet must be presented to the animal appropriately (e.g., feeding diurnal animals during daylight hours, offering prey on land vs. in the water or vice versa).
- Clients should be notified that offering live food items to anorectic animals could result in rapid, serious injury to their pet secondary to prey attacks.
- In most cases, live prey (rodents) should not be offered to lizards without direct supervision.

MEDICATIONS

DRUG(S) OF CHOICE

- Commercial, high-calorie formulations designed for nutritional support in birds and reptiles are recommended when feeding anorectic lizards.
- Alternatively, a slurry can also be made with a commercial pelleted diet.

PRECAUTIONS/INTERACTIONS

- Exercise caution when force-feeding, to prevent dental or mandibular trauma.
- Be careful not to administer too large a volume of nutritional formula in small patients.
- Feed 1–3% f body weight initially to ensure that the animal will tolerate the feedings.

FOLLOW-UP

PATIENT MONITORING

- Individuals should be monitored for resolution of anorexia following correction of any husbandry and dietary deficiencies.
- Serial imaging and blood chemistry evaluation may be considered to monitor for development or resolution of secondary liver diseases such as hepatic lipidosis.
- In patients with esophagostomy tubes, the tube should be monitored for clogging and the stoma regularly evaluated for signs of infection.

EXPECTED COURSE AND PROGNOSIS

- Anorexia may continue until the underlying reason is identified and treated.
- Prognosis for resolution of anorexia depends on the severity of the underlying cause.

MISCELLANEOUS

COMMENTS

- Simply providing appropriate husbandry will help prevent many causes of anorexia in lizards.
- Supportive care should be continued while an underlying cause for the anorexia is identified and corrected.
- Prompt diagnosis of true anorexia enables initiation of proper nutritional support and may prevent formation of hepatic lipidosis, which can perpetuate the lack of appetite.
- Gravid individuals may decrease their amount of food consumption from lack of coelomic space for GI distension.
- Animals that are anorectic from an underlying pathologic condition may cease or abort reproductive activity due to preferential allotment of energy for other physiologic functions.
- Male lizards may drop substantial body weight during the active breeding season.

ZOONOTIC POTENTIAL

N/A

SYNONYMS

- Anophagia
- Aphagia
- Inappetence

ABBREVIATIONS

- AST = aspartate aminotransferase
- BCS = body condition score
- CBC = complete blood count
- CT = computed tomography
- GI = gastrointestinal
- PCV = packed cell volume
- TS = total solids
- UVB = ultraviolet B

Suggested Reading

De Voe RS. Nutritional support of reptile patients. *Vet Clin North Am Exot Anim Pract* 2014;17:249–261.

Divers SJ, Stahl S, eds. *Mader's Reptile and Amphibian Medicine and Surgery*. 3rd ed. St. Louis, MO: Elsevier; 2019.

Author Grayson Doss, DVM, DACZM

BALANTIDIUM

BASICS

DEFINITION/OVERVIEW

Balantidium is a genus of large ciliated protozoal organisms that resides within the GI tract. The trophozoite is elliptical in shape and ranges in size from 30–300 × 25–120 µm. It is densely covered with cilia along its surface. At the tapered front end lies the cytostome (mouth). Cysts have a thick wall; they are spherical in shape and have a kidney bean-shaped macronucleus. *Balantidium* spp. have been reported from green iguanas (*Iguana iguana*) and spiny-tailed lizards (*Uromastyx dispar*). They are typically found in herbivorous reptiles and rarely in carnivorous reptiles.

ETIOLOGY/PATHOPHYSIOLOGY

- Transmission is through the fecal–oral route.
- Cysts are ingested and then undergo excystation in the intestinal tract.
- Trophozoites inhabit the large colon and replicate by binary fission.
- Trophozoites undergo encystation, in which infective cysts are formed and then excreted in feces.
- *Balantidium* spp. are facultative parasites and only become pathogenic when other virulence factors such as hyaluronidase are present. This then allows them to penetrate the intestinal mucosa and cause extensive hemorrhage and necrosis.
- It is generally limited to the large intestinal tract. In severe infections, the protozoal organisms migrate to the liver and cause abscessation.

SIGNALMENT/HISTORY

Uncommon in lizards

CLINICAL PRESENTATION

- Diarrhea
- Tenesmus
- Inappetence
- Weight loss

RISK FACTORS

Husbandry

Improper husbandry

Others

Immunocompromised animals with active parasitic/bacterial infections are more predisposed for the protozoan to become pathogenic.

DIAGNOSIS

DIFFERENTIAL DIAGNOSIS

Nyctotherus spp.

DIAGNOSTICS

- Microscopic evaluation of fresh fecal material to visualize trophozoites and cysts.
- SAF technique can be used for better visualization.

PATHOLOGICAL FINDINGS

Hemorrhagic necrotizing colitis

TREATMENT

APPROPRIATE HEALTH CARE

N/A

NUTRITIONAL SUPPORT

N/A

CLIENT EDUCATION/HUSBANDRY RECOMMENDATIONS

- Practice proper hygiene
- Wash fruits and vegetables before being fed out.

MEDICATIONS

DRUG(S) OF CHOICE

- Metronidazole 50 mg/kg PO q24h for 7 days
- Nimorazole 125 mg/kg PO q24h for 4 days
- Tetracyclines 5–10 mg/kg q24h for 5–8 days

PRECAUTIONS/INTERACTIONS

N/A

FOLLOW-UP

PATIENT MONITORING

Recheck feces on a routine basis.

EXPECTED COURSE AND PROGNOSIS

- Treatment with antiprotozoal drugs should be started only if clinical disease is observed.
- Since most cases do not require therapy, prognosis is usually good as long as it does not have effects beyond the intestines.

MISCELLANEOUS

COMMENTS

N/A

ZOONOTIC POTENTIAL

B. coli is the only known species to infect humans.

SYNONYMS

N/A

ABBREVIATIONS

- GI = gastrointestinal
- PO = per os
- SAF = sodium acetate acetic acid formalin

INTERNET RESOURCES

- De Bosschere H, Roels S. Balantidium sp. and Nyctotherus sp.: Two Common Members of the Digestive-Tract Flora in Mediterranean Tortoises. Tortoise Trust. https://www.tortoisetrust.org/articles/balantidium.htm
- Divers SJ. Parasitic Diseases of Reptiles. MSD Manual Veterinary Manual, June 2020. http://www.merckvetmanual.com/exotic-and-laboratory-animals/reptiles/parasitic-diseases-of-reptiles

Suggested Reading

Hnizdo J, Pantchev N. Protozoa (digestive tract). In: *Medical Care of Turtles and Tortoises.* Diagnosis. Surgery. Pathology. Parasitology. Frankfurt, Germany: Edition Chimaira; 2011: 194–195.

Jacobson ER. Parasites and parasitic diseases of reptiles. In: Jacobson ER, ed. *Infectious Diseases and Pathology of Reptiles: Color Atlas and Text.* Boca Raton, FL: CRC Press; 2007:571–665.

Rataj AV, Lindtner-Knific R, Vlahovic K, et al. Parasites in pet reptiles. *Acta Vet Scand* 2011;53(1):33.

Author Elsburgh O. Clarke III, DVM, DACZM

BUPHTHALMOS

BASICS

DEFINITION/OVERVIEW
Buphthalmos is an enlarged globe that is positioned normally in the socket.

ETIOLOGY/PATHOPHYSIOLOGY
An increase in IOP causing enlargement and distention of the globe secondary to chronic glaucoma.

SIGNALMENT/HISTORY
- There is no standard signalment for this disease.
- Common findings in the history may include tearing and squinting noted by the owners, as well as an asymmetry of the globes and loss of vision on the affected side(s).

CLINICAL PRESENTATION
- While it can be bilateral, most cases in lizards are unilateral.
- The corneal diameter of the affected eye is increased due to globe stretching.
- There may be blepharospasm and epiphora.
- Unlike exophthalmia, the conjunctiva and position of the nictitans is usually normal.
- There may be a red ciliary flush (red ring around the cornea) and congested episcleral vessels.
- There may be lens luxation and/or cataracts in the affected eye(s).
- Retropulsion of the globe is normal but the globe itself may feel more firm than normal.

RISK FACTORS
Husbandry
- Diet and environmental factors are likely to have an effect on the development of cataracts.
- Cataract development in brumating lizards has been associated with damage from freezing temperatures.

Others
- Trauma, especially if there is corneal penetration, can induce uveitis and cataract formation.
- The presence of a cataract may increase the chance of lens luxation and/or lens induced uveitis, both of which can lead to glaucoma.

DIAGNOSIS

DIFFERENTIAL DIAGNOSIS
- It is important to first differentiate between exophthalmia, buphthalmos, and pesudobuphthalmos, which occurs in species of lizards with spectacles, such as many geckos.
- Glaucoma in lizards is usually secondary to outflow obstruction of the aqueous humor, which is most often caused by uveitis, lens luxation, or intraocular neoplasia.

DIAGNOSTICS
- Physical examination findings should raise suspicion of buphthalmos, which is confirmed by finding elevated IOP.
- Normal IOP in two lizard species has been reported to be 5.61–6.44 mmHg (*Pogona vitticeps*) and 4.89±1.73 mmHg (*Cyclura cychlura cychlura*).
- Since most cases are unilateral, a significant difference in IOP between eyes may be most indicative of a problem.
- Ocular examination and ultrasound are helpful in further evaluating the root cause, although scleral ossicles, if present, can limit visualization.

PATHOLOGICAL FINDINGS
Chronically elevated IOP will lead to pain and blindness.

TREATMENT

APPROPRIATE HEALTH CARE
N/A

NUTRITIONAL SUPPORT
- Additional nutritional support is not necessary in most cases if the IOP can be brought down.
- If needed, syringe feeding can be used to provide nutritional support.

CLIENT EDUCATION/HUSBANDRY RECOMMENDATIONS
- While buphthalmos can occur in any animal, those with husbandry deficiencies may be at increased risk.
- In addition to medical and surgical therapy, maximizing husbandry will improve prognosis.

SURGICAL CONSIDERATIONS
Enucleation of the diseased globe

MEDICATIONS

DRUG(S) OF CHOICE
- If acute glaucoma is suspected, it is important to start medical treatment immediately.
- As most of these cases present in a chronic state, vision is often already lost and medications are used to control pain and slow the disease process during diagnostic evaluation, but enucleation as a salvage procedure is usually indicated.
- If acute glaucoma is suspected: topical β-adrenergic blockers (e.g., timolol) and carbonic anhydrase inhibitors (e.g., dorzolamide) b.i.d. to t.i.d. and mannitol (1–2 g/kg IV slowly over 20–30 minutes) to try to reduce the IOP and preserve vision.
- If uveitis is suspected, systemic and topical antibiotics (e.g., ceftazadime 20 mg/kg IM or SC q48–72h) and steroids (prednisolone 0.25–0.5 mg/kg daily or dexamethasone 0.04–0.08 mg/kg daily) should also be instituted.

PRECAUTIONS/INTERACTIONS
N/A

FOLLOW-UP

PATIENT MONITORING
Serial IOPs are useful to determine whether there has been a response to therapy.

EXPECTED COURSE AND PROGNOSIS
- Prognosis is related to the underlying cause of the glaucoma, which is not always readily identifiable.
- Enucleation of the diseased globe will resolve the issue in most cases.

MISCELLANEOUS

COMMENTS
N/A

ZOONOTIC POTENTIAL
Depends on the cause of the buphthalmos but low to most often no zoonotic potential.

SYNONYMS
N/A

ABBREVIATIONS
- IM = intramuscular
- IOP = intraocular pressure
- IV = intravenous
- SC = subcutaneous

Suggested Reading

Hochleithner C, Holland M. Ultrasonography. In: Mader, DR, Divers SJ, eds. *Current Therapy in Reptile Medicine and Surgery*. Saint Louis, MO: Elsevier; 2014:93–106.

Lawton, MPC. Reptilian Ophthalmology. In: Mader DR, ed. *Reptile Medicine and Surgery*. 2nd ed. St. Louis, MO: Saunders/Elsevier; 2006: 323–342.

Schuster EJ, Strueve J, Fehr MJ, Mathes KA. Measurement of intraocular pressure in healthy unanesthetized inland bearded dragons (*Pogona vitticeps*). *Am J Vet Res* 2015;76(6):494–499.

Wojick KB, Naples L, Knapp CR. Ocular health assessment, tear production, and intraocular pressure in the Andros Island iguana (*Cyclura cychlura cychlura*). *J Zoo Wildl Med* 2013;44(1):116–123.

Author Christopher S. Hanley, DVM, DACZM

CARDIAC DISEASE

BASICS

DEFINITION/OVERVIEW

Cardiovascular disease is a group of disorders of the heart and blood vessels that include cardiomyopathy, septic endocarditis, valvular insufficiency (with no current evidence of primary degenerative endocardiosis), myocarditis, pericardial effusion, infarct, atherosclerosis, aneurysm (rupture of aortic or carotid aneurysm), gout, arterial calcification, thrombus, parasitic infestations, congenital heart defects, and tumors.

ETIOLOGY/PATHOPHYSIOLOGY

Infectious

• Often secondary to systemic infections in captive reptiles.
• Bacterial: aerobic Gram-negative bacteria: *Salmonella* spp., *Corynebacterium* spp., *Pseudomonas* spp. (endocarditis). *Mycobacterium* spp. in in a frilled lizard (*Chlamydosaurus kingii*; granulomatous myocarditis).
• Viral: *Adenovirus*: acute death of a Savannah monitor (*Varanus exanthematicus*) with myocarditis.
• Parasitic: encapsulated cestodes have been reported within the heart of wild whiptail lizards (*Cnemidophorus* spp.). Filarial nematodes (*Macdonaldius oschei*) within the cardiovascular system can cause edema, thrombosis, and necrosis.

Non-Infectious

• Neoplastic (primary neoplasia is uncommon in reptiles): hemangioma, hemangiosarcoma, cardiac rhabdomyosarcoma, fibrosarcoma. Metastasis to the heart: metastatic chondrosarcoma, metastasis of oviductal adenocarcinoma, disseminated mast cell tumor, multicentric lymphoblastic lymphoma and lymphoblastic malignant lymphoma.
• Metabolic: visceral gout can cause urate crystal deposition in the pericardium. Cardiomyopathy is of undetermined origin in reptiles. Myocardial degeneration can be the consequence of gout (of metabolic, nutritional or iatrogenic origin) and/or vitamin E and selenium deficiencies. The myocardium and the major arteries may also be subject to mineralization (calcification) with a diet of excessive levels of calcium and vitamin D3. Aortic rupture associated with mineralization of the aorta attributed to secondary nutritional hyperparathyroidism is reported in lizards.
• Pericardial effusion is reported in many species but a small amount of fluid within the pericardial sac may also be normal. The etiology of pathologic pericardial effusion is unknown.

SIGNALMENT/HISTORY

• There are no known species, sex, or age predilections.
• Owners may report weakness and dyspnea.
• Peripheral edema may be also present.

CLINICAL PRESENTATION

Similar to that in mammals, but certain differences exist due to differing cardiovascular physiology and anatomy. These include:
• Non-specific clinical signs such as lethargy, depression, anorexia, weight loss, weakness, dyspnea, bilateral exophthalmia, and sudden death.
• Cyanosis
• Peripheral edema (e.g., in gular region)
• Pulmonary edema, ascites
• Neurological signs, such as ataxia and head tilt, in case of brain anoxia.
• Peripheral thrombosis and necrosis in case of filarial infestation of the cardiovascular system.
• Coughing is not a feature of congestive heart failure as observed in mammals.

RISK FACTORS

Husbandry

Inadequate husbandry, resulting in chronic stress, immune suppression and malnutrition, is the most likely common predisposing factor for the development of cardiovascular conditions in captive reptiles.

Others

Atherosclerosis and viral diseases can also be predisposing factors.

DIAGNOSIS

DIFFERENTIAL DIAGNOSIS

All other diseases that induce lethargy and/or respiratory distress.

DIAGNOSTICS

Ambient temperature can influence cardiopulmonary parameters in reptiles so must be considered during examination.

Auscultation

• Use a pressure sensitive acoustic stethoscope.
• A continuous Doppler ultrasonic probe (8 MHz) can also be used for cardiac "auscultation". It allows determination of heart rate and rhythm but only indicates blood flow (not valve closure). This may be difficult in some species due to anatomic specificities (pectoral girdle, scutes, osteoderms).

Ultrasound

• The most practical diagnostic tool for antemortem evaluation of reptilian heart diseases.
• Allows visualization of blood flow within the heart. In varanids, the heart can be easily accessed via a ventral approach. In other lizards, the probe can be placed in the left or right axillary region in sternal or lateral recumbency.

Hematology and Biochemistry

Blood pressure measurement and pulse oximetry are not reliable in reptiles.

Clinical Pathology

• CK and LDH may increase with conditions affecting cardiac muscle in reptiles such as myocarditis or infarct. However, these are non-specific and may also increase with skeletal muscle damage from traumatic injuries, loss of body condition and intramuscular injections.
• Currently, cardiac troponins have not been assessed in lizards.
• Leukocytosis, lymphocytosis, and heterophilia may be present and are suggestive of underlying infection or hematopoietic neoplasia with secondary cardiac effects.

Electrocardiography

• Low electric amplitudes (usually < 1.0 mV) and standard parameters have not been established for many species.
• Common findings in the normal reptilian ECG include P-wave pleomorphism, very small Q and S deflections and prolonged Q-T intervals compared with similar-sized mammals.
• Correct electrode placement (challenging in reptiles) is essential to avoid erroneous ECG readings.

Radiography

Challenging to produce images of high diagnostic value in lizards.

CT and MRI

• Apart from obvious cardiomyopathy, neither CT nor MRI (unless using a very high magnetic field
• strengths) are of use for visualizing intracardiac structures and large vessels.
• Evaluate for concurrent disease to determine whether cardiac issue is primary or secondary (neoplastic, infectious).

PATHOLOGICAL FINDINGS

• Hemoculture can be helpful in case of bacterial endocarditis.
• Gross and histopathologic findings depend on the type of heart disease.

TREATMENT

APPROPRIATE HEALTH CARE

• Little information
• Actions of cardiac drugs in reptiles are poorly understood and few data are available in the literature (pharmacokinetics, toxicity, etc.).

NUTRITIONAL SUPPORT

No specific nutritional support considerations and/or recommendations.

CLIENT EDUCATION/HUSBANDRY RECOMMENDATIONS

Reduce stress by minimizing handling, separating from cage mates, and maintaining the reptile at its preferred optimal temperature zone.

MEDICATIONS

DRUG(S) OF CHOICE

- Beta-blockers: of unknown effectiveness in reptile patients.
- Methylatropine: administration results in an increase in resting heart rate of iguanas (*Iguana iguana*).
- Enalapril: inhibited angiotensin I conversion in alligators 0.5–0.7 mg/kg once q24h (combined with spironolactone and furosemide). No data available in lizards.
- Furosemide: possible diuretic effect in chelonians and ophidians despite lacking the loop of Henle. No data available in lizards.
- Hydrochlorothiazide: has been used as a diuretic in lizards with renal disease.
- Methylated xanthines (aminophylline and theophylline) have successfully induced diuresis.
- Nothing is known about the potential use of spironolactone in reptiles.

PRECAUTIONS/INTERACTIONS

N/A

FOLLOW-UP

PATIENT MONITORING

Repeated echocardiographic examinations

EXPECTED COURSE AND PROGNOSIS

As no specific treatment is available, fast deterioration can be expected.

MISCELLANEOUS

COMMENTS

N/A

ZOONOTIC POTENTIAL

Can be zoonotic in case of salmonellosis and other Gram-negative bacteria.

SYNONYMS

- Cardiovascular disease
- Heart disease

ABBREVIATIONS

- CK = creatine kinase
- CT = computed tomography
- ECG = electrocardiogram
- LDH = lactate dehydrogenase
- MRI = magnetic resonance imaging

Suggested Reading

Beaufrère H, Schilliger L, Pariaut R. Cardiovascular system In: Mitchell MA, Tully TN, eds. *Current therapy of exotic animal practice*. St. Louis, MO: Elsevier; 2016:151–220.

Mitchell MA. Reptile cardiology. *Vet Clin North Am Exot Anim Pract* 2009;12:65–79.

Schilliger L, Girling S. Cardiology. In: Divers S, Stahl S, eds. *Mader's Reptile and Amphibian Medicine and Surgery*. St. Louis, MO: Elsevier; 2019:669–698.

Author Lionel Schilliger, DVM, DECZM (Herpetology), DABVP (Reptile & Amphibian Practice)

CAROTID ANEURYSM

BASICS

DEFINITION/OVERVIEW

A carotid aneurysm is a bulging or ballooning of the carotid artery wall. It can be extracranial, intracranial or both. It is caused when a portion of the artery wall weakens. As the wall of the artery grows progressively thinner, it expands, increasing the likelihood that the aneurysm will burst.

ETIOLOGY/PATHOPHYSIOLOGY

- The etiology is unknown
- The carotid artery is somewhat unprotected by its shallow position in the dorsolateral oropharynx, as it runs over the ventral aspect of the skull and neck. Thus, it might be exposed to trauma during feeding.
- Possible causes may include a congenital arterial defect, hypertension, and atherosclerosis with dyslipidemia but no specific cause has been reported.

SIGNALMENT/HISTORY

- Carotid aneurysm has been reported in bearded dragons (*Pogona vitticeps*).
- Animals usually behave normally and continue to eat.
- They may cease to feed, as the aneurysm can be large enough to potentially affect normal jaw abduction and food prehension.

CLINICAL PRESENTATION

- Typically, lizards present with a large soft or firm swelling up to 5 cm in diameter on the dorsolateral neck, caudally to the skull.
- Mucous membranes may be pale in case of blood loss.

RISK FACTORS

Husbandry

- Unknown
- Husbandry is an unlikely cause

Others

Unknown

DIAGNOSIS

DIFFERENTIAL DIAGNOSIS

- Abscess
- Trauma
- Granuloma
- Cystic mass
- Hematoma
- Mycetoma
- Tumor

DIAGNOSTICS

- Ultrasound and Doppler examination of the concerned swelling may confirm blood accumulation.
- Angiography can also be useful
- CT and MRI are indicated to determine the exact size and shape of the aneurysm (can be bilobed, expanding dorsally and nasally, and can be contained within the skull).
- Aneurysms generally arise from the internal carotid artery near where it branches off the aorta or from the aorta itself.
- Aspiration with a needle and syringe can yield several cubic centimeters of whole blood, after which the mass is rapidly refilled with blood, indicating communication with a large and/or high-pressure blood vessel.

PATHOLOGICAL FINDINGS

- Extracranial aneurysms arise from the internal carotid artery near its origin from the aorta.
- The walls of the artery become fibrous and lack the elasticity of a normal artery.
- Thus, the lack of compliance of the high-pressure vessel predisposes it to bursting and hemorrhage.

TREATMENT

APPROPRIATE HEALTH CARE

- If untreated, the blood collected coagulates, which predisposes the animal to carotid obstruction and/or thromboembolism.
- Carotid aneurysm can be surgically removed, although intraoperative blood loss can require a transfusion from a donor bearded dragon.

NUTRITIONAL SUPPORT

If associated with hyperlipidemia and potentially atherosclerosis, diet should be balanced and feeding insect larvae (yellow mealworms, kingworm beetles and greater wax moth larvae) should be avoided.

CLIENT EDUCATION/HUSBANDRY RECOMMENDATIONS

N/A

MEDICATIONS

DRUG(S) OF CHOICE

No medical treatment known

PRECAUTIONS/INTERACTIONS

N/A

FOLLOW-UP

PATIENT MONITORING

If not treated surgically, follow-up ultrasound may be useful to evaluate the amount of blood collected in the region of the aneurysm.

EXPECTED COURSE AND PROGNOSIS

This condition generally carries a poor prognosis.

MISCELLANEOUS

COMMENTS

Aneurysms can also be encountered on the limbs, over the hips, in the mouth and in the aorta, close to the heart.

ZOONOTIC POTENTIAL

N/A

SYNONYMS

Aneurysm syndrome

ABBREVIATIONS

- CT = computed tomography
- MRI = magnetic resonance imaging

INTERNET RESOURCES

Mader D. Bearded Dragon Aneurysms. Reptiles Magazine, January 5, 2016. http://www.reptilesmagazine.com/Bearded-Dragon-Aneurysms

Suggested Reading

Barten SL, Wyneken J, Mader DR, Garner M. Aneurysm in the dorsolateral neck of two bearded dragons (*Pogona vitticeps*). *Proceedings of the Association of Reptilian and Amphibian Veterinarians* 2006:43–44.

Sweet CR, Linnetz E, Golden E, Mayer J. What Is Your Diagnosis? *J Am Vet Med Assoc* 2009;234(10):1259–1260.

Author Lionel Schilliger, DVM, DECZM (Herpetology), DABVP (Reptile & Amphibian Practice)

CLOACAL PROLAPSE

BASICS

DEFINITION/OVERVIEW

A prolapse is the moving or slipping of a body part from its usual position or anatomic relation. In the reptile, a prolapse from the vent may be of cloacal, rectal, phallus/hemipenal, oviductal, or bladder in origin.

ETIOLOGY/PATHOPHYSIOLOGY

- The underlying cause for prolapse is often unknown.
- See Differential Diagnosis for a list of possible etiologies.

SIGNALMENT/HISTORY

- There appears to be no specific signalment or predilections noted for the various reptilian prolapses.
- Female reptilians may be overrepresented due to occurrences of dystocia.

CLINICAL PRESENTATION

- A prolapse is easy to visualize as abnormal tissue protruding from the cloacal/ vent region.
- In reptiles housed outdoors and in case of small prolapses, the owners may not notice a problem until days after it has occurred. For this reason, a prolapse should be considered an emergency and evaluated promptly.
- The tissue should be kept moist either through gentle washing of the area with water and loosely wrapping in a damp cloth or paper towel until the animal can be evaluated by a veterinarian.
- The extruded tissue should be identified to the tissue(s) involved (e.g., cloacal with/ without bladder, oviduct, proctodeum, colon, hemipenis).
- Once the issues are identified, the clinician may be able to narrow the differential diagnoses (see below) to determine the course of diagnostics and therapeutics.

RISK FACTORS

- In cases of NSHP, the muscle tone around the cloacal opening is decreased, leading to potential tissue exposure.
- Any generalized physical straining of the patient can lead to tissue exposure through the cloaca, such as dyspnea, obstipation, parasites, infection.
- Space-occupying lesions located in the coelomic cavity such as uroliths, neoplasia, hepato/renomegaly, eggs, may also cause increase straining and cloacal prolapse.

Husbandry

- Several factors of husbandry may lead to one of the clinical conditions that may be responsible for the prolapse.
- Correction of the deficient aspects of the husbandry can lead to reversal of some conditions.

Others

- Iatrogenic prolapses may occur when owners attempt to manually manipulate ova in suspected cases of dystocia or feces in constipated animals.
- Some cloacal tissue may prolapse during normal oviposition.

DIAGNOSIS

DIFFERENTIAL DIAGNOSIS

- Parasites
- Hypocalcemia
- Dehydration
- Metabolic disease
- Neoplasia
- Impaction
- Obstruction
- Trauma
- Coelomic space-occupying lesion
- Obesity
- Bacterial infection
- Intoxication

DIAGNOSTICS

- Radiography and ultrasound may be useful in determining internal abnormalities (e.g., impactions, masses, obstructions).
- The small size of some reptiles may lead to reduced imaging detail, which makes interpretation challenging.
- Dental radiography may be a better alternative in smaller species (< 100 g).
- A fecal examination should be performed in all cases. This can be directly from the feces, a saline cloacal wash, or a direct impression smear of the prolapsed tissue may reveal the presence of parasites such as nematode larvae or eggs.
- A complete blood count and chemistry panel may assist in the determination of underlying physiologic abnormalities.

PATHOLOGICAL FINDINGS

- Protozoal infections affecting the gastrointestinal tract may be diagnosed on histopathology.
- Other findings will be consistent with the underlying cause but often no specific cause or pathology can be identified.

TREATMENT

APPROPRIATE HEALTH CARE

- Treatment often involves direct replacement of the tissue back into normal anatomic position either by manual or surgical means in combination with correction of the underlying etiology.
- The patient should be fully evaluated for general health status and treated accordingly.
- The prolapsed tissue should be evaluated for presence of devitalization, which must be surgically or medically addressed prior to prolapse reduction.
- In cases of reproductive system prolapse (i.e., oviduct), the tissue may be replaced but damage to the suspensory ligaments and internal vasculature may be present.
- In some cases, the internal reproductive structures may be medically or surgically repaired; however, further reproductive events could result in dystocia.
- The prolapse may be reduced in size by coating with a hyperosmotic solution such as 2–5% ophthalmic saline or a concentrated sugar solution.
- Direct application of dry salt or sugar may be attempted, but the extreme osmolar difference could lead to direct tissue damage and should be closely monitored. After several minutes of application, the prolapsed tissue should become less edematous and capable of reduction back into the body cavity.
- A moistened and lubricated (water soluble) cotton tip applicator or metal probe is used to gently push the tissue back inside the body cavity aligning the lumen.
- A pursestring suture around the cloaca or lateral sutures across the cloacal margin may be placed for 10–14 days to allow for the tissue swelling to resolve in place.

NUTRITIONAL SUPPORT

The reptilian patient may need weight and body condition monitoring to determine whether additional caloric supplementation is needed.

CLIENT EDUCATION/HUSBANDRY RECOMMENDATIONS

- If surgical correction of the prolapse was undertaken, the client should be directed on postoperative care of any surgical sites, suture, etc.
- A detailed log of activity, as well as food intake/defecations, should be maintained and related back to the veterinarian.
- If any changes to the husbandry were determined, the owner should correct those prior to the patient returning home, such as changes to temperature and/or humidity, exposure ultraviolet lighting, etc.
- Surgical options such as resection of the diseased tissue and double-layer closure can be performed prior to tissue replacement.
- In more extensive cases, a coeliotomy may be performed with the tissue resection performed within the coelomic cavity where the tissue is in approximate "normal" anatomic position.
- Colonic prolapses may require a colopexy where sutures are placed to facilitate the "tacking" of the colon to the dorsolateral body wall.

CLOACAL PROLAPSE (CONTINUED)

• In severe oviductal prolapses, discussion with the owner about desired reproductive status should take place, with a potential for coeliotomy and ovariosalpingectomy.

MEDICATIONS

DRUG(S) OF CHOICE

• NSAIDs or opioids may be used in management of the inflammation and pain associated with the physical discomfort of the prolapse or surgery.
• Depending on the determined etiology, antibiotics or anti-parasiticides may be indicated.

PRECAUTIONS/INTERACTIONS

• When replacing the prolapse, extreme care must be taken not to tear or perforate the delicate, inflamed tissue.
• After the sutures are removed, the tissue may re-prolapse if swelling/inflammation are still present or the underlying etiology has not been corrected.
• Placement of additional sutures may be required.
• Hydration status of the patent must be considered before use of NSAIDs.

FOLLOW-UP

PATIENT MONITORING

• The patient should be followed-up daily after clinical repair of the prolapse for reoccurrence.
• The owner should monitor and record all food intake and defecations during this time.
• Any abnormal changes should be related back to the veterinarian to determine any further changes to the therapy.

EXPECTED COURSE AND PROGNOSIS

• Prolapses of the oviduct and bladder tend to have a guarded to grave prognosis due to the degree of underlying physical damage to the affected tissues and cloaca.
• Rectal and cloacal prolapses tend to have a fair prognosis if treated promptly.
• Phallus/hemipenal prolapses have excellent to good prognosis, as these are purely copulatory organs.
• The length of time the prolapse presents has an inverse effect on the prognosis.
• When treated early in the disease process and the tissue appears viable, cloacal prolapse replacement may lead to clinical resolution if the underlying etiology is addressed.
• Once the tissue begins to desiccate and become devitalized, there is a guarded to grave prognosis.

MISCELLANEOUS

COMMENTS

N/A

ZOONOTIC POTENTIAL

N/A

SYNONYMS

N/A

ABBREVIATIONS

• NSAIDs = nonsteroidal anti-inflammatory drugs
• NSHP = nutritional secondary hyperparathyroidism

Suggested Reading

Barten, SL. Penile prolapse. In: Mader DR, ed. *Reptile Medicine and Surgery*. 2nd ed. St. Louis, MO: Elsevier Saunders; 2006:862–864.

Bennett, RA. Cloacal prolapse. In: Mader DR, ed. *Reptile Medicine and Surgery*. 2nd ed. St. Louis, MO: Elsevier Saunders; 2006:751–755.

Author Rob L. Coke, DVM, DACZM, DABVP (Reptile & Amphibian), CVA

CONJUNCTIVITIS

BASICS

DEFINITION/OVERVIEW

Conjunctivitis is defined as inflammation of the conjunctiva. In reptiles, conjunctivitis often presents concurrently with blepharoedema, which is edema and swelling of the eyelids. In many cases, the blepharedema is severe enough to impede proper evaluation of the eye and identification of conjunctivitis. Blepharoconjunctivitis is a common presentation.

ETIOLOGY/PATHOPHYSIOLOGY

- In lizards, conjunctivitis is more often associated with noninfectious causes such as squamous metaplasia, due to hypovitaminosis A, or dysecdysis. Infectious etiologies may include viral, bacterial, fungal, or parasitic.
- In bearded dragons, a microsporidial keratoconjunctivitis has been reported.
- Poor air quality, environmental irritants, or toxins can also be etiologies, although they are less likely.
- Trauma should be considered, especially in cases of unilateral conjunctivitis.

SIGNALMENT/HISTORY

- There is no specific signalment for the occurrence of conjunctivitis.
- The main focus should be on obtaining a thorough history of the husbandry.

CLINICAL PRESENTATION

- In addition to the conjunctivitis itself, lizards may present with blepharedema, blepharospasm, and/or periocular swelling usually affecting both eyes and causing blepharoconjunctivitis.
- Animals may also present with anorexia, depression, and lethargy, due to either the systemic effects of the underlying etiology or simply from their inability to see properly.

RISK FACTORS

Husbandry

- Poor diet, dehydration, and low humidity should be considered as possible predisposing factors.
- Poor cleanliness and hygiene of the enclosure can also lead to increased environmental bacterial load, which can contribute to conjunctivitis.

Others

N/A

DIAGNOSIS

DIFFERENTIAL DIAGNOSIS

- Hypovitaminosis A
- Dehydration
- Trauma
- Microsporidian infection

DIAGNOSTICS

- A complete ophthalmic examination with the use of magnification by direct or indirect ophthalmoscopy, including fluorescein test to detect corneal ulcers.
- Sampling of the conjunctiva for bacterial culture and sensitivity.
- Biopsy of the conjunctiva, especially when non-responsive to treatment.

PATHOLOGICAL FINDINGS

- Blepharoconjunctivitis is a common presentation.
- Plaques or caseous material may be observed within the fornix or even covering the corneal surface.
- Mucopurulent discharge

TREATMENT

APPROPRIATE HEALTH CARE

- The treatment will be based on the underlying etiology, but anti-inflammatories and analgesics should be considered in most cases.
- Correction of diet and husbandry are essential for response to therapy.
- Concurrent systemic and ophthalmic therapy is recommended for best response in cases of infectious etiologies.
- Treatment of viral infections is often unrewarding.
- Flushing and cleaning of the eyes is also necessary to remove any adhered material or plaques that may be harboring organisms.
- A solution of 1 part povidone iodine to 50 parts saline can be used. When blepharoedema is present, a pipette tip, tomcat catheter, or intravenous catheter can be inserted between the eyelids to flush the eyes.

NUTRITIONAL SUPPORT

- In cases of anorectic animals, force-feeding with easily digestible proteins should be initiated.
- Direct feeding by stomach tube or gavage needle can be performed in some species.
- Placement of an esophagostomy tube should be considered for chronic management.
- In addition, supportive fluid therapy should be provided.

CLIENT EDUCATION/HUSBANDRY RECOMMENDATIONS

- Remove and isolate sick individuals and reduce stress by providing optimal living conditions, and hygiene.
- Thoroughly clean the cage to reduce environmental load of infectious organisms.
- Ensure that quarantine protocols have been implemented for all new arrivals.
- Treatment compliance is key for response to therapy.

MEDICATIONS

DRUG(S) OF CHOICE

Systemic Therapy

- Meloxicam 0.5 mg/kg IM, PO q24h
- Dexamethasone sodium phosphate 0.1–0.3mg/kg IM, SC, IV q24h for 3 days.
- Ceftazidime 22 mg/kg IM q72h
- Ceftiofur crystalline free acid 30 mg/kg SC q5d.
- Amikacin 5 mg/kg IM q48h
- Enrofloxacin 5–10 mg/kg IM, PO q24–48h.
- Oxytetracycline 5–10 mg/kg IM q24h, 10 mg/kg IM q5d for long-acting formulation.
- Itraconazole 5 mg/kg PO q24h
- Fenbendazole 50 mg/kg PO q24h for 3–5 days.
- Vitamin A: parenteral treatment or oral supplementation of retinol forms to herbivores should be avoided. Use dietary carotenoids (non-beta-carotene) instead. For omnivorous, carnivorous, and insectivorous reptiles, parenteral vitamin A (usually has vitamin D3 as well): 500–5000 iu/kg IM q7–14d for up to 4 treatments. Dosing must be done carefully to avoid over-supplementation with vitamin A in the retinol form.

Ophthalmic Therapy

- Ophthalmic antibiotics applied 3–4 times daily
- Ophthalmic anti-inflammatory applied 3–4 times daily
- Ophthalmic itraconazole applied 3–4 times daily

PRECAUTIONS/INTERACTIONS

Parenteral administration of vitamin A must be done only in cases with clear indication of hypovitaminosis A, otherwise there is a risk of causing hypervitaminosis A.

FOLLOW-UP

PATIENT MONITORING

Weekly to every 2-week re-evaluation is recommended to determine response to therapy.

EXPECTED COURSE AND PROGNOSIS

- Course and prognosis will vary according to the etiology.
- Prognosis for viral infections is grave, as these animals typically become progressively worse over time.
- For other etiologies prognosis is good to excellent.

MISCELLANEOUS

COMMENTS

N/A

ZOONOTIC POTENTIAL

Low for the most common etiologies

SYNONYMS

N/A

ABBREVIATIONS

- IM = intramuscular
- IV = intravenous
- PO = per os
- SC = subcutaneous

Suggested Reading

Lawton, MPC. Reptilian Ophthalmology. In: Mader DR, ed. *Reptile Medicine and Surgery*. 2nd ed. St. Louis, MO: Elsevier Saunders; 2006:334–336.

Martel-Arquettee A, Chen S, Hempstead J, et al. Microsporidial keratoconjunctivitis in a pet bearded dragon (*Pogona vitticeps*). *J Exot Pet Med* 2017;26(4):257–262.

Author Javier G. Nevarez, DVM PhD DACZM DECZM (Herpetology)

CRYPTOSPORIDIUM

BASICS

DEFINITION/OVERVIEW

Cryptosporidia are apicomplexan parasites typified by possessing an apical complex, and with four naked sporozoites within each oocyte. *Cryptosporidium* spp. can be distinguished from other coccidian parasites by the location that they occupy within the host cell membrane, their capacity for autoinfection, and their resistance to anti-parasitic medication. Possessing a durable oocyst wall consisting of a double layer of a protein–lipid–carbohydrate matrix, cryptosporidia are highly resistant to environmental degradation and chemical disinfection. Historically, oocyst morphology has been used for species identification, but this is considered unreliable and species assignment is now determined by molecular characteristics (Plutzer & Karanis, 2009). *Cryptosporidium* spp. are ubiquitous in the environment and are globally distributed.

ETIOLOGY/PATHOPHYSIOLOGY

- *Cryptosporidium* infections are common in reptiles and have been reported in at least 57 different species (Pedraza-Diaz et al., 2009).
- *C. varanii* (syn. *C. saurophilum*) is the most common in lizards and is typically an intestinal parasite (Fayer, 2010). Cross-infection of other reptilian taxa has been reported with this species.
- An additional *Cryptosporidium*, *C. ducismarci* has been isolated from intestinal lesions in asymptomatic chameleons (Fayer, 2010).
- Transmission is direct, with reptiles becoming infected after ingesting oocysts that have been shed in feces.
- Autoinfection may also occur with some oocysts releasing their sporozoites within the host's body.
- No prepatent period has been determined (Scullion et al., 2009).

SIGNALMENT/HISTORY

Infected animals usually have a history of chronic wasting accompanied by diarrhea and inappetence.

CLINICAL PRESENTATION

- Subclinical (carrier state): animals may appear healthy and are able to shed oocysts intermittently for years.
- Enteritis: a chronic debilitating enteritis without gastric involvement, which may be accompanied by concurrent disease.
- Atypical presentations, such as aural polyps, may also be seen but these are rare (Uhl et al., 2001).

RISK FACTORS

Husbandry

The greatest risk factor for developing infection is poor quarantine of new animals entering a collection.

Others

N/A

DIAGNOSIS

DIFFERENTIAL DIAGNOSIS

Enteritis—bacterial or other protozoal disease.

DIAGNOSTICS

- Examination of feces, unstained smears is useful, but sensitivity of detection increases with an acid-fast stain and is greatest with an IFA stain. Sensitivity may be increased if performed postprandially. An important limitation of these tests is their lack of specificity to differentiate *Cryptosporidium* spp. False positive results can occur in animals that have ingested food items (i.e., mice) infected with other *Cryptosporidium* spp. that are not pathogenic to reptiles.
- Serum antibody titers can be assessed using an ELISA but it takes 6 weeks for antibodies to develop. Best if combined with fecal samples.
- ELISA positive, fecal positive—animal infected and shedding.
- ELISA negative, fecal negative—not infected.
- ELISA negative, fecal positive—recent infection (< 6 weeks) or passing non-reptilian *Cryptosporidium* spp.
- ELISA positive, fecal negative—has been infected at some point but not shedding or shedding at undetectable levels.
- PCR on fecal samples is the only method to differentiate between *Cryptosporidium* spp.

PATHOLOGICAL FINDINGS

- Gross: intestinal lesions may include mucosal thickening with mucus accumulation.
- Histopathology: intestinal lesions consist of a mixed inflammatory response with up to 80% of epithelial cells containing parasites.

TREATMENT

APPROPRIATE HEALTH CARE

Elimination of *Cryptosporidium* from reptiles is difficult and rarely rewarding.

NUTRITIONAL SUPPORT

- Force-feeding with easily digestible proteins.
- Direct feeding by stomach tubing can be performed in some species; placement of an esophagostomy tube should be considered for chronic management.
- Supportive fluid therapy should be provided.

CLIENT EDUCATION/HUSBANDRY RECOMMENDATIONS

- Clients should be made aware of the insidious nature of infection, the unlikelihood of successful treatment, and the risks that affected animals pose to the remaining collection.
- Owners should be reminded that while *C. varanii* has no zoonotic potential, prey items fed to reptiles might harbor *Cryptosporidium* that can pose a risk to immunocompromised individuals.

MEDICATIONS

DRUG(S) OF CHOICE

- Trimethoprim sulfonamide 30 mg/kg PO q24h for 14 days, then 1–3 times weekly for 3 months may reduce oocyst shedding but does not eliminate *Cryptosporidium* organisms from the gastrointestinal mucosa (Shahiduzzaman & Daugschies, 2012).
- Paromomycin 100 mg/kg PO q24h for 7 days; then twice weekly for 6 weeks; and 360 mg/kg q48h for 10 days has resulted in complete resolution in experimentally infected bearded dragons (*Pogona vitticeps*; Grosset et al., 2011).
- Hyperimmune bovine colostrum 1% body weight by volume PO once weekly for 6 weeks (currently not available commercially; Shahiduzzaman & Daugschies, 2012).

PRECAUTIONS/INTERACTIONS

- Euthanasia should be strongly considered for affected animals to limit spread.
- If this is not an option, then diseased reptiles should be separated from the remaining collection and strict barrier nursing protocols enacted to prevent spread.

FOLLOW-UP

Regular fecal examination and ELISA assays for suspected at risk animals.

PATIENT MONITORING

Monitor for signs of disease: wasting, diarrhea, persistent regurgitation.

EXPECTED COURSE AND PROGNOSIS

Grave prognosis, likely chronic wasting and death.

MISCELLANEOUS

COMMENTS

N/A

ZOONOTIC POTENTIAL

- *C. varanii* has no zoonotic potential (Fayer et al., 1995).
- *C. ducismarci* shows genetic similarities to other zoonotic *Cryptosporidium* spp.
- It should be remembered that prey items fed to reptiles may harbor cryptosporidium that can pose a risk to immunocompromised individuals.

CRYPTOSPORIDIUM (CONTINUED)

SYNONYMS

N/A

ABBREVIATIONS

- ELISA = enzyme-linked immunosorbent assay
- IFA = immunofluorescent antibody
- PCR = polymerase chain reaction

Suggested Reading

Cranfield MR, Graczyk TK. *Cryptosporidiosis*. In: Mader DR, ed. *Reptile Medicine and Surgery*. 2nd ed. St. Louis, MO: Elsevier Saunders; 2006: 756–762.

Fayer R. Taxonomy and species delimitation in *Cryptosporidium*. *Exp Parasitol* 2010;124(1):90–97.

Fayer R, Graczyk TK, Cranfield MR. Multiple heterogenous isolates of *Cryptosporidium serpentis* from captive snakes are not transmissible to neonatal BALB/c mice (*Mus musculus*). *J Parasitol* 1995;81(3):482–484.

Graczyk TK, Owens R, Cranfield MR. Diagnosis of subclinical cryptosporidiosis in captive snakes based on stomach lavage and cloacal sampling. *Vet Parasitol* 1996;67:143–151.

Grosset C, Villeneuve A, Brieger A, Lair S. Cryptosporidiosis in juvenile bearded dragons (*Pogona vitticeps*) effects of treatment with paromomycin. *J Herp Med Surg* 2011;21:10–15.

Pedraza-Diaz S, Ortega-Mora LM, Carrion BA, Navarro V, Gomez-Bautista M. Molecular characterisation of *Cryptosporidium* isolates from pet reptiles. *Vet Parasitol* 2009;160(3–4):204–210.

Scullion FT, Scullion MG. Gastrointestinal Protozoal Diseases in Reptiles. *J Exot Pet Med* 2009;18(4):266–278.

Shahiduzzaman M, Daugschies A. Therapy and prevention of cryptosporidiosis in animals. *Vet Parasitol* 2012;188(3–4):203–214.

Uhl EW, Jacobson E, Bartick TE, et al. Aural-pharyngeal polyps associated with *Cryptosporidium* infection in three iguanas (*Iguana iguana*). *Vet Path* 2001;38:239–242.

Author T. Franciscus Scheelings, BVSc, MVSc, PhD, MANCVSc (Wildlife Health), DECZM (Herpetology)

DIARRHEA

BASICS

DEFINITION/OVERVIEW

Diarrhea is the production of unformed or liquid fecal matter, often associated with increased fecal volume and frequency of defection.

ETIOLOGY/PATHOPHYSIOLOGY

- Diarrhea is usually associated with enteritis due to primary infectious (e.g., endoparasites) or non-infectious (e.g., dietary) causes.
- In herbivorous lizards (e.g., green iguanas) ingestion of diets high in fermentable carbohydrates (e.g., fruits) and/or insufficient fiber ingestion can result in dysbacteriosis, which can cause diarrhea.
- Environmental factors, such as low temperatures, lead to decreased GI motility, dysbacteriosis and diarrhea due overgrowth of opportunistic pathogens.
- Endoparasites can cause diarrhea in lizards.
- Nematodes: oxyurids (pin worms) are common in insectivorous and herbivorous lizards. Ascarids and *Strongyloides* nematodes are uncommon.
- Coccidia: *Isospora amphiboluri* in bearded dragons and other agamids. *I. jaracimrmani* in veiled chameleons. Less frequently, *Eimeria* spp. in geckos. Coccidia are usually host specific.
- Ciliated protozoa: *Balantidium* spp. (opportunistic pathogen). Common in green iguanas. Not host specific; considered part of normal GI flora.
- Flagellates: *Trichomonas* spp. are common in chameleons.
- *Cryptosporidium saurophilium* is common in leopard geckos. Diarrhea is not always observed; emaciation and anorexia are more common, in particular in leopard geckos.
- Bacteria: *Shigella*, *Proteus*, and *Salmonella* spp. are often asymptomatic carriers but can lead to diarrhea.

SIGNALMENT/HISTORY

- Diarrhea is more common in young lizards.
- Inappropriate husbandry: low environmental temperatures and overcrowding (stress) can lead to enteritis and diarrhea.
- Owners report liquid feces, frequently malodorous, and increased frequency of defecation.
- Possible straining to defecate, weight loss, anorexia, and cloacal prolapse.

CLINICAL PRESENTATION

- Depending on duration (acute vs. chronic), severity and etiology of diarrhea.
- Fecal staining around cloaca and ventral aspects of proximal hind limbs and tail base.
- Presence of abnormally soft or liquid fecal matter in transport container.
- Herbivorous lizards with diarrhea caused by inappropriate diet might show no other clinical signs or may show unspecific clinical signs, such as lethargy, reduced food intake, or dehydration.
- Chronic diarrhea can lead to weight loss and cachexia due to malabsorption of nutrients.
- Cloacal prolapse

RISK FACTORS

Husbandry

- Herbivorous lizards: diet low in fiber and/or high in fermentable simple carbohydrates (e.g., fruits).
- Change in diet
- Poor sanitation often leads to high endoparasite load because of the direct life cycle of many intestinal parasites.
- Overcrowding resulting in stress
- Inappropriate (too low or to high) environmental temperatures.

Others

- Young age. Coccidiosis causes higher morbidity and mortality in young lizards.
- Lack of fecal parasitology screening after acquisition of lizards.

DIAGNOSIS

DIFFERENTIAL DIAGNOSIS

- Fecal consistency varies physiologically between reptile species and mainly depends on their diet.
- It is therefore important to be aware of the species-specific fecal consistency to avoid misinterpretation of normal fecal consistency as diarrhea.
- Polyuria

DIAGNOSTICS

- Fecal direct wet mount to evaluate for motile protozoa.
- Fecal flotation to evaluate for helminths and protozoa (coccidian, amoeba cysts).
- Diagnostic imaging (radiographs, CT, ultrasound) as needed.

PATHOLOGICAL FINDINGS

- Enteritis
- Malodorous and liquid intestinal content.
- Emaciation

TREATMENT

APPROPRIATE HEALTH CARE

N/A

NUTRITIONAL SUPPORT

- Correct diet to ensure sufficient fiber intake in herbivorous lizards.
- Provide nutritional support to emaciated and/or anorexic animals.
- Provide fluid therapy to dehydrated animals.

CLIENT EDUCATION/HUSBANDRY RECOMMENDATIONS

N/A

MEDICATIONS

DRUG(S) OF CHOICE

- Coccidiostats are indicated
- Toltazuril (Baycox®, Bayer Inc., Mississauga, ON, 2.5%) 10 mg/kg PO once or q7d for 2–3 treatments.
- Sulfonamides, e.g., trimephoprim/sulfamethoxazole 30 mg/kg PO q24h.
- Metronidazole 25 mg/kg PO q24h for 5–10 days is effective against motile protozoal organisms.
- Fenbendazole 10–20 mg/kg PO q24h for 3–5 days is effective against nematodes and flagellates.
- Ivermectin 0.2 mg/kg PO, SC, IM is effective against nematodes.
- Emodepside/praziquantel (Profender®, Bayer Inc., Mississauga, ON): 1 ml/kg topical on skin. Repeat after 14 days. Effective against nematodes, trematodes, and cestodes.
- Prevention of reinfection is critically important during and following treatment against parasites with a direct life cycle. Keep on newspaper until treatment is completed and recheck fecal exams.
- Immediate removal of feces to prevent ingestion, bathing the lizard, and cleaning of the pericloacal region to remove feces and eggs or cysts is recommended.

PRECAUTIONS/INTERACTIONS

- Fenbendazole has been shown in other reptiles to cause bone marrow suppression and temporary pancytopenia. Avoid using doses greater than 20 mg/kg.
- Do not use ivermectin in skinks.

FOLLOW-UP

PATIENT MONITORING

- Return to normal fecal consistency
- Weight gain and maintenance of hydration.
- Repeat fecal exams to ensure that treatment is effective.

EXPECTED COURSE AND PROGNOSIS

- If dietary causes are responsible for the diarrhea, prognosis is excellent to good.
- Animals in good body condition with no concurrent morbidities have an excellent to good prognosis.

DIARRHEA (CONTINUED)

- Animals in poor body condition with signs of systemic illness (dehydration, lethargy, etc.) have a guarded to poor prognosis.
- There is currently no effective treatment against *Cryptosporidium* spp.

MISCELLANEOUS

COMMENTS

- Diarrhea is a clinical sign associated with an underlying disease, improper husbandry or nutrition.
- Identification of the underlying cause is necessary to improve outcome and reduce the risk of reoccurrence.
- Correction of husbandry is always recommended to in help improve the outcome.

ZOONOTIC POTENTIAL

Salmonella spp. are commonly shed by lizards with and without diarrhea.

SYNONYMS

N/A

ABBREVIATIONS

- CT = computed tomography
- GI = gastrointestinal
- IM = intramuscular
- PO = per os
- SC = subcutaneous

INTERNET RESOURCES

Divers SJ. Parasitic Diseases of Reptiles. MSD Manual Veterinary Manual, June 2020. http://www.merckvetmanual.com/exotic-and-laboratory-animals/reptiles/parasitic-diseases-of-reptiles

Suggested Reading

Funk RS. Diarrhea. In: Mader DR, ed. *Reptile Medicine and Surgery*. 2nd ed. St. Louis, MO: Elsevier Saunders; 2006:772–773.

Greiner EC, Mader DR. Parasitology. In: Mader DR, ed. *Reptile Medicine and Surgery*. 2nd ed. St. Louis, MO: Elsevier Saunders; 2006:343–364.

Author Christoph Mans, Dr. med. vet., DACZM

DYSECDYSIS

BASICS

DEFINITION/OVERVIEW

Dysecdysis means difficult or abnormal shedding. It is a common presentation for reptile species. True dysecdysis implies that the lizard has retained shed that requires assistance for removal or that the shed has come off in an abnormal pattern, which could lead to further problems.

ETIOLOGY/PATHOPHYSIOLOGY

- In lizards, shedding is a discontinuous process through a well-described ecdysis cycle.
- For simplicity, the ecdysis cycle can be split into a resting phase and a renewal phase, which has up to five stages. During the beginning of the renewal phase, the skin begins to appear duller as regeneration of cells and enzymatic separation of the skin layers becomes activated. This period lasts approximately 5 ± 2 days. Afterwards the skin becomes even duller.
- In species lacking eyelids, the spectacles turn opaque in what is commonly described being in "blue". This appearance is in large part due to lymphatic fluid accumulation which helps to separate the old and new skin layers.
- This second period lasts 5 ± 2 days, and is followed by the last stage during which lymphatic fluid resorption occurs leading to a clearing of the skin and spectacle. At this time, the skin regains some of its sheen and shedding typically occurs 5 ± 2 days later.
- The pattern of ecdysis in lizards varies from a single piece of skin starting at the head and progressing to the tip of the tail (similar to snakes) in some geckos, to a seemingly random, multifocal shed in other species.
- Those shedding in a single piece usually use a rough surface to help break the skin at the snout and aid in the skin removal.
- In lidless species, the shed skin should be inspected to ensure that both spectacles have been shed appropriately.

SIGNALMENT/HISTORY

- There is no typical signalment for dysecdysis.
- Lizards presenting with dysecdysis typically have a history of taking a longer time to shed, have delayed shedding stages, or having shed stuck in specific areas.

CLINICAL PRESENTATION

- Lizards with dysecdysis can present with patches of retained skin through the body or segmental dysecdysis in a specific region.
- The eyes, digits, and tip of the scales and tail must be examined carefully, as dysecdysis at these sites is common and can lead to further complications such as subspectacular abscess and avascular necrosis.
- It is also possible to see focal dysecdysis in areas of previous injuries or surgical incisions that have scarred over.
- In some instances, there will always be an abnormal shed observed over these areas, even in well-hydrated patients.

RISK FACTORS

Husbandry

- Inappropriate humidity, temperature, and access to water are common husbandry deficiencies.
- A lack of a rough surface within the enclosure may also be the cause of dysecdysis.
- Dehydration is a key contributor to dysecdysis because dehydrated animals may not be able to mobilize enough lymphatic fluid, which is an essential part of the renewal phase.

Others

- Ecdysis is under pituitary–thyroid control.
- In lizards, it is reported that thyroid hormones help to stimulate the ecdysis process.
- It could be speculated that lizards with increased shedding frequency may have overproduction of thyroid hormones, but there are no reports to support this theory.
- Skin disease (bacterial or fungal) may also lead to dysecdysis or even increased shedding frequency.

DIAGNOSIS

DIFFERENTIAL DIAGNOSIS

Bacterial or fungal dermatitis

DIAGNOSTICS

- Dysecdysis is easily diagnosed at physical examination.
- Any lizard presenting with retained, incomplete, or abnormal shedding, is suffering from dysecdysis.
- Careful examination of the spectacle with an ophthalmoscope should be performed to diagnose retained spectacles.
- Retained spectacles tend to have more dull appearance, and irregular pieces of skin may be observed in the periocular/perispectacular area.
- Fluid accumulation may also be present in the subspectacular space unilaterally or bilaterally.
- Leopard geckos (*Eublepharis macularius*) often get accumulation of material over the cornea with the appearance of a retained spectacle. However, since they have eyelids, it in proposed that this accumulation into a pseudospectacle is rather the result of retained skin within the periocular space leading to secondary infections and tissue metaplasia.

PATHOLOGICAL FINDINGS

- The different stages of ecdysis can be identified microscopically.
- It may be possible to obtain a histologic diagnosis, although this is seldom required.
- Histological examination would be beneficial in cases where an underlying bacterial or fungal infection is suspected.
- Microscopic examination can help to identify organisms that are present in between skin layers or deep within the dermis, which would be more indicative of true pathology, as opposed to organisms on the epidermis layer alone, which may be suggestive of superficial contamination.
- In cases of retained spectacles, grossly there will be opacity of the spectacle. Microscopically, layering of retained skin with bacterial and or fungal contamination may be observed.

TREATMENT

APPROPRIATE HEALTH CARE

N/A

NUTRITIONAL SUPPORT

There are no specific nutritional requirements other than ensuing proper hydration.

CLIENT EDUCATION/HUSBANDRY RECOMMENDATIONS

- Ensuring access to water and proper temperature and humidity is essential for prevention of dehydration.
- In lizard species originating from habitats with low environmental humidity, a humidity box consisting of a plastic container with sphagnum moss or moist paper towels should be provided so the animal can seek additional humidity as needed.
- Water bowls must also be large enough for the lizard to soak in if they chose to do so.
- Prey items can also be soaked in water prior to feeding to provide additional moisture.
- The lizards should be inspected after every shed to ensure there is no retained skin and assist in the removal of any leftover pieces.

MEDICATIONS

DRUG(S) OF CHOICE

- Because dysecdysis is often associated with poor husbandry, any deficiencies must be corrected.
- Retained skin must not be removed if still firmly adhered to the animal.
- The treatment approach should consist of subcutaneous fluid therapy (20–30 ml/kg SC) since dehydration is a significant contributor to dysecdysis.
- The lizard should be misted and/or soaked in water, or covered with a wet towel to increase the moisture of the skin and aid in the shedding process.

- In lizards with firmly adhered skin, it may take up to a week of daily soaking before the retained shed can be peeled off easily.
- In cases of retained spectacles, the spectacle must not be forcibly removed unless it is loosely adhered.
- In addition to the treatments mentioned above, topical treatment with artificial tears q6–8h should be performed to help soften the spectacle. This can be done until it can either be removed or until the next shed occurs.
- If waiting until the next shed, the frequency of applying artificial tears can be decreased once the husbandry is corrected and the animal is properly hydrated.

PRECAUTIONS/INTERACTIONS

N/A

FOLLOW-UP

PATIENT MONITORING

- The character of future sheds should be recorded to determine if the issue has been resolved.
- It may take 1–2 shed cycles for the animals to shed properly again.
- Remember that retained shed over scars and old incisions may occur despite appropriate husbandry.

EXPECTED COURSE AND PROGNOSIS

- Dysecdysis has a good to excellent prognosis as long as husbandry is corrected, and lizards are provided with enough access to water.
- Even lizards with retained spectacles have a good prognosis due to the eye's ability to heal.

MISCELLANEOUS

COMMENTS

Subspectacular abscesses may occur as a result of retained spectacles but also have other etiologies.

ZOONOTIC POTENTIAL

N/A

SYNONYMS

Retained shed

ABBREVIATIONS

SC = subcutaneous

Suggested Reading

Cooper, JE. Dermatology. In: Mader DR, ed. *Reptile Medicine and Surgery*. 2nd ed. St. Louis, MO: Elsevier Saunders; 2006:196–199.

Jacobson ER. Overview of reptile biology, anatomy, and histology. In: Jacobson ER, ed. *Infectious Diseases and Pathology of Reptiles: Color Atlas and Text*. Boca Raton, FL: CRC Press; 2007:4–6.

Author Javier G. Nevarez, DVM PhD DACZM DECZM (Herpetology)

DYSTOCIA

BASICS

DEFINITION/OVERVIEW

Dystocia is difficulty laying eggs or giving birth.

ETIOLOGY/PATHOPHYSIOLOGY

- The reproductive hormone mechanism in reptiles is not as well understood as in mammals.
- It is suspected that a multitude of environmental and behavioral factors, as well as underlying diseases, contribute to an abnormal function of the endocrine system, which in turn leads to dystocia.
- It is also possible that a lack of breeding and exposure to males may be contributing factors.
- In addition to basic husbandry aspects such as UVB light, temperature, humidity and a proper diet, female reptiles also have a need for appropriate substrate and environment that is conductive for egg laying or birthing in the case of viviparous species.
- Dystocia is less commonly reported in viviparous species.

SIGNALMENT/HISTORY

- Dystocia occurs in female lizards of reproductive age or size.
- Most animals have a history of inadequate nutrition and husbandry lacking an appropriate area for laying eggs or giving birth.

CLINICAL PRESENTATION

- Signs of dystocia may include coelomic distention, straining with or without vocalization, decreased fecal production, cloacal prolapse, lethargy and anorexia.
- In some instances, the eggs may be grossly visible during physical exam.
- Palpation of the coelomic cavity must be done gently to avoid rupturing the eggs.
- In the majority of cases, the owners are not aware of the fact that their lizard is in dystocia.
- Other abnormalities identified in physical exam may include dehydration, poor body condition score, and pliable bones.

RISK FACTORS

Husbandry

- Inappropriate husbandry is likely a significant contributing factor to the occurrence of dystocia.
- Beyond temperature and humidity, inadequate UVB light exposure and calcium supplementation is key in the development of NSHP, which in turn can have a significant impact in calcium availability, egg calcification, and contractions of the reproductive tract.
- Many lizards presenting for dystocia also have concurrent NSHP.
- An often-forgotten aspect of the husbandry of reproductive female lizards is the provision of an adequate substrate for nesting/oviposition and parturition.
- Reptiles that may not perceive the environmental conditions are adequate for successful oviposition may not have the proper stimuli to lay their eggs.

Others

- A less discussed topic is the effect that lack of exposure to males may have on the reproductive cycle of reptiles.
- Many reptiles display courtship and breeding behaviors that likely influence the proper hormonal stimulation of prospective females.
- Many female lizards in captivity are kept alone without the benefit of behavioral cues from a male counterpart.
- This possibility of a behavioral effect must be considered, especially when animals are maintained in proper husbandry and are otherwise healthy.

DIAGNOSIS

DIFFERENTIAL DIAGNOSIS

- Follicular stasis
- Neoplasia
- Egg yolk coelomitis
- Ovarian cysts
- GI obstruction

DIAGNOSTICS

Radiography

- Eggs can appear as minimally calcified to calcified, round to ovoid, depending on the species of lizard.
- In viviparous species, the skeletons of the offspring may be observed.

Ultrasound

- The calcification of the egg varies widely across lizard species; appearance on ultrasound varies from a well-delineated hyperechogenic eggshell membrane to significant acoustic shadowing.
- In those with poorly calcified eggshell, ultrasound may be more sensitive than radiography at diagnosing broken eggs, which may be associated with egg yolk coelomitis.
- In viviparous species, ultrasound can help to determine viability of the fetuses by documenting heart rate and blood flow.

CT and MRI

Both these modalities are extremely sensitive at identifying eggs and can better assess their structure, integrity, and location.

Coelioscopy

- Coelioscopic examination allows for confirmation of the presence of eggs and ruling out egg yolk coelomitis. However, the presence of eggs makes coelioscopy more difficult due to their space occupying nature. It can also be used to assess the viability of the oviduct based on appearance and coloration.

Hematology and Biochemistry

- A chemistry panel is essential to help identify other possible underlying disease processes such as dehydration and NSHP. In addition to Ca and P, Mg levels should be documented as Mg also plays an important role in Ca homeostasis. Levels of Mg below 1 mg/dl and/or ionized Ca below 1 mmol/l should be considered deficient. Hypercalcemia and hyperphosphatemia are common findings in reproductively active female lizards.
- CBC: a leukocytosis indicates a significant inflammatory response that may suggest an additional underlying disease like egg yolk coelomitis.

PATHOLOGICAL FINDINGS

- Grossly, dystocia can be identified by the presence of eggs or fetuses within the oviduct.
- Pathologic findings may include variation in eggs size, calcification, malformations, broken eggshells, and oviduct torsions.
- Healthy eggs should be smooth, uniform in shape and white in color.
- A deviation from this appearance (i.e., dark, shriveled) is indicative of pathology.

TREATMENT

APPROPRIATE HEALTH CARE

- The treatment approach to dystocia is based on the species of lizard, clinical condition at presentation, amount and appearance of the eggs based on imaging or coelioscopy, and ability to provide a suitable environment for egg laying.
- All lizards will benefit from medical treatment even if surgery is ultimately required.
- Medical therapy consists of correcting the husbandry, providing an appropriate nesting area, and supportive therapy with emphasis on correcting calcium deficiencies.
- Oxytocin or arginine vasotocin can be administered as long as an obstructive process is not suspected.
- Some recommend the use of beta-adrenergic blockers such as propranolol or atenolol before administration of oxytocin, as these have been shown to potentiate the effects of oxytocin in humans due to their ability to increase uterine activity.

DYSTOCIA (CONTINUED)

- It is critical to provide an appropriate nesting box.
- A plastic container with a 12–16-inch (30–40 cm) deep mixture of equal parts sand and soil can be used.
- If the lizard appears to be stable, medical therapy alone can be attempted and the animal monitored for evidence of egg laying/ parturition.
- There are no specific timelines as to how quickly egg laying/parturition should occur once medical therapy is initiated.
- Many lizards, especially chameleons, will ultimately require surgical intervention.
- Surgery is best performed before dystocia progresses while the animal is metabolically stable.
- Surgery should be an immediate consideration for lizards with documented chronic dystocia, metabolic derangements, and when egg yolk coelomitis is suspected.
- The goal of surgery is to remove the eggs and perform an ovariosalpingectomy to avoid recurrence.
- Extreme care must be taken to not rupture the eggs in the coelomic cavity, as the yolk is extremely antigenic and will cause a severe inflammatory response.
- If leakage occurs, the coelomic cavity should be thoroughly lavaged before closure.

NUTRITIONAL SUPPORT

Dietary deficiencies must be corrected with special emphasis on UVB light and oral Ca supplementation.

CLIENT EDUCATION/HUSBANDRY RECOMMENDATIONS

- Clients should be encouraged to seek veterinary care of lizards early on to establish individual baseline values and confirm the sex of the animal.
- Dystocia likely has a multifactorial cause, so all husbandry deficiencies must be corrected with emphasis on UVB light, calcium supplementation, nutrition, temperature, humidity, and provision of adequate nesting substrate for oviparous species.
- Lizards should be weighed at least weekly to document any sudden weight increases that may be indicative of egg development.

MEDICATIONS

DRUG(S) OF CHOICE

- Propranolol 1 mg/kg PO once, at least 3 hours prior to oxytocin administration.
- Atenolol 7 mg/kg PO once, at least 3 hours prior to administration of oxytocin or arginine vasotocin.
- Arginine vasotocin 0.5–1 µg/kg IV, IO, IM, ICe q12–24h. Should be administered 30–60 minutes after IM or SC injection of calcium gluconate.
- Oxytocin 5–10 iu/kg IM, IV, IO q4–8h. IV administration may be more efficacious but must be done slowly.
- Calcium—start with calcium gluconate (100 mg/kg IM, SC q12–24h) followed by calcium glubionate (10–100 mg/kg PO q4–24h) long term.
- Magnesium sulfate 20 mg/kg IM, SC q24–72h, or magnesium lactate (Rescue Cal+, Repashy Ventures, Saskatoon, SK) 20 mg/kg PO q24h.
- Crystalloid fluids 20–30 ml/kg SC, IV, IO q24h.
- Meloxicam 0.5 mg/kg PO, IM, SC q24–48h.

PRECAUTIONS/INTERACTIONS

- There is scant information about the safety and efficacy of oxytocin and arginine vasotocin when used for prolonged periods over 2–3 days.
- Intravenous administration of both these drugs should be done slowly, as they can cause life threatening hypotension.
- Beta-adrenergic blockers also may cause bradycardia and hypotension.

FOLLOW-UP

PATIENT MONITORING

- If performing medical therapy alone, especially with oxytocin or arginine vasotocin, the lizard should be monitored closely to identify any signs of distress, although this is a rare occurrence.
- If an underlying disease process was diagnosed, appropriate follow-up diagnostics should be performed to determine improvement of that condition or the need to alter therapy.
- For those undergoing surgery, a re-evaluation within 1–2 weeks is recommended to evaluate the surgical site and overall recovery.

EXPECTED COURSE AND PROGNOSIS

- Ultimately the prognosis will depend on the underlying cause of dystocia and the response to therapy.
- Cases with underlying infectious or metabolic disease that respond to medical therapy have a good prognosis.
- Many cases requiring surgical therapy have a good to guarded prognosis.

MISCELLANEOUS

COMMENTS

- The ultimate diagnosis of dystocia is based on interpretation of clinical signs, history, and results of physical exam and diagnostics.
- In all cases it is essential to have at least one confirmatory test that there are indeed eggs present in the coelomic cavity.
- It must be mentioned that the sex of the animals must be confirmed as female before surgery is performed.
- While this may seem obvious, in some lizard species sex determination can be quite challenging and males may present with coelomic neoplasias or GI obstructions that clinically appear very similar to dystocia.

ZOONOTIC POTENTIAL

N/A

SYNONYMS

- Egg bound
- Post-ovulatory follicular stasis

ABBREVIATIONS

- Ca = calcium
- CT = computed tomography
- GI = gastrointestinal
- ICe = intracoelemic
- IM = intramuscular
- IO = intraosseous
- IV = intravenous
- Mg = magnesium
- MRI = magnetic resonance imaging
- NSHP = nutritional secondary hyperparathyroidism
- P = phosphorus
- PO = per os
- SC = subcutaneous
- UVB = ultraviolet B

Suggested Reading

Hochleithner C, Holland M. Ultrasonography. In: Mader DR, Divers SJ, eds. *Current Therapy in Reptile Medicine and Surgery*. St. Louis, MO: Elsevier Saunders, 2014:107–127.

Jacobson ER. Overview of reptile biology, anatomy, and histology. In: Jacobson ER, ed. *Infectious Diseases and Pathology of Reptiles: Color Atlas and Text*. Boca Raton, FL: CRC Press; 2007:14–17.

Knotek Z, Cermakova E, Oliveri M. Reproductive medicine in lizards. *Vet Clin North Am Exot Anim Pract* 2007;20(2):411–438.

Author Javier G. Nevarez, DVM PhD DACZM DECZM (Herpetology)

EGG YOLK COELOMITIS

BASICS

DEFINITION/OVERVIEW

Egg yolk coelomitis occurs when yolk material is released into the coelomic cavity as a result of a ruptured follicle or egg due to oophoritis, follicular stasis, dystocia, salpingitis, or aggressive palpation. Egg yolk coelomitis has been identified as a significant cause of mortality in Fiji island banded iguanas (*Brachylophus fasciatus*) and Komodo dragons (*Varanus komodensis*).

ETIOLOGY/PATHOPHYSIOLOGY

- In all cases, yolk coelomitis is a result of yolk material free within the coelomic cavity overwhelming the body's activity to resorb the material.
- This leads to an intense inflammatory response that is often sterile but can also be associated with secondary bacterial infection.
- It can progress to adhesions throughout the coelomic cavity, septicemia, and death.

SIGNALMENT/HISTORY

- Egg yolk coelomitis occurs in female lizards of reproductive age or size, usually older than 1 year.
- In some species, such as veiled chameleons (*Chamaeleo calyptratus*), it can occur in animals younger than 1 year.
- Most animals have a history of inadequate husbandry, being housed alone without access to a male, and lacking an appropriate area for laying eggs or giving birth.

CLINICAL PRESENTATION

- Lizards with yolk coelomitis often present for non-specific clinical signs like anorexia, lethargy, and coloration changes.
- Some animals may present with coelomic distention.
- Other abnormalities identified in physical exam may include hind-limb weakness/paresis, dehydration, poor body condition score, and pliable bones.
- Some animals may present obtunded due to rapid progression of the disease.

RISK FACTORS

Husbandry

- Any factors that may result in follicular stasis or dystocia are also contributing factors to yolk coelomitis.
- These factors include inadequate husbandry, nutrition, brumation, and nesting environment.

Others

- A less discussed topic is the effect that lack of exposure to males may have on the reproductive cycle of reptiles.
- Many reptiles display courtship and breeding behaviors that likely influence the proper hormonal stimulation of prospective females.
- Many female lizards in captivity are kept alone without the benefit of behavioral cues from a male counterpart.
- This possibility of a behavioral effect must be considered, especially when animals are maintained in proper husbandry and are otherwise healthy.

DIAGNOSIS

DIFFERENTIAL DIAGNOSIS

- Follicular stasis
- Dystocia
- Neoplasia
- Ovarian cysts
- GI obstruction
- Septicemia

DIAGNOSTICS

Cytology

- Evaluation of free fluid in the coelomic cavity will confirm yolk coelomitis.
- In acute cases, fluid is yellow to white with high amount of proteinaceous material and inflammatory cells.
- In chronic cases, the fluid may appear cloudier. Blood and bacteria may also be observed with either presentation.

Imaging

- Radiographic findings may include free fluid, follicles, or ruptured eggs.
- Ultrasound: aspiration of any free fluid can be used to diagnose egg yolk coelomitis.
- CT and MRI are extremely sensitive for evaluation of the reproductive tract. These modalities can also help to assess damage to other organs.

Coelioscopy

Coelioscopic examination allows for confirmation of yolk coelomitis but may be confounded by changes in anatomy due to adhesions.

Hematology and Biochemistry

- A chemistry panel is essential to help identify other possible underlying disease processes such as dehydration and NSHP.
- In addition to Ca and P, Mg levels should be documented as it also plays an important role in Ca homeostasis.
- Levels of Mg below 1 mg/dl and/or ionized Ca below 1 mmol/L should be considered deficient.
- Hypercalcemia and hyperphosphatemia are common findings in reproductively active female lizards. Hyperproteinemia, anemia, and hypoglycemia may also be identified.
- On CBC, a leukocytosis may be observed but does not always occur, especially in chronic cases. Leukopenia may be present if sepsis has ensued.

PATHOLOGICAL FINDINGS

- During the acute stages, egg yolk coelomitis presents as yellow to white, viscous, free fluid within the cavity.
- Fragments of more solid yolk may also be free floating within the cavity.
- Chronically, more adhesions develop and form a white fibrinous to fibrotic membrane on the serosal surfaces of the organs.
- The lesions are often severe enough that surgical repair is not possible.
- Many cases are diagnosed postmortem

TREATMENT

APPROPRIATE HEALTH CARE

- Any underlying abnormalities (e.g., NSHP, dehydration, anemia) must be treated accordingly.
- These animals must also receive anti-inflammatories and analgesia, as the reaction to the yolk and subsequent adhesions are extremely painful.
- Animals with yolk coelomitis must undergo surgery in an attempt to correct the condition, which can be fatal.
- The goal of exploratory coeliotomy is to determine the severity of the diseases and whether successful lavage and cleaning of the cavity can be performed.
- Any free-floating material must be removed and the cavity lavaged copiously to remove the protein.
- If this can be accomplished, an ovariosalpingectomy is performed.

NUTRITIONAL SUPPORT

Dietary deficiencies must be corrected with special emphasis on UVB light and oral Ca supplementation.

CLIENT EDUCATION/HUSBANDRY RECOMMENDATIONS

- Clients should be encouraged to seek veterinary care of lizards early on to establish individual baseline values and to confirm the sex of the animal.
- Egg yolk coelomitis occurs as a sequel to multifactorial causes, so all husbandry deficiencies must be corrected with emphasis on UVB light, Ca supplementation, nutrition, temperature, humidity, and provision of adequate nesting substrate for oviparous species.
- Lizards should be weighed at least weekly to document any sudden weight increases, which may be indicative of follicular development that may lead to yolk coelomitis.

MEDICATIONS

DRUG(S) OF CHOICE

• Meloxicam 0.5 mg/kg PO, IM, SC q24–48 h.
• Morphine 1–10 mg/kg IM, SC q24h
• Hydromorphone 0.2–0.5 mg/kg IM, SC q 2–24h.

PRECAUTIONS/INTERACTIONS

• Morphine and hydromorphone can cause sedation and respiratory depression.
• Dose and frequency of administration should be refined based on the patient's response.

FOLLOW-UP

PATIENT MONITORING

• If an underlying disease process was diagnosed, appropriate follow-up diagnostics should be performed to determine improvement of that condition or the need to alter therapy.
• A re-evaluation within 1–2 weeks of surgery is recommended to evaluate the surgical site and overall recovery.

EXPECTED COURSE AND PROGNOSIS

• The overall prognosis will depend on the speed with which the disease is recognized by the owners and diagnosed and treated by the veterinarian.
• Per acute to acute cases have a fair prognosis.
• Chronic cases have a grave prognosis.

MISCELLANEOUS

COMMENTS

N/A

ZOONOTIC POTENTIAL

N/A

SYNONYMS

• Egg coelomitis/peritonitis
• Yolk coelomitis/peritonitis

ABBREVIATIONS

• Ca = calcium
• CBC = complete blood count
• CT = computed tomography
• GI = gastrointestinal
• IM = intramuscular
• Mg = magnesium
• MRI = magnetic resonance imaging
• NSHP = nutritional secondary hyperparathyroidism
• P = phosphorus
• PO = per os
• SC = subcutaneous
• UVB = ultraviolet B

INTERNET RESOURCES

Pollock C. Reproductive Disease in Reptiles: Twelve Key Facts. Lafeber Vet, September 23, 2012. https://lafeber.com/vet/reproductive-disease-in-reptiles-twelve-key-facts

Suggested Reading

Gardner BR, Barrows MG. Yolk coelomitis in w white throated monitor lizard (Varanus albigularis). *J S Afr Vet Assoc* 2010;81(2):121–122.

Knotek Z, Cermakova E, Oliveri M. Reproductive medicine in lizards. *Vet Clin North Am Exot Anim Pract* 2007;20(2):411–438.

Stacy BA, Howard L, Kinkaid J, et al. Yolk coelomitis in Fiji island banded iguanas (*Brachylophus fasciatus*). *J Zoo Wildl Med* 2008;39(2):161–169.

Author Javier G. Nevarez, DVM PhD DACZM DECZM (Herpetology)

EIMERIA

BASICS

DEFINITION/OVERVIEW

Eimeria are apicomplexan parasites characterized by oocytes having four sporocysts that each contain two sporozoites. *Eimeria* are typically intracytoplasmic parasites, although some have been described as having intranuclear development. They rarely cause disease and commonly form a normal component of the gastrointestinal flora of reptiles.

ETIOLOGY/PATHOPHYSIOLOGY

- Over 200 species of *Eimeria* have been described in reptiles, and with the advent of molecular techniques, the rate of species discovery is increasing exponentially.
- *Eimeria* have a direct lifecycle with infective stages passed in the feces of the host.
- *Eimeria* can be found in the gallbladder, bile ducts, and intestinal epithelium of snakes, lizards and crocodilians.
- Most reports of illness associated with *Eimeria* infection are from captive animals that have been housed under suboptimal conditions.
- Virulence may be exacerbated by a range of intrinsic and extrinsic factors such as concurrent disease and infective dose.

SIGNALMENT/HISTORY

Disease usually occurs under circumstances of high stocking density, unsanitary conditions, and maladaptation of wild animals entering captive situations.

CLINICAL PRESENTATION

- Most animals are asymptomatic carriers but, when disease occurs, clinical signs are reflective of host cell destruction and are dependent on the site of infection.
- Typically, signs are related to GI disorder and may include anorexia, weight loss, dehydration, diarrhea, and in severe cases death.

RISK FACTORS

Husbandry

New (captive or wild) animals entering a collection with poor hygiene and high stocking densities.

Others

Concurrent disease or excessive stress may cause immunosuppression, thus increasing risks of disease expression.

DIAGNOSIS

DIFFERENTIAL DIAGNOSIS

Other GI disease such as bacterial or protozoal infections (i.e., *Isospora*).

DIAGNOSTICS

- Examination of feces for presence of oocysts using light microscopy is the most reliable test.
- Molecular techniques such as PCR may aid in species delineation but are unlikely to improve treatment efficacy or prognosis.
- Protozoa may also be seen in biopsy or necropsy samples.
- For preservation of coccidia for future diagnostics, fecal samples should be stored in 2–3% aqueous (w/v) potassium dichromate ($K_2Cr_2O_7$).

PATHOLOGICAL FINDINGS

- Lesions may include proliferation of connective tissue and erosions of epithelial cells lining the intestines, gallbladder, and extra hepatic ducts.
- There may also be an accompanying catarrhal or diphtheroid inflammatory response in the small and large intestines of affected animals.

TREATMENT

APPROPRIATE HEALTH CARE

- Supportive fluid therapy should be provided.
- Ensure that animals are well hydrated, especially if medicating with sulfa drugs.

NUTRITIONAL SUPPORT

- Ensure that animals are well hydrated, especially if medicating with sulfa drugs.
- In cases of anorectic animals, force-feeding with easily digestible proteins should be initiated.
- Direct feeding by stomach tubing can be done in most species, but placement of an esophagostomy tube should be considered for chronic management.
- Supportive fluid therapy should be provided.

CLIENT EDUCATION/HUSBANDRY RECOMMENDATIONS

- Remove and isolate sick individuals and reduce stress by providing optimal living conditions and hygiene.
- Thorough cleaning of cage to reduce environmental contamination of oocysts.
- Ensure that quarantine protocols are adopted for all new arrivals.
- During quarantine, all animals should be subjected to repeated clinical and fecal examinations.

MEDICATIONS

DRUG(S) OF CHOICE

- Ponazuril 30 mg/kg PO q48h for 2 treatments, or 30 mg/kg PO q24h for 4 treatments, then repeat for 2–4 treatments 2 weeks apart.
- Toltrazuril 15 mg/kg PO q48h for 30 days
- Sulfadimethoxine 50 mg/kg q24h for 21 days.
- Trimethoprim-sulfa 30 mg/kg daily for 5 days, then q48h until the coccidia are eliminated.
- Because *Eimeria* spp. are rarely pathogenic, prophylactic therapy or treatment should not be based on the identification of *Eimeria* spp. alone, to avoid development of resistance.
- Treatment should only be given after *Eimeria* has been confirmed to be causing clinical signs.

PRECAUTIONS/INTERACTIONS

Sulfa drugs are known to be nephrotoxic and care should be taken with their use, particularly in dehydrated or severely compromised individuals.

FOLLOW-UP

PATIENT MONITORING

Repeat fecal examination at monthly intervals.

EXPECTED COURSE AND PROGNOSIS

- Treatment may have variable efficacy as many protozoa are resistant to a range of anti-coccidial medication.
- Prognosis is good to guarded and is determined primarily by the state of the animal at initial presentation and the presence or absence of concurrent disease.

MISCELLANEOUS

COMMENTS

N/A

ZOONOTIC POTENTIAL

Due to their high host-specificity, there is no known zoonotic risk with any *Eimeria* species.

SYNONYMS

N/A

ABBREVIATIONS

- GI = gastrointestinal
- PCR = polymerase chain reaction
- PO = per os

EIMERIA (CONTINUED)

Suggested Reading

Gibbons PM. Advances in Reptile Clinical Therapeutics. *J Exot Pet Med* 2014;23(1):21–38.

Helke KL, Cooper TK, Mankowski JL, Poynton SL. Disseminated visceral coccidiosis in Indo-gangetic flap-shelled turtles, *Lissemys punctata andersonii*. *J Wildl Dis* 2006;42(4):788–796.

Jacobson ER. Parasites and parasitic diseases of reptiles. In: Jacobson ER, ed. *Infectious Diseases and Pathology of Reptiles: Color Atlas and Text.* Boca Raton, FL: CRC Press; 2007:571–665.

Scullion FT, Scullion MG. Gastrointestinal protozoal diseases in reptiles. *J Exot Pet Med* 2009;18(4):266–278.

Vetterling JM, Widmer EA. *Eimeria cascabeli* sp. n. (*Eimeriidae, Sporozoa*) from rattlesnakes, with a review of the species of *Eimeria* from snakes. *J Parasitol* 1968;54(3):569–576.

Author T. Franciscus Scheelings, BVSc, MVSc, PhD, MANCVSc (Wildlife Health), DECZM (Herpetology)

ENTAMOEBA

BASICS

DEFINITION/OVERVIEW

Entamoeba is considered to be one of the most significant parasites in reptilian species, and are capable of forming pseudopodia. *Entamoeba* species are characterized into two groupings based on morphology (number of nuclei present). *Entamoeba* species in the group containing four nuclei are considered to be pathogenic and are the main concern for reptilian species. *Entamoeba* species in the group containing eight nuclei are considered to be noninvasive. *Entamoeba invadens* is the most common pathogenic species seen in reptiles and has been known to cause significant mortality. Virulence can differ between strains of *E. invadens*. Infectious cysts are 11–20.2 µm with four nuclei and a small central karyosome. Trophozoites are 17.5–50 µm in length (average 36.18 µm), 10–25 µm in width (average 12 µm), and average diameter of 24.1 µm. Trophozoites also possess a single nuclei with a large central karyosome that is 5–7.5 µm (average 5.65 µm) in diameter.

ETIOLOGY/PATHOPHYSIOLOGY

- *E. invadens* has a direct life cycle and transmission is the through fecal–oral route.
- Cysts are ingested and then undergo excystation in the intestinal tract.
- Once in systemic circulation, trophozoites can spread to virtually all other organs within the body including, lungs, kidneys, pancreas, and brain.
- The parasite can migrate to the brain, causing abscessation and meningoencephalitis.
- The motile feeding trophozoite can also encyst and then be passed through the host's GI tract and out in the feces.
- Trophozoites undergo encystation in which infective cysts are formed and then excreted in feces.
- Cysts can remain infective for 14 days or more at temperatures of 8 degrees C and several days at 37 degrees C. Secondary bacterial infections with *Salmonella* spp. are common occurrences with the infection.

SIGNALMENT/HISTORY

- All ages can be affected
- Animals consistently kept in temperatures 25–33 degrees C.
- Carnivorous lizards appear to be more susceptible than herbivorous lizards.
- Clinical infection appears to be not as common in lizard species.

CLINICAL PRESENTATION

- Anorexia
- Diarrhea
- Dehydration
- Weight loss
- Bloody and mucoid stools
- Hardening of the large intestinal tract that can be palpated
- Intussusception
- Vomiting
- Convulsions
- Listlessness
- Sudden death
- Diffuse necrotizing enterohepatitis is the most common clinical presentation in afflicted animals
- Myositis has also been observed in varanids

RISK FACTORS

Husbandry

- Improper hygiene
- Diarrhea
- Housing uninfected with infected animals
- Decreased immune status
- Temperatures held between 25–33 degrees C
- Invertebrates (i.e., roaches and flies) act as mechanical vectors
- Being housed with chelonian species

Others

- *E. invadens* can easily be transmitted between reptilian species, with chelonian species being the most notorious carriers.
- Lizards housed with chelonians may be at higher risk of exposure.

DIAGNOSIS

DIFFERENTIAL DIAGNOSIS

- Salmonellosis
- Gastrointestinal helminths

DIAGNOSTICS

- Microscopic evaluation of fresh fecal material to visualize trophozoites and cysts.
- Trophozoites may be seen in fresh fecal material but die rapidly within 20–30 minutes once outside the host.
- SAF technique can be used for better visualization.
- Fecal material/cysts can be placed within a petri dish with water and trophozoites will emerge from the dissolved envelope within several hours.
- Polymerase chain reaction assays can be used to distinguish *Entamoeba* spp.

PATHOLOGICAL FINDINGS

- Amoeba can be observed in tissues using hematoxylin and eosin.
- Trophozoites can be observed using Periodic acid–Schiff stain.

TREATMENT

APPROPRIATE HEALTH CARE

N/A

NUTRITIONAL SUPPORT

Nutritional supplementation may be indicated if diarrhea or dehydration is severe.

CLIENT EDUCATION/HUSBANDRY RECOMMENDATIONS

- Practice proper hygiene
- Wash fruits and vegetables before being fed.
- Refrain from housing chelonians and squamates within the same enclosure/exhibit.

MEDICATIONS

DRUG(S) OF CHOICE

Metronidazole 25 mg/kg PO q24h for 5–7 days.

PRECAUTIONS/INTERACTIONS

N/A

FOLLOW-UP

PATIENT MONITORING

- Monitor for weight gain
- Take fecal samples

EXPECTED COURSE AND PROGNOSIS

Good, with early diagnosis and treatment.

MISCELLANEOUS

- *E. invadens* in culture dies at 37°C, so the owner can raise the temperature to 37°C if it is within the animal's preferred optimum temperature range.
- *E. histolytica* and *E. dispar* which are found in humans GI tracts are morphologically similar to *E. invadens* but considered to be non-pathogenic.

COMMENTS

N/A

ZOONOTIC POTENTIAL

E. histolytica and *E. dispar* are species found in humans; they are morphologically similar to *E. invadens* but are not considered to be pathogenic.

SYNONYMS

Amebiasis

ABBREVIATIONS

- GI = gastrointestinal
- PO = per os
- SAF = sodium acetate acetic acid formalin

ENTAMOEBA (CONTINUED)

INTERNET RESOURCES

- de Cardenas C. Amebiasis in Reptiles. PetMD, October 1, 2008. https://www.petmd.com/reptile/conditions/digestive/c_rp_amebiasis
- Divers SJ. Parasitic Diseases of Reptiles. MSD Manual Veterinary Manual, June 2020. http://www.merckvetmanual.com/exotic-and-laboratory-animals/reptiles/parasitic-diseases-of-reptiles

Suggested Reading

Chia M-Y, Jeng C-R, Hsiao S-H, et al. *Entamoeba invadens* myositis in a common water monitor lizard (*Varanus salvator*). *Vet Pathol* 2009;47:673–676.

Denver MC. Reptile protozoa. In: Fowler M, Miller E, eds. *Zoo and Wildlife Medicine: Current Therapy 6.* St. Louis, MO: Elsevier Saunders ; 2008:154–159.

Hnizdo J, Pantchev N. Protozoa (digestive tract). In: *Medical Care of Turtles and Tortoises.* Diagnosis. Surgery. Pathology. Parasitology. Frankfurt, Germany: Edition Chimaira; 2011:194–195.

Jacobson ER. Parasites and parasitic diseases of reptiles. In: Jacobson ER, ed. *Infectious Diseases and Pathology of Reptiles: Color Atlas and Text.* Boca Raton, FL: CRC Press; 2007:571–665.

Author Elsburgh O. Clarke III, DVM, DACZM

EXOPHTHALMIA

BASICS

DEFINITION/OVERVIEW

Exophthalmia is the anterior protrusion of a normal-sized globe.

ETIOLOGY/PATHOPHYSIOLOGY

A space-occupying swelling or mass in the orbit placing pressure on the globe, displacing it anteriorly.

SIGNALMENT/HISTORY

- There is no standard signalment for this disease.
- Gradual protrusion of the eye, possibly preventing blinking, and potentially anorexia are common findings in the history.

CLINICAL PRESENTATION

- While it can be bilateral, exophthalmia is more commonly unilateral.
- The displacement of the globe will often push the eyelids forward, and cause protrusion of the nictitans, and excessive conjunctiva will be visible.
- Retropulsion of the globe is met with resistance due to the presence of the retrobulbar swelling.

RISK FACTORS

Husbandry

Inadequate husbandry, especially dietary deficiencies and hypothermia, may predispose animals to this condition due to decreased immune function leading to retrobulbar cellulitis and/or abscess.

Others

N/A

DIAGNOSIS

DIFFERENTIAL DIAGNOSIS

- It is important to first differentiate between exophthalmia and buphthalmos.
- The most common cause for exophthalmia in lizards is retrobulbar abscessation.
- Other differentials include cellulitis, trauma, granulomas, neoplasia, mucoceles, and sialadenitis.

DIAGNOSTICS

- Physical examination will confirm exophthalmia, but additional diagnostics are necessary to determine the cause.
- Ocular ultrasound is helpful in evaluating the problem, and can assist in fine-needle aspiration, although the scleral ossicles, when present, can limit visualization.
- Advanced imaging, such as CT or MRI, is most helpful in determining the extent of the mass and whether resection is possible.
- Exploratory surgery of the retrobulbar space to collect biopsies and resect any masses present is the most definitive way to reach a diagnosis, but many cases require enucleation to reach the retrobulbar space. Histopathology is always recommended for definitive diagnosis.
- Fine-needle aspiration, cytology, culture, and sensitivity panel can help to identify bacterial or fungal elements.
- A CBC may provide information on the severity of the infection/inflammation.

PATHOLOGICAL FINDINGS

Histology and culture are most useful to diagnose the cause of the exophthalmia and allow the clinician to form an appropriate treatment plan.

TREATMENT

APPROPRIATE HEALTH CARE

- Enucleation may be required if medical therapy is unsuccessful.
- Advanced imaging is recommended to determine the full extent of damage to surrounding tissues as this will be directly correlated with expected prognosis.
- Some species may not feed on their own after enucleation and will require hand-feeding thereafter.

NUTRITIONAL SUPPORT

- Additional nutritional support is not necessary if the animal is eating.
- It may be necessary to syringe-feed or place an esophagostomy tube if anorexia is occurring.

CLIENT EDUCATION/HUSBANDRY RECOMMENDATIONS

- While exophthalmia can occur in any animal, those with husbandry deficiencies may be at increased risk.
- Improved hygiene is critical to minimize contamination and source of bacteria.

MEDICATIONS

DRUG(S) OF CHOICE

- Treatment should be based on results of culture, histology, and/or fine-needle aspiration.
- Starting an appropriate broad-spectrum antibiotic with a good Gram-negative spectrum (e.g., ceftazidime 20 mg/kg IM or SC q48–72h) and anti-inflammatory (e.g., meloxicam 0.2–0.3 mg/kg IM or SC q24–48h) can be helpful while test results are pending.

PRECAUTIONS/INTERACTIONS

N/A

FOLLOW-UP

PATIENT MONITORING

Serial CBCs, especially if the first one was abnormal, may provide an indication of response to treatment.

EXPECTED COURSE AND PROGNOSIS

- Prognosis is related to the underlying cause of the exophthalmia.
- Cellulitis and trauma have the most favorable outcomes.
- Retrobulbar abscesses can be extensive and therefore carry a more guarded prognosis.
- Retrobulbar neoplasia usually carries a poor prognosis because of their location and the inability to get clean margins.

MISCELLANEOUS

COMMENTS

N/A

ZOONOTIC POTENTIAL

Depends on the cause of the retrobulbar swelling, but generally low to no zoonotic potential.

SYNONYMS

- Exophthalmos
- Proptosis—severe case of exophthalmia

ABBREVIATIONS

- CBC = complete blood count
- CT = computed tomography
- IM = intramuscular
- MRI = magnetic resonance imaging
- SC = subcutaneous

Suggested Reading

Hochleithner C, Holland M. Ultrasonography. In: Mader, DR, Divers SJ, eds. *Current Therapy in Reptile Medicine and Surgery*. Saint Louis, MO: Elsevier Saunders; 2014: 93–106.

Lawton MPC. Reptilian ophthalmology. In: Mader DR, ed. *Reptile Medicine and Surgery*. 2nd ed. St. Louis, MO: Elsevier Saunders; 2006: 323–342.

Author Christopher S. Hanley, DVM, DACZM

FOLLICULAR STASIS

BASICS

DEFINITION/OVERVIEW

Follicular stasis is the retention of ovarian follicles. Normally, follicles ovulate into the oviduct or undergo atresia. If neither happens, then the reptile is considered to be in follicular stasis. Identifying whether the presence of follicles is pathologic or physiologic is difficult given that, most of the time, the stage of the reproductive cycle in an individual animal is unknown. A diagnosis of follicular stasis is often made once the animal starts showing clinical signs of illness or follicles are present for a longer period than expected for the species. Follicular stasis can occur in either oviparous or viviparous species and is a common presentation in lizards. Among lizard species, chameleons tend to present more commonly for follicular stasis.

ETIOLOGY/PATHOPHYSIOLOGY

- Follicles can fail to ovulate and undergo atresia for a number of reasons but in most cases an abnormal hormonal status can be assumed.
- The reproductive hormone mechanism in reptiles is not as well understood as it is in mammals.
- It is suspected that a multitude of environmental and behavioral factors, as well as underlying diseases, contribute to an abnormal function of the endocrine system, which in turn leads to follicular stasis.
- It is also possible that a lack of breeding and exposure to males may have a negative impact on reptiles' ability to properly ovulate.
- Inappropriate or lack of brumation may also be a contributing factor.
- In addition to basic husbandry aspects such as UVB light, temperature, humidity, and a proper diet, female reptiles also have a need for appropriate substrate and environment that is conductive for egg laying or birthing in the case of viviparous species.

SIGNALMENT/HISTORY

- Follicular stasis occurs in female lizards of reproductive age or size, usually older than 1 year.
- In some species (e.g., veiled chameleons, *Chamaeleo calyptratus*), follicular stasis can occur in animals younger than 1 year.
- Most animals have a history of inadequate husbandry, being housed alone without access to a male, and lacking an appropriate area for laying eggs or giving birth.

CLINICAL PRESENTATION

- Lizards with follicular stasis often present for non-specific clinical signs like anorexia and lethargy.
- These could be due to the pathologic effects of the retained follicles, an underlying disease, or both.
- Some animals may present with coelomic distention.
- In some instances, the follicles may be grossly visible during physical exam as irregular nodular masses on the mid to caudal coelom.
- Palpation of the coelomic cavity must be done gently to avoid rupturing the follicles.
- In the majority of cases, the owners are not aware of the fact that their lizard is in follicular stasis.
- Other abnormalities identified in physical exam may include dehydration, poor body condition score, and pliable bones.

RISK FACTORS

Husbandry

- Inappropriate husbandry is likely a significant contributing factor to the occurrence of follicular stasis.
- Beyond temperature and humidity, inadequate UVB light exposure and Ca supplementation is key in the development of NSHP, which in turn can have a significant impact on Ca availability and follicular development.
- Many lizards presenting with follicular stasis also have concurrent NSHP.
- An often-forgotten aspect of the husbandry of reproductive female lizards is the provision of an adequate substrate for nesting/oviposition.
- It is often accepted that reptiles that may not perceive that environmental conditions are adequate for successful reproduction will resorb the follicles through atresia.
- In captivity, there may be a combination of factors that do not allow for normal follicular atresia.

Others

- A less discussed topic is the effect that lack of exposure to males may have on the reproductive cycle of reptiles.
- Many reptiles display courtship and breeding behaviors that likely influence the proper hormonal stimulation of prospective females.
- Many female lizards in captivity are kept alone without the benefit of behavioral cues from a male counterpart.
- This possibility of a behavioral effect must be considered, especially when animals are maintained in proper husbandry and are otherwise healthy.

DIAGNOSIS

DIFFERENTIAL DIAGNOSIS

- Dystocia
- Neoplasia
- Egg yolk coelomitis
- Ovarian cysts
- GI obstruction

DIAGNOSTICS

Imaging

- Radiography: follicles appear as non-calcified, round to ovoid, variably sized soft tissue opacities in the mid to caudal coelom. At times, the follicles may either be large enough or of large enough numbers to encompass over 50% of the coelomic cavity.
- Ultrasound: early follicles appear as anechoic and progress to have more echogenicity as they mature or fail to ovulate. Follicles with a more heterogeneous distribution within the lumen should be highly suspicious of being retained follicles as the material within becomes firmer and inspissated. Ultrasound examination and aspiration of any free fluid can also be used to rule out egg yolk coelomitis.
- CT and MRI are both extremely sensitive at identifying follicles and can better assess the differences in size, shape and content of the follicles.
- Coelioscopic examination allows for confirmation of the presence of follicles and evaluation of their color and size to help in making a determination of whether the presentation may be pathologic.

Hematology and Biochemistry

- A chemistry panel is essential in identifying other possible underlying disease processes such as dehydration and NSHP. In addition to Ca and P, Mg levels should be documented as it also plays an important role in Ca homeostasis. Levels of Mg below 1 mg/dl should be considered deficient. Hypercalcemia and hyperphosphatemia are common findings in reproductively active female lizards.
- CBC: a leukocytosis indicates a significant inflammatory response that may suggest an additional underlying disease like egg yolk coelomitis.

PATHOLOGICAL FINDINGS

- Grossly, follicular stasis can be differentiated from dystocia by the presence of follicles outside of the oviduct.
- At times, the follicles may be large enough to appear to be in chains but are surrounded by the ovarian membrane rather than the oviduct.
- Healthy follicles should be smooth and white to yellow in color.
- A deviation from this appearance (i.e., dark, shriveled, or cystic follicles) is indicative of pathology.

TREATMENT

APPROPRIATE HEALTH CARE

- The treatment approach to follicular stasis is based on diagnosis and treatment of contributing factors leading to the stasis and treatment of the stasis itself.

- The species of lizard, clinical condition at presentation, amount and appearance of the follicles based on imaging or coelioscopy, and ability to provide a suitable environment all contribute to the decision-making process.
- All lizards will benefit from medical treatment even if surgery is ultimately required.
- Medical therapy consists of correcting the husbandry, providing an appropriate nesting area, and supportive therapy with emphasis on correcting calcium deficiencies.
- If the lizard appears to be stable, medical therapy alone can be attempted and the animal monitored for evidence of follicular atresia.
- There are no timelines as to how quickly atresia can be expected.
- Many lizards, especially chameleons, will ultimately require surgical intervention.
- Surgery is best performed before stasis progresses while the animal is metabolically stable.
- Surgery should be an immediate consideration for lizards with documented chronic stasis, metabolic derangements, and when egg yolk coelomitis is suspected.
- The goal of surgery is to remove the follicles and to perform an ovariectomy, to avoid reoccurrence.
- Follicular stasis is commonly associated with follicles on both ovaries but, even if only one is affected, bilateral ovariectomy is recommended.
- Extreme care must be taken to not rupture the follicles in the coelomic cavity, as the yolk is extremely antigenic and will cause a severe inflammatory response.
- If leakage occurs, the coelomic cavity should be thoroughly lavaged before closure.

NUTRITIONAL SUPPORT

Dietary deficiencies must be corrected with special emphasis on UVB light and oral Ca supplementation.

CLIENT EDUCATION/HUSBANDRY RECOMMENDATIONS

- Clients should be encouraged to seek veterinary care of lizards early on to establish individual baseline values and confirm the sex of the animal.
- Follicular stasis likely has a multifactorial cause, so all husbandry deficiencies must be corrected, with emphasis on UVB light, calcium supplementation, nutrition, temperature, humidity, and provision of adequate nesting substrate for oviparous species.
- Lizards should be weighed at least weekly to document any sudden weight increases that may be indicative of follicular development.

MEDICATIONS

DRUG(S) OF CHOICE

- Calcium: start with calcium gluconate 100 mg/kg IM, SC q2–24h followed by calcium glubionate 10–100 mg/kg PO q4–24h long term.
- Magnesium sulfate 20 mg/kg IM, SC q24–72h, or magnesium lactate (Rescue Cal+, Repashy Ventures, Saskatoon, SK) 20 mg/kg PO q24h.
- Crystalloid fluids 20–30 ml/kg SC, IV q24h.
- Meloxicam: 0.5 mg/kg PO, IM, SC q24–48h.
- Morphine: 1–10 mg/kg IM, SC q24h.
- Hydromorphone: 0.2–0.5 mg/kg IM, SC q12–24h.

PRECAUTIONS/INTERACTIONS

- Morphine and hydromorphone can cause sedation and respiratory depression.
- Dose and frequency of administration should be refined based on the patient's response.

FOLLOW-UP

PATIENT MONITORING

- If performing medical therapy alone, the weight of the lizard should be recorded daily to every other day to provide an early indication that follicle atresia may be occurring.
- Any acute weight losses beyond 10% of the body weight should prompt re-evaluation by a veterinarian.
- If an underlying disease process was diagnosed, appropriate follow-up diagnostics should be performed to determine improvement of that condition or the need to alter therapy.
- For those undergoing surgery, a re-evaluation within 1–2 weeks is recommended to evaluate the surgical site and overall recovery.

EXPECTED COURSE AND PROGNOSIS

- Ultimately the prognosis will depend on the underlying cause of follicular stasis and the required therapy.
- Cases with underlying infectious or metabolic disease that respond to medical therapy have a good prognosis.
- Many cases requiring surgical therapy have a good to guarded prognosis.

MISCELLANEOUS

COMMENTS

- The ultimate diagnosis of follicular stasis is based on interpretation of clinical signs, history, and results of physical exam and diagnostics.
- Before ovariectomy is performed, it is essential to have at least one confirmatory test that there are indeed follicles present in the coelomic cavity.
- It must be mentioned that the sex of the animals must be confirmed as female before surgery is performed.
- While this may seem obvious, in some lizard species sex determination can be quite challenging and males may present with coelomic neoplasias or GI obstructions that clinically appear very similar to follicular stasis.

ZOONOTIC POTENTIAL

N/A

SYNONYMS

Preovulatory follicular stasis

ABBREVIATIONS

- Ca = calcium
- CBC = complete blood count
- CT = computed tomography
- GI = gastrointestinal
- IM = intramuscular
- Mg = magnesium
- MRI = magnetic resonance imaging
- P = phosphorus
- NSHP = nutritional secondary hyperparathyroidism
- PO = per os
- SC = subcutaneous
- UVB = ultraviolet B

Suggested Reading

Jacobson ER. Overview of reptile biology, anatomy, and histology. In: Jacobson ER, ed. *Infectious Diseases and Pathology of Reptiles: Color Atlas and Text.* Boca Raton, FL: CRC Press; 2007:14–17.

Knotek Z, Cermakova E, Oliveri M. Reproductive medicine in lizards. *Vet Clin North Am Exot Anim Pract* 2007;20(2):411–438.

Author Javier G. Nevarez, DVM PhD DACZM DECZM (Herpetology)

GASTRIC NEUROENDOCRINE CARCINOMAS

BASICS

DEFINITION/OVERVIEW

Neuroendocrine tumors are rare neoplasms in any species arising from dispersed neuroendocrine cells found throughout the body but primarily the GI tract and bronchopulmonary system. Classification of these tumors is complicated because of the varied morphologic and biologic behavior. Currently they are categorized as well-differentiated neuroendocrine neoplasms, neuroendocrine carcinomas, poorly differentiated carcinomas, and mixed endocrine/exocrine carcinomas. Subclassification is based on hormone production as identified by IHC. Neoplasms may be nonfunctional, may secrete a single product, or exhibit multihormonal expression. In reptiles, these tumors have only been identified in young bearded dragons. They have all been neuroendocrine gastric carcinomas, generally high grade, associated with alterations in blood glucose, and, based on IHC, subclassified as somatostatinomas.

ETIOLOGY/PATHOPHYSIOLOGY

- In humans and rodents, the association between atrophic gastritis, hypergastrinemia, and the development of gastric neuroendocrine neoplasia is well documented. A similar condition has not been described in bearded dragons.
- It is speculated, based on findings in humans, that decreased functional neurofibromin may play a role in the pathogenesis of somatostatinomas in bearded dragons.
- Somatostatinomas in humans are commonly associated with neurofibromatosis type 1 (Von Recklinghausen's disease), caused by a mutation in the tumor suppressor gene NF1, which results in decreased expression of neurofibromin.
- The most common alteration in clinical chemistry, hyperglycemia, in bearded dragons with gastric neuroendocrine tumors is most likely due to increased levels of somatostatin.
- Somatostatin inhibits pancreatic hormones (such as insulin and glucagon) and GI hormones.

SIGNALMENT/HISTORY

- The tumors typically occur in young bearded dragons, aged 1–3 years.
- There is no apparent sex predilection.

CLINICAL PRESENTATION

- Bearded dragons commonly present with anorexia, vomiting, weakness, weight loss, melena, hyperglycemia, and anemia.
- Anemia is reported to range from 4% to 24% (normal value 30% ± 6%).
- Blood glucose is generally over 900 mg/dl (normal 60–100 mg/dl).
- In some animals, hyperglycemia is less severe but persistently elevated above 350 mg/dl over multiple samplings.

RISK FACTORS

Husbandry

N/A

Others

- The prevalence of developing a gastric neuroendocrine tumor is low in bearded dragons: 1.5% (Ritter et al., 2009) and 0.9% (Reavill, unpublished data).
- Cases have not been reported in other reptiles.

DIAGNOSIS

DIFFERENTIAL DIAGNOSIS

- Diagnosis is based on biopsy and/or necropsy histopathology of the affected stomach.
- Given the high metastatic potential, evaluation of the liver, intestines, kidney, pancreas, spleen, and lung is recommended.
- A CBC, PCV, and chemistry panel should be performed.
- Hyperglycemia and anemia are the most frequently reported abnormalities.
- Persistent hyperglycemia is highly suggestive of disease even in the absence of other clinical signs.

Gastric Mass

- Gastric squamous cell carcinoma or other gastric tumor.
- Gastritis due to microsporidia, bacteria, fungus, cryptosporidia.

Hyperglycemia

- Pancreatitis
- Stress-associated hyperglycemia
- Sepsis
- Granulomatous disease

DIAGNOSTICS

- Physical examination: a palpable anterior coelomic mass, may be present.
- Chemistry panel: persistent hyperglycemia above 350 mg/dl or single glucose above 900 mg/dl.
- Imaging: radiography with or without contrast, MRI, and ultrasound. These studies may highlight mass lesions in the stomach and other organs if there have been metastases.
- Endoscopy: either oral or coelomic entry for evaluation of the gastric sections and biopsy samples.
- Biopsy and histopathology are the gold standard investigations.

PATHOLOGICAL FINDINGS

- On gross evaluation, some animals have decreased body condition.
- Inconsistently, a mass can be identified in the stomach, as well as foci in the liver, pancreas, kidney, and other organs.
- There may be gastric mucosal ulceration.
- The gastric masses are variably sized, multinodular, but well-circumscribed, pale tan to white, and firm.
- The tumors arise in the submucosa and are infiltrative, frequently extending through the muscular tunics to the gastric serosa.
- They may be supporting an overlying ulcerative gastritis.
- Neoplastic cells are closely placed and arranged in packets, acini, and trabecular cords, separated by a fine fibrovascular stroma.
- They may form rosettes and pseudorosettes.
- Cells are relatively monomorphic with round euchromatic nuclei and scant cytoplasm.
- The liver is the most common site for metastasis.
- With immunohistochemistry, most have cells that stain positive for somatostatin, and uncommonly gastrin, synaptophysin, pancreatic polypeptide, Chromogranins A and B, and glucagon.

TREATMENT

APPROPRIATE HEALTH CARE

- Treatment has rarely been described
- Surgical removal of the tumor via gastrotomy has been attempted but survival was less than 24 hours.

NUTRITIONAL SUPPORT

General nutritional support to maintain body condition.

CLIENT EDUCATION/HUSBANDRY RECOMMENDATIONS

N/A

MEDICATIONS

DRUG(S) OF CHOICE

Supportive care with antibiotics, analgesics, insulin, and possibly antiemectics as needed to control clinical signs.

PRECAUTIONS/INTERACTIONS

N/A

FOLLOW-UP

PATIENT MONITORING

N/A

EXPECTED COURSE AND PROGNOSIS

- The diagnosis is generally made shortly after clinical signs develop.
- The reported interval from presentation to death (natural and/or euthanasia) is 1–3 weeks.
- The prognosis is grave, given the frequent metastasis and disease progression.

MISCELLANEOUS

COMMENTS

N/A

ZOONOTIC POTENTIAL

N/A

SYNONYMS

- Gastric carcinoids
- Gastric tumor

ABBREVIATIONS

- CBC = complete blood count
- GI = gastrointestinal
- IHC = immunohistochemistry
- MRI = magnetic resonance imaging
- NF1 = neurofibromatosis type 1
- PCV = packed cell volume

Suggested Reading

Kiupel M, Capen C, Miller M, Smedley R. Tumors of the islets of Langerhans and tumors of dispersed endocrine cells. In: Schulman FY, ed. *Histological Classification of Tumors of the Endocrine System of Domestic Animals. 2nd series (XII).* Washington, DC: Armed Forces Institute of Pathology; 2008:49–68.

Levine BS. Gastric endoneurocrine carcinoma (somatostatinoma) in a bearded dragon, *Pogona vitticeps. Proc ARAV* 2011:149–151.

Lyons JA, Newman SJ, Greenacre CB, Dunlap J. A gastric neuroendocrine carcinoma expressing somatostatin in a bearded dragon (*Pogona vitticeps*). *J Vet Diagn Invest* 2010;22:316–320.

Ritter J, Garner MM, Chilton JA, et al. Gastric neuroendocrine carcinomas in bearded dragons (*Pogona vitticeps*). *Vet Path* 2009;46:1109–1116.

Author Drury R. Reavill, DVM, DABVP (Avian and Reptile & Amphibian Practice), DACVP

GIARDIA

BASICS

DEFINITION/OVERVIEW

The parasitic organism *Giardia* can be carried by reptiles, especially wild-caught animals, in the GI tract. However, unlike in mammalian species, infection and clinical disease are rare.

ETIOLOGY/PATHOPHYSIOLOGY

- *Giardia varani* is the species that may affect lizards. Infection occurs by the fecal–oral route through ingestion of cysts in contaminated water or food, or exploration of the environment (tongue flicking).
- In the small intestine, the cysts release trophozoites, which multiply in the lumen of the proximal small intestine, where they can be free or attached to the mucosa by a ventral sucking disk. Encystation occurs as the parasites move toward the colon.
- Cysts are shed in the feces and are infectious immediately when passed.

SIGNALMENT/HISTORY

- *Giardia* can be present in animals of any age and either sex.
- It is more commonly seen in wild-caught animals.

CLINICAL PRESENTATION

- Typically, the animal will have no clinical signs but the organism is found incidentally on a fecal exam.
- Alternatively, the animal could have signs of enteritis.

RISK FACTORS

Husbandry

- Clinical disease would be more likely to be seen in any reptile that is stressed, which can occur with any deficiencies in husbandry.
- These deficiencies can include low temperatures, improper lighting, improper diet or feeding regimen, failure to clean the cage regularly or thoroughly.
- The organism can survive longer in moist conditions, so proper cage cleaning is essential.

Others

The organism is found most commonly in wild-caught animals.

DIAGNOSIS

DIFFERENTIAL DIAGNOSIS

Other protozoal organisms, both identified incidentally on fecal exam and/or as cause of clinical disease and similar symptoms:
- *Trichomonas*
- *Hexamita*
- *Nyctotherus*
- *Balantidium*
- Amoeba

Infectious enteritis:
- Bacterial
- Fungal
- Viral
- Parasitic

DIAGNOSTICS

- Fecal flotation and saline direct wet mount (include both plain saline and Lugol's iodine stain).
- Zinc sulfate flotation
- ELISAs are typically species specific, so may not be reliable for *G. varani.*

PATHOLOGICAL FINDINGS

- This condition typically does not have clinical disease associated with it.
- *Giardia* in other species can cause loss of intestinal brush border surface area, villous flattening and atrophy.
- There is also an increase in crypt length and crypt cell proliferation.

TREATMENT

APPROPRIATE HEALTH CARE

N/A

NUTRITIONAL SUPPORT

- Nutritional support is typically not needed, as clinical disease is rarely if ever reported from this organism.
- If clinical disease is present and the patient is not eating, or is weak or lethargic, supportive feeding may be indicated.
- Most lizards can be fed at 1–2% of body weight once or twice daily of an appropriate carnivore, omnivore, or herbivore feeding formula.

CLIENT EDUCATION/HUSBANDRY RECOMMENDATIONS

- Giardia cysts are infective immediately when shed in the feces, therefore proper hygiene is necessary to prevent reinfection.
- At the initiation of treatment, the entire enclosure and its contents should be cleaned with hot soapy water, rinsed, then disinfected with dilute bleach or an ammonia-based cleaner.
- Use minimal cage furnishings and non-particulate substrate such as newspaper or paper towels for the duration of treatment.
- Alternatively, place the animal in a clean environment free of cysts for 24 hours after each treatment.
- Each time the animal defecates, the feces need to be removed as soon as possible and the cage disinfected again, especially in the case of insectivores, where prey items may walk through fecal material before being ingested.

MEDICATIONS

DRUG(S) OF CHOICE

- Metronidazole—many dosing regimens exist. Consider each animal on a case by case basis: 50 mg/kg PO q24h for 5–10 days, or 50–100 mg/kg PO q14d for 3 treatments. Use a lower dose for unfamiliar or sensitive species. Daily dosing is used more often in lizards.
- Fenbendazole is the drug of choice for mammals, but no reports exist of using this drug to treat *Giardia* in reptiles.

PRECAUTIONS/INTERACTIONS

- Metronidazole: neurologic signs possible with higher doses, death reported at 100 mg/kg in indigo snakes and mountain king snakes.
- Fenbendazole: toxicity has been reported with higher doses in ball pythons; bone marrow suppression has also been described.

FOLLOW-UP

PATIENT MONITORING

Repeat fecal exam at the end of treatment to confirm that the organism has been cleared.

EXPECTED COURSE AND PROGNOSIS

- Typically, reptiles do not have clinical disease.
- If *Giardia* is found on a fecal exam, treatment if needed, together with good hygiene, will likely clear the organism.

MISCELLANEOUS

COMMENTS

- The only case report described in the literature is that of a water monitor (*Varanus salvator*) with *G. varani*-like organisms found on a fecal exam.
- This report lists several other instances of identification of *Giardia* organisms in reptiles, none associated with clinical disease.
- If protozoal organisms are identified on a fecal exam, it is far more likely that they are another species.

ZOONOTIC POTENTIAL

- *G. varani* has not been known to affect humans, but other species of *Giardia* can, so zoonotic potential can be assumed.
- Since transmission is via fecal–oral route, prevention relies on washing hands after

handling a reptile or cleaning the cage and practicing good overall hygiene measures.
• The animal should never come in contact with areas where human food is prepared or eaten.
• In the case of an active infection, the owner should wear gloves and the cage should be thoroughly cleaned and disinfected after each time the animal defecates, to help avoid infection or reinfection of the animal.

SYNONYMS

N/A

ABBREVIATIONS

• ELISA = enzyme-linked immunosorbent assay
• GI = gastrointestinal
• PO = per os

INTERNET RESOURCES

• Centers for Disease Control and Prevention. *Giardia* and pets. July 25, 2015. https://www.cdc.gov/parasites/giardia/prevention-control-pets.html
• Center for Food Security and Public Health. Giardiasis (Technical Factsheet). http://www.cfsph.iastate.edu/DiseaseInfo/disease.php?name=giardiasis&lang=en
• Giardiasis. Medscape, October 1, 2018. http://emedicine.medscape.com/article/176718-overview#a3

Suggested Reading

Divers SJ. Parasitic diseases of reptiles. In: *Merck Veterinary Manual, 11th ed. Whitehouse Station, NJ*: Merck & Co., Inc; 2016.
Greiner EC, Mader DR. Parasitology. In: Mader DR, ed. *Reptile Medicine and Surgery*. 2nd ed. St. Louis, MO: Elsevier Saunders; 2006:343–364.
Upton SJ, Zien CA. Description of a *Giardia varani*-like flagellate from a water monitor, *Varanus salvator*, from Malaysia. *J Parasitol* 1997;83:970–971.

Author Stacey Leonatti Wilkinson, DVM DABVP (Reptile and Amphibian)

GOUT

BASICS

DEFINITION/OVERVIEW

Gout is a common disease seen in reptiles. It occurs due to the buildup of uric acid crystals deposited in or around the joints or throughout visceral organs.

ETIOLOGY/PATHOPHYSIOLOGY

- Increased production of uric acid may occur due to excessive levels of dietary proteins or potentially due to an inherited enzyme defect, as occurs in humans.
- Excretion may be compromised, for example by dehydration, starvation, nephrotoxic drugs or renal pathology.
- Uric acid is a relatively insoluble substance so, when levels are elevated in the blood or in other body fluids, crystallization will occur and deposits will form.
- Uric acid crystals may deposit in the joints (articular gout), around the joints (periarticular gout) or throughout other internal organs (visceral gout).
- Common sites for visceral gout include the kidneys, liver, spleen, pericardial sac, lungs, and subcutaneous tissue.

SIGNALMENT/HISTORY

- Often seen in lizards with a history of husbandry or diet deficits.
- Sometimes may have been previously treated with potentially nephrotoxic drugs.

CLINICAL PRESENTATION

- Animals with articular or periarticular gout usually present with obvious joint swellings.
- One or more joints may be affected, and the animal may be lame.
- Animals with visceral gout may be asymptomatic or have non-specific signs such as lethargy and reduced appetite.
- Sometimes white nodules may be visualized on examination of the oral cavity or subcutaneously.

RISK FACTORS

Husbandry

- Inappropriate environmental temperatures
- Inappropriate water provision (e.g., low humidity or water not supplied in a way recognizable to the lizard)
- High-protein diets

Others

Administration of potentially nephrotoxic drugs (e.g., aminoglycosides), especially to dehydrated patients.

DIAGNOSIS

DIFFERENTIAL DIAGNOSIS

For articular swellings, differentials include pseudogout, septic arthritis, trauma, and metabolic bone diseases.

DIAGNOSTICS

- Gout may be suspected on history and clinical examination, but diagnostic testing will be necessary for definitive diagnosis.
- Cytologic examination of aspirates from affected joints for articular or periarticular gout.
- For visceral gout, biopsies need to be taken for histopathology.
- Demonstration of uric acid (usually monosodium urate) crystals is necessary for definitive diagnosis.
- Blood uric acid levels may be elevated, but this is not always a consistent finding, as the level depends on the stage in the disease process.
- On radiography of affected limbs, lytic lesions may be seen in and around joints. Crystals are radiolucent so will not be detected.
- Ultrasound of the coelomic organs may reveal echodense areas of precipitates within internal organs in cases of visceral gout.

PATHOLOGICAL FINDINGS

- On gross postmortem examination, small white nodules (tophi) can be seen scattered throughout visceral organs, within or around joints.
- On histopathological examination, tophi are often surrounded by granulomatous inflammation.

TREATMENT

APPROPRIATE HEALTH CARE

- Treatment aims to lower blood uric acid levels and promote uric acid excretion.
- Supportive treatment should always include appropriate analgesia, as in other species this is known to be a painful condition.
- Euthanasia may be considered in severe cases.
- Surgical removal of tophi may be considered if only one joint is affected, but permanent damage to the joint may already have occurred.

NUTRITIONAL SUPPORT

- Some patients may be anorexic and severely dehydrated on presentation. Fluid deficits should always be corrected, and nutritional support provided.
- Care should be taken to provide an appropriate diet low in dietary purines to minimize further uric acid production.

CLIENT EDUCATION/HUSBANDRY RECOMMENDATIONS

- Husbandry should be reviewed to identify any predisposing factors such as inappropriate temperatures or low humidity, and these should be corrected.
- Clean fresh water should always be available in a recognizable form for the species.
- A water drip system must be provided for chameleons.
- Diet should be reviewed to ensure that it is appropriate for the species and not too high in protein.
- Clients should be advised that this condition will require long-term management and can potentially be very painful if allowed to progress.

MEDICATIONS

DRUG(S) OF CHOICE

- Allopurinol is the most common choice for treating gout. It is a xanthine oxidase-inhibiting drug which works by inhibiting the conversion of hypoxanthine and xanthine to uric acid in the liver, consequently reducing blood uric acid levels. If blood uric acid levels remain consistently low, then existing deposits may potentially dissolve. Doses of 10–20 mg/kg PO q24h are recommended for most species, although in iguanas around 25 mg/kg has been used successfully. Long-term medication will be necessary to prevent relapses.
- Other drugs to promote uric acid excretion, such as probenecid, can theoretically be used, but are contraindicated in dehydrated patients. In cases of visceral gout, it should also be avoided as it increases uric acid excretion by the kidneys and could theoretically make the condition worse.

PRECAUTIONS/INTERACTIONS

Allopurinol and probenecid may potentially interact, although the clinical significance of this in reptiles is unknown.

FOLLOW-UP

PATIENT MONITORING

- Response to therapy is usually monitored by physical examination findings (e.g., increase in activity levels or no progression in joint swellings).
- Repeat blood samples can also be taken to recheck uric acid levels, which would be expected to start reducing within 7 days of allopurinol treatment.

EXPECTED COURSE AND PROGNOSIS

- The prognosis for patients with severe widespread disease is poor, but if diagnosed early the condition could be managed successfully.
- If left untreated, the disease will progress, with widespread uric acid deposition ultimately resulting in organ failure and death.

MISCELLANEOUS

COMMENTS

Figures 1, 2 and 3 – see web image supplementary content for Section III (Lizards).

ZOONOTIC POTENTIAL

N/A

SYNONYMS

N/A

ABBREVIATIONS

PO = per os

INTERNET RESOURCES

Veterinary Information Network: www.vin.com

Suggested Reading

Dallwig R. Allopurinol. *J Exot Pet Med* 2010;19(3):255–257.

Jones YL, Fitzgerald SD. (2009). Articular gout and suspected pseudogout in a basilisk lizard (*Basilicus plumifrons*). *J Zoo Wildl Med* 2009;40(3):576–578.

Mader DR. Gout. In: Mader DR, ed. *Reptile Medicine and Surgery*. 2nd ed. St. Louis, MO: Elsevier Saunders; 2006:374–379.

Author Joanna Hedley BVM&S, DZooMed (Reptilian), DECZM (Herpetology), MRCVS

HEMIPENE PROLAPSE

BASICS

DEFINITION/OVERVIEW

A prolapse is the moving or slipping of a body part from its usual position or anatomic relation. A prolapse of one or both paired hemipenes may occur in lizards.

ETIOLOGY/PATHOPHYSIOLOGY

- The underlying causes for prolapse is often unknown.
- See Differential Diagnosis for a list of possible etiologies.

SIGNALMENT/HISTORY

- There appears to be no specific signalment or predilections noted.
- Prolapse may occur more commonly in breeding animals.

CLINICAL PRESENTATION

- A prolapse is easy to visualize as abnormal tissue protruding from the vent region.
- Sometimes the owners may not notice a problem until days after it has occurred.
- A prolapse should be considered an emergency and evaluated promptly.
- The tissue should be kept moist either through gentle washing the area with water and loosely wrapped in a damp cloth or paper towel until the animal can be evaluated by a veterinarian.
- The anatomy of the extruded tissue should be confirmed.
- In the case of the hemipenis, the tissue may be pink to purple, although some species have black pigmentation normally.
- Some species of lizards may have "ornate" hemipenes with a flower-like end and/or small spike-shaped papilla.
- Exposure of the prolapsed tissue may result in further damage due to desiccation and trauma.
- The act of crawling and walking exposes the prolapsed organ to mechanical damage from the ground, branches, etc.

RISK FACTORS

- In cases of NSHP, the muscle tone around the cloacal opening is decreased leading to potential tissue exposure.
- Any generalized physical straining by the patient (e.g., dyspnea, obstipation, parasites, infection) can lead to tissue exposure through the vent.
- Space-occupying lesions located in the coelomic cavity such as uroliths, neoplasia, hepato/renomegaly, may also cause increase straining and hemipenal prolapse.
- Seminal plugs are produced normally in male lizards. The plugs are white to brown structures emerging from the cloacal area and may be mistaken for parasites. These are waxy discharges mixed with semen that form a "plug" inside the inverted hemipenes. Manual rubbing or pressure often removes these structures. In some cases, the plug enlarges to a point where it is not able to be expressed without causing damage.
- The patient may continue to rub the area and inadvertently prolapse the hemipenes in the process. On occasions, attempting to remove these plugs may also lead to a prolapse.

Husbandry

- Several factors of husbandry may lead to one of the clinical conditions listed under Differential Diagnosis below.
- Corrections of the deficient aspects of the husbandry can lead to reversal of some conditions.
- The act of copulation may result in trauma to the hemipenis, resulting in swelling and the inability to invert the organ.
- Any eversion of the organ may result in direct trauma with the environment (i.e., ground, dirt, etc.) or bite wounds from a cage mate.

Others

- A prolapse of the hemipenes may be iatrogenic through sex determination where a probe is placed inside the inverted hemipenis and torn.
- The act of "popping" the hemipenes through digital pressure to evert the tissue to determine sex may cause direct damage.

DIAGNOSIS

DIFFERENTIAL DIAGNOSIS

- Trauma
- Sexual activity
- Constipation
- Cloacal impaction (urates, cystic calculi, cage substrate)
- Neurological deficits
- Coelomic masses
- Parasites
- Hypocalcemia
- Metabolic disease
- Bacterial infection

DIAGNOSTICS

- Radiography and ultrasound may be useful in determining internal abnormalities (e.g., impactions, masses, obstructions).
- The small size of some reptiles may lead to reduced imaging detail, which makes interpretation challenging.
- Dental radiographs may be a better alternative in smaller species (< 100 g).
- A fecal examination should be performed in all cases. This can be directly from the feces, a saline cloacal wash, or direct impression smear of the prolapsed tissue may reveal the presence of parasites such as nematode larvae or eggs.
- A complete blood count and chemistry panel may assist in the determination of underlying physiologic abnormalities.

PATHOLOGICAL FINDINGS

- The length of time the prolapse presents has an inverse effect on the prognosis.
- The longer an internal mucosal tissue is exposed to the outside environment, the higher the risk for the tissue to desiccate and potentially devitalize.
- Any devitalized tissue must be removed.
- The greater the amount of tissue devitalized, the lower the prognosis to save the organ.

TREATMENT

APPROPRIATE HEALTH CARE

- Treatment often involves direct replacement of the tissue back into normal anatomic position either by manual or surgical means in combination with correction of the underlying etiology.
- The patient should be fully evaluated for general health status and treated accordingly.
- The prolapsed tissue should be evaluated for presence of devitalization, which must be surgically or medically addressed prior to prolapse reduction.
- The prolapsed hemipenis may be reduced in size by coating it with a hyperosmotic solution, such as 2–5% ophthalmic saline or concentrated sugar solution.
- Direct application of dry salt or sugar may be attempted, but the extreme osmolar difference could lead to direct tissue damage and should be closely monitored. After several minutes of application, the prolapsed tissue should become less edematous and capable of reduction back into the body cavity.
- A moistened and lubricated (water soluble) cotton tip applicator or metal probe is used to gently push the tissue by inversion back inside the body cavity aligning the lumen.
- Lateral sutures across the cloacal margin may be placed for 10–14 days to allow for the tissue swelling to resolve in place.
- If the tissue is devitalized or traumatized, or the prolapsed tissue cannot be easily replaced, the best option may be amputation.
- Since the hemipenis is not associated with the urinary system, the tissue can be amputated with no long-term effects.
- To perform amputation the exteriorized tissue should be further removed to identify and isolate the base of the organ.
- The base should be ligated with a transfixation and/or mattress suture.

- A double ligation is warranted due to the well-developed vascular system, as well as the vascular stimulation secondary to the prolapse.
- The remaining surgical stump should be replaced back into the hemipenal pocket at the base of the tail.

NUTRITIONAL SUPPORT

The reptilian patient may need weight and body condition monitoring to determine whether additional caloric supplementation is needed.

CLIENT EDUCATION/HUSBANDRY RECOMMENDATIONS

- If surgical correction of the prolapse was undertaken, the client should be directed on postoperative care of any surgical sites, suture, etc.
- A detailed log of activity, as well as food intake and defecations, should be maintained and related back to the veterinarian.
- If any changes to the husbandry were determined, the owner should correct those prior to the patient returning home such as changes to temperature and/or humidity, exposure to ultraviolet lighting.

MEDICATIONS

DRUG(S) OF CHOICE

- NSAIDs or opioids may be used in management of the pain and inflammation associated with the physical discomfort of the prolapse or surgery.
- Depending on the underlying etiology, antibiotics or antiparasiticides may be indicated.

PRECAUTIONS/INTERACTIONS

- When replacing the prolapse, extreme care must be taken not to tear or perforate the delicate, inflamed tissue.
- After the sutures are removed, the tissue may re-prolapse if swelling/inflammation are still present or the underlying etiology has not been corrected.
- Placement of additional sutures may be required, or amputation may be considered at this time.
- Hydration status of the patent must be considered before use of NSAIDs.

FOLLOW-UP

PATIENT MONITORING

- The patient should be followed up daily after clinical repair of the prolapse for reoccurrence.
- The owner should monitor and record all food intake and defecations during this time.
- Any abnormal changes should be related back to the veterinarian to determine any further changes to the therapy.

EXPECTED COURSE AND PROGNOSIS

- Hemipenal prolapses have excellent to good prognosis, as these are purely copulatory organs, therefore even in if amputation is required, there are rarely any ill effects on the patient.
- Even if one hemipene is amputated, the animal could still breed with the contralateral organ.

MISCELLANEOUS

COMMENTS

N/A

ZOONOTIC POTENTIAL

N/A

SYNONYMS

N/A

ABBREVIATIONS

- NSAIDs = nonsteroidal anti-inflammatory drugs
- NSHP = nutritional secondary hyperparathyroidism

Suggested Reading

Barten, SL. Penile prolapse. In: Mader DR, ed. *Reptile Medicine and Surgery*. 2nd ed. St. Louis, MO: Elsevier Saunders; 2006:862–864.

Bennett, RA. Cloacal prolapse. In: Mader DR, ed. *Reptile Medicine and Surgery*. 2nd ed. St. Louis, MO: Elsevier Saunders; 2006:751–755.

Author Rob L. Coke, DVM, DACZM, DABVP (Reptile & Amphibian), CVA

HEPATIC LIPIDOSIS

BASICS

DEFINITION/OVERVIEW

Hepatic lipidosis is the excessive accumulation of triglycerides in the hepatocytes, which can result in altered hepatic function. It is a common lesion diagnosed in reptiles. It is expected to be a reversible lesion if the underlying cause is corrected.

ETIOLOGY/PATHOPHYSIOLOGY

- Triglyceride accumulation in hepatocytes can occur due to disturbances of lipid metabolism from primary metabolic liver disease, toxins, protein malnutrition, diabetes mellitus, obesity, anorexia (increased fatty acid mobilization from peripheral stores), extrahepatic visceral inflammation, and anoxia (inhibits fatty acid oxidation).
- In female reptiles, the change can be associated with folliculogenesis.
- The common factor for each of these possible etiologies is a negative balance between the rates of deposition and dispersal of fat from the liver, resulting in an accumulation of triglycerides in the liver.
- In reptiles, obesity from rich diets can result in hepatic lipidosis and enlargement of the coelomic fat bodies.
- Reduced activity will also contribute to increased fat deposits and is a common presentation in monitors and turtles.
- Reproductive activity is commonly associated with hepatic lipidosis in iguanas.

SIGNALMENT/HISTORY

- Data from one laboratory (D Reavill, unpublished) found the percentages of hepatic lipidosis in the reptile groups with the liver submitted for evaluation, to be: chelonians (turtles and tortoises) 14% (97/676); lizards 20% (304/1485); snakes 5.4% (91/1672).
- There is a reported difference in tolerance to the condition with Old World chameleons and monitors being very sensitive to metabolic derangements.

CLINICAL PRESENTATION

- The clinical signs are generally non-specific. These include weakness, depression, pale oral mucous membranes, and non-specific neurologic signs.
- Green to blue urates are reported, and clay-like, tan, or watery feces may also be noted.

RISK FACTORS

Husbandry

- Inappropriate diet and overfeeding such as savannah monitors fed only mice.
- Chronic stress: inappropriate captive husbandry conditions (POTZ, cage size, feeding strategies).
- Inactivity: restricted physical activity due to space or adequate stimulation.
- Inappropriate support for reproduction
- Inappropriate hibernation conditions
- Anorexia/hyporexia

Others

N/A

DIAGNOSIS

Although the presumptive diagnosis is based on history, clinical signs, laboratory data, and imaging, the definitive diagnosis is made by microscopic evaluation of a liver biopsy or necropsy examination.

DIFFERENTIAL DIAGNOSIS

- Vascular congestion: underlying cardiovascular disease.
- Toxins: mycotoxins, pesticides, heavy metals.
- Infectious diseases: herpesvirus, adenovirus, salmonella, mycobacteria, Gram-negative bacterial infections, abscesses/granulomas, protozoa.
- Tumor: lymphoma, hepatoma.

DIAGNOSTICS

Imaging

- Radiographs ± contrast, ultrasound, CT, and MRI
- There may an enlarged hepatic silhouette on radiography
- Ultrasound may reveal a brightly reflective, enlarged, rounded liver
- CT provides measurements of radiodensity of the liver

Hematology and Biochemistry

- Serum biochemistry: lack of species-specific reference ranges make interpretation challenging.
- In general, decreased plasma proteins; increased triglycerides, cholesterol, AST, and LDH; glucose and bile acid levels vary; blood is often noticeably lipemic.

PATHOLOGICAL FINDINGS

- The gross appearance is of an enlarged, friable liver, pale tan to yellow, and it typically has a greasy feel.
- Biopsy and/or necropsy histopathology: the hepatocytes will be variably enlarged, and supporting cytoplasmic vacuolization with HE stains.
- Additional stains will demonstrate the prominent oil-red O-positive lipid droplets in all the hepatocytes.

TREATMENT

APPROPRIATE HEALTH CARE

N/A

NUTRITIONAL SUPPORT

- Maintain at appropriate temperature and humidity
- Allow exercise
- Caloric reduction with a nutritionally complete, low-fat, high-quality protein, liquid diet (Lafeber's EmerAid Sustain®, EmerAid, LLC, Cornell, IL; Oxbow Critical Care® or Oxbow Carnivore Care®, Oxbow Animal Health, Omaha, NE); hydration.
- Placement of an esophagostomy tube for feeding and administering oral medications is recommended.

CLIENT EDUCATION/HUSBANDRY RECOMMENDATIONS

N/A

MEDICATIONS

DRUG(S) OF CHOICE

- Nutraceuticals such as silymarin, milk thistle. This is reported to be an anti-inflammatory and antioxidant, although there are no studies to support its claim for hepatic benefits.

PRECAUTIONS/INTERACTIONS

Avoid hepatotoxic agents use in reptiles:

- Antibiotics: doxycycline, clindamycin, erythromycin
- Antivirals: acyclovir
- Antifungals: itraconazole, ketoconazole
- Antiparasitic: metronidazole, dichlorvos, tiabendazole, ivermectin

FOLLOW-UP

PATIENT MONITORING

Regular checkups to assess body weight, change in serum biochemistries, and possibly repeat biopsy.

EXPECTED COURSE AND PROGNOSIS

After support through any acute crisis, the long-term prognosis depends on associated conditions and whether these can be changed.

MISCELLANEOUS

COMMENTS

N/A

ZOONOTIC POTENTIAL

N/A

SYNONYMS

Fatty liver
Vacuolar hepatopathy

ABBREVIATIONS

- AST = aspartate aminotransferase
- CT = computed tomography
- HE = hematoxylin and eosin
- LDH = lactate dehydrogenase
- MRI = magnetic resonance imaging
- POTZ = preferred optimal temperature zone

Suggested Reading

Divers SJ, Cooper JE. Reptile hepatic lipidosis. *Semin Avian Exot Pet* 2000;9(3):153–164.

Knotková Z, Dorrestein GM, Jekl V, et al. Fasting and postprandial serum bile acid concentrations in 10 healthy female red-eared terrapins (*Trachemys scripta elegans*). *Vet Rec* 2008;163(17):510–514.

Marchiori A, da Silva ICC, de Albuquerque Bonelli M, et al. Use of computed tomography for investigation of hepatic lipidosis in captive *Chelonoidis carbonaria* (spix, 1824). *J Zoo Wildl Med* 2015;46(2):320–324.

Martínez-Silvestre A. *Hepatic Lipidosis in reptiles*. Proc SEVC, October 2013, Barcelona, Spain.

West G. Endoscopic hepatic biopsy in Coahuilan box turtles, *Terrapene coahuila*. *J Herpetol Med Surg* 2001;11(2):28–29.

Author Drury R. Reavill, DVM, DABVP (Avian and Reptile & Amphibian Practice), DACVP

HYPERGLYCEMIA

BASICS

DEFINITION/OVERVIEW

Hyperglycemia is abnormally high blood glucose concentration. In most species, glucose concentrations fluctuate.
Normal glucose concentration ranges from 60 mg/dl to 200 mg/dl (3.3–11 mmol/l).

ETIOLOGY/PATHOPHYSIOLOGY

- The etiology is largely unknown
- Transient hyperglycemia may be postprandial or stress induced.
- Elevated glucose may be seen during ovulation/gestation.
- Gastric neuroendocrine carcinomas have been associated with hyperglycemia in *Pogona vitticeps*.
- Iatrogenic from prior glucose or glucocorticosteroid administration.
- It is speculated that endocrine pancreas disease may lead to insulin deficiency, resulting in a diabetes mellitus-like syndrome, but this has not been documented.

SIGNALMENT/HISTORY

N/A

CLINICAL PRESENTATION

Possibly increased water consumption, increased urine (urate) production, and weight loss.

RISK FACTORS

Husbandry

- Largely unknown
- Stress from handling or improper housing may predispose.

Others

Unknown

DIAGNOSIS

Blood glucose levels above 200 mg/dl (11 mmol/l) indicate hyperglycemia.

DIFFERENTIAL DIAGNOSIS

Gastric neuroendocrine carcinomas in bearded dragons (*Pogona vitticeps*).

DIAGNOSTICS

- Blood glucose measurements should be repeated, as a single elevated value is likely insignificant.
- Persistent hyperglycemia is a more relevant finding.
- Glucosuria should be evaluated to identify chronic hyperglycemia.
- Underlying causes should be investigated: ovarian activity, neoplasia (particularly stomach and pancreas), metabolic disease.

PATHOLOGICAL FINDINGS

The etiology for persistent hyperglycemia is unknown, but endocrine pancreas should be thoroughly evaluated.

TREATMENT

APPROPRIATE HEALTH CARE

N/A

NUTRITIONAL SUPPORT

N/A

CLIENT EDUCATION/HUSBANDRY RECOMMENDATIONS

N/A

MEDICATIONS

DRUG(S) OF CHOICE

- In cases with persistent hyperglycemia, where systemic disease has been ruled out, experimental insulin treatment may be attempted.
- Suggested starting dose 5–10 iu q24–48h.

PRECAUTIONS/INTERACTIONS

N/A

FOLLOW-UP

PATIENT MONITORING

Follow up with repeated glucose measurements and monitor the general health of the patient.

EXPECTED COURSE AND PROGNOSIS

Transient hyperglycemia is likely insignificant, while chronically elevated levels carry a poor prognosis.

MISCELLANEOUS

COMMENTS

N/A

ZOONOTIC POTENTIAL

N/A

SYNONYMS

N/A

ABBREVIATIONS

N/A

INTERNET RESOURCES

Kaplan M. Hypoglycemia and Hyperglycemia in Reptiles. Melissa Kaplan's Herp Care Collection, January 1, 2014. http://www.anapsid.org/diabetes.html

Suggested Reading

Campbell TW. Clinical pathology. In: Mader DR, Divers SJ, eds. *Current Therapy in Reptile Medicine and Surgery*. St. Louis, MO: Elsevier; 2014:70–92.

Ritter JM, Garner MM, Chilton JA, et al. Gastric neuroendocrine carcinomas in bearded dragons (*Pogona vitticeps*). *Vet Pathol* 2009;46(6):1109–1116.

Stahl SJ. Hyperglycemia in reptiles. In: Mader DR, ed. *Reptile Medicine and Surgery*. 2nd ed. St. Louis, MO: Elsevier Saunders; 2006:822–830.

Author Mads F. Bertelsen, DVM DVSc DACZM DECZM (ZHM)

HYPERVITAMINOSIS A

BASICS

DEFINITION/OVERVIEW

Hypervitaminosis A is a well-recognized health concern in lizard species such as chameleons and crested geckos. It can be caused by OTC supplements provided by well-meaning owners, parenteral overdosing by veterinarians, or diets with high animal compared with plant-based (beta carotene) vitamin A levels.

ETIOLOGY/PATHOPHYSIOLOGY

- In vertebrates, the vitamin A forms are trans-retinyl esters, trans-retinol, -retinal and -retinoic acid (99% of all vitamin A present in body), while most dietary provitamin A carotenoid is beta carotene.
- The all-trans-vitamin A isomers are the only forms used physiologically.
- The liver absorbs and stores preformed vitamin A; however, at a certain point, storage capacity is reached and toxicity occurs.
- Other storage sites include adipose, lung, and kidney.
- In humans, retinoid delivery pathway to tissues involves primarily retinol-bound to retinol-binding protein; however, chylomicrons, very low density lipoprotein, low density lipoprotein, and albumin, also provide transport.
- Adverse effects in humans include increased bone turnover by suppression of osteoblast activity and stimulation of osteoclast formation. This can lead to hypercalcemia, osteoporosis, pathologic fractures, altered skeletal development in children, and skeletal pain.
- Vitamin A is fat soluble and high levels can affect metabolism of other fat-soluble vitamins (D, E, and K), with the effects on vitamin D contributing to the aforementioned bone pathology, although stimulation of bone resorption by vitamin A is reported independent of effects on vitamin D.
- Vitamin A can have a toxic effect on mitochondrial function and is reported to cause hypothyroidism in mice.

SIGNALMENT/HISTORY

- First-time owner of reptiles/species and young animals.
- Owner using OTC vitamin A drops, OTC multivitamin with vitamin A in formulation other than beta carotene, using cod liver oil or feeding liver to carnivorous/omnivorous animal.
- Occasional issues with extruded diets with inadvertent toxic levels of non-beta carotene vitamin A.

CLINICAL PRESENTATION

- The animal presents with vague signs such as anorexia, dehydration, lethargy.
- Usually has a dermatological component including: dysecdysis, epidermal flakiness, ulceration, and sloughing.
- Bilateral epiphora and periorbital edema may be noted.
- Ulcerative stomatitis can be seen
- Secondary bacterial and fungal infections can occur.
- Based on pathophysiology, suspect metabolic bone diseases may have interplay with hypervitaminosis A.

RISK FACTORS

- Juvenile animal
- Reproductively active female
- Liver disease

Husbandry

N/A

Others

Iatrogenic dietary or parenteral over supplementation of non-beta carotene vitamin A.

DIAGNOSIS

DIFFERENTIAL DIAGNOSIS

- Hypovitaminosis A
- Infection
- Hepatic/renal disease
- UVB/thermal burns
- Poor overall husbandry/diet
- Improper conspecific arrangement
- Metabolic bone diseases

DIAGNOSTICS

- Liver biopsy for histopathology and testing vitamin A levels (need normal values for the species).
- Presumptive diagnosis based upon history and clinical presentation.

PATHOLOGICAL FINDINGS

- Hepatic fibrosis
- Osteoporosis
- Decreased/abnormal bony growth in juvenile animals
- Epidermal ulceration

TREATMENT

APPROPRIATE HEALTH CARE

- Discontinuing supplementation of non- beta carotene vitamin A.
- Pain management can be important
- Systemic fluid therapy may be needed but with the goal of transitioning to oral fluids or passive soaking.
- Vitamins E and K and taurine administration have all been shown to help mitigate hypervitaminosis A in rat studies, but no studies are available in reptiles.

NUTRITIONAL SUPPORT

- Often need assist-feeding
- An esophageal feeding tube is often recommended, especially when skin sloughing is present.

CLIENT EDUCATION/HUSBANDRY RECOMMENDATIONS

- Proper education about the correct diet and formulation of vitamin A for the species.
- Education about differences between water- and fat-soluble vitamins.

MEDICATIONS

DRUG(S) OF CHOICE

- Other treatment focuses on supportive therapy and managing secondary infections.
- Judicious topical use of silver sulfadiazine cream for epidermal ulcers can help.

PRECAUTIONS/INTERACTIONS

Interacts with other fat-soluble vitamins (D, E, K).

FOLLOW-UP

PATIENT MONITORING

- Reassessment of clinical manifestation
- Review of current diet plan
- Repeat liver biopsy if feasible

EXPECTED COURSE AND PROGNOSIS

- In the acute form, generally resolves quickly and clinical manifestation uncommon (excepting very high overdosing).
- Chronic form most common, clinical resolution can take many months, with most dermatological manifestations resolving, although skeletal and hepatic damage may be permanent.

MISCELLANEOUS

COMMENTS

N/A

ZOONOTIC POTENTIAL

N/A

SYNONYMS

N/A

ABBREVIATIONS

- OTC = over the counter
- UVB = ultraviolet B

HYPERVITAMINOSIS A (CONTINUED)

Suggested Reading

Chen LP, Huang CH. Effects of dietary β-carotene levels on growth and liver vitamin A concentrations of the soft-shelled turtle, *Pelodiscus sinensis* (Wiegmann). *Aquacult Res* 2011;42:1848–1854.

Chen LP, Huang CH. Estimation of dietary vitamin A requirement of juvenile soft-shelled turtle, *Pelodiscus sinensis*. *Aquacult Nutr* 2015;21:457–463.

Mans C, Braun J. Update on common nutritional disorders of captive reptiles. *Vet Clin North Am Exot Anim Pract* 2014;17(3):369–395.

Author Eric Klaphake, DVM DACZM

HYPOGLYCEMIA

BASICS

DEFINITION/OVERVIEW

Hypoglycemia is an abnormally low blood glucose concentration. In most species, glucose concentrations fluctuate. Normal concentrations range from 60 mg/dl to 200 mg/dl (3.3–11 mmol/l), but lower values could be normal.

ETIOLOGY/PATHOPHYSIOLOGY

- Exhaustion, starvation, malnutrition
- Septicemia
- Hepatobiliary disease
- Pancreatic disease

CLINICAL PRESENTATION

- Weakness
- Tremors
- Loss of righting reflex
- Torpor
- Unresponsiveness

RISK FACTORS

- Systemic disease
- Poor nutritional status

Husbandry

N/A

Others

N/A

DIAGNOSIS

Blood glucose levels below 20 mg/dl (1.1 mmol/l) indicate hypoglycemia.

DIFFERENTIAL DIAGNOSIS

N/A

DIAGNOSTICS

- Detection of hypoglycemia in a clinically healthy animal should not cause concern.
- In animals with clinical signs and hypoglycemia, attempts should be made to rule out septicemia, hepatobiliary disease, and pancreatic neoplasia.
- Glucose may be artificially low in blood samples that have been stored for a prolonged period prior to separation of plasma/serum.

PATHOLOGICAL FINDINGS

- Depends on underlying etiology
- The pancreas should be thoroughly evaluated.

TREATMENT

APPROPRIATE HEALTH CARE

N/A

NUTRITIONAL SUPPORT

Consider energy-rich nutritional support by stomach tube in cases of anorexia.

CLIENT EDUCATION/HUSBANDRY RECOMMENDATIONS

If related to poor nutrition and management, educate clients on appropriate feeding practices.

MEDICATIONS

DRUG(S) OF CHOICE

- Treat underlying disease.
- Supportive administration of glucose or dextrose parenterally (e.g., 2.5% in 0.45% saline, 20–40 ml/kg SC) or orally (3 g/kg PO) may be indicated.

PRECAUTIONS/INTERACTIONS

N/A

FOLLOW-UP

PATIENT MONITORING

Follow-up entirely depends on the underlying cause.

EXPECTED COURSE AND PROGNOSIS

- If the hypoglycemia is related to nutritional status, the prognosis is good.
- If it is secondary to severe systemic disease, the prognosis is poor.

MISCELLANEOUS

COMMENTS

N/A

ZOONOTIC POTENTIAL

- Animals with severe systemic disease may be predisposed.
- Long-lasting anorexia

SYNONYMS

N/A

ABBREVIATIONS

- PO = per os
- SC = subcutaneous

INTERNET RESOURCES

Kaplan M. Hypoglycemia and Hyperglycemia in Reptiles. Melissa Kaplan's Herp Care Collection, January 1, 2014. http://www.anapsid.org/diabetes.html

Suggested Reading

Campbell TW. Clinical pathology. In: Mader DR, Divers SJ, eds. *Current Therapy in Reptile Medicine and Surgery*. St. Louis, MO: Elsevier; 2014:70–92.

Stahl SJ. Hyperglycemia in reptiles. In: Mader DR, ed. *Reptile Medicine and Surgery*. 2nd ed. St. Louis, MO: Elsevier Saunders; 2006:822–830.

Author Mads F. Bertelsen, DVM DVSc DACZM DECZM (ZHM)

HYPOVITAMINOSIS A

BASICS

DEFINITION/OVERVIEW

Hypovitaminosis A is a well-recognized health concern in pet carnivorous, insectivorous, and omnivorous lizard species such as chameleons and crested geckos. The primary cause is feeding food items deficient in the correct form of vitamin A for the species or in under or incorrectly supplementing vitamin A.

ETIOLOGY/PATHOPHYSIOLOGY

- In vertebrates, vitamin A forms are trans-retinyl esters, trans-retinol, -retinal and -retinoic acid (99% of all vitamin A present in body), while the major dietary provitamin A carotenoid is beta carotene.
- The all-trans-vitamin A isomers are the only forms used physiologically.
- Carnivores, insectivores, and possibly omnivores, need these forms in their diet, while reptile herbivores can convert the carotenoids lutein and canthaxanthin into trans-retinyl esters, beta carotene does not convert as well.
- Hypovitaminosis A in herbivores is extremely unlikely, except after long periods of anorexia.
- The liver absorbs and stores preformed vitamin A. Other storage sites include adipose tissue, lung, and kidney.
- In humans, the retinoid delivery pathway to tissues involves primarily retinol bound to retinol-binding protein; however, chylomicrons, very low density lipoprotein and low density lipoprotein, and albumin, also provide transport.
- Adverse effects in humans include night blindness, impaired immune function, cancer, and birth defects.

SIGNALMENT/HISTORY

- First time owner of reptiles/species.
- Supplementing with beta carotene-based vitamin A or no supplementation.

CLINICAL PRESENTATION

- Most present with non-specific signs such as anorexia, dehydration, and lethargy.
- Upper respiratory signs include bilateral nasal–ocular discharge, blepharedema, conjunctivitis, "pus" in conjunctival sacs (actually desquamated debris), swelling and closure of palpebral fissures due to squamous metaplasia and glandular hypertrophy, and secondary bacterial infections.
- Ulcerative stomatitis, glossal plaques, and glossitis may also be observed.
- In panther chameleons, periocular edema, ocular discharge, gular and lip edema, tail tip necrosis, reduced reproduction, skeletal abnormalities have been noted.
- Dysecdysis and impacted hemipenile may occur.
- In advanced cases, multifocal metaplasia in the renal system and pancreas can become systemic.

RISK FACTORS

Husbandry

N/A

Others

- Incorrect diet
- Insectivore, carnivore not receiving vertebrate prey with liver.

DIAGNOSIS

DIFFERENTIAL DIAGNOSIS

- Bacterial infection
- Hepatic/renal disease
- Ultraviolet B/thermal burns
- Ocular trauma
- Water-based toxins
- Poor overall husbandry/diet
- Improper conspecific arrangement
- Metabolic bone diseases

DIAGNOSTICS

- Presumptive diagnosis is based upon history and clinical presentation, and response to correct supplementation.
- Liver biopsy for histopathology and testing vitamin A levels can be performed but there is a lack of normal values.
- Hepatic vitamin A levels are normally extremely high in carnivores, much lower in herbivores, and intermediate in insectivores and omnivores.
- Sex of animal, testing methodology, and reported units can affect results.

PATHOLOGICAL FINDINGS

- Squamous metaplasia
- Epidermal ulceration

TREATMENT

APPROPRIATE HEALTH CARE

N/A

NUTRITIONAL SUPPORT

- Omnivores/carnivores can be fed whole prey still containing liver, or for semiaquatic turtles, can offer extruded diet with correct form of vitamin A.
- Supportive feeding, including esophageal feeding tubes, may be needed until the reptile feels better and can actually see the food.
- For herbivores, feed plenty of leafy greens and red/orange/yellow vegetables.
- For insectivores, it becomes more complex.
- Invertebrates store retinols in the retina only, so invertebrates (or juvenile forms) without eyes have no vitamin A.
- Dusting invertebrates must be done immediately before feeding, as the vitamin powder is usually often self-groomed off the invertebrate before the reptile has ingested it.
- Gut-loading guidelines are still controversial but seem to still be the best option—especially consider the Li diet (see Suggested Reading).
- Consider feeding non-toxic, wild-caught invertebrates, as they generally have much higher levels of vitamin A than captive-raised invertebrates.

CLIENT EDUCATION/HUSBANDRY RECOMMENDATIONS

- Proper education about correct diet for the species.
- Discuss correct formulation of vitamin A for the species.
- Correct invertebrates to offer and how to supplement them.
- Clear explanation of differences between water-soluble and fat-soluble vitamins.

MEDICATIONS

DRUG(S) OF CHOICE

- Parenteral treatment or oral supplementation of retinol forms to herbivores should be avoided.
- Use dietary carotenoids (non-beta carotene) instead.
- For omnivorous, carnivorous, and insectivorous reptiles, parenteral vitamin A (usually has vitamin D3 as well): 500–5000 iu/kg IM q7–14d for up to 4 treatments.
- Dosing must be done carefully to avoid over supplementation with vitamin A in the retinol form.
- Manage secondary infections with systemic antibiotics or antifungals.
- Judicious topical use of silver sulfadiazine cream for epidermal ulcers can help.
- Removal of conjunctiva plugs or flushing nasolacrimal ducts (when present) can be a beneficial symptomatic treatment.

PRECAUTIONS/INTERACTIONS

Vitamin A interacts with other fat-soluble vitamins (D, E, K).

FOLLOW-UP

PATIENT MONITORING

- Re-evaluate for improvement of clinical signs.
- Review diet plan by owner
- Repeat liver biopsy if feasible

EXPECTED COURSE AND PROGNOSIS

Usually chronic; clinical resolution can take several months with most manifestations resolving, although renal damage may be permanent.

MISCELLANEOUS

COMMENTS

N/A

ZOONOTIC POTENTIAL

N/A

SYNONYMS

N/A

ABBREVIATIONS

IM = intramuscular

INTERNET RESOURCES

Vitamin A deficiency. Wikipedia, October 5, 2020. https://en.wikipedia.org/wiki/Vitamin_A_deficiency

Suggested Reading

Chen LP, Huang CH. Estimation of dietary vitamin A requirement of juvenile soft-shelled turtle, *Pelodiscus sinensis. Aquacult Nutr* 2015;21:457–463.

Li H, Vaughan MJ, Browne RK. A complex enrichment diet improves growth and health in the endangered Wyoming toad (*Bufo baxteri*). *Zoo Biol* 2009;28:197–213.

Mans C, Braun J. Update on common nutritional disorders of captive reptiles. *Vet Clin North Am Exot Anim Pract.* 2014;17(3):369–395.

Miller EA, Green SL, Otto GM, Bouley DM. Suspected hypovitaminosis A in a colony of captive green anoles (*Anolis carolinensis*). *Contemp Top Lab Anim Sci* 2001;40:18–20.

Author Eric Klaphake, DVM, DACZM

HYPOVITAMINOSIS B

BASICS

DEFINITION/OVERVIEW

Hypovitaminosis B generally refers to hypothiaminosis. It is a health concern in reptiles that are fed fish—whether live or frozen thawed. Other cases have been reported in herbivorous reptiles and those fed vitamin supplements lacking thiamine.

ETIOLOGY/PATHOPHYSIOLOGY

- In humans, thiamine deficiency can occur rapidly and can advance to metabolic coma and death; causes are malnutrition, a diet high in thiaminase-rich foods (raw freshwater fish, raw shellfish, ferns), chronic gastrointestinal diseases, and diabetes mellitus.
- Thiamine derivatives and thiamine-dependent enzymes are present in all cells, but the nervous system is very sensitive, leading to nerve fiber myelin sheath degeneration, which causes necrotizing encephalopathy and peripheral neuritis.
- Bilateral vision loss due to optic neuropathy can occur.
- Thiamine is a water-soluble vitamin synthesized by bacteria, fungi, and plants.
- Captive fish-eating garter snakes, semi-aquatic turtles, and captive and free-ranging crocodilians are most commonly affected.
- Feeding fish high in thiaminase (goldfish and fathead minnow), improperly thawed fish (thawing too slowly), or fish that has been frozen a long time can all be factors.
- Some frozen thawed vegetables containing phytothiaminases have led to thiamine deficiency in green iguanas.
- Insectivorous anoles have developed thiamine deficiency due to lack of any thiamine in the multivitamin supplement because of extensive storage before use.
- Thiamine is a rapidly deteriorating vitamin, so it is important to ensure that supplements are stored and used properly.

SIGNALMENT/HISTORY

- Fish as primary diet
- Thawed frozen vegetables
- Using same container of vitamin supplement/powder beyond expiration date or past 6 months after opening.

CLINICAL PRESENTATION

- Can present with non-specific signs such as anorexia, dehydration, and lethargy.
- Suspicions of thiamine deficiency are greater with torticollis, opisthotonus, muscle tremors, incoordination, blindness, jaw gaping, and sudden death.

RISK FACTORS

Husbandry

Thawed frozen vegetables

Others

Piscivores

DIAGNOSIS

DIFFERENTIAL DIAGNOSIS

- Trauma
- Infectious encephalitis
- Toxins
- Metabolic bone diseases
- Hepatoencephalopathy
- Neoplasia
- Cardiac disease
- Renal disease
- Ruptured aneurysm

DIAGNOSTICS

Diagnosis is usually based upon history, clinical signs, and response to parenteral thiamine (B-complex vitamins).

PATHOLOGICAL FINDINGS

Cerebral cortical necrosis and peripheral neuritis.

TREATMENT

APPROPRIATE HEALTH CARE

N/A

NUTRITIONAL SUPPORT

- Avoid feeding fish known to have high thiaminase levels, such as goldfish and fathead minnows.
- Avoid feeding too many thawed frozen vegetables.
- Proper storage of frozen fish by not keeping beyond six months of death/freezing.
- Rapid thawing for five minutes in 80 degrees C (175 degrees F) water denatures thiaminase.
- Thawing in a refrigerator also avoids thiaminase activation.
- An added level of protection would be to add 25 mg thiamine/kg fish.
- Do not use vitamin supplements beyond expiration date or 6 months after opened.

CLIENT EDUCATION/HUSBANDRY RECOMMENDATIONS

- Proper education about expiration dates/opening dates of vitamin supplements, avoiding certain live fish species and carrying out proper thawing techniques for frozen fish.
- Avoidance of too many thawed frozen vegetables.

MEDICATIONS

DRUG(S) OF CHOICE

- Thiamine administered at 50–100 mg/kg IM, SC, or PO q24 hours until resolution of clinical signs.
- A vitamin B complex formulation is less ideal but can be used if thiamine only supplement is not available.

PRECAUTIONS/INTERACTIONS

N/A

FOLLOW-UP

PATIENT MONITORING

Reassess diet, diet processing/handling, supplementation at every visit.

EXPECTED COURSE AND PROGNOSIS

- If there is thiamine deficiency without concurrent issues, should have immediate response to therapy, but repeated treatments may be needed.
- In non-piscivores, often not considered and diagnosed postmortem on histopathology.

MISCELLANEOUS

COMMENTS

N/A

ZOONOTIC POTENTIAL

N/A

SYNONYMS

Thiamine deficiency

ABBREVIATIONS

- IM = intramuscular
- PO = per os
- SC = subcutaneous

INTERNET RESOURCES

Thiamine deficiency. Wikipedia, October 5, 2020. https://en.wikipedia.org/wiki/Thiamine_deficiency

Suggested Reading

Mans C, Braun J. Update on common nutritional disorders of captive reptiles. *Vet Clin North Am Exot Anim Pract* 2014;17(3):369–395.

Author Eric Klaphake, DVM DACZM

IRIDOVIRUSES

BASICS

DEFINITION/OVERVIEW

Viruses in the family *Iridoviridae* are large, double-stranded DNA viruses that contain a lipid component and can be enveloped. Iridoviruses that have been described in reptiles include ranaviruses, erythrocytic viruses (named hemocytiviruses) and IIV. The ranaviruses are the most commonly described, and have the greatest clinical importance. They can infect a wide range of ectothermic vertebrates including reptiles, amphibians, and bony fish. In reptiles, they are most commonly described in chelonians, but have also been found in a wide range of squamate species. Hemocytiviruses have also been described in a wide range of species, while invertebrate iridoviruses have been described mostly in insectivorous squamates.

ETIOLOGY/PATHOPHYSIOLOGY

- Ranaviruses have occasionally been described in pet lizards.
- Numerous ranavirus strains can be transmitted between different animal classes.
- In North America, the ranaviruses described in reptiles have all been closely related to *Frog virus 3*, the type species of the genus, while ranaviruses found in reptiles in other parts of the world (particularly Europe) have been more genetically diverse.
- In infected reptiles, ranaviruses can cause severe disease, often associated with lesions in the mouth, liver, blood vessels, and skin.
- Hemocytiviruses have mostly been described in wild-caught reptiles, as well as amphibians and fish. They lead to the development of intracytoplasmic inclusions in blood cells, mostly erythrocytes, and can cause anemia and systemic disease in infected animals.
- Invertebrate iridoviruses are relatively common in insects bred as feed for the pet trade, where they can cause increased mortality rates. They have been detected in insectivorous reptiles, and appear able to replicate in these, although they may only be associated with disease under certain circumstances.

SIGNALMENT/HISTORY

Ranaviruses

- The majority of ranavirus strains detected in reptiles have been closely related to amphibian ranaviruses.
- Multiple studies have indicated that many of these viruses can switch between a wide range of ectothermic hosts.
- In lizards, outbreaks have often been associated with movement of groups of animals, generally through the pet trade.

Hemocytiviruses

Erythrocytic viruses have been detected in lizards, snakes, and turtles from various parts of the world, often in blood smears from wild-caught animals.

Invertebrate Iridoviruses

- These viruses have been detected in a number of species of captive lizards, generally insectivorous species.
- Since feeder insects may be infected and contain high numbers of virus particles, IIV detection in swabs from live, healthy animals should not be considered as proof that the animal is infected, as it may be the result of contamination.

CLINICAL PRESENTATION

Ranaviruses

- In squamates, ranaviral disease has been described in association with oral lesions, increased erythema of the skin and mucous membranes, and liver lesions.
- In these animals, skin lesions have been frequently reported.

Hemocytiviruses

- Erythrocytic viruses have been found in animals with no apparent signs of disease, in animals with anemia, and in animals with systemic fatal disease.
- Affected animals may become lethargic and lose weight.
- In some cases, infection has been associated with oral lesions and hepatic necrosis.
- The temperature appears to play a role in the course of infection.

Invertebrate Iridoviruses

- It is not known if IIVs play a role in disease in reptiles.
- They may be involved in multisystemic disease processes.
- Skin lesions are the most common clinical sign observed.

RISK FACTORS

Husbandry

- Close contact with infected amphibians, many of which can be inapparent carriers, can lead to virus transmission.
- Contaminated water can also lead to transmission.
- Ranaviruses do not replicate at high temperatures, so keeping animals at low temperatures may increase the risk of infection.
- Hemocytiviruses are likely transmitted by hematophagous invertebrates, so keeping biting insects away from animals is important.
- Feeding of infected invertebrates (e.g., crickets) may lead to IIV infection of reptiles.

Others

N/A

DIAGNOSIS

DIFFERENTIAL DIAGNOSIS

- Oral lesions can also be caused by various bacterial and/or fungal infections.
- Skin lesions (and in some cases oral lesions) in lizards can also be caused by bacteria and fungi, especially members of the order Onygenales (e.g., *Nannizziopsis* spp.) and the order Hypocreales (e.g. *Metarhizium* spp., formerly *Chamaeleomyces*).

DIAGNOSTICS

Ranaviruses

- In the United States, all the ranaviruses described in reptiles to date have been genetically closely related, and a highly sensitive real-time PCR is available for their detection.
- In other parts of the world, ranaviruses found in reptiles have been more genetically diverse, and PCRs capable of detecting these should be used.
- These viruses can also be relatively easily isolated in cell culture.
- Skin has been used for virus detection in lizards with skin lesions.
- Liver and kidney should also be tested if possible.

Hemocytiviruses

- Infections have most often been initially diagnosed by cytological examination of blood smears, with confirmation of etiology carried out by electron microscopy.
- Genomic information is now available from several members of this proposed genus, and PCRs for virus detection are likely to become more available.
- Virus detection is generally carried out from blood samples, but the liver can also be used.

Invertebrate Iridoviruses

- Can be detected in the skin and multiple internal organs (e.g., liver) of infected lizards.
- Portions of the digestive tract should not be tested, as virus in these organs may represent contamination from feeder animals.
- In insects, the fat body generally contains large numbers of virus particles.
- This statement is true for all of the viruses mentioned (ranaviruses, hemocytiviruses, and invertebrate iridoviruses). It should therefore be clearly separate from the previous bullet points which only refer to the diagnosis of invertebrate iridoviruses.

PATHOLOGICAL FINDINGS

- Oral necrotic plaques, granulomatous lesions in the liver, liver necrosis, skin ulcers, hemorrhage, and edema have all been described in infected lizards.

IRIDOVIRUSES (CONTINUED)

- In some, but not all cases, infection may be associated with basophilic intracytoplasmic inclusions in affected cells.

TREATMENT

APPROPRIATE HEALTH CARE

- There is no specific treatment available for iridovirus infections in reptiles.
- All the viruses in this family replicate at temperatures below 32 degrees C (89.6 degrees F); environmental temperature has been shown to influence the pathogenicity of ranaviruses in turtles.
- It is, however, important to keep the POTZ of the affected species in mind when adjusting environmental temperature.

NUTRITIONAL SUPPORT

N/A

CLIENT EDUCATION/HUSBANDRY RECOMMENDATIONS

- Ranaviruses can be transmitted between various ectothermic vertebrate classes, and care should be taken not to mix species.
- Quarantine procedures for all ectothermic vertebrates in a collection should include testing for ranaviruses.
- Since wild reptiles and amphibians can be infected, and ranaviruses may survive for some period in the environment, especially under cold conditions, introduction of virus into a collection via the environment (e.g., water, soil), should be avoided.
- Conversely, in the case of an outbreak, special care should be taken to avoid contamination of the environment, and all water and substrate that comes into contacted with infected animals should be disinfected before it is disposed of, as should all husbandry items.
- Carcasses from dead animals should be disposed of appropriately and must not come in contact with other animals.
- Since ectoparasites may play a role in the transmission of various iridoviruses, effective measures for parasite control should be implemented.

MEDICATIONS

DRUG(S) OF CHOICE

N/A

PRECAUTIONS/INTERACTIONS

- Affected animals should be barrier nursed.
- Viruses can cross species and class barriers, so contact with any other ectothermic vertebrates should be avoided.
- In has been suggested that ranaviruses and hemocytiviruses may be transmitted by hematophagus invertebrates, so control of mosquito populations may be helpful.

EXPECTED COURSE AND PROGNOSIS

Animals that survive infection may remain carriers and should be kept separate from susceptible animals including reptiles, amphibians, and fish.

FOLLOW-UP

PATIENT MONITORING

- The time to development of disease in contact animals can vary depending on the route of infection, amount of infectious material, virus strain and host species, so monitoring should be continued for several weeks to months in an affected collection.
- Surviving infected animals can become carriers.

EXPECTED COURSE AND PROGNOSIS

N/A

MISCELLANEOUS

COMMENTS

N/A

ZOONOTIC POTENTIAL

Viruses in the family *Iridoviridae* are generally temperature restricted and can only replicate at temperatures below 32 degrees C (89.6 degrees F). These viruses are therefore unable to infect mammals or birds.

SYNONYMS

- Erythrocytic necrosis virus
- Ranavirus

ABBREVIATIONS

- IIV = invertebrate iridovirus
- PCR = polymerase chain reaction
- POTZ = preferred optimal temperature zone

INTERNET RESOURCES

Gray MJ, Chinchar VG. Ranaviruses: Lethal Pathogens of Ectothermic Vertebrates. Heidelberg: Springer Nature; 2015. http://link.springer.com/book/10.1007%2F978-3-319-13755-1

Suggested Reading

Alves de Matos AP, Paperna I, Crespo E. Experimental infection of lacertids with lizard erythrocytic viruses. *Intervirology* 2002;45:150–159.

Marschang RE. Virology. In: Divers SJ, Stahl SJ, eds. *Mader's Reptile and Amphibian Medicine and Surgery*. St. Louis, MO: Elsevier; 2019:247–269.

Stöhr AC, Blahak S, Heckers KO, et al. Ranavirus infections associated with skin lesions in lizards. *Vet Res* 2013;44:84.

Wellehan JF Jr, Strik NI, Stacy BA, et al. Characterization of an erythrocytic virus in the family Iridoviridae from a peninsula ribbon snake (*Thamnophis sauritus sackenii*). *Vet Microbiol* 2008;131:115–122.

Author Rachel E. Marschang, PD, Dr. med. vet., DECZM (Herpetology), FTÄ Mikrobiologie

ISOSPORA

BASICS

DEFINITION/OVERVIEW

Isospora is a genus of apicomplexan parasites with two sporocysts containing four sporozoites. Isospora is typically an intracytoplasmic parasite, but some species may have intranuclear development.

ETIOLOGY/PATHOPHYSIOLOGY

- *Isospora* spp. have a direct life cycle, with infective stages passed in the feces of the host. Infections are confined to the intestines.
- Most reports of illness associated with *Isospora* infection are from captive animals that have been housed under suboptimal conditions, with infection often further complicated by concurrent disease such as dependoviruses and adenoviruses.
- The most significant species is *I. amphiboluri*, from juvenile and neonate captive-bred bearded dragons (*Pogona* spp.).
- Up to 23% of adult bearded dragons have been shown to shed oocytes in feces.
- Importantly, animals shedding oocytes may not have clinical coccidiosis and many may shed occytes intermittently.

SIGNALMENT/HISTORY

- High stocking density
- Unsanitary conditions
- Maladaptation of wild animals entering captivity.

CLINICAL PRESENTATION

Typically, signs are related to GI disorder and may include anorexia, weight loss, dehydration, diarrhea, and in severe cases death.

RISK FACTORS

Husbandry

- Breeding colonies at high stocking density are at greatest risk.
- Poor hygiene and stress are likely to predispose to infection and disease.

Others

Concurrent disease or excessive stress may cause immunosuppression, increasing risks of disease expression.

DIAGNOSIS

DIFFERENTIAL DIAGNOSIS

Other GI disease such as bacterial or protozoal infections (i.e. *Eimeria*).

DIAGNOSTICS

- Examination of feces for presence of oocysts using light microscopy.
- Molecular techniques such as PCR may aid in species delineation but are unlikely to improve treatment efficacy or prognosis.
- Protozoa may also be seen in biopsy or necropsy samples.
- Fecal samples should be stored in 2–3% aqueous (w/v) potassium dichromate ($K_2Cr_2O_7$).

PATHOLOGICAL FINDINGS

- Gross lesions may be mild and unapparent in many cases.
- Histologically, there may be small intestinal villous atrophy with intracytoplasmic coccidia within enterocytes.

TREATMENT

APPROPRIATE HEALTH CARE

Medical therapy with appropriate drugs (see below).

NUTRITIONAL SUPPORT

- Ensure animals are well hydrated, especially if medicating with sulfa drugs.
- In cases of anorectic animals, force-feeding with easily digestible proteins should be initiated.
- Direct feeding by stomach tubing can be performed in most species, but placement of an esophagostomy tube should be considered for chronic management.
- In addition, supportive fluid therapy should be provided.

CLIENT EDUCATION/HUSBANDRY RECOMMENDATIONS

- Remove and isolate sick individuals and reduce stress by providing optimal living conditions, and hygiene.
- Thorough cleaning of cage to reduce environmental contamination of oocysts.
- Ensure that quarantine protocols have been adopted for all new arrivals.
- During quarantine, all animals should be subjected to repeated clinical and fecal examinations.
- Keep stocking densities as low as possible, especially in stressful conditions such as breeding colonies.

MEDICATIONS

DRUG(S) OF CHOICE

- Ponazuril 30 mg/kg PO q48h for 2 treatments, or 30 mg/kg PO q24h for 4 treatments, then repeat for 2–4 treatments 2 weeks apart.
- Toltrazuril 15 mg/kg PO q48h for 30 days.
- Sulfadimethoxine 50 mg/kg q24h for 21 days.
- Trimethoprim-sulfa 30 mg/kg daily for 5 days, then q48h until the coccidia are eliminated.

PRECAUTIONS/INTERACTIONS

Sulfa drugs are known to be nephrotoxic.

FOLLOW-UP

PATIENT MONITORING

Repeat fecal examination at monthly intervals.

EXPECTED COURSE AND PROGNOSIS

- Treatment may have variable efficacy, as many protozoa are resistant to a range of anti-coccidial medication.
- Prognosis is good to guarded and is determined primarily by the state of the animal at initial presentation and the presence or absence of concurrent disease.

MISCELLANEOUS

COMMENTS

N/A

ZOONOTIC POTENTIAL

N/A

SYNONYMS

N/A

ABBREVIATIONS

- GI = gastrointestinal
- PCR = polymerase chain reaction

Suggested Reading

Gibbons PM. Advances in Reptile Clinical Therapeutics. *J Exot Pet Med* 2014;23(1):21–38.

Jacobson ER. Parasites and parasitic diseases of reptiles. In: Jacobson ER, ed. *Infectious Diseases and Pathology of Reptiles: Color Atlas and Text.* Boca Raton, FL: CRC Press; 2007:571–665.

Kim DY, Mitchell MA, Bauer RW, et al. An outbreak of adenoviral infection in inland bearded dragons (*Pogona vitticeps*) coinfected with depndovirus and coccidial protozoa (*Isospora* sp.). *J Vet Diagn Invest* 2002;14:332–334.

Scullion FT, Scullion MG. Gastrointestinal protozoal diseases in reptiles. *J Exot Pet Med* 2009;18(4):266–278.

Walden M, Mitchell MA. Evaluation of Three Treatment Modalities against Isospora amphiboluri in Inland Bearded Dragons (Pogona vitticeps). *J Exot Pet Med* 2012; 21(3): 213-218.

Wolf D, Vrhovec MG, Failing K, et al. Diagnosis of gastrointestinal parasites in reptiles: comparison of two coprological methods. *Acta Vet Scand* 2014;56:1–13.

Author T. Franciscus Scheelings, BVSc, MVSc, PhD, MANCVSc (Wildlife Health), DECZM (Herpetology)

LEUKEMIA

BASICS

DEFINITION/OVERVIEW

Leukemia is a neoplasia of the white blood cells, which starts in the bone marrow.

ETIOLOGY/PATHOPHYSIOLOGY

- Although radiation at a dose of 3000 R induced experimentally leukemia in Indian spiny-tailed lizards (*Saara hardwickii*), no confirmed etiology has been proved for any cases described in reptiles, including viral etiology.
- Leukemias are classified as myeloid or lymphoid, depending upon the neoplastic blood cell.
- It is generally accepted, on the basis of previously reported cytochemical staining characteristics, that reptilian granulocytes, monocytes, and azurophils are from the myeloid cell lineage, whereas reptilian lymphocytes are from the lymphoid cell lineage.
- Leukemias are commonly graded as acute or chronic, depending on the number of blast cells in peripheral circulation.
- Blast cells predominate in acute leukemia, whereas mature forms predominate in chronic onset leukemia, with less than 30% of the peripheral leukocytes being blast cells.
- Acute leukemias are rapidly fatal in untreated patients.

SIGNALMENT/HISTORY

The majority of reported cases are in bearded dragons, but this may simply be due to their numbers in the pet trade rather than species predisposition.

CLINICAL PRESENTATION

- Anorexia and lethargy are frequently reported.
- Weight loss is common in chronic leukemia.

RISK FACTORS

Husbandry

N/A

Others

N/A

DIAGNOSIS

DIFFERENTIAL DIAGNOSIS

- Multiple myeloma or plasma cell myeloma
- Monoclonal gammopathy

DIAGNOSTICS

- Hemogram: a marked leukocytosis characterized by lymphocytosis/monocytosis (depending upon the type of leukemia) is observed in many cases.
- Cytological evaluation of blood smears and/or bone marrow aspirates.
- Necropsy and subsequent histopathology
- Cytochemical and immunocytochemical stains to confirm cell lineage.
- Peroxidase activity, chloroacetate esterase activity, and α-naphthyl butyrate esterase activity can be used as markers to distinguish myeloid or lymphoid origin; it is important to study comparison samples from both clinically healthy and affected animals of the same species because of the paucity of cytochemical characterization of blood cells for most reptiles.
- L1-calprotectin antibody identifies myeloid cells, whereas CD3 antibody identifies T-cell lymphocytes, and CD79 antibody identifies B-cell lymphocytes.
- Transmission electron microscopy can be attempted to determine histogenesis and to identify viral particles.

PATHOLOGICAL FINDINGS

- Cytological evaluation of blood smears and/or bone marrow aspirates can reveal abnormal cell morphology of the neoplastic cells, abnormal nuclear to cytoplasm ratio, and anisokaryosis; mitotic figures are frequently detected.
- Histopathologic examination of tissue samples can reveal infiltration of neoplastic cells in several organs and occasional mitotic figures.

TREATMENT

APPROPRIATE HEALTH CARE

Medical therapy (see below)

NUTRITIONAL SUPPORT

An esophagostomy tube should be considered in anorexic animals or for long-term administration of medications.

CLIENT EDUCATION/HUSBANDRY RECOMENDATIONS

An early diagnosis can maximize the success of therapy.

MEDICATIONS

DRUG(S) OF CHOICE

- Because cytosine arabinoside is the most frequently used treatment for mammals with chronic monocytic leukemia, Jankowski et al. treated an initially diagnosed chronic monocytic leukemia in a bearded dragon (*Pogona vitticeps*) with cytosine arabinoside at a dose of 100 mg/m^2.
- Normosol®-R was used to dilute the solution of 12.5 mg/ml cytosine arabinoside to a 0.78 mg/ml solution, which was administered IV at a rate of 0.3 ml/hour for 48 hours.
- 44 hours into the treatment, the dragon became acutely unresponsive and died within 1 hour.
- Prednisone therapy is widely used and accepted for patients with lymphoid leukemia and lymphoma, not being effective for myeloid leukemias.

PRECAUTIONS/INTERACTIONS

Although suspected cytosine arabinoside toxicity characterized by renal failure has been reported when treating a rhinoceros viper, no evidence of renal failure or other organ failure related to administration of the drug were observed by Jankowski et al. in a bearded dragon.

FOLLOW-UP

PATIENT MONITORING

Complete blood count must be done for monitoring the overall WBC count and different leukocyte counts to gauge response to the drugs.

EXPECTED COURSE AND PROGNOSIS

The prognosis of the disease, especially in acute leukemia, is poor.

MISCELLANEOUS

COMMENTS

N/A

ZOONOTIC POTENTIAL

N/A

SYNONYMS

N/A

ABBREVIATIONS

- IV = intravenous
- WBC = white blood cells

Suggested Reading

Jankowski G, Sirninger J, Borne J, Nevarez JG. Chemotherapeutic treatment for leukemia in a bearded dragon (*Pogona vitticeps*). *J Zoo Wildl Med* 2011;42:322–325.

Mauldin GN, Done LB. Oncology. In: Mader DR, ed. *Reptile Medicine and Surgery*. 2nd ed. St. Louis, MO: Elsevier Saunders; 2006:299–322.

Tocidlowski M, McNamara PL, Wojcieszyn JW. Myelogenous leukemia in a bearded dragon (*Acanthodraco vitticeps*). *J Zoo Wildl Med* 2001;32:90–95.

Author Jorge Orós, DVM, PhD, DECZM

LOWER RESPIRATORY TRACT DISEASE

BASICS

DEFINITION/OVERVIEW

Diseases of the respiratory tract are common and are often responsible for considerable morbidity and mortality in reptiles. LRTD often occurs concurrently with disease of the URT. In lizards, the LRT consists of the glottis, larynx, trachea, paired bronchi, and, depending on the species, single-chambered, transitional, or multichambered lungs. The site of the glottis may vary considerably. The trachea is composed of incomplete (C-shaped) cartilaginous rings in most lizards. Chameleons have an inflatable gular sac extending ventrally from the trachea. In lizards, the bronchial anatomy follows one of two patterns. The bronchus either enters the cranial pole of the lung, from which it extends caudally a very short distance (e.g., in chameleons), or it traverses the entire length of the lung (e.g., in monitor lizards). Tuataras lack bronchi and have a single-chambered lung. In most lizards, the left and right lungs are almost the same size and are situated within the cranial half of the coelomic cavity. The lungs of chameleons extend along the dorsal and lateral body cavity and have internal separations and tentacular diverticula. The intercostal muscles move the dorsal and ventral ribs to control ventilation. Gular pumping can also be used to ventilate.

ETIOLOGY/PATHOPHYSIOLOGY

- There is a wide range of etiologies associated with LRTD, but infectious causes are some of the most common.
- LRTD may also be secondary to other diseases such as stomatitis.

Infectious

- Bacteria (*Mycobacteria*; Gram-negatives such as *Bordetella* spp., *Pseudomonas* spp., *Salmonella* spp., *Morganella morganii*, *Acinetobacter* spp., *Klebsiella* spp., *Serratia marcescens*, *Proteus* spp., *Aeromonas* spp., *Providencia rettgeri*; Gram-positive *Streptococcus* spp.)
- Fungi (*Paecilomyces* spp., *Penicillium* spp., *Chrysosporium* spp., *Candida* spp.)
- Viruses (ferlavirus associated primarily with in caiman lizards, adenovirus in chameleons, reovirus and iridovirus).
- Parasites may cause physical damage to epithelium and may serve as vectors for other infections, sometimes a combination of parasitic and bacterial or viral.
- *Pneumonema tiliquae* in the lung of *Tiliqua scincoides*.
- Pentastomids (in the oral cavity, pharynx, trachea, bronchi, lung), sometimes exiting via the glottis and then through the mouth and nares.
- *Armillifer* spp.; *Rallietiella* spp., *Raillietiellia* spp., and *Sambonia* spp.

Non-infectious

- Neoplasia (lymphosarcoma in a Savannah monitor lizard, plasma cell tumor in the lung of an East Indian water lizard; hepatic spindle-cell sarcoma metastasizing to the lung in a Savannah monitor lizard, malignant lymphoma of an East Indian water lizard and a generalized lymphosarcoma in a Malayan monitor).
- Foreign bodies within the oral cavity, trachea, bronchus or lung.
- Physical trauma/injuries
- Improper husbandry

SIGNALMENT/HISTORY

No age, sex or species predisposition.

CLINICAL PRESENTATION

- Depending on the underlying cause and lizard species.
- Nonspecific signs, such as anorexia, lethargy, inactivity.
- Sometimes nasal discharge/exudate and obstructed external nares.
- Tachypnea or dyspnea
- Respiratory distress (intermittent or persistent).
- Open-mouth breathing (in severe cases).
- Gaping of the mouth with extended glottis.
- Elevated head and forced breathing/increased respiratory efforts.
- Stridor, gurgling, or wheezing
- Excess salivation/oral exudate
- Simultaneous occurrence of stomatitis (sometimes necrotizing).
- Sometimes glottal discharge, reddening and/or edema of the glottis.
- Cyanosis in severe cases
- Excessive air-filled digestive tract (aerophagia) due to increased and forced inspiration.
- Acute death due to blockage with plug (sometimes mucopurulent) or tissue (hyperplasia or neoplasia).

RISK FACTORS

Husbandry

- Inadequate husbandry
- Stressors
- Poor hygiene
- Inappropriate temperatures and humidity
- Stagnant water
- Substrate with irritating compounds (e.g., cedar shavings)
- Poor ventilation

Others

- Immunosuppression, which may be caused by stress, overcrowding, relocation, concurrent disease or inappropriate husbandry.
- Sudden changes in temperature or humidity.
- Improper diet (including starvation) and endoparasitism may also be predisposing factors.

DIAGNOSIS

DIFFERENTIAL DIAGNOSIS

- Infectious diseases (bacterial, viral, fungal, parasitic)
- Trauma
- Neoplasia
- Foreign bodies
- Inhalation of irritating substances

DIAGNOSTICS

- Physical examination, including thorough exam of the oral cavity and choana. The use of magnification may aid in identifying subtle lesions.
- Bacterial culture and sensitivity (aerobic and anaerobic) and/or fungal culture of tracheal or lung lavage is critical for proper diagnosis.
- Cytology of oral mucus and tracheal or lung lavage.
- Diagnostic imaging (radiography, CT, MRI)
- Endoscopy, including nasal lavage and biopsy for further diagnostics such as cytology, histopathology, virology, and electron microscopy.
- Biopsy, cytology, and histopathology of the affected lung(s) may be beneficial in refractory cases.
- In cases of virus infections, virus isolation and/or PCR using tracheal or lung lavage, nasal flush or nasal swab, choanal, oral, esophageal swabs, or lung tissue; detection of antibodies in blood samples (serology).
- In case of suspected *Mycobacteria*: immunohistochemistry and PCR.
- Fecal exam

PATHOLOGICAL FINDINGS

- Pathologic findings will vary according to the underlying cause and may range from mild to severe.
- Histopathology in an adenovirus infection in a Jackson's chameleon revealed proliferation of the mucosal epithelium lining the trachea and esophagus, and intranuclear inclusions in cells of the trachea and esophagus.
- Histological changes associated with paramyxovirus infections in caiman lizards consisted of a proliferative heterophilic and histiocytic pneumonia with mucoid fluid in both lungs and flocculent material in the central airway.

LOWER RESPIRATORY TRACT DISEASE (CONTINUED)

TREATMENT

APPROPRIATE HEALTH CARE

N/A

NUTRITIONAL SUPPORT

- Nutritional supplementation for anorexic animals is essential for recovery.
- Carnivore critical care diets can be fed until the lizard starts eating on its own.
- Fluid therapy at a fluid rate of 10–30 ml/kg/day as supportive care.
- Placement of an esophagostomy tube is recommended to facilitate administration of food, medications, and decrease stress of handling.

CLIENT EDUCATION/HUSBANDRY RECOMMENDATIONS

- Correct any husbandry deficiencies with special attention to temperature, humidity, and ventilation.
- Isolate animal from others in collection, especially when viral etiology is suspected.
- It is important to ensure a full course of treatment to avoid recurrence of disease.

MEDICATIONS

DRUG(S) OF CHOICE

- In case of confirmed mycobacterial infection – no treatment, euthanasia.
- Individual housing of affected animals, sanitation and strict quarantine.
- Separating collections into smaller groups and minimizing intergroup contact to prevent the spread of infections in large collections.
- Foreign body within the URT/LRT/adjacent organs (e.g., gastrointestinal tract): extraction (including possible surgery).
- Injuries affecting larynx, glottis, trachea, bronchus, lung(s): adequate wound treatment.
- Oxygen cage therapy in severe cases.
- Neoplasia: surgical removal if feasible, followed by radiation or chemotherapy
- Depends on the underlying cause and the affected lizard species.
- Bacteria: systemic or nebulized antibiotics (enrofloxacin, cephalosporin, oxytetracycline, amikacin, doxycycline, ceftazidime, tylosin, trimethoprim-sulfadiazine), preferably according to sensitivity panel for at least 4–6 weeks. Local instillation of antibiotics (injectable or ophthalmic solutions) in the nasal passage may also be effective.
- Fungi: systemic, local, nebulized antifungals (e.g., terbinafine, voriconazole, amphotericin B). Systemic use of itraconazole may cause severe side effects in some lizards.
- Nebulization with acetylcysteine for the elimination of exudates in severe cases.
- Viral: separation, strict quarantine, and intensive supportive therapy. Antiviral therapy has had low success and euthanasia is often required depending on the state of the animal and the disease.
- Parasites: antiparasitic treatment according the species. In some cases, physical removal of the parasites via surgery or endoscopy may be performed.

PRECAUTIONS/INTERACTIONS

- Many systemic antibiotics (e.g., gentamycin or enrofloxacin) are excreted through the kidney or show renal toxicity.
- Adequate hydration and regular monitoring of renal values is recommended.

FOLLOW-UP

PATIENT MONITORING

- Improvement of clinical signs should be expected within 1–2 weeks for bacterial and fungal infections when definitive diagnosis and treatment are employed.
- It is critical to continue treatment until clinical signs are fully resolved and repeating cultures to confirm resolution of infection if unsure.
- In cases that do not show any improvement or worsen during the first 1–2 weeks of treatment, it should be considered that the etiology and/or treatment are not accurate.
- Viral infections should also be considered in cases that do not respond to therapy or have chronic, intermittent recurrence of disease.
- Repeat diagnostics may be needed to assess resolution or progression of disease.

EXPECTED COURSE AND PROGNOSIS

- Depends on the etiology
- Bacterial: good prognosis depending on response to antibiotics.
- Fungal: guarded to poor prognosis
- Viral: poor to grave prognosis, especially when showing clinical signs.
- Parasitic: good prognosis
- Neoplastic: poor to grave prognosis
- Others: depends on severity and involvement of other tissues.

MISCELLANEOUS

COMMENTS

N/A

ZOONOTIC POTENTIAL

- Depends on the causative agent
- Mycobacteria, salmonella, pentastomids (rare), and other etiologies have zoonotic potential.

SYNONYMS

Pneumonia

ABBREVIATIONS

- CT = computed tomography
- LRT = lower respiratory tract
- LRTD = lower respiratory tract disease
- MRI = magnetic resonance imaging
- PCR = polymerase chain reaction
- URT = upper respiratory tract

Suggested Reading

Flach EJ, Riley J, Mutlow AG, McCandlish IA. Pentastomiasis in Bosc's monitor lizards (*Varanus exanthematicus*) caused by an undescribed *Sambonia* species. *J Zoo Wildl Med* 2000;31(1):91–95.

Jacobson E. Diseases of the respiratory system in reptiles. *Vet Med Small Anim Clin* 1978;73(9):1169–1175.

Jacobson ER, Gardiner CH. Adeno-like virus in esophageal and tracheal mucosa of a Jackson's chameleon (*Chamaeleo jacksoni*). *Vet Path* 1990;27(3):210–212.

Jacobson ER, Origgi F, Pessier AP, et al. Paramyxovirus infection in caiman lizards (*Draecena guianensis*). *J Vet Diagn Invest* 2001;13(2):143–151.

Junge RE, Miller RE. Reptile respiratory diseases. In: Kirk RW, Bonagura JD, eds. *Kirk's Current Veterinary Therapy XI. Small Animal Practice*. 11th ed. Philadelphia, PA: W.B. Saunders; 1992:1204–1210.

Schumacher J. Respiratory medicine of reptiles. *Vet Clin North Am Exot Anim Pract* 2011;14(2):207–224.

Wyneken J, Witherington D. Respiratory anatomy: form and function in reptiles. *Exotic DVM* 2001;3:17–22.

Author Karina A. Mathes, DVM, Dr. med. vet., DECZM (Herpetology), European Veterinary Specialist in Zoological Medicine (Herpetology), Certified Specialist in Reptiles (Fachtieraerztin fuer Reptilien), Certified Specialist in Reptiles and Amphibians (ZB Reptilien und Amphibien)

LYMPHOMA

BASICS

DEFINITION/OVERVIEW

Lymphoma is a lymphoid neoplasia that originates in the lymphocyte cells.

ETIOLOGY/PATHOPHYSIOLOGY

- An infectious etiology was suspected in an unusually high incidence of lymphoid neoplasia in a collection of Egyptian spiny-tailed lizards (*Uromastyx aegyptius*), but no viral etiology has been identified in most cases of lymphoid neoplasias in reptiles.
- Lymphoid neoplasias are more frequent in lizards and snakes than in other reptiles, and they most commonly have a multicentric distribution.
- There is insufficient information about lymphoma in reptiles to be able to meaningfully stage this entity.
- In some of the reptile lymphomas, immunohistochemistry was attempted to determine the cellular origin, but no correlation to the biological behavior of the tumor was made.

SIGNALMENT/HISTORY

Lymphoma has been reported in numerous lizard species representing several families.

CLINICAL PRESENTATION

- Anorexia and lethargy are frequently reported.
- In many cases, the complete blood count reveals marked lymphocytosis.
- Physical examination can reveal single or multiple tumor nodules.

RISK FACTORS

Husbandry

N/A

Others

N/A

DIAGNOSIS

DIFFERENTIAL DIAGNOSIS

- Other tumors
- Inflammatory reactions (abscesses, granulomas, etc.)

DIAGNOSTICS

- Hemogram: a marked leukocytosis characterized by lymphocytosis is observed in many cases.
- In advanced stages of the disease, it is unclear whether the neoplasia originated within the bone marrow or whether leukemia is a feature of disseminated, end-stage lymphoma.
- Histological examination of direct smears from a fine-needle aspirate of the nodular masses and/or of the biopsy specimen can reveal the presence of neoplastic lymphoid cells.
- Necropsy and subsequent histopathology
- Transmission electron microscopy can be attempted to identify viral particles.

PATHOLOGICAL FINDINGS

- Gross lesions include white and firm nodules in several organs, not limited to lymphoid organs.
- Splenomegaly is also frequently observed
- Histologically, unencapsulated masses or monotonous sheets composed of hyperchromatic neoplastic lymphoid cells are observed.
- Mitotic figures are variable

TREATMENT

APPROPRIATE HEALTH CARE

Chemotherapy (see below)

NUTRITIONAL SUPPORT

An esophagostomy tube should be considered in anorexic animals or for long-term administration of medications.

CLIENT EDUCATION/HUSBANDRY RECOMMENDATIONS

N/A

MEDICATIONS

DRUG(S) OF CHOICE

- Lymphoma in a green iguana (*Iguana iguana*) has been successfully treated with a single 10-Gy fraction of radiation directed at the tumor, and a 29-month modified canine CHOP chemotherapy protocol (the dosages were scaled down to one-third the dose administered to dogs).
- During the course of treatment, there were two modifications in the chemotherapy protocol; at 161 days of therapy, cyclophosphamide was given every other week, vincristine and doxorubicin were eliminated, and prednisone was continued as before; at 525 days of therapy, cyclophosphamide was eliminated, and doxorubicin was initiated at 3-week intervals (dosage gradually increased until 0.75 mg/kg).

PRECAUTIONS/INTERACTIONS

A heterophil count threshold of 1500 cells/μl as an indicator of drug toxicity in green iguana has been used.

FOLLOW-UP

PATIENT MONITORING

Monitor the overall WBC and lymphocyte counts to gauge response to the drugs, together with reduction in tumor size, weight gain, and quality-of-life assessment.

EXPECTED COURSE AND PROGNOSIS

- Because little is known about most chemotherapeutic agents in reptiles, the prognosis of the disease is poor.
- Most cases are diagnosed postmortem

MISCELLANEOUS

COMMENTS

N/A

ZOONOTIC POTENTIAL

Unknown

SYNONYMS

- Lymphoid neoplasm
- Lymphosarcoma

ABBREVIATIONS

- CHOP = doxorubicin, vincristine, cyclophosphamide, and prednisone
- WBC = white blood cell

Suggested Reading

Folland DW, Johnston MS, Thamm DH, Reavill D. Diagnosis and management of lymphoma in a green iguana (*Iguana iguana*). *J Am Vet Med Assoc* 2011;239:985–991.

Gyimesi ZS, Garner MM, Burns RB, et al. High incidence of lymphoid neoplasia in a colony of Egyptian spiny-tailed lizards (*Uromastyx aegyptius*). *J Zoo Wildl Med* 2005;36:103–110.

Hernandez-Divers SM, Orcutt SJ, Stahl SJ, et al. Lymphoma in lizards: 3 case reports. *J Herp Med Surg* 2003;13:14–22.

Mauldin GN, Done LB. Oncology. In: Mader DR, ed. *Reptile Medicine and Surgery*. 2nd ed. St. Louis, MO: Elsevier Saunders; 2006:299–322.

Schultze AE, Mason GL, Clyde VL. Lymphosarcoma with leukemic blood profile in a savannah monitor lizard (Varanus exanthematicus). *J Zoo Wildl Med* 1999;30:158–164.

Author Jorge Orós, DVM, PhD, DECZM

METARHIZIUM INFECTION

BASICS

DEFINITION/OVERVIEW

Metarhizium infection is a severe disseminated systemic granulomatous fungal infection of chameleons. It has been reported from Europe, New Zealand, and North America, but may occur worldwide.

ETIOLOGY/PATHOPHYSIOLOGY

- Usually *Metarhizium granulomatis*, less often the closely related *M. viridis*. These fungi were formerly in a novel genus, *Chamaeleomyces*, but have been reassigned to *Metarhizium*.
- Dimorphic fungi, with yeast morph in tissues.
- Fungal spores/conidia ingested or inhaled.
- Dissemination to lung, liver, spleen, and other organs.
- Miliary, densely packed, whitish granulomas throughout infected tissues.
- Source of infection poorly understood but *M. viridis* is a known insect pathogen, so possibly infected feeder insects.

SIGNALMENT/HISTORY

- In chameleons, sex and age irrelevant.
- Very sporadic, and cases often clustered.
- Bearded dragons susceptible to *M. viridis* infection.

CLINICAL PRESENTATION

- Anorexia, weight loss, depression, death.
- Conspicuous miliary granulomatous glossitis and pharyngitis often present.
- Sometimes cutaneous lesions
- Often diagnosed at necropsy, based on systemic granulomatous infection.

RISK FACTORS

Husbandry

- Predisposing factors unknown
- Optimal husbandry to minimize stress and immune suppression.

Others

N/A

DIAGNOSIS

DIFFERENTIAL DIAGNOSIS

- Bacterial abscesses
- Mycobacteriosis
- Other fungal infection
- Neoplasia

DIAGNOSTICS

- Fairly characteristic lesions
- Culture from lesions
- PCR needed to distinguish *M. granulomatis* from *M. viridis*

PATHOLOGICAL FINDINGS

- White, spherical, granulomatous glossitis and pharyngitis, and liver and splenic lesions highly suggestive.
- Yeast-like elements in granulomas on histopathology.

TREATMENT

APPROPRIATE HEALTH CARE

- Difficult; disease almost always diagnosed when dissemination has occurred.
- Systemic antifungal, and topical if applicable.

NUTRITIONAL SUPPORT

- Assist-feeding if needed
- Fluids and thermal support may be indicated.

CLIENT EDUCATION/HUSBANDRY RECOMMENDATIONS

- Isolation of sick animals and thorough hygiene.
- Critical review of husbandry

MEDICATIONS

DRUG(S) OF CHOICE

M. granulomatis is susceptible in vitro to terbinafine and nystatin, but not to triazoles.

PRECAUTIONS/INTERACTIONS

- Some chameleons treated with terbinafine succumbed soon after, but probably from disease rather than a reaction to drug.
- Liver often massively compromised, replaced by granulomas, in chameleons with *Metarhizium* infection, so drug toxicity may be potentiated.

FOLLOW-UP

PATIENT MONITORING

- Monitor appetite, demeanor, and improvement with treatment.
- Blood work to assess hepatic function.

EXPECTED COURSE AND PROGNOSIS

Prognosis poor to grave because of the insidious and invasive nature of the infection.

MISCELLANEOUS

COMMENTS

M. anisopliae is an entomopathogenic fungus that can cause opportunistic but severe fungal pneumonia in tortoises and crocodilians, and almost always secondarily after these were subjected to cold captive environments.

ZOONOTIC POTENTIAL

- None identified to date
- These fungi do not grow at 37 degrees C.

SYNONYMS

N/A

ABBREVIATIONS

PCR = polymerase chain reaction

Suggested Reading

Schmidt V, Plenz B, Pfaff M, Pees M. Disseminated systemic mycosis in veiled chameleons (*Chamaeleo calyptratus*) caused by *Chamaeleomyces granulomatis*. *Vet Microbiol* 2012;161:145–152.

Schmidt V, Klasen L, Schneider J, et al. Fungal dermatitis, glossitis and disseminated visceral mycosis caused by different *Metarhizium granulomatis* genotypes in veiled chameleons (*Chamaeleo calyptratus*) and first isolation in healthy lizards. *Vet Microbiol* 2017;207:74–82.

Sigler L, Gibas CFC, Kokotovic B, Bertelsen MF. Disseminated mycosis in veiled chameleons (*Chamaeleo calyptratus*) caused by *Chamaeleomyces granulomatis*, a new fungus related to *Paecilomyces viridis*. *J Clin Microbiol* 2010;48:3182–3192.

Author Jean A. Paré, DMV, DVSc, DACZM, DECZM (Zoo Health Management)

MICROSPORIDIOSIS

BASICS

DEFINITION/OVERVIEW

Microsporidiosis is a disease caused by single-celled eukaryotes closer to fungi than protozoa. While this is not considered a common disease of reptiles, there are several reports of unidentified, and recently identified microsporidia infecting various reptile species. More recent reports have focused on *Encephalitozoon* sp. infections of bearded dragons (*Pogona vitticeps*).

ETIOLOGY/PATHOPHYSIOLOGY

- Within the Microsporidia, *Encephalitozoon* sp. are the most commonly reported from reptiles.
- *Encephalitozoon pogonae* was recently described as a new species causing disease in bearded dragons.
- *E. lacerate* has been described from an African skink and a common wall lizard (*Podacris muralis*).

SIGNALMENT/HISTORY

- No predisposing age or sex, but most cases in bearded dragons have been females.
- Yellow masses in the oral mucosa have been reported from an infected bearded dragon in Japan.

CLINICAL PRESENTATION

- Infected animals present with non-specific signs of chronic disease. Weight loss and/or poor body condition are commonly reported across most cases.
- Other common clinical signs include lethargy, anorexia, and death.

RISK FACTORS

At this time, risk factors for occurrence of this disease are unknown.

DIAGNOSIS

- There is no antemortem diagnosis reported at this time.
- Biopsies from infected organs obtained during coelioscopy should be tested if microsporidiosis is suspected.

DIFFERENTIAL DIAGNOSIS

- Mycobacteriosis
- Fungal infection

DIAGNOSTICS

- Histopathology
- Electron microscopy
- PCR and sequencing

PATHOLOGICAL FINDINGS

Multifocal necrotizing and/or granulomatous disease affecting various organs.

TREATMENT

APPROPRIATE HEALTH CARE

- There is no reported treatment as all cases have been diagnosed postmortem.
- Coelioscopy of surviving animals may be a consideration, to biopsy any apparent lesions and attempt antemortem diagnosis.

NUTRITIONAL SUPPORT

N/A

CLIENT EDUCATION/HUSBANDRY RECOMMENDATIONS

- Any reptiles that were housed with infected animals should be examined for evidence of weight loss.
- While the mode of transmission is unknown at this time, proper hygiene and husbandry practices should be implemented.

MEDICATIONS

DRUG(S) OF CHOICE

N/A

PRECAUTIONS/INTERACTIONS

N/A

FOLLOW-UP

PATIENT MONITORING

N/A

EXPECTED COURSE AND PROGNOSIS

Prognosis is grave as all cases of infected animals have died.

MISCELLANEOUS

COMMENTS

N/A

ZOONOTIC POTENTIAL

- Unknown for the reptile species.
- Other *Encephalitozoon* spp. infecting animals are reported as zoonotic; thus, infected reptiles should be handled with caution.

SYNONYMS

N/A

ABBREVIATIONS

PCR = polymerase chain reaction

Suggested Reading

Ritcher B, Csokai J, Graner I, et al. Encephalitozoonosis in two inland bearded dragons (*Pogona vitticeps*). *J Comp Pathol* 2013;148(2–3):278–282.

Shibasaki K, Tokiwa T, Sukegawa A, et al. First report of fatal disseminated microsporidiosis in two inland bearded dragons *Pogona vitticeps* in Japan. *JMM Case Rep* 2017;12(4):e005089.

Sokolova YY, Sakaguchi K, Paulsen DB. Establishing a new species *Encephalitozoon pogonae* for the microsporidian parasite of inland berdaed dragon *Pogona vitticeps* Ahl 1927 (Reptilia, Squamata, Agamidae). *J Eukaryot Microbiol* 2016;63(4):524–535.

Author Javier G. Nevarez, DVM PhD DACZM,DECZM (Herpetology)

MITES

BASICS

DEFINITION/OVERVIEW

Both wild and captive lizards can be affected by external parasites (ticks and mites). The lizard mite (*Hirstiella trombidiiformis*) and the chigger mites (Trombiculidae family) are the most commonly encountered. Although snakes are the usual hosts of the snake mite, *Ophionyssus natricis*, captive lizards may also become infested (in particular *Pogona* spp. lizards).

ETIOLOGY/PATHOPHYSIOLOGY

- *O. natricis* belongs to the sub-order Mesostigmata of the Macronyssidae family.
- It has a life span of about 40 days, irrespective of feeding.
- The life cycle is relatively short, at 7–16 days.
- The female (up to 1.5 mm in length) is larger than the male and takes 2–3 blood meals lasting 4–8 days at an interval of 1–2 weeks.
- A clutch of about 20 eggs is laid on the inner surfaces of the terrarium.
- When the humidity rises above 85% and the temperature ranges between 68–86 degrees F (20–30 degrees C), larvae hatch in 1–4 days.
- The free-living larvae measure about 400 μm, are whitish in color and possess three pairs of legs.
- When the temperature reaches 77–86 degrees F (25–30 degrees C) with a humidity above 75%, the larvae molt into protonymphs within 24 hours.
- The protonymphs, which possess four pairs of legs, take a single blood meal, which enables them to survive 3–7 days at 77 degrees F (25 degrees C).
- 12–48 hours following their meal, 90% molt into deutonymphs.
- Like larvae, the deutonymph stage is a free-living non-parasitic stage. At 77 degrees F (25 degrees C), the deutonymphs molt into adults, a process that takes approximately 24 hours.
- Adults are highly mobile; following mating, females lay eggs that hatch into females only.
- If the eggs are not fertilized, they hatch into males only by arrhenotokous parthogenesis.
- Nymphs and adults of trombiculid mites (*Eutrombicula* spp., *Neotrombicula* spp., *Vatacarus* spp.) are free living but their larval stage is parasitic in lizards (chiggers). Their meal consists of lymph and tissue debris, rather than blood.
- *Hirstiella* spp. is a mite that can be parasitic in different species of lizards, together with other members of the family Pterygosomatidae (*Cyclurobia* spp., *Geckobia* spp., *Geckobiella* spp., *Ixoderma* spp., *Pterygosoma* spp., *Scaphotrix* spp., *Tequisistlana* spp. and *Zonurobia* spp.).

SIGNALMENT/HISTORY

- Infected lizards are often asymptomatic.
- Mite infestation is relatively obvious, but owners may notice infestation only when they find mites on their own skin after handling infested lizards.
- Chigger-causing mites can congregate and appear as red or orange spots on the skin.

CLINICAL PRESENTATION

Lizard mites are usually red to orange and can be easily seen with the naked eye.

RISK FACTORS

Husbandry

- Mites are usually introduced into a collection with substrate, pieces of wood, plants and prey (e.g., crickets) in a cage.
- A newly acquired infested lizard can transmit parasites to a whole collection.

Others

- The lizard mites prefer darkness and are prone to climbing.
- Crevasses and corners (particularly those at the top of the cages) must be regularly inspected and cleaned.

DIAGNOSIS

DIFFERENTIAL DIAGNOSIS

- Microscopic examination is used to differentiate between species: snake mites (*O. natricis*), trombiculid mites (chiggers) and lizard mites (e.g., *H. trombidiiformis*).
- Other acarids such as ticks (*Amblyomma* spp., *Hyalomma* spp., *Ornithodoros* spp.) can be encountered. They differ markedly from mites in size and shape.

DIAGNOSTICS

- Scrupulous examination of the integument is necessary.
- In heavy infestations, mites can be easily visible on the body surface moving on the chin shields, tympanic scales, axillary folds, dorsal and lateral surface of the tail (*Hirstiella* spp.), or around the head.
- Swab the sides of the body of the animal with a moistened cotton swab and then examined microscopically.
- The difference between juvenile chiggers (6 legs) and adults (8 legs) can be appreciated under the microscope.

PATHOLOGICAL FINDINGS

N/A

TREATMENT

APPROPRIATE HEALTH CARE

The predatory mite *Cheyletus* eruditus (Taurrus®, APPI Biological Control, Haverhill, UK) is a good candidate for the biological control of *O. natricis*. It has strong predatory potential, good environmental survival, and a temperature range adapted to captive snake conditions. It can only be used only if substrate is present in the enclosure.

NUTRITIONAL SUPPORT

N/A

CLIENT EDUCATION/HUSBANDRY RECOMMENDATIONS

- Environmental treatment involves removal of all objects in the terrarium.
- The terrarium should be washed and scrubbed with hot water (> 122 degrees F; 50 degrees C) and then thoroughly sprayed with an acaricide.
- Decorations can be treated in the same manner, but bark and soil should be discarded.
- Quarantine new specimens before introducing them into a collection.
- Freeze or soak in hot water the bedding material, decorations (wood, stones, bowls, plastic plants), before introducing them into a terrarium.

MEDICATIONS

DRUG(S) OF CHOICE

- Many insecticidal and acaricidal compounds used in dogs, cats and other mammals can be used.
- Pyrethrins, pyrethroids (0.5% spray) and fipronil can be applied on the animal and used for environmental treatment.
- Enclosures, bowls, and other inanimate objects should be thoroughly rinsed after using these compounds.
- Ivermectin 0.2 mg/kg IM, SC, or PO q14d. Prepare a diluted topical spray of 5–10 mg/l water applied q3–5d weekly or every other week for 6 to 8 weeks.
- Fipronil: apply directly to the animal and wipe off within 5 minutes q7d as needed; alternatively, can spray on gauze or cloth and then wipe the lizard with it to spread over the skin.

PRECAUTIONS/INTERACTIONS

- Toxicity may occur if the lizards soak or drink from a water bowl that has not been carefully rinsed after application of an acaricide.
- Ivermectin should not be used in skinks, as suspected toxicity has been reported.

FOLLOW-UP

PATIENT MONITORING

Repeated, thorough examinations of the entire tegument of the lizard.

EXPECTED COURSE AND PROGNOSIS

Total elimination is only successful if coupled with rigorous environmental treatment.

MISCELLANEOUS

COMMENTS

- *Hirstiella* spp. may serve as vector for hemogregarines.
- Figure 4 – see web image supplementary content for Section III (Lizards)

ZOONOTIC POTENTIAL

Lizard mites do not infest humans.

SYNONYMS

N/A

ABBREVIATIONS

- IM = intramuscular
- PO = per os
- SC = subcutaneous

Suggested Reading

Fitzgerald KT, Vera R. Acariasis. In: Mader DR, ed. *Reptile Medicine and Surgery*. 2nd ed. St. Louis, MO: Elsevier Saunders; 2006:720–738.

Jacobson ER. Parasites and parasitic diseases of reptiles. In: Jacobson ER, ed. *Infectious Diseases and Pathology of Reptiles*. Boca Raton, FL: CRC Press; 2007:571–665.

Author Lionel Schilliger, DVM, DECZM (Herpetology), DABVP (Reptile & Amphibian Practice)

MYCOBACTERIOSIS

BASICS

DEFINITION/OVERVIEW

Mycobacteriosis is a cosmopolitan disease that affects all classes of vertebrates. In reptiles, atypical or non-tuberculosis *Mycobacterium* spp. are most common. *Mycobacterium* spp. are more fastidious in ectothermic animals, and thus can appear as latent or chronic infections. While the apparent prevalence of mycobacteriosis in reptiles is low, it is likely underdiagnosed. Systemic and localized infections of *Mycobacterium* spp. have been documented in lizards.

ETIOLOGY/PATHOPHYSIOLOGY

- Aerobic, acid-fast+, Gram-positive rod bacteria.
- *Mycobacterium chelonae, M. szulgai, M. marinum, M. fortuitum, M. ulcerans, M. leprae, M. haemophilum, M. avium, M. lepraemurium, M. kansasii, M. terrae, M. intracellulare, M. genavense, M. kumamotonense, M. fuscus, M. nonchromogenicum, M. smegmatis, M. confluentis, M. hiberniae.*
- The epidemiology of mycobacteriosis in reptiles is not well documented.
- Transmission of *Mycobacterium* spp. in reptiles is most likely through direct and indirect contact with infected animals and materials in the captive environment.
- Infected animals can shed the organisms through various body excretions (e.g., respiratory, skin, GI), contaminating the environment and directly exposing conspecifics.
- Non-tuberculosis mycobacterial species are ubiquitous within the environment; thus water, soil, dust, and plants can all serve as sources of exposure.
- Stress likely plays a role in the dissemination of this disease, as animals with compromised immune systems are more susceptible to infection.

SIGNALMENT/HISTORY

- No species, age, or sex predilection.
- Animals are typically housed under poor husbandry conditions: inappropriate environmental temperature, high organic loads, and poor water quality.

CLINICAL PRESENTATION

- Affected animals may be clinically inapparent or may show clinical signs that include emaciation and weight loss with or without anorexia.
- Draining or nodular skin lesions may be present.
- Animals with systemic mycobacteriosis may be dyspneic.
- Fecal production and consistency may vary in animals with lesions in their GI tract.

RISK FACTORS

Husbandry

- Inappropriate husbandry, such as a low environmental temperature, can lead to immunosuppression, making individuals more susceptible to infection.
- An absence of a quarantine program can lead to the introduction of an infected animal to a collection.
- High stocking densities in a production system may lead to an increased risk of exposure in a closed system.
- Mycobacterial infections are more common in aquatic species.
- High organic load and poor water quality likely contribute to the buildup and dissemination of the bacteria in these systems.
- Inappropriate nutrition

Others

- Stress
- Chronic disease
- Captive wild animals: wild-caught or imported animals.

DIAGNOSIS

DIFFERENTIAL DIAGNOSIS

- Any chronic disease process
- Systemic infection
- Organ dysfunction—liver failure, renal failure
- Tachypnea—pulmonary disease
- Malabsorptive GI disease
- Infectious—parasitism, viral disease, other bacterial disease
- Neoplasia

DIAGNOSTICS

Polymerase Chain Reaction

- PCR testing for *Mycobacterium* spp. does exist and is a more sensitive test than historical methodologies.
- The most common PCR primer used to diagnose *Mycobacterium* spp. in most laboratories is the 16s ribosomal RNA primer; however, a nested PCR assay targeting a 65 kDA heat shock protein has also been used as a diagnostic tool.
- Sensitives and specificities for these diagnostics have yet to be evaluated in reptiles. Sequencing is important to confirm the species of *Mycobacterium.*

Cytology

- Cytologic examination of skin lesions can be a useful first line diagnostic tool for diagnosing a *Mycobacterium* sp. infection. Cytology can be used to provide direct evidence of chronic inflammation in the lesions and demonstrate the presence of bacteria. Gram stain and acid-fast staining can be used to further characterize the presence of the bacteria, directing the clinician to other more sensitive diagnostics such as PCR and histopathology.
- Tissue biopsy and histopathology are considered the gold standard for diagnosing a *Mycobacterium* sp. infection. In addition to granulomatous lesions being present in the microscopic tissue architecture, acid-fast stains, including Ziehl–Neelsen and the Fite method, can be used to confirm the presence of acid-fast bacteria within the lesions. The sensitivity of these stains is considered low for *Mycobacterium* spp.

Microbiological Culture

- Microbiological culture has fallen out of favor for clinical samples because of the special media required to culture *Mycobacterium* spp. and the long culture times associated with growing these organisms.
- Speciation can be performed on cultured samples.
- Antibacterial sensitivities can also be performed on cultured *Mycobacterium* spp. if therapy is elected.

Hematology and Biochemistry

- Hematology and biochemistry testing can be used to characterize the physiologic status of the reptile patient.
- A chronic inflammatory leukogram characterized by a heterophilia and monocytosis may be observed.
- Anemia of chronic disease is also common.
- Biochemistry testing typically reveals dehydration (hyperproteinemia, hyperuricemia, hypernatremia, hyperchloremia).
- If the liver is involved, elevated bile acids may be identified.

PATHOLOGICAL FINDINGS

- Gross necropsy findings can range from a single white to gray focal lesion/nodule to multifocal to coalescing white lesions/nodules within any organ system.
- Granulomatous inflammation is the most common histopathological finding in reptile mycobacteriosis cases.
- Granulomas can range from compact nests of macrophages containing intracellular acid-fast bacilli to complex granulomas containing caseated centers.
- Acute mycobacteriosis can have extracellular proliferation of acid-fast organisms with associated caseous necrosis and infiltrative heterophils and macrophages.

TREATMENT

APPROPRIATE HEALTH CARE

N/A

NUTRITIONAL SUPPORT

- If treatment is pursued, nutritional support should be considered.
- Mycobacteriosis in reptiles often leads to weight loss because of the negative energy balance that develops in these patients.
- Placement of an esophagostomy tube is indicated to provide critical care diets and medications.

CLIENT EDUCATION/HUSBANDRY RECOMMENDATIONS

- Disease exposure and dissemination can be limited by quarantine and testing (PCR) new arrivals.
- Implementing husbandry practices that reduce organic loads in both aquatic and terrestrial vivariums is highly recommended.
- Regular water changes can minimize pathogen buildup in a closed system.
- Husbandry recommendations should be species specific to minimize stress and the potential for compromising the immune system of a reptile.
- Clients and veterinary staff should follow standard hygiene practices to minimize zoonotic potential.

MEDICATIONS

DRUG(S) OF CHOICE

- No proven or approved treatments exist for mycobacteriosis in reptiles.
- Treatment is controversial due to the lack of clinical data on appropriate therapy, poor response to therapy, and the implications that treating reptiles may have in the increase of multidrug-resistant *Mycobacterium* spp., which may have implications for human health.
- Euthanasia should be considered to mitigate zoonotic potential and further dissemination of the organism within a collection.
- In human medicine, *Mycobacterium* infections are treated based on culture and sensitivity results, with a multi drug-treatment protocol including macrolides, aminoglycosides, ethambutol, and/or rifamycins.
- Treatment is long term until there is no evidence of disease for at least 12 months.

PRECAUTIONS/INTERACTIONS

If treatment is elected, owner compliance is critical to minimize the development of multidrug resistance.

FOLLOW-UP

PATIENT MONITORING

- Humane euthanasia is recommended for these cases.
- If treatment is pursued, regular examinations and blood work (hematology and biochemistry testing) are necessary to evaluate the patient's quality of life and physiologic status.

EXPECTED COURSE AND PROGNOSIS

- Reptiles diagnosed with *Mycobacterium* spp. have a grave prognosis.
- The likelihood for mycobacterial transmission to other reptiles and the zoonotic potential of these organisms present a challenge.
- Therapeutic options, if pursued, are long term and are not commonly reported to be successful in reptiles.
- Animals that do not undergo therapy often develop disseminated mycobacteriosis, which includes chronic weight loss, cachexia, and emaciation.
- Because of these challenges, euthanasia is recommended.

MISCELLANEOUS

COMMENTS

N/A

ZOONOTIC POTENTIAL

- *Mycobacterium* spp. can be zoonotic.
- Atypical mycobacteria are most commonly isolated from reptiles, and while not the most common forms found in humans, they are known to infect humans.
- Atypical *Mycobacterium* spp. are classified as the Runyon group IV and are characterized as antibiotic resistant.
- Preventive measures that should be followed to reduce the zoonotic potential of these organisms include minimizing direct contact with infected animals, wearing appropriate personal protective equipment (e.g., gloves, face mask) when handling infected animals, and following strict personal hygiene practices such as hand washing and not using human wash basins to clean these animals or materials from their environment.
- Immunocompromised individuals and children should avoid contact with infected animals and their environment.

SYNONYMS

- Atypical mycobacterium
- Granulomatous disease
- Vivarium granuloma

ABBREVIATIONS

- GI = gastrointestinal
- PCR = polymerase chain reaction

Suggested Reading

Ebani VV, Fratini F, Bertelloni F, et al. Isolation and identification of mycobacteria from captive reptiles. *Res Vet Sci* 2012;93:1136–1138.

Jacobson ER. Bacterial diseases of reptiles. In: Jacobson ER, ed. *Infectious Diseases and Pathology of Reptiles: Color Atlas and Text.* Boca Raton, FL: CRC Press; 2007:461–526.

Mitchell MA. Mycobacterial infections in reptiles. *Vet Clin North Am Exot Anim Pract* 2012;15(1):101–111.

Authors Sean M. Perry, DVM, PhD, and Mark A. Mitchell, DVM, MS, PhD, DECZM (Herpetology)

NANNIZZIOPSIS MYCOSES

BASICS

DEFINITION/OVERVIEW

Dermatomycosis of captive lizards worldwide. Sometimes disseminates to internal structures.

ETIOLOGY/PATHOPHYSIOLOGY

- *Nannizziopsis guarroi*, and less often *N. draconii* and *N. chlamydospora*, cause YFD, a focal to extensive dermatomycosis of inland bearded dragons (*Pogona vitticeps*), but also other agamids, iguanas, and other taxa.
- *N. barbata* infects coastal bearded dragons (*P. barbata*) and was recovered from free-ranging Eastern water dragons (*Physignathus lesueurii*) with dermatitis.
- *N. dermatitidis* causes severe dermatitis in chameleons, geckos, and probably other lizards. *N. crocodili* infects young farmed saltwater crocodiles in Australia.
- Spores/conidia from infected animals on intact skin or cutaneous breaches lead to hyphal proliferation in epidermal stratum corneum and necrosis and hyphae in the dermis and deeper structures.
- Rarely disseminates to internal structures.

SIGNALMENT/HISTORY

- YFD is a contagious cutaneous infection of pet bearded dragons, common in North America and Europe and possibly elsewhere.
- Focal to multifocal, progressive necrosis and crusting, and even full-thickness sloughing of the epidermis over the head, body, or limbs.
- Deeper infection may cause granulomatous inflammation in muscles and bones.

CLINICAL PRESENTATION

- Focal/multifocal often extensive necrotic skin lesions.
- Discolored and/or thickened scales, coalescing necrotic and/or crusty scales, ulcers.
- Most often over the head/face/rostrum, but also over the body.
- Facial features may be distorted from deeper infection.
- It is often ultimately fatal

RISK FACTORS

Husbandry

- *N. dermatitidis* is a primary pathogen, as probably are other lizard-associated *Nannizziopsis* spp.
- Can occur even when captive husbandry seems adequate.
- Proper quarantine of incoming animals is warranted.
- Close inspection of skin of any new pet lizard.

Others

Most often seen in bearded dragons purchased from large pet store chains.

DIAGNOSIS

DIFFERENTIAL DIAGNOSIS

- Trauma, thermal injuries/burns
- Papillomas
- Dermatophilosis
- *Devriesea agamarum* infection
- Other bacterial dermatitides
- Abscesses, parasites, and tumors when presenting with dermal and/or deep granulomas

DIAGNOSTICS

- Presentation is often suggestive.
- When present, arthroconidia on stained impression smears of skin lesions are highly suggestive.
- A combination of histopathology and culture of skin biopsies are essential for definitive diagnosis.
- PCR on fungal isolate or on biopsy/tissue sections required.
- Molecular tools are needed to identify any *Nannizziopsis* isolate to species.

PATHOLOGICAL FINDINGS

- Epidermal/dermal hyalohyphomycosis with extensive epidermal necrosis, often hyperkeratosis, heterophilic and then mixed inflammatory cell infiltration, with or without dermal or deeper granulomas.
- PAS or silver stains may be needed to identify fungal elements.
- Rarely, systemic involvement

TREATMENT

APPROPRIATE HEALTH CARE

- Review and improvement of captive husbandry.
- Supportive measures (fluids, thermal support).
- Topical antiseptic or antifungal
- Systemic antifungal drugs are almost always indicated.

NUTRITIONAL SUPPORT

Assist-feeding if needed

CLIENT EDUCATION/HUSBANDRY RECOMMENDATIONS

- Awareness when purchasing a lizard to inspect the integument
- Quarantine all new lizards
- Isolate sick animals and use strict hygiene
- Thorough review of husbandry and adjustments when needed.

SURGICAL CONSIDERATIONS

Surgical debridement of necrotic/crusty lesions is indicated to decrease fungal load.

MEDICATIONS

DRUG(S) OF CHOICE

- *N. dermatitidis* and *N. crocodili* equally susceptible in vitro to itraconazole, terbinafine, and voriconazole.
- Minimal inhibitory concentrations for itraconazole are higher for *N. guarroi*.
- Itraconazole and terbinafine may be synergistic, and both accumulate and persist in the epidermal corneum.

PRECAUTIONS/INTERACTIONS

- Interactions of triazoles and/or allylamines with other drugs possible.
- Itraconazole and terbinafine may be synergistic.

FOLLOW-UP

PATIENT MONITORING

- Monitor appetite, demeanor, and skin improvement with treatment.
- Bloodwork to monitor liver enzymes while on antifungals.

EXPECTED COURSE AND PROGNOSIS

- Variable
- Good if lesions are mild and/or superficial and addressed early.
- Guarded or poor if deeper lesions (e.g., myositis, osteomyelitis) present or in chronic and/or severe cases.

MISCELLANEOUS

COMMENTS

N/A

ZOONOTIC POTENTIAL

- None identified to date
- *Nannizziopsis* isolates from humans belong to species distinct from those infecting reptiles.

SYNONYMS

Practically all the *Chrysosporium* anamorph of *N. vriesii* lizard isolates deposited over decades in fungal collections were reassigned to the above novel *Nannizziopsis* species when molecular probes were used. *Nannizziopsiosis* is a better term for the disease.

ABBREVIATIONS

- PAS = periodic acid–Schiff
- PCR = polymerase chain reaction
- YFD = yellow fungus disease

Suggested Reading

Paré JA, Sigler L. An overview of reptile fungal pathogens in the genera *Nannizziopsis*, *Paranannizziopsis*, and *Ophidiomyces*. *J Herp Med Surg* 2016;26:46–53.

Sigler L, Hambleton S, Paré JA. Molecular characterization of reptile pathogens currently known as members of the *Chrysosporium* anamorph of *Nannizziopsis vriesii* complex and relationship with some human-associated isolates. *J Clin Microbiol* 2013;51:3338–3357.

Author Jean A. Paré , DMV, DVSc, DACZM, DECZM (Zoo Health Management)

LIZARDS

NUTRITIONAL SECONDARY HYPERPARATHYROIDISM

BASICS

DEFINITION/OVERVIEW

NSHP is one of the most common disorders in captive reptiles. The disease is characterized by hypocalcemia caused by deficiency of calcium and/or vitamin D in the diet or a lack of UVB light exposure. This results in increased PTH production leading to increased calcium resorption from the bones. Affected reptiles typically present with functional and morphological bone changes including pathological fractures and/or with tetany, seizure-like activity and muscle tremors.

ETIOLOGY/PATHOPHYSIOLOGY

- Etiology of NSHP is considered multifactorial.
- In herbivorous/omnivorous reptiles, a diet poor in calcium and high in phosphorus is a common cause of NSHP.
- Briefly, the low calcium intake in the diet results in low blood calcium concentrations.
- Blood calcium concentrations below 2.3 mmol/l trigger parathyroid glands to produce PTH to raise calcium concentrations.
- PTH stimulates the osteoclastic activity, resulting in different degrees of bone depletion. It also stimulates calcium reabsorption in the kidneys.
- The lack of UVB light exposure from the sun or UVB bulbs is another critical factor in the development of NSHP.
- The active form of vitamin D3 is 1,25 dihydroxycholecalciferol, which is mediated in most species by exposure to UVB light in the range of 280–315 nm. The 1,25-dihydroxycholecalciferol increases intestinal calcium absorption and renal calcium reabsorption.

SIGNALMENT/HISTORY

- NSHP is the most common nutritional disorder of captive reptiles, especially lizards.
- It is most commonly observed in herbivorous, omnivorous, or insectivorous species.
- Carnivores offered whole prey are rarely affected by NSHP because whole vertebrate prey contains adequate amounts of calcium and vitamin D3.
- Reptiles in life stages experiencing intensive growth are most affected from the chronic form of the disease (i.e., skeletal deformities), due to the increased demands of calcium during these periods.
- Reptiles in life stages experiencing high demands of calcium for a short period (e.g., reproductive females), are usually presented with the acute form of the disease (i.e., hypocalcemia and tetany).

CLINICAL PRESENTATION

- Clinical signs vary depending on the severity of the disease.
- In lizards, clinical signs of NSHP include softening of the mandible (rubber jaw), deformation of long bones, tetany, seizure-like activity, muscle tremors, decreased activity, and anorexia.

RISK FACTORS

Husbandry

- Diets that lead to NSHP generally present a combination of insufficient calcium intake, excessive phosphorus intake, insufficient vitamin D intake, excessive vitamin A intake.
- Husbandry errors that lead to NSHP include insufficient exposure to UVB radiation in the range of 280–315 nm, lack of brumation in applicable species, which results in excessive growth rates.

Others

Concurrent parasitism may exacerbate NSHP

DIAGNOSIS

DIFFERENTIAL DIAGNOSIS

- Renal secondary hyperparathyroidism
- Primary hyperparathyroidism

DIAGNOSTICS

- In most cases, NSHP is diagnosed based on clinical presentation and history of inappropriate diet and/or management.
- Radiography, blood work and fecal exams are indicated to confirm the clinical suspicion, determine the severity of the disease and to formulate a prognosis.
- These diagnostic tests are also useful to rule out concomitant conditions like urinary bladder overdistension, egg dystocia, endoparasitism, and constipation.

Radiography

- Decreased bony cortices and pathologic fractures may be observed.
- Depending on the duration of the disease, lizards may present long-bone deformities.
- Animals with multiple fractures and decreased cortices across the majority of the long bones tend to have a worse prognosis for recovery.

Chemistry

- Hypocalcemia is usually observed in the early and late stages of the disease; it is common to have animals with NSHP be normocalcemic or even hypercalcemic due to the active resorption of calcium from the bones.
- Hyperphosphatemia may be observed concurrently, especially when hypocalcemia is present.
- A chemistry panel is particularly indicated in reptiles presenting with seizure-like activity or muscle tremors. It is also useful for monitoring response to therapy.
- Analysis should include measurement of ionized calcium. In general, values of ionized calcium lower than 1.0–1.2 mmol/l are abnormal.
- The calcium to phosphorus ratio is expected to be 1 : 5 to 2 : 1, and a decrease is suggestive of calcium depletion (e.g., NSHP, renal secondary hyperparathyroidism, or renal disease).

Fecal Exams

Endoparasites may be a confounding factor in the development of this disease as they can contribute to depletion of nutrients.

PATHOLOGICAL FINDINGS

- Gross pathological findings include deformity and softening of bone tissue, including jaws and/or long bones in lizards.
- Alterations of parathyroid glands may be present in form of generalized or focal enlargements.
- Histopathological lesions may range from increased osteoclastic resorption of otherwise well-formed and mineralized bone laminae, to thinning of laminae and widening of medullary cavities, with scalloped endosteal surfaces due to massive resorptive activity.
- The cortices may be thinned and layers of osteoblasts and unmineralized osteoid on the periosteal surface may be present.

TREATMENT

APPROPRIATE HEALTH CARE

N/A

NUTRITIONAL SUPPORT

- Reptiles with chronic NSHP are often anorectic.
- The anorexia is usually transient and improves once the management is corrected.
- Reptiles with severe NSHP may not be able to ingest food due to the changes in the mandibular bones or concurrent diseases.
- In such cases, gavage feeding or placement of an esophagostomy tube is indicated.

• CLIENT EDUCATION/HUSBANDRY RECOMMENDATIONS

- NSHP is caused by improper husbandry and diet.
- Despite the efforts made in order to educate owners on adequate husbandry practices, NSHP is still one of the most common disorders of captive reptiles.
- Husbandry issues to consider in order to prevent NSHP are provision of unfiltered sunlight (or as an alternative UVB through a UVB-emitting lamp), and provision of an environment adequate for brumation in brumating species.

• Dietary issues to consider in order to prevent NSHP are provision of a diet that is naturally high in calcium and is low in phosphorus, and provision of a diet that has the proper quantity of vitamins, especially vitamin A and D.

MEDICATIONS

DRUG(S) OF CHOICE

• In reptiles presented with acute hypocalcemic crisis, calcium should be administered intravenously, or intramuscularly when an intravenous line is not available.
• There is no dosage that has been evaluated for effectiveness and safety in reptiles.
• In general, dosages of 50–100 mg/kg of calcium gluconate are considered effective.
• Monitoring of calcium, heart activity through an ECG, and other electrolytes is highly suggested during seizure-like crisis.
• Fluid administration is also required, as reptiles presenting with this condition are usually severely dehydrated.
• In reptiles presented with chronic NSHP, the mainstay of the therapy is an improvement in husbandry and diet.
• Exposure to unfiltered sunlight for basking species is preferred over artificial UVB lights.
• When sunlight exposure is not possible or ideal (e.g., winter time), proper selection and use of UVB lights is necessary.
• A gradual change to a diet that contains the appropriate levels of calcium, vitamin D, and fibers, with low level of phosphorus is also required.
• Administration of oral calcium may assist in the recovery, but it must not be used as a standalone treatment.
• Calcium supplements containing vitamin D should be carefully dosed to avoid hypervitaminosis D.
• Calcium gluconate 50–100 mg/kg SC, IM, IV q6–24h
• Calcium glubionate 50–360 mg/kg PO q12–24h

PRECAUTIONS/INTERACTIONS

• It is presumed that, as in other vertebrates, parenteral calcium administration may provoke cardiac arrhythmias.
• Administration of exogenous vitamin D3 may result in excessive concentrations, resulting in intoxication and metastatic calcification of tissues.
• The only cases where exogenous vitamin D3 should be administered are where renal and/or hepatic functions are impaired, and endogenous vitamin D3 cannot be produced.
• The absorption of dietary vitamin D can be variable across species of reptiles.
• In all the other cases, the exposure to unfiltered sunlight or UVB-emitting lamps is considered a safer approach.

FOLLOW-UP

PATIENT MONITORING

• In cases of acute hypocalcemic crisis, the reptile requires intensive care and monitoring of ionized calcium levels and ECG activity.
• In cases of chronic NSHP, if the reptile is eating on its own, a physical exam once every 7–14 days, accompanied by radiography and blood work, is usually adequate to assess response to therapy.

EXPECTED COURSE AND PROGNOSIS

• The prognosis of the disease is strictly dependent on the chronicity of the improper husbandry and on the severity of clinical signs and pathology upon presentation.
• For example, young iguanas, even if presented with hypocalcemic crisis, may have a favorable outcome if treated aggressively.
• Older animals, that present with chronic bone tissue depletion, may have a worse prognosis.
• Different species also have different prognoses.
• Geckos and chameleons in general are very sensitive to calcium deficiencies and have a poor prognosis once NSHP has developed.

MISCELLANEOUS

COMMENTS

Currently, there is a lack of information as to the proper amounts of calcium, vitamin D and other nutrients required for proper health of reptiles. The source of these nutrients may also influence their ability to be properly absorbed through the intestinal tract. It is possible that supplementation of these nutrients is not as effective as the natural ingestion via proper foods.

ZOONOTIC POTENTIAL

N/A

SYNONYMS

• Fibrous osteodystrophy
• Metabolic bone disease
• Nutrition-related metabolic bone disease

ABBREVIATIONS

• ECG = electrocardiogram
• IM = intramuscular
• IV = intravenous
• NSHP = nutritional secondary hyperparathyroidism
• PO = per os
• PTH = parathyroid hormone
• SC = subcutaneous
• UVB = ultraviolet B

INTERNET RESOURCES

• Additional information on reptile endocrinology from Carl Gans Collections: Biology of the Reptilia. http://carlgans.org/bor-view/?borv=3&borp=7
• Information on secondary hyperparathyroidism in humans: Kim L. Hyperparathyroidism. Medscape, August 18, 2020. http://emedicine.medscape.com/article/127351-overview?pa=mcKd1JF66kULHOzxxIxn2fK%2Bx5xE5kE6dUeU7dvJSrcnjyhACchqCtq5rNZR2UhkQPQxex%2Bo7mr5pATtx84gCBXKySxof3ndUJD5aivxmIc%3D#a4

Suggested Reading

Fledelius B, Jorgensen GW, Jensen HE, Brimer L. Influence of the calcium content of the diet offered to leopard tortoises (*Geochelone pardalis*). *Vet Rec* 2005;156(26):831–835.

Hoby S, Wenker C, Robert N, et al. Nutritional metabolic bone disease in juvenile veiled chameleons (*Chamaeleo calyptratus*) and its prevention. *J Nutr* 2010;140:1923–1931.

Mans C, Braun J. Update on common nutritional disorders of captive reptiles. *Vet Clin North Am Exot Anim Pract* 2014;17(3):369–395.

Authors Paolo Selleri, DMV, PhD, SpecPACS, DECZM (Herpetology & Small Mammals), and Nicola Di Girolamo, DMV, MSc (EBHC), PhD, DECZM (Herpetology)

NYCTOTHERUS

BASICS

DEFINITION/OVERVIEW

Nyctotherus is a large ciliated protozoal organism that resides within the gastrointestinal tract. The trophozoite is dorsoventrally flattened like a bean and ranges in size from 60–200 µm. It has peristomal cilia, which is characteristic for the organism. The cystostome (mouth) is long and curved. Cysts are brown, have a thick wall, are ovoid in shape, and have a polar cap.

ETIOLOGY/PATHOPHYSIOLOGY

- Transmission is through fecal–oral route.
- Cysts are ingested and then undergo excystation in the intestinal tract.
- Trophozoites hatch and emerge in the small intestine.
- They then migrate and manifest in the large colon and replicate by cell division.
- They feed on the chyme, bacteria, fiber, and other ingesta within the intestinal tract.
- Trophozoites undergo encystation in which infective cysts are formed and then excreted in feces.
- If in a moist environment, cysts remain infective for several weeks.
- *Nyctotherus* spp. are generally not considered pathogens.
- Animals with diarrhea have been observed to large amounts of trophozoites within fecals, but this is believed to be secondary due to the more liquid environment within the large intestine.

SIGNALMENT/HISTORY

All ages can be affected

CLINICAL PRESENTATION

- Diarrhea, dehydration, weight loss
- Clinical signs are only likely to occur in severely immunocompromised individuals.

RISK FACTORS

Husbandry

Improper husbandry

Others

N/A

DIAGNOSIS

DIFFERENTIAL DIAGNOSIS

- Oxyurid nematodiasis
- Trematodes

DIAGNOSTICS

- Microscopic evaluation of fresh fecal material to visualize trophozoites and cysts.
- SAF technique can be used for better visualization.
- Fecal/cysts can be placed within a petri dish with water and trophozoites will emerge from the dissolved envelope within several hours.

PATHOLOGICAL FINDINGS

- Diarrhea
- Dehydration
- Weight loss

TREATMENT

APPROPRIATE HEALTH CARE

Treatment is rarely required because *Nyctotherus* spp. are mostly non-pathogenic.

NUTRITIONAL SUPPORT

Nutritional supplementation may be indicated if diarrhea and dehydration are severe.

CLIENT EDUCATION/HUSBANDRY RECOMMENDATIONS

- Practice proper hygiene
- Wash fruits and vegetables before being fed.
- House infected animals separately

MEDICATIONS

DRUG(S) OF CHOICE

Metronidazole 25 mg/kg PO q24h for 5–7 days.

PRECAUTIONS/INTERACTIONS

N/A

FOLLOW-UP

PATIENT MONITORING

- Monitor for weight gain
- Take fecal samples

EXPECTED COURSE AND PROGNOSIS

Good

MISCELLANEOUS

COMMENTS

N/A

ZOONOTIC POTENTIAL

Unknown

SYNONYMS

N/A

ABBREVIATIONS

- PO = per os
- SAF = sodium acetate acetic acid formalin

INTERNET RESOURCES

- De Bosschere H, Roels S. *Balantidium* sp. and *Nyctotherus* sp: two common members of the digestive-tract flora in Mediterranean tortoises. Tortoise Trust. https://www.tortoisetrust.org/articles/balantidium.htm
- Divers SJ. Parasitic Diseases of Reptiles. MSD Manual Veterinary Manual, June 2020. http://www.merckvetmanual.com/exotic-and-laboratory-animals/reptiles/parasitic-diseases-of-reptiles

Suggested Reading

Hnizdo J, Pantchev N. Protozoa (digestive tract). In: *Medical Care of Turtles and Tortoises*. Diagnosis. Surgery. Pathology. Parasitology. Frankfurt, Germany: Edition Chimaira; 2011: 194–195.

Jacobson ER. Parasites and parasitic diseases of reptiles. In: Jacobson ER, ed. *Infectious Diseases and Pathology of Reptiles: Color Atlas and Text*. Boca Raton, FL: CRC Press; 2007:571–665.

Author Elsburgh O. Clarke III, DVM, DACZM

OTHER HYALOHYPHOMYCOSES

BASICS

DEFINITION/OVERVIEW

Hyalohyphomycoses refers to any infection with non-pigmented (hyaline) filamentous fungi such as *Aspergillus*, *Purpureocillium lilacinum* (formerly *Paecilomyces lilacinus*), *Fusarium*, and many other genera. Hyalohyphomycoses caused by other hyaline molds, such as *Metarhizium*, *Nannizziopsis*, *Paranannizziopsis*, *Ophidiomyces*, and *Emydomyces* are addressed separately.

ETIOLOGY/PATHOPHYSIOLOGY

- Ubiquitous environmental fungi that act as opportunistic pathogens in stressed/immunocompromised, or otherwise sick or debilitated animals.
- Some, like *Fusarium incarnatum* (formerly *F. semitectum*) in Texas tortoises or *Schizangiella serpentis* in snakes, may act as true pathogens while others, like *Purpureocillium lilacinum* or *F. solani*, seem to need little help in causing infection.
- Some are known insect pathogens, like *Metarhizium anisopliae* or *Beauveria bassiana*.

SIGNALMENT/HISTORY

- Any reptile, any age, any sex.
- History usually discloses substandard to outright deficient husbandry, poor hygiene, concurrent disease or infection, climactic extreme conditions (e.g., cold stunning in sea turtles) or life-support system failure in captive animals (e.g. loss of heat from power failure) that result in immune suppression.

CLINICAL PRESENTATION

- Reflects the organ system affected
- Systemic, disseminated disease also often a serious consequence of prior hypothermia.

RISK FACTORS

Husbandry

- Climactic events in wild reptiles
- Poor or deficient husbandry is probably the single most important predisposing factor.

Others

Chronic debilitating disease process, concurrent bacterial or other infections, prolonged antibiotic therapy.

DIAGNOSIS

DIFFERENTIAL DIAGNOSIS

- Differential depends on presentation and targeted organ system.
- Bacterial/mycobacterial, viral, and parasitic diseases.
- Neoplasia when disseminated granulomas

DIAGNOSTICS

- Culture and cytology of material/clinical samples.
- Biopsy of lesions and histopathology to confirm causation.
- Blood work and imaging to determine extent of disease/lesions.

PATHOLOGICAL FINDINGS

Hyaline hyphae or other fungal elements within inflamed and/or necrotic tissue or within granulomas, consistent in morphology (e.g., diameter, septation, branching) to those of hyaline fungus isolated from the lesion.

TREATMENT

APPROPRIATE HEALTH CARE

- Broad-spectrum antifungal drugs
- Fluids, antibiotic coverage, thermal and nutritional support.
- Correct perceived husbandry deficiencies

NUTRITIONAL SUPPORT

Assist-feeding if needed

CLIENT EDUCATION/HUSBANDRY RECOMMENDATIONS

- Quarantine of incoming animals
- Thorough and meticulous captive husbandry

SURGICAL CONSIDERATIONS

Debulking of lesions, when possible

MEDICATIONS

DRUG(S) OF CHOICE

- Ideally based on fungal identification and known susceptibility of the causative fungus to the various antifungal drugs.
- In vitro assays might be available.
- Broad-spectrum antifungals that are efficacious against molds (itraconazole, voriconazole, terbinafine) probably indicated pending culture and sensitivity results.

PRECAUTIONS/INTERACTIONS

- Triazole antifungal and terbinafine possibly synergistic.
- Interactions with other drugs possible.

FOLLOW-UP

PATIENT MONITORING

- Monitor appetite, demeanor, and skin improvement with treatment.
- Bloodwork to monitor liver enzymes and other parameters while on antifungals, and/or to assess immune status indicated.

EXPECTED COURSE AND PROGNOSIS

- Often diagnosed late in the course of disease.
- Early infection often subclinical in reptiles, which tend to be stoic, and fungal etiology often unsuspected by clinicians.
- Prognosis is therefore usually guarded to very poor, but may vary depending on duration, severity, and extent of lesions, and on the sensitivity pattern of the offending fungus.

MISCELLANEOUS

COMMENTS

The isolation of Aspergilli or Penicillia from reptile skin is practically expected because they are normal constituents of the reptile cutaneous mycobiota, and is clinically irrelevant if not supported by histopathology.

ZOONOTIC POTENTIAL

- Many *Fusaria* and *Aspergillus* spp. carry some mild zoonotic potential.
- Dermatomycosis with *Trichophyton mentagrophytes var. interdigitale*, a human pathogen, has been reported from green iguanas in Iran.

SYNONYMS

Necrotizing scute disease refers to *F. incarnatum* infection of the shell in Texas tortoises, and likely other tortoises (e.g., *Testudo* spp.).

Suggested Reading

Paré JA, Jacobson ER. Mycotic diseases of reptiles. In: Jacobson ER, ed. *Infectious Disease and Pathology of Reptiles, Color Atlas and Text.* Boca Raton, FL: CRC Press; 2007:527–570.

Author Jean A. Paré, DMV, DVSc, DACZM, DECZM (Zoo Health Management)

OXYURIDS

BASICS

DEFINITION/OVERVIEW
Oxyurids (pinworms) have a direct life cycle and are host specific. They are common in many reptilian species, particularly in herbivorous animals. They are considered non-pathogenic in animals without clinical signs.

ETIOLOGY/PATHOPHYSIOLOGY
- Animals are usually asymptomatic
- Parasites inhabit the lower intestinal tract.
- Severe infestations may cause secondary problems, especially in debilitated and dehydrated animals.

SIGNALMENT/HISTORY
Oxyurids are most commonly found in herbivorous reptiles as commensal organisms of the lower intestinal tract.

CLINICAL PRESENTATION
- Disease caused by oxyurids is usually a secondary complication due to an underlying disease.
- Anorexia
- Lethargy
- Diarrhea
- Dehydration

RISK FACTORS
Husbandry
- Inadequate husbandry may lead to stress, immunosuppression, and a myriad of secondary conditions.
- Poor hygiene, high fecal loads, and overcrowding may contribute to higher infection rates.

Others
N/A

DIAGNOSIS

DIFFERENTIAL DIAGNOSIS
- Rule out prey-item source in carnivorous, insectivorous, and omnivorous lizards.
- Commensals of the rodent cecum
- Insects have species specific pinworms in their gut flora.

DIAGNOSTICS
- Eggs vary in shape, can be ovoid, elongate, or D-shaped, and lack the thick wall of ascarid eggs.
- The eggs measure approximately 130 × 40 μm.
- Some eggs can be larvated
- Adult worms are visible in fecal material.
- Oxyurid eggs are commonly seen in feces of herbivorous reptiles.

PATHOLOGICAL FINDINGS
Impaction of the intestinal tract may be observed in sick animals with severe pinworm infection.

TREATMENT

APPROPRIATE HEALTH CARE
Excessive numbers of these organisms in sick animals may require medical treatment.

NUTRITIONAL SUPPORT
- In ill animals, nutritional support after rehydration is needed to maintain positive nitrogen balance.
- Feed small amounts more frequently
- Use high protein and fat diets for carnivores and complex carbohydrate diets for herbivores.

CLIENT EDUCATION/HUSBANDRY RECOMMENDATIONS
- Follow proper husbandry guidelines for the species at hand.
- Environmental temperature, proper housing, and feeding regimen all play a crucial role in the wellbeing of reptilian species kept in captivity.

MEDICATIONS

DRUG(S) OF CHOICE
- Fenbendazole 25–50 mg/kg PO q24h for 5 days; 50–100 mg/kg PO q14d.
- Oxfendazole 66 mg/kg PO once, may repeat in 14 days as needed.
- Pyrantel pamoate 25 mg/kg PO sid for 3 days, repeat in 3 weeks.
- Ivermectin 0.2 mg/kg IM, SC, PO, once, then repeat in 14 days.

PRECAUTIONS/INTERACTIONS
- Avoid fenbendazole and oxfendazole in severely debilitated and dehydrated animals to minimize the risk of the potential adverse effects (bone marrow suppression, intestinal cell damage) associated with these drugs.
- Lower doses of these drugs should also be considered in species of critical conservation status if previous; safe use is unknown.

FOLLOW-UP

PATIENT MONITORING
- Evaluate hydration frequently after starting treatment.
- Make husbandry changes to provide proper environment and nutrition.

EXPECTED COURSE AND PROGNOSIS
- Oxyurids are non-pathogenic in healthy, immunocompetent animals.
- In sick animals, treatment is aimed at decreasing the parasite load in the gut to minimize chance of impaction.
- Prognosis is excellent to good if the underlying source of illness is identified and treated effectively (husbandry mismanagement, primary disease process).

MISCELLANEOUS

COMMENTS
N/A

ZOONOTIC POTENTIAL
N/A

SYNONYMS
N/A

ABBREVIATIONS
- IM = intramuscular
- PO = per os
- SC = subcutaneous
- sid = once a day

Suggested Reading

Mader DR, ed. *Reptile Medicine and Surgery*. 2nd ed. St Louis, MO: Saunders Elsevier, 2006.

Rataj AV, Lindtner-Knific R, Vlahović K, et al. Parasites in pet reptiles. *Acta Vet Scand* 2011;53(1):33.

Author Sam Rivera, DVM, MS, DABVP (avian), DACZM, DECZM (Zoo Health Management)

PAPILLOMAVIRUS

BASICS

DEFINITION/OVERVIEW

Papillomaviruses cause mucocutaneous and cutaneous epithelial proliferative lesions in several vertebrate hosts, including reptiles.

ETIOLOGY/PATHOPHYSIOLOGY

- The members of the family Papillomaviridae are non-enveloped, icosahedral viral particles with a diameter of 50–55 nm and a small (7–8 kb), circular, double-stranded DNA.
- Papillomavirus-like particles were identified on electron microscopy in two European green lizards (*Lacerta viridis*) with cutaneous proliferative lesions.
- No genomic characterization of papillomaviruses in lizards has been reported.

SIGNALMENT/HISTORY

Among lizards, the only species in which papillomavirus-like particles have been identified associated with cutaneous proliferative lesions is the European green lizard (*Lacerta viridis*).

CLINICAL PRESENTATION

The first documented cases of papillomavirus-like particles in lizards showed gray, raised, spherical (1–4 mm diameter) dermal masses multifocally distributed.

RISK FACTORS

Husbandry

Because transmission is likely by direct contact, absence of quarantine for new admitted lizards can contribute to widespread the disease.

Others

The presence of papillomaviral lesions may be an indication of immuno-suppression.

DIAGNOSIS

DIFFERENTIAL DIAGNOSIS

- Herpesvirus and/or reovirus infection
- In a green lizard, herpesvirus-like and reovirus-like particles have also been also detected.

DIAGNOSTICS

Although TEM can be used for detecting intranuclear aggregates of virions consistent in morphology with papillomavirus, a definitive diagnosis of papillomavirus in suspected samples must be by PCR.

PATHOLOGICAL FINDINGS

- Gross lesions resemble very early papillomavirus lesions in mammals.
- Histologically, the lesions are benign in appearance and consist of epidermal hyperplasia with prominent anisocytosis and anisokaryosis of keratinocytes and severe parakeratotic hyperkeratosis.

TREATMENT

APPROPRIATE HEALTH CARE

No drug therapy has been reported in reptiles.

NUTRITIONAL SUPPORT

N/A

CLIENT EDUCATION/HUSBANDRY RECOMMENDATIONS

Affected lizards should be isolated, and their cages should be cleaned and disinfected to minimize virus transmission and secondary infections.

SURGICAL CONSIDERATIONS

Surgical removal may be performed when lesions affect quality of life or normal function of the animal.

MEDICATIONS

DRUG(S) OF CHOICE

Antiviral drugs (cidofovir and imiquimod) have been effective in mammalian papillomavirus infections but efficacy in reptiles is uknown.

PRECAUTIONS/INTERACTIONS

N/A

FOLLOW-UP

PATIENT MONITORING

N/A

EXPECTED COURSE AND PROGNOSIS

- In most cases of papillomavirus infection in reptiles the lesions are benign and regression of lesions is expected.
- Secondary bacterial infections can be observed.

MISCELLANEOUS

COMMENTS

N/A

ZOONOTIC POTENTIAL

- Papillomaviruses are highly species-specific pathogens.
- There is no evidence for zoonosis from papillomaviruses affecting reptiles.

SYNONYMS

N/A

ABBREVIATIONS

- PCR = polymerase chain reaction
- TEM = transmission electron microscopy

Suggested Reading

Cooper JE, Gschmeissner S, Holt PE. Viral particles in a papilloma from a green lizard (*Lacerta viridis*). *Lab Anim* 1982;16:12–13.

Raynaud A, Adrian M. [Cutaneous lesions with papillomatous structure associated with viruses in the green lizard *(Lacerta viridis Laur.)] C R Acad Hebd Sceances Acad Sci D* 1976;283(7):845–847.

Author Jorge Orós, DVM, PhD, DECZM

PARANANNIZZIOPSIS MYCOSES TUATARA

BASICS

DEFINITION/OVERVIEW

Paranannizziopsis mycoses infection is caused by any of five fungal species in the genus *Paranannizziopsis.* It is an important disease of tuataras in New Zealand.

ETIOLOGY/PATHOPHYSIOLOGY

P. australasiensis causes fungal skin disease in captive tuataras.

SIGNALMENT/HISTORY

- No age or sex predilection is reported.
- Contagious and often affects most to all animals in a captive setting.
- *P. australasiensis* can infect acrochordid snakes, tuataras, coastal bearded dragons, and probably other lizards but, up until recently, has only been reported from Australia and New Zealand.

CLINICAL PRESENTATION

- Outcome is often fatal
- In tuataras, dermatitis with raised, yellow to brown crusts can progress to necrosis and ulcers.
- Similar disease was seen in one coastal bearded dragon housed near diseased tuataras.

RISK FACTORS

Husbandry

Substandard husbandry

Others

N/A

DIAGNOSIS

DIFFERENTIAL DIAGNOSIS

Caustic, thermal, bacterial, viral, or even parasitic dermatitides or dermatoses should be ruled out.

DIAGNOSTICS

- Crusting dermatitis in tuataras should evoke *P. australasiensis* infection.
- Arthroconidia may be seen on stained impression smears of lesions.
- Culture of clinical samples (crusts, sloughed skin or shed skin, lesion biopsies) is required.
- PCR is needed to identify *Paranannizziopsis* isolates to genus and species.
- Histopathology should always be performed to support causality.

PATHOLOGICAL FINDINGS

Hyphae or other fungal elements within inflamed and/or necrotic epidermis and in the underlying dermis.

TREATMENT

APPROPRIATE HEALTH CARE

- Correct perceived husbandry deficiencies.
- Assess water quality parameters, especially pH.
- Fluids, antibiotics, thermal and nutritional support as needed.
- *P. crustacea* is susceptible in vitro to itraconazole, voriconazole, and terbinafine.
- Itraconazole yielded clinical cure in many tuataras infected with *P. australasiensis.*

NUTRITIONAL SUPPORT

Assist-feeding if needed

CLIENT EDUCATION/HUSBANDRY RECOMMENDATIONS

- Quarantine of incoming animals.
- Thorough and meticulous review of captive husbandry.
- Close monitoring of water-quality parameters.

SURGICAL CONSIDERATIONS

Debulking of lesions and/or sloughed skin, when possible.

MEDICATIONS

DRUG(S) OF CHOICE

Wide-spectrum antifungals (itraconazole, voriconazole, terbinafine) are indicated pending culture and sensitivity results.

PRECAUTIONS/INTERACTIONS

- Triazole antifungal and terbinafine possibly synergistic.
- Interactions with other drugs possible

FOLLOW-UP

PATIENT MONITORING

- Monitor appetite, demeanor, and skin improvement with treatment.
- Bloodwork to monitor liver enzymes and other parameters while on antifungals.

EXPECTED COURSE AND PROGNOSIS

- Often diagnosed late in the course of disease.
- Progression of lesions may be rapid, and disease may spread.

MISCELLANEOUS

COMMENTS

N/A

ZOONOTIC POTENTIAL

None identified to date

SYNONYMS

Used to be referred to as *Chrysosporium* anamorph of *Nannizziopsis vriesii* (CANV) complex before reassignment based on molecular studies to the genus *Paranannizziopsis.*

ABBREVIATIONS

PCR = polymerase chain reaction

Suggested Reading

Bertelsen MF, Crawshaw GJ, Sigler L, Smith DA. Fatal cutaneous mycosis in tentacled snakes (*Erpeton tentaculatum*) caused by the *Chrysosporium* anamorph of *Nannizziopsis vriesii. J Zoo Wildl Med* 2005;36:82–87.

Paré JA, Sigler L. An overview of reptile fungal pathogens in the genera *Nannizziopsis, Paranannizziopsis,* and *Ophidiomyces. J Herp Med Surg* 2016;26:46–53.

Sigler L, Hambleton S, Paré JA. Molecular characterization of reptile pathogens currently known as members of the *Chrysosporium* anamorph of *Nannizziopsis vriesii* complex and relationship with some human-associated isolates. *J Clin Microbiol* 2013;51:3338–3357.

Author Jean A. Paré, DMV, DVSc, DACZM, DECZM (Zoo Health Management)

PENTASTOMIDS

BASICS

DEFINITION/OVERVIEW

Pentastomids are crustacean endoparasites of the respiratory system. Approximately 90% of pentastomids use carnivorous reptiles as their definitive hosts, with 70% being found in snakes. Pentastomiasis occurs on all continents except Antarctica.

ETIOLOGY/PATHOPHYSIOLOGY

- Pentastomid infections may be asymptomatic, but adult and larval pentastomids can cause severe pathology resulting in the death of their intermediate and definitive hosts, usually via obstruction of airways or secondary bacterial infections.
- Adult pentastomids live in the lungs or air sacs of lizards, where they breed and feed. Females are larger than males and longer lived (up to up to 8 years in some species).
- A single female can produce millions of eggs, which remain viable for months in the environment.
- Eggs are coughed up from the lungs and passed out into the environment when the lizard drinks or expels fluid orally. Alternatively, eggs are ingested and passed in feces.
- Intermediate hosts, such as insects (especially cockroaches), fish, anurans, reptiles, birds, or mammals, ingest pentastomid eggs, which hatch, and go through two instars (growth periods between molts), before becoming encysted somewhere in the intermediate host's body.
- When the intermediate host is eaten by the definitive host, third-stage larvae emerge from the cyst and migrate to the host's lungs, where they feed on blood through the lung wall (hematophagous).
- Pentastomids damage the lungs, which may lead to secondary bacterial or fungal colonization, pneumonia, septicemia or death.
- Heavy infestations can occlude the lungs or trachea.
- Several pentastomid genera parasitize lizards, including *Raillietiella*, *Elaenia* and *Sambonia*. Nymphs of *Waddycephalus* have been recorded in several lizard species, but they are probably not a definitive host, as adult pentastomes have yet to be found.

SIGNALMENT/HISTORY

- *Raillietiella* infect numerous tropical lizard genera, including agamids (*Pogona*, *Japalura*), gekkonids (*Gecko*, *Gehyra*, *Hemidactylus*, *Lepidodactylus*, *Nephrurus*, *Oedura*, *Phyllopezus*), iguanids (*Anolis*, *Tropidurus*, *Furcifer*), scincids (*Mabuya*, *Micrablepharus*, *Tiliqua*), and teiids (*Cnemidophorus*).
- *Elaenia* and *Sambonia* both infect monitors and goannas, *Varanus* spp.
- About 30% of free-living Tokay geckos necropsied in the early 1980s from the tropical habitat building at the Kansas City Zoo had a *Raillietiella* spp. in their lungs. Several species of cockroaches were thought to be the intermediate hosts.
- At the Federal University of Paraiba in João Pessoa, Brazil, 20% of wild *Hemidactylus mabouia* had *Raillietiella frenatus* in their lungs.

CLINICAL PRESENTATION

Can be subclinical or have subcutaneous swellings, respiratory tract disease, pneumonia, dyspnea, weight loss, or poor growth.

RISK FACTORS

Husbandry

Yet another compelling reason for quarantine and fecal examinations.

Others

Wild-caught or free-living lizards (especially *Hemidactylus* spp.) with access to intermediate hosts such as insects or rodents.

DIAGNOSIS

- Detection of pentastomid eggs on fecal flotation, lung or colonic washes, or tracheal discharge.
- Adult pentastomids are sometimes visible on radiography or via pulmonoscopy. Adults may also be found on exploratory surgery, necropsy, or histopathology.

DIFFERENTIAL DIAGNOSIS

Respiratory signs may also be caused by other parasites, viruses, bacterial, fungi, neoplasia, trauma or foreign bodies.

DIAGNOSTICS

- Fecal examination revealing thin-walled, large (up to 130 µm in diameter), distinct ova, containing larvae with four claw-like hooklets.
- A complete blood count might reveal anemia or eosinophilia.

PATHOLOGICAL FINDINGS

- Pentastomids are medium to large (0.25–15 cm), superficially segmented, wormlike parasites, with two compound pairs of hooks surrounding the mouth.
- Adults may be recovered from the mouth, trachea, lungs, and air sacs.
- Encysted instars may be found throughout the body.
- In tissues, pentastomids are identified histologically by the presence of acidophilic glands adjacent to the intestine, and black sclerotized openings in the body wall.
- Inflammatory response in the lung may be mild with pentastomids because all life stages secrete surfactant very similar to that of the host surfactant, which is thought to help them evade the host's immune system.
- Degrading molted pentastomid cuticles shed into the lung lumen may induce putrid pneumonia. Feed attachment sites on the lung surface can cause multiple crateriform ulcers.
- Pentastomids can be identified by morphological and molecular techniques.

TREATMENT

APPROPRIATE HEALTH CARE

- Stabilize the patient first with antibiotics, fluids and nutritional support, if indicated.
- If medical therapy is unsuccessful consider benign neglect or transpulmonary laparoscopic removal.

NUTRITIONAL SUPPORT

- EmerAid™ Sustain Carnivore (EmerAid, LLC, Cornell, IL) or Oxbow Critical Care Carnivore® (Oxbow Animal Health, Omaha, NE) via gavage feeding once daily if indicated.
- Not indicated if in good body condition or still eating on their own.

CLIENT EDUCATION/HUSBANDRY RECOMMENDATIONS

- Zoonotic, therefore biosecurity methods, including wearing gloves and washing hands, should be employed when working with infected animals.
- Wash hands after handling lizards or wear gloves.

MEDICATIONS

DRUG(S) OF CHOICE

- Treatment of a Savannah monitor with 0.2 mg/kg ivermectin SC, repeated in 10 days was apparently successfully.
- A tokay gecko, *Gecko gecko*, kept shedding pentastomid ova in feces after fenbendazole, praziquantel, and ivermectin treatments 2 weeks apart.
- A higher dose of ivermectin, 0.4 mg/kg PO, q14d for 3 treatments, failed, but a single treatment of 1 mg/kg caused indefinite cessation of ova shedding with no signs of ivermectin toxicity.
- Ivermectin, again at 1 mg/kg, PO q14d for 2 treatments, also stopped ova shedding in 4 Standing's day geckos, *Phelsuma standingi*, with no obvious ill effects.
- The lungs were not available in any of these geckos to confirm the death of the adult parasites.

PRECAUTIONS/INTERACTIONS

• Living pentastomids secrete surfactant that helps them to evade the host's immune system, but upon their death in tissue or lungs a severe antigenic release, or putrefaction, with serious and potential lethal complications can occur.

FOLLOW-UP

PATIENT MONITORING

Perform serial fecal examinations post-treatment to gauge effectiveness.

EXPECTED COURSE AND PROGNOSIS

Highly variable, dependent on parasitic burden, chronicity, condition of patient, and response to therapy.

MISCELLANEOUS

COMMENTS

Several species of house geckos, *Hemidactylus* spp., are thought to be spreading *Raillietiella* spp. worldwide via cargo transport.

ZOONOTIC POTENTIAL

• Species infecting humans belong to the families Linguatulidae, Armilliferidae, Porocephalidae, and Raillietiellidae; only the last has been reported in lizards.
• Rare human cases from Raillietiellidae were associated with eating raw snake (Democratic Republic of Congo) or live geckos as part of alternative medicine in Asia.
• All pentastomids should be considered potentially zoonotic.
• In the intermediate hosts, pentastome larvae often hatch and bore through the stomach wall and encyst in nearby mesentery, serosa, or viscera.

SYNONYMS

• Pentastomiasis
• Tongue worms

ABBREVIATIONS

• PO = per os
• SC = subcutaneous

INTERNET RESOURCES

Wildlife Health Australia. Pentastomiasis in Australian reptiles. https://www.wildlifehealthaustralia.com.au/FactSheets.aspx

Suggested Reading

Flach EJ, Riley J, Mutlow AG, McCandlish IA. Pentastomiasis in Bosc's monitor lizards (*Varanus exanthematicus*) caused by an undescribed Sambonia species. *J Zoo Wildl Med* 2000;31:91–95.

Jacobson ER. Parasites and parasitic diseases of reptiles. In: Jacobson ER, ed. *Infectious Disease and Pathology of Reptiles*. Boca Raton, FL: CRC Press; 2007:571–665.

Micinilio J. Ivermectin for the treatment of pentastomids in a tokay gecko, *Gekko gecko. Bull Assoc Rept Amphib Vet* 1996;6(2):5–6.

Paré JA. An overview of pentastomiasis in reptiles and other vertebrates. *J Exot Pet Med* 2008;17:285–294.

Wright K. Ivermectin for treatment of pentastomids in the Standing's day gecko, *Phelsuma standingi. Bull Assoc Rept Amphib Vet* 1997;7(1):5.

Author Thomas H. Boyer, DVM, DABVP (Reptile and Amphibian Practice)

PHAEOHYPHOMYCOSES

BASICS

DEFINITION/OVERVIEW

Phaeohyphomycoses refers to any infection with dematiaceous (pigmented) fungi, such as *Exophiala*, *Cladosporium*, *Ochroconis*, *Ulocladium*, *Trichoderma*. The cell walls of these fungi contain variable amounts of melanin, and hyphae are therefore easily seen on routine H&E histological sections. These infections are relatively uncommon in reptiles.

ETIOLOGY/PATHOPHYSIOLOGY

- All are environmental fungi often found in soil and/or water, and usually infect cutaneous wounds or, less often, sick or debilitated animals.
- These opportunistic pathogens typically cause deep granulomatous infections of the feet and rarely disseminate.
- *Exophiala* species, in particular, have been isolated with some regularity from reptiles with phaeohyphomycosis.

SIGNALMENT/HISTORY

Any reptile, any age or sex.

CLINICAL PRESENTATION

- Swellings, nodules, wounds, often on the feet or ventrum (body parts in contact with soil).
- Slow progression
- Tends to not disseminate

RISK FACTORS

Husbandry

- Substandard or otherwise deficient husbandry.
- Soil substrate
- Poor water quality

Others

Open wounds or other cutaneous breaches may facilitate invasion by these opportunistic fungi.

DIAGNOSIS

DIFFERENTIAL DIAGNOSIS

- Other fungal infections
- Mycobacteriosis
- Abscesses
- Neoplasia

DIAGNOSTICS

- Biopsy and histopathology
- Culture of biopsy tissue or PCR.
- Pigmented fungi associated with inflammation/necrosis in histological section, and morphology of fungi in tissues consistent with morphology of putative isolate cultured from biopsy.

PATHOLOGICAL FINDINGS

Pigmented hyphae or other fungal elements within inflamed and/or necrotic tissue or within granulomas, consistent in morphology (e.g., pigmentation, diameter, septation, branching) with those of fungal isolate from the lesion.

TREATMENT

APPROPRIATE HEALTH CARE

- Fluids, antibiotic coverage, thermal and nutritional support.
- Correct perceived husbandry deficiencies.

NUTRITIONAL SUPPORT

Assist-feeding if needed

CLIENT EDUCATION/HUSBANDRY RECOMMENDATIONS

- Quarantine of incoming animals
- Thorough and meticulous captive husbandry

SURGICAL CONSIDERATIONS

- Debulking of lesions, when possible
- Amputation may be indicated when deep lesion located on/in feet.

MEDICATIONS

DRUG(S) OF CHOICE

- Ideally based on fungal identification and known susceptibility of the causative fungus to the various antifungal drugs.
- In vitro assays might be available.
- Many, if not most, pigmented fungi display resistance to triazoles and allylamines.

PRECAUTIONS/INTERACTIONS

N/A

FOLLOW-UP

PATIENT MONITORING

- Monitor appetite, demeanor, and skin improvement with treatment.
- Bloodwork to monitor liver

EXPECTED COURSE AND PROGNOSIS

- Often diagnosed late in the course of disease when lesions are chronic and/or extensive.
- Prognosis is usually guarded, but may vary depending on duration, severity, and extent of lesions, and on the sensitivity pattern of the offending fungus.
- Enzymes and other parameters while on antifungals and/or assess immune status indicated.

MISCELLANEOUS

COMMENTS

N/A

ZOONOTIC POTENTIAL

- Minimal
- Some pigmented fungi can cause local infections and onychomycosis in humans, and rarely fungemia and disseminated disease.

SYNONYMS

N/A

ABBREVIATIONS

- H&E = hematoxylin and eosin
- PCR = polymerase chain reaction

Suggested Reading

Paré JA, Jacobson ER. Mycotic diseases of reptiles. In: Jacobson ER, ed. *Infectious Disease and Pathology of Reptiles, Color Atlas and Text.* Boca Raton, FL: CRC Press; 2007:527–570.

Author Jean A. Paré, DMV, DVSc, DACZM, DECZM (Zoo Health Management)

PSEUDOGOUT

BASICS

DEFINITION/OVERVIEW

Pseudogout is a condition that occurs due to the deposition of crystals, other than uric acid, in or around the joints.

ETIOLOGY/PATHOPHYSIOLOGY

- Crystals may be deposited for a variety of reasons.
- In humans, these include previous joint damage, hyperparathyroidism or hereditary factors.
- In reptiles, the exact etiology is unclear but deposition of calcium crystals in and around joints may be seen, especially CPPD.
- This can result in an acute inflammatory response in the affected joint.

SIGNALMENT/HISTORY

- Pseudogout may be seen in lizards with a history of inappropriate husbandry or diet.
- Signs may also be seen in combination with true gout.

CLINICAL PRESENTATION

- Animals with pseudogout usually present with obvious joint swellings.
- One or more joints may be affected.
- The animal may be lame

RISK FACTORS

Husbandry

Excessive calcium and vitamin D supplementation may be a predisposing factor.

Others

Previous joint damage, previous metabolic bone disease or renal disease are all thought to predispose to the development of pseudogout.

DIAGNOSIS

DIFFERENTIAL DIAGNOSIS

- Gout
- Septic arthritis
- Trauma
- Metabolic bone diseases

DIAGNOSTICS

- Pseudogout may be suspected based on history and clinical examination, but diagnostic testing will be necessary for definitive diagnosis.
- On radiography of affected limbs, calcified lesions may be seen in and around the joints.
- Metastatic calcification on whole-body radiography may also be seen concurrently affecting internal organs, but is not always a feature.
- Demonstration of calcium crystals in joints or within diseased tissue is necessary for definitive diagnosis.
- Aspirates may be taken from affected joints and examined microscopically for the presence of crystals or the whole joint may be submitted for histopathology if amputation is performed.
- Von Kossa or Alizarin red S staining may help in the identification of calcium crystals.

PATHOLOGICAL FINDINGS

- On gross postmortem examination, pale nodules can be seen within or around joints.
- On histopathological examination, nodules are often surrounded by granulomatous inflammation.

TREATMENT

APPROPRIATE HEALTH CARE

- Amputation of the affected digit or limb may be considered if signs are localised.
- If signs are mild, NSAIDs can be given to reduce inflammation and pain.
- Euthanasia may be considered in severe cases.
- Fluid therapy may help dissolve the crystals.

NUTRITIONAL SUPPORT

N/A

CLIENT EDUCATION/HUSBANDRY RECOMMENDATIONS

- Diet should be reviewed to ensure that it is appropriate for the species and not does not contain excessive levels of calcium or vitamin D3.
- Clients should be advised that this is a condition that will require long-term management and can potentially be very painful if allowed to progress.

MEDICATIONS

DRUG(S) OF CHOICE

N/A

PRECAUTIONS/INTERACTIONS

N/A

FOLLOW-UP

PATIENT MONITORING

Response to therapy is usually monitored by physical examination findings (e.g., increase in activity levels or no progression in joint swellings).

EXPECTED COURSE AND PROGNOSIS

- The prognosis for patients with severe widespread signs is poor, but if diagnosed early the condition can often be managed successfully.
- If the underlying cause is not addressed, disease can progress to affect multiple joints.

MISCELLANEOUS

COMMENTS

N/A

ZOONOTIC POTENTIAL

N/A

SYNONYMS

- Chondrocalcinosis
- CPPD crystal deposition disease

ABBREVIATIONS

- CPPD = calcium pyrophosphate dihydrate
- NSAIDs = non-steroidal anti-inflammatories

INTERNET RESOURCES

Veterinary Information Network: www.vin.com

Suggested Reading

Jones YL, Fitzgerald SD. Articular gout and suspected pseudogout in a Basilisk lizard (*Basilicus plumifrons*). *J Zoo Wildl Med* 2009;40(3):576–578.

Mader DR. Gout. In: Mader DR ed. *Reptile Medicine and Surgery*. 2nd ed. Philadelphia, PA: Elsevier Saunders; 2006:374–379.

Rosenthal AK, Ryan LM. Calcium pyrophosphate deposition disease. *N Engl J Med* 2016;374(26):2575–2584.

Author Joanna Hedley BVM&S, DZooMed (Reptilian), DECZM (Herpetology), MRCVS

REGURGITATION

BASICS

DEFINITION/OVERVIEW

Regurgitation is passive discharge through the mouth of undigested food or other contents within a short time after eating.

ETIOLOGY/PATHOPHYSIOLOGY

- Regurgitation usually originates as an esophageal or pharyngeal problem.
- The origin may be gastric if the gastroesophageal sphincter is incompetent or the stomach is markedly diseased.

SIGNALMENT/HISTORY

- All species, ages, sexes may be affected.
- The owner may report observing regurgitation or only that regurgitated material was found.
- Lethargy, anorexia, weight loss, respiratory distress, or increased basking frequency.
- Ingestion of foreign material

CLINICAL PRESENTATION

- No clinical signs are specific to regurgitation, and physical exam may be normal.
- Presentation varies depending on the underlying cause and chronicity.
- Dehydration and/or emaciation/cachexia
- Hard mass on palpation of the coelomic cavity due to an obstructive lesion or organomegaly.
- Skeletal abnormalities that may include pathological fractures or abnormal growth patterns.
- Lethargy and/or obtunded mentation
- Ulceration and accumulation of caseous material in the oral cavity.
- Secondary respiratory disease (e.g., oral/nasal discharge, abnormal respiratory sounds) or enteritis (e.g., diarrhea).

RISK FACTORS

Husbandry

- Too much disturbance or lack of hiding places (increases stress/anxiety).
- Poor sanitation, overcrowding, hyper- or hypothermia, lack of quarantine for new individuals (increases stress, possibility of secondary infections, and disease transmission).
- Toxin exposure (cleaning chemicals, pesticides, heavy metals).
- Excessive/inappropriate handling (especially soon after feeding).
- Inadequate diet (incorrect calcium/phosphorus ratio, improper prey items, excessive feeding).
- Inappropriate substrate (may be accidentally ingested).

Others

Concomitant infectious or parasitic disease

DIAGNOSIS

DIFFERENTIAL DIAGNOSIS

- Stomatitis
- Esophagitis
- Esophageal stricture
- Gastritis
- Handling/stress (e.g., excessive pressure to coelom)
- Obstructive lesions (e.g., GI foreign body, intussusception, neoplasia, abscess, granuloma)
- Metabolic disease (e.g., NSHP, renal or hepatic dysfunction)
- Toxicoses (e.g., zinc)
- Iatrogenic (e.g., enrofloxacin, xylazine, levamisole)
- Trauma to esophagus or stomach
- Parasites (e.g., *Cryptosporidium*, amoebiasis, ascaridiasis, cestodiasis)
- Viruses
- Bacteria/septicemia (e.g., *Chlamydophila*)
- Congenital GI defects

DIAGNOSTICS

- Husbandry review
- Physical examination
- Complete blood count and plasma biochemistries.
- Radiography with or without contrast
- Ultrasonography
- Fecal parasite exam
- Bacterial cultures from oral lesions
- GI endoscopy or coeliotomy (direct tissue evaluation and biopsy).

Suspected Cryptosporidiosis

- Acid-fast staining and/or IFA of feces, regurgitated material, or gastric wash (best collected 3 days after feeding in carnivorous species).
- PCR of feces, regurgitated material, gastric wash, or biopsy from affected tissues (e.g., stomach).

PATHOLOGICAL FINDINGS

- Dependent on underlying cause
- Cryptosporidiosis in lizards primarily affects the intestinal tract, but could also potentially affect the stomach.

TREATMENT

APPROPRIATE HEALTH CARE

The primary goal is to identify and address the underlying cause.

NUTRITIONAL SUPPORT

- Correct fluid deficits and maintain hydration. Intracoelomic, subcutaneous, or intravenous routes for administration of a reptile Ringer's solution are most effective. Maintenance rate is 10–30 ml/kg/day.
- Tube or assist-feeding liquid or gel diets (e.g., EmerAid®, Hill's® Prescription Diet® a/d®; Mazuri® Amphibian & Carnivorous Reptile Gel; Oxbow Professional Line™®) may be beneficial during initial treatment/recovery. Gradually add normal diet items as animal improves.

CLIENT EDUCATION/HUSBANDRY RECOMMENDATIONS

- Review husbandry and correct any problems.
- Avoid overfeeding and disturbing carnivorous lizards 1–2 days after feeding.
- Institute quarantine procedures for new animals, including 30–60-day period, veterinary evaluation, and 1–3-weekly fecal exams for parasites.

MEDICATIONS

DRUG(S) OF CHOICE

- Cimetidine 4 mg/kg IM, PO q8–12h, or famotidine 0.25–0.5 mg/kg SC, PO q24–72h.
- Metoclopramide 0.06 mg/kg PO q24h for 7 days, or cisapride 0.5–2 mg/kg PO q24h.
- Sucralfate 500-1000 mg/kg PO q 6-8 h.

PRECAUTIONS/INTERACTIONS

N/A

FOLLOW-UP

PATIENT MONITORING

Monitor for continued signs of regurgitation and possible complications.

EXPECTED COURSE AND PROGNOSIS

- Dependent on underlying cause
- Prognosis for subclinical cryptosporidiosis is fair to good.
- Prognosis for clinical disease is poor to grave, and euthanasia is often indicated.

MISCELLANEOUS

COMMENTS

N/A

ZOONOTIC POTENTIAL

N/A

SYNONYMS

Reflux

ABBREVIATIONS

- GI = gastrointestinal
- IFA = immunofluorescence antibody assay
- IM = intramuscular

- NSHP = nutritional secondary hyperparathyroidism
- PCR = polymerase chain reaction
- PO = per os
- SC = subcutaneous

Suggested Reading

Funk RS. Vomiting and regurgitation. In: Mader DR, ed. *Reptile Medicine and Surgery*. 2nd ed. St. Louis, MO: Elsevier Saunders; 2006:939–940.

Gibbons PM, Klaphake E, Carpenter JW. Reptiles. In: Carpenter JW, Marion CJ, eds. *Exotic Animal Formulary*. 4th ed. St. Louis, MO: Elsevier Saunders; 2013:83–182.

Mitchell MA, Diaz-Figueroa O. Clinical reptile gastroenterology. *Vet Clin N Am Exot Anim Pract* 2005;8:277–298.

Author Tamara Kruse, DVM, MS, and Trevor T. Zachariah, DVM, MS, DACZM

RENAL SECONDARY HYPERPARATHYROIDISM

BASICS

DEFINITION/OVERVIEW

RSHP can be a common occurrence in captive reptiles. It is a consequence of late-stage chronic renal failure, where calcium and vitamin D levels are depleted. The decrease in blood calcium triggers an overproduction of PTH, which stimulates resorption of bone tissue. Prognosis for this disease is poor to guarded, because even if calcium imbalances can be corrected, the renal function is rarely improved by means of current treatments.

ETIOLOGY/PATHOPHYSIOLOGY

- RSHP develops in reptiles suffering of chronic renal failure.
- Reduction in renal mass results in diminished elimination of phosphorus with a consequent increase in serum phosphate concentrations, and decreased 1,25-dihydroxycholecalciferol (vitamin D3) formation.
- Both these perturbations lead to a decrease of blood calcium, which is followed by an uncontrolled, diffuse proliferation of parathyroid cells (polyclonal proliferation) in the initial stages of the disease, and subsequently in nodular proliferation (monoclonal proliferation) in patients with higher stages of chronic kidney disease.
- The consequent increase in PTH concentrations result in increased osteoclastic activity and severe bone resorption.
- In humans, the cardiovascular system is also affected as a consequence of the increased PTH levels, with increased risk of congestive heart failure and coronary artery disease.
- Chronic renal failure may be triggered by degenerative disease, as caused by diets with excess in proteins, and infectious diseases, including picornavirus infection.

SIGNALMENT/HISTORY

- Compared with NSHP, RSHP is more commonly seen in older animals, where a chronic decline in kidney function lead to the aforementioned metabolic disturbances.
- Less commonly, an entire group of young reptiles is presented with clinical signs related with metabolic bone disease with no history of poor diet or improper husbandry.
- An infectious agent affecting the kidneys should be considered in these cases.

CLINICAL PRESENTATION

- Compared with NSHP, reptiles with RSHP do not have significant bone resorption when presented for clinical examination.
- Most reptiles with RSHP are presented for clinical signs caused by renal failure, including celomic effusion, anorexia and lethargy.
- Alternatively, they may present with the acute consequence of hypocalcemia, which includes seizures-like crisis, muscle tremors, depression and collapse.
- Reptiles with RSHP and chronic renal failure may present with increase in kidney size.

RISK FACTORS

Husbandry

- Lizards that develop RSHP during adulthood typically have a chronic history of poor husbandry and diet.
- Excess in dietary protein intake
- Low fiber content in the diet
- Low environmental humidity resulting in chronic dehydration.
- Inappropriate environmental temperatures resulting in inadequate metabolism.
- Lack of brumation in brumating species resulting in excessive growth rates.

Others

- Toxic exposure
- Neoplasia
- Infectious disease
- Degenerative renal changes including fluid-filled and epidermoid cyst formation.

DIAGNOSIS

DIFFERENTIAL DIAGNOSIS

- Differential diagnoses for seizure-like activity and muscle tremors include other causes of hypocalcemia, particularly NSHP and primary hyperparathyroidism.
- Differential diagnoses for increased renal size include gout and neoplasia.
- Other forms of renal failure may mimic the clinical signs of RSHP.

DIAGNOSTICS

- In most cases, a clinical suspicion of chronic kidney disease is made based on history of long-term inappropriate diet and/or husbandry and clinical signs.
- Diagnosis of RSHP is supported by hyperphosphatemia with concurrent hypocalcemia. Increased uric acid and/or urea may also be observed.
- Alterations in phosphorus, calcium and uric acid/urea due to RSHP typically do not improve with fluid therapy.
- PTH levels may be measured but reference intervals are lacking for most reptile species.
- Radiographs can be used to evaluate bone cortices.
- Ultrasound can be used to evaluate renal and parathyroid parenchyma.
- If coelomic effusion is present, perform standard cytological and microbiological analyses.

PATHOLOGICAL FINDINGS

- Grossly, the kidneys may be enlarged and may present superficial and/or parenchymal alterations.
- Depending on the severity of the RSHP, bone softening or deformity may be observed, including jaws and/or long bones in lizards.
- Alterations of parathyroid glands may be present as generalized or focal enlargements.
- Histopathology of kidneys may reveal different degrees and types of renal alterations.
- Histopathological bone lesions may range from increased osteoclastic resorption of otherwise well-formed and mineralized bones, to thinning of lamina and widening of medullary cavities, with scalloped endosteal surfaces due to increased resorptive activity.
- Long bones may show thinned cortices with layers of osteoblasts and unmineralized osteoid on the periosteal surface.

TREATMENT

APPROPRIATE HEALTH CARE

N/A

NUTRITIONAL SUPPORT

- Reptiles with RSHP are often anorectic.
- The anorexia is usually associated with the concurrent renal failure and may persist for long period.
- Lizards with severe bone depletion may not be able to ingest food due to the changes in the mandibular bones.
- In either case, nutritional support in form of periodic gavage feeding or placement of an esophagostomy tube must be implemented.

CLIENT EDUCATION/HUSBANDRY RECOMMENDATIONS

- Chronic renal failure is more common in animals that had improper husbandry and diet during their life.
- Owners should be informed that at the very first signs of renal failure (e.g., limb/coelomic swelling, anorexia, decreased activity), a thorough veterinary assessment is required for early diagnosis and to limit phosphorus increase, calcium depletion, and consequent PTH increase.
- Owners should be advised to feed diets low in proteins and high in fiber.
- For non-aquatic species, a low environmental humidity may result in chronic dehydration, which exacerbates renal failure.
- It is believed that either excessive or insufficient environmental temperatures may worsen renal disease.

• In brumating species, the procedure of systematic skipping brumation by artificial provision of heat during the winter can lead to physiologic strain on the organs.

MEDICATIONS

DRUG(S) OF CHOICE

• In reptiles with RSHP, both the hyperparathyroidism and the renal disease should be corrected.
• Treatment of RSHP includes therapy designed to minimise the clinical and pathophysiological consequences of reduced kidney function and at correcting the primary cause of the renal impairment, including bacterial, fungal, and parasitic disease.
• The main goal of therapy is to correct calcium, phosphorus, and uric acid/urea levels.
• In cases where renal disease has been caused by improper husbandry, the mainstay of the therapy is an improvement in husbandry and diet.
• Exposure to UVB light daily
• Fluid therapy 20–30 ml/kg/day IV, IO, SC, ICe.
• Phosphate binders (lanthanum carbonate octahydrate) 120–200 mg/kg mixed with feed q24h.
• Calcium gluconate 50–100 mg/kg SC, IM, IV q6–24h followed by calcium glubionate at 50–360 mg/kg PO q12–24h.
• Allopurinol 100 mg/kg q24h if hyperuricemic.
• Angiotensin-converting enzyme inhibitors and antihypertensive therapy may also be considered on a case-by-case basis.

PRECAUTIONS/INTERACTIONS

• Lanthanum carbonate octahydrate has been tested as a feed additive (120–200 mg/kg/day in food) in bearded dragons and chameleons with renal disease.
• In most reptiles, blood phosphorus levels decreased but in chameleons, vomiting was a frequent occurrence. The use of this phosphate binder in chameleons is currently discouraged.

FOLLOW-UP

PATIENT MONITORING

• If reptiles are presented in acute hypocalcemic crisis, intensive care and frequent monitoring of phosphorus and calcium levels (ionized and total), as well as other electrolytes and ECG activity is essential.
• Also, in young reptiles with RSHP as a consequence of bacterial or viral renal infection, intensive care should be provided until the infection is resolved.
• In cases of chronic RSHP, if the reptile is eating on its own, a physical exam once every 7–14 days, accompanied by blood work (hematocrit, uric acid/urea, calcium and phosphorus), is recommended to assess response to therapy.

EXPECTED COURSE AND PROGNOSIS

• The prognosis for animals suffering RSHP is poor.
• Even if calcium and phosphorus imbalances can be corrected via fluid therapy, exogenous supplementation, and phosphate binder administration, there is currently no effective treatment for renal failure in reptiles.

MISCELLANEOUS

• Currently, it seems that intestinal phosphate binders have a species-specific activity and their use is discouraged in chameleons.
• There is a need to develop novel diets that may reduce the protein intake in carnivorous/omnivorous reptiles suffering of renal disease but at the same time provide the correct amount of nutrients.

COMMENTS

N/A

ZOONOTIC POTENTIAL

N/A

SYNONYMS

Renal-related metabolic bone disease

ABBREVIATIONS

• ECG = electrocardiogram
• ICe = intracoelomic
• IO = intraosseous
• IV = intravenous
• NSHP = nutritional secondary hyperparathyroidism
• PTH = parathyroid hormone
• RSHP = renal secondary hyperparathyroidism
• SC = subcutaneous
• UVB = ultraviolet B

INTERNET RESOURCES

• Additional information on reptile renal physiology from Carl Gans Collections: Biology of the Reptilia. http://carlgans.org/bor-view/?borv=5&borpage=447&borp=459
• Information on secondary hyperparathyroidism in humans: Kim L. Hyperparathyroidism. Medscape, August 18, 2020. http://emedicine.medscape.com/article/127351-overview?pa=mcKd1JF66kULHOzxxIxn2fK%2Bx5xE5kE6dUeU7dvJSrcnjyhACchqCtq5rNZR2UhkQPQxex%2Bo7mr5pATtx84gCBXKySxof3ndUJD5aivxmIc%3D#a4

Suggested Reading

Hernandez-Divers SJ, Martinez-Jimenez D, Bush S, et al. Effects of allopurinol on plasma uric acid levels in normouricaemic and hyperuricaemic green iguanas (*Iguana iguana*). *Vet Rec* 2008;162(4):112–115.
Heuser W, Pendl H, Knowles NJ, et al. Soft plastron, soft carapace with skeletal abnormality in juvenile tortoises: Histopathology and isolation of a novel picornavirus from *Testudo graeca* and *Geochelone elegans*. *Tierarztl Prax Ausg K Kleintiere Heimtiere.* 2014;42(5):310–320.
Selleri P, Hernandez-Divers SJ. Renal diseases of reptiles. *Vet Clin North Am Exot Anim Pract* 2006;9(1):161–174.

Author Paolo Selleri, DMV, PhD, SpecPACS, DECZM (Herpetology & Small Mammals), and Nicola Di Girolamo, DMV, MSc (EBHC), PhD, DECZM (Herpetology)

SALMONELLOSIS

BASICS

DEFINITION/OVERVIEW

Salmonellosis is a cosmopolitan disease that can infect all vertebrates. While salmonellosis can occur in lizards, most serve as latent carriers or reservoirs of *Salmonella* spp. and pose a zoonotic concern for pet owners. Historically, green iguanas (*Iguana iguana*) were considered an important reservoir for reptile-associated salmonellosis; however, due to changes in the reptile trade, bearded dragons (*Pogona vitticeps*) have now taken over in popularity and as important potential reservoirs for this pathogen. Lizards that are affected may develop gastroenteritis (e.g., diarrhea) or systemic disease (e.g., abscesses). *Salmonella* spp. should be considered a component of the indigenous microflora of lizards. Because these animals can naturally harbor this pathogen, clients should be made aware of the risks of ownership and provided information regarding best hygiene practices to minimize their exposure.

ETIOLOGY/PATHOPHYSIOLOGY

- Anaerobic, Gram-negative, straight rods, flagellated.
- Species: *Salmonella bongori* and *S. enterica*, subsp. *enterica* [1], *salamae* [II], *arizonae* [IIIa], *diarizonae* [IIIb], *houtenae* [IV], and *indica* [VI].
- Reptiles are most likely to be carriers of *S. arizonae* [IIIa] and *S. diarizonae* [IIIb].
- There are over 2,637 extant *Salmonella* serovars. All *Salmonella* serovars should be considered pathogenic. Serovars are characterized by their somatic (O) and flagellar (H) antigens. Common serovars identified in lizards include Newport, Poona, Saint-Paul, Typhimurium, and Pomona. It is not uncommon to have multiple serotypes in the same lizard. Serovar identification is still used to identify sources of salmonellosis. Additionally, antimicrobial resistance patterns and pulse-field gel electrophoresis are used to confirm the sources of salmonellosis for human patients.
- The prevalence of *Salmonella* spp. in wild and captive lizards can vary between 0% and 100%. Captive raised animals have a higher prevalence because of stocking densities leading to increased exposure, and poor hygiene practices. The low prevalence reported in wild lizards may be associated with the sampling method; single samples are typically collected for prevalence studies and may misclassify animals due to intermittent shedding.
- The epidemiology of *Salmonella* infection in lizards has been evaluated using the green iguana as a model. Green iguanas raised at a breeding farm were found to be exposed through both horizontal and vertical routes of transmission. Horizontal transmission can occur via contaminated sources of food, water, and soil. Similarly, animals housed in captivity may be exposed or re-exposed through these sources. It is for this reason that clients should be made aware of the importance of removing feces from an enclosure on a regular basis. Vertical transmission is likely at the level of the follicle, as *Salmonella* spp. has been isolated from the ovary of green iguanas, and during the time of egg deposition. When eggs pass through the cloaca, they are potentially contaminated by *Salmonella* spp. shed through the colon. Lizards can serve as a source of *Salmonella* spp. in their captive environment by serving as both direct and indirect sources of contamination.

SIGNALMENT/HISTORY

- Because many of the cases of lizard associated salmonellosis are from latent carriers, all animals should be considered *Salmonella* spp. positive.
- More specifically, bearded dragons and iguanas are species of concern because their pet owners often allow them free roam in the household or place them on surfaces where food is prepared.

CLINICAL PRESENTATION

- Lizards that are carriers of *Salmonella* spp. typically appear healthy on physical examination or present for another illness; thus, it is important to recognize that these animals may serve as a potential source of infection to the veterinary staff working with them or that the treatment used (e.g., antibiotics) could alter the pathogenicity of the *Salmonella* spp.
- Lizards presenting with primary salmonellosis may present with the following clinical signs: lethargy, anorexia, weakness, failure to thrive, weight loss, decreased body condition, neurological abnormalities, coelomic swelling or mass, or osteomyelitis.

RISK FACTORS

Husbandry

- Inappropriate husbandry conditions can potentiate the likelihood of infection for conspecifics and the human caretakers of lizards.
- Environmental temperatures should be appropriate for the species, as low or high temperatures can lead to stress and the potential for increased shedding of the organism.
- Substrate should be changed regularly as high organic loads can increase the growth rate of *Salmonella* spp.
- Animal density and mixing of lizards can increase stress levels and *Salmonella* spp. shedding.
- Routine cleaning and disinfection of a lizard's enclosure is necessary to prevent dissemination of *Salmonella* spp.

Others

- Source of animals: confiscated or imported animals have an increased risk associated with clinical illness and zoonotic potential because of the increased likelihood of shedding *Salmonella* spp.
- Stress: shipping, overcrowding, and suboptimal husbandry conditions can lead to infection or increased shedding of *Salmonella* spp.

DIAGNOSIS

DIFFERENTIAL DIAGNOSIS

- Enteritis (other species of Enterobacteriaceae)
- Renal disease
- Liver disease
- Primary and secondary bacterial infections
- Fungal infections
- Neoplasia
- Osteomyelitis

DIAGNOSTICS

- Microbiological culture of a gastrointestinal sample or abscess can be used to confirm the presence of *Salmonella* spp. Positive fecal cultures in clinically normal animals are not uncommon. These animals should not be treated for *Salmonella* spp., as this can lead to the development of antimicrobial resistance in the *Salmonella* spp.
- Culture of *Salmonella* spp. requires special consideration, as the organism can be outcompeted by other Enterobacteriaceae under standard culture methods. Thus, it is important to specifically request a *Salmonella* spp. culture from your diagnostic laboratory if the organism is suspected. Enrichment with selenite or tetrathionate is required. Samples are then plated onto specific agars such as XLD, SS, or XLT-4 agars. XLD and XLT-4 agars have a hydrogen sulfide indicator system to detect lactose fermenting *Salmonella* spp.
- Factors that influence the reliability of culture include the collection method, quantity and/or type of sample collected, temporal variation in shedding, and culture methods. Time to perform culture can delay appropriate antimicrobial therapy and control/mitigation procedures.
- PCR testing can be used to confirm the presence of *Salmonella* spp. in a sample. This test is considered more sensitive than culture and provides faster turnaround times. One limitation is that it cannot provide an antibiotic sensitivity profile to guide treatment.
- Parallel testing with PCR and culture is recommended to increase the sensitivity of the testing methods.
- Complete blood counts can be used to confirm an inflammatory leukogram or toxic changes that might occur with salmonellosis.

• Radiography can be used to examine the coelomic cavity for organomegaly and bony structures for osteomyelitis.
• Ultrasound can be used to improve visualization of the coelomic organs.
• Fine-needle aspiration of coelomic fluid or osteomyelitis and cytologic review of the sample can be used to confirm the presence of Gram-negative bacteria and inflammatory cells.

PATHOLOGICAL FINDINGS

• *Salmonella* spp. are commonly isolated from the gastrointestinal tract of lizards on postmortem examinations as an incidental finding.
• Lizards that have clinical salmonellosis will have typical inflammatory signs associated with the pathogen causing an enteritis, osteomyelitis, or systemic infection.

TREATMENT

APPROPRIATE HEALTH CARE

• Lizards that are clinically normal and not showing signs of disease should never be treated for *Salmonella* spp.
• Treating animals that are latent carriers could potentiate antimicrobial resistance.
• Animals that are clinically affected by *Salmonella* spp. should only be treated if an antibiotic sensitivity profile is available. This will help to minimize the likelihood of resistance.
• Some clinicians elect to not treat affected animals with antibiotics but instead provide supportive care and allow the infection to run its course.
• As with any bacterial disease, therapy should be driven by culture and antibiotic sensitivity testing.
• Minimum inhibitory concentration information is valuable in these cases to increase the likelihood for treatment success.
• Because *Salmonella* spp. are indigenous in lizards, treatment with antibiotics for other ailments may impact their resistance patterns.

NUTRITIONAL SUPPORT

• Nutritional support should be implemented in patients that have concurrent weight loss, hyporexia, or anorexia; however, fluid support should be provided first to ensure the gastrointestinal tract is functioning properly.
• In animals with diarrhea, nutritional support can exacerbate the diarrhea.
• Assist-feeding can support the daily nutritional requirements of these patients with a highly digestible diet, which should be based on the species life history and nutritional requirements.

CLIENT EDUCATION/HUSBANDRY RECOMMENDATIONS

• Clients should be educated on the risks of keeping lizards and provided information on the most appropriate husbandry and sanitation procedures.
• Owners should be made aware that it is not recommended to allow their lizard to free roam in their household. This can serve as a source of indirect exposure for children.
• To minimize the zoonotic potential of lizards, it is important to practice strict hygiene and biosecurity.
• Hand washing with soap and warm water is one of the simplest and most effective methods of eliminating exposure to *Salmonella* spp.
• Individuals handling these animals or any part of their captive habitat should wash their hands thoroughly after working with them.
• The water removed from the enclosures of these animals should be discarded outside or down a toilet. It should never be discarded down a sink used for cooking or cleaning food or where water is obtained for drinking or a bathtub.
• The enclosure and its contents should be cleaned outside, if at all possible, and never in an area where food or drink is prepared.
• Separate washing receptacles, such as a plastic container, are recommended.
• Dilute bleach solution can be used to clean the environment and food and water bowls; however, it is important that the client rinse these thoroughly to minimize the potential for bleach toxicity.

MEDICATIONS

DRUG(S) OF CHOICE

Salmonella spp. isolated from lizards are typically susceptible to the following antibiotics:
• Ceftiour sodium 5 mg/kg IM, SC q24h.
• Ceftiofur crystalline-free acid 30 mg/kg q10–12d.
• Amikacin 5 mg/kg IM loading then 2.5 mg/kg q72h.
• Enrofloxacin 5–10 mg/kg IM, PO q24–48h.

PRECAUTIONS/INTERACTIONS

N/A

FOLLOW-UP

PATIENT MONITORING

• Serial culture and PCR testing can be done to monitor the *Salmonella* spp. status and antimicrobial sensitivity profile of a patient or captive population of lizards.
• Complete blood counts to monitor responses to treatment.
• Repeat radiographs to monitor for progression or resolution of osseous lesions.

EXPECTED COURSE AND PROGNOSIS

• Lizards diagnosed with salmonellosis from culture or PCR may not require any intervention.
• Many lizards test positive for *Salmonella* spp., but these animals are often latent carriers and do not show signs of disease.
• Animals that test negative for *Salmonella* spp. on a single test may still be positive because intermittent shedding is common.

MISCELLANEOUS

COMMENTS

N/A

ZOONOTIC POTENTIAL

• Lizards have and continue to serve as a source of reptile-associated salmonellosis for humans.
• Because these animals serve as reservoirs and latent carriers of *Salmonella* spp., clients are often unaware as to the risks associated with maintaining these animals as pets.
• To minimize the zoonotic potential of lizards, it is important to practice strict hygiene and biosecurity.

SYNONYMS

Typhoid fever

ABBREVIATIONS

• IM = intramuscular
• PCR = polymerase chain reaction
• SC = subcutaneous
• SS = Salmonella–Shigella
• XLT = xylose lysine desoxycholate
• XLT-4 = xylose lysine-Tergitol 4

INTERNET RESOURCES

Centers for Disease Control and Prevention, National Center for Emerging and Zoonotic Infectious Diseases. Reptiles and Amphibians. October 28, 2019. https://www.cdc.gov/features/salmonellafrogturtle/index.html

Association of Reptile and Amphibian Veterinarians: http://www.ARAV.org

Center for Food Security and Public Health. Reptile Associated Salmonellosis. January 2013. http://www.cfsph.iastate.edu/DiseaseInfo/factsheets.php

Suggested Reading

Clancy MM, Davis M, Valitutto MT, et al. Salmonella infection and carriage in reptiles in a zoological collection. *J Am Vet Med Assoc* 2016;248(9):1050–1059.

Gray TZ. Update: reptiles and salmonella. *J Exot Pet Med* 2011;20(1):14–17. https://doi.org/10.1053/j.jepm.2010.11.005

Authors Sean M. Perry, DVM, PhD, and Mark A. Mitchell, DVM, MS, PhD, DECZM (Herpetology)

SQUAMOUS CELL CARCINOMA

BASICS

DEFINITION/OVERVIEW

SCCs are malignant epithelial cell tumors, most commonly associated with cutaneous or mucocutaneous regions of the body. In reptiles, SCCs are most commonly found on the skin or associated with oropharyngeal tissues. They tend to be well differentiated with some evidence of local infiltration of adjacent tissues, and limited evidence of metastatic behavior. SCCs are not uncommon in reptile species, and have been identified in a variety of lizards (including one tuatara).

ETIOLOGY/PATHOPHYSIOLOGY

- An underlying cause of SCCs in reptiles is unknown.
- Published hypotheses with respect to risk factors and etiology include those based on mammalian or avian examples: overexposure to ultraviolet radiation, including exposure at higher altitudes, light skin color, chronic hypovitaminosis A, and possibly chronic viral infections. However, there is no evidence that any of these risk factors are associated with reptile SCCs.
- No viruses have been associated with SCCs in reptiles.
- Most reptile SCCs are locally invasive; metastasis is uncommon.

SIGNALMENT/HISTORY

- In the reptile neoplasia literature, there is no clear predisposition with respect to species or sex.
- There may be an association between the presence of SCCs and increasing age of the reptile, but this has not been evaluated systematically.
- Historically, reptiles diagnosed with SCC are observed to have a focal mass or masses anywhere on the skin, within the oral cavity, or at other mucocutaneous junctions.
- The raised tissue may become hemorrhagic, ulcerative and/or necrotic.
- With chronicity, bacterial abscessation may develop within or in close association with the tumor. Most commonly, the neoplastic cells invade adjacent tissues.
- Depending on the site of the tumor, the animal may become hyporexic/anorexic, exhibit a depressed attitude, and/or favor a limb/eye or other anatomical sites that may be involved.
- If the eyes are involved, vision may become impaired and the animal may, uncharacteristically, fall from cage furniture or not be able to find food.

CLINICAL PRESENTATION

- The clinical signs may be somewhat variable depending on the anatomic locations of the mass.
- Discrete skin lesions tend to appear raised, with erythema, hemorrhage, and/or ulceration, or appear as chronic nonhealing wounds.
- If the lesions involve the digits, there may be more diffuse swelling and some degree of lameness.
- With SCCs of the oropharynx, hyporexia, or anorexia may be present, in addition to masticatory dysfunction and mild oral hemorrhage.

RISK FACTORS

Husbandry

- Purely hypothetical risk factors in reptiles are based on mammalian or avian risk factors.
- In the case of husbandry, hypovitaminosis A or excessive ultraviolet light exposure could be predisposing risk factors but there is no evidence documenting a link between these factors and SCCs.

Others

N/A

DIAGNOSIS

DIFFERENTIAL DIAGNOSIS

- Bacterial abscesses
- Fungal granulomas (especially *Chrysosporium* species)
- Viral papillomatous lesions
- Chronic traumatic wounds with fibrosis
- Cloacal prolapse
- Other neoplastic diseases (e.g., melanomas, fibrosarcomas, cutaneous papillomas, fibropapillomas, lipomas, spindle cell sarcomas, and chromatophormas).

DIAGNOSTICS

- Histopathology of the lesion is the gold standard for diagnosis, through complete surgical excision or biopsy of the mass.
- A fine-needle aspirate with cytologic evaluation may or may not be diagnostic.
- Imaging modalities, such as radiography or CT may be helpful in detecting local soft tissue or bone involvement.
- Contrast CT may be useful when trying to evaluate for metastases.

PATHOLOGICAL FINDINGS

- In domestic mammals, histologic subtypes of SCCs are typically described as poorly differentiated, moderately differentiated, or well differentiated.
- In general, SCCs are histopathologically characterized as round to polygonal cells with varying amounts of basophilic cytoplasm and keratinization.
- The nuclei tend to be round, with significant variation in size and chromatin pattern; from coarsely stippled to pyknotic, and commonly with perinuclear vacuoles. Frequently, there is marked variation in nucleus to cytoplasm ratio because the cells vary in degree of differentiation.
- In reptiles, the histologic description of SCC is similar. Typically, there are anastomosing cords and nests of polygonal cells with abundant eosinophilic cytoplasm, distinct intercellular bridges, and round to oval nuclei with finely stippled chromatin and multiple nucleoli, with occasional mitotic figures.
- Neoplastic cells are described as having differing levels of anisokaryosis, and frequently form circular keratinized foci consistent with keratin pearls and usually invade and/or replace adjacent tissues.

TREATMENT

APPROPRIATE HEALTH CARE

N/A

NUTRITIONAL SUPPORT

- Non-specific nutritional support may include regular force-feeding of an appropriate commercial diet and/or placement of an esophagostomy tube to facilitate administering nutritional supplements, especially to patients in which the oral cavity is not easily accessible.

CLIENT EDUCATION/HUSBANDRY RECOMMENDATIONS

N/A

MEDICATIONS

DRUG(S) OF CHOICE

- Surgical excision with histopathologic evidence of clean margins is the treatment of choice.
- In birds and mammals, focal SCCs have been treated with surgical debulking and intralesional platinum-based chemotherapeutic agents (e.g., cisplatin or carboplatin-impregnated beads).
- SCC was diagnosed in a panther chameleon, with raised lesions on the skin of the lateral body wall.
- Some lesions were surgically debulked, but those that could not be debulked were implanted with cisplatin impregnated beads. The masses implanted with beads shrunk in size.
- Antimicrobial drugs may be used as needed for secondary bacterial infections.

• NSAIDs may help with any discomfort, but there are no systematically derived data with respect to efficacy of NSAIDs in any reptile species.
• There are also no data demonstrating negative adverse effects, such as renal impairment and/or gastrointestinal bleeding.
• Depending on the species, meloxicam may be administered orally or subcutaneously (0.2–0.5 mg/kg).

PRECAUTIONS/INTERACTIONS

• With surgical excision of a SCC, recurrence should be considered and discussed with the owner.
• Should the owner elect intralesional chemotherapy, the possible outcomes include lack of therapeutic response; systemic absorption of the chemotherapeutic agent causing hyporexia/anorexia, depressed attitude, anemia or other blood cell changes, and necrosis of surrounding healthy tissues.

FOLLOW-UP

PATIENT MONITORING

• SCCs are likely to recur with incomplete surgical excision and may recur regardless of complete surgical excision.
• In addition, there are a few documented cases of local tissue invasion and/or metastasis.
• The patient should be monitored for recurrence of the tumor, and contrast CT may be of some use in monitoring for local invasion or metastatic disease.
• If treatment is recommended and accepted by the owner (partial excision and intralesional chemotherapy or electrochemotherapy), the treatment site should be monitored for secondary microbial infection or self-trauma.
• The owner should be instructed to report any signs of skin discoloration, discharge, or dysfunction of the anatomical region of the original tumor.
• Because of possible systemic absorption of locally administered chemotherapeutic agents, a complete blood count and biochemical profile should be evaluated prior to the start of chemotherapy, and serially evaluated during and after the course of chemotherapy.

EXPECTED COURSE AND PROGNOSIS

• With complete surgical excision and clean tissue margins as evidenced by histopathology, the prognosis is good to guarded, with the possibility of recurrence.
• With recent published cases documenting metastatic disease, a guarded prognosis is wise until we know more about the behavior of SCCs across multiple reptile species.
• There may be some promising new intralesional chemotherapeutic techniques or refined radiation therapy techniques applied to future cases of SCCs in reptiles, which may improve prognostic factors.

MISCELLANEOUS

COMMENTS

N/A

ZOONOTIC POTENTIAL

N/A

SYNONYMS

N/A

ABBREVIATIONS

• CT = computed tomography
• SCC = squamous cell carcinoma
• NSAIDs nonsteroidal anti-inflammatory drugs

Suggested Reading

Christman J, Devau M, Wilson-Robles H, et al. Oncology of reptiles: diseases, diagnosis, and treatment. *Vet Clin North Am Exot Anim Pract* 2017;20(1):87–110.
Hannon DE, Garner MM, Reavill DR. Squamous cell carcinomas in inland bearded dragons (*Pogona vitticeps*). *J Herp Med Surg* 2011;21(4):101–106.
Johnson J, Naples LM, Chu C, et al. Cutaneous squamous cell carcinoma in a panther chameleon (*Furcifer pardalis*) and treatment with carboplatin implantable beads. *J Zoo Wildl Med* 2016;47(3):931–934.
Sykes JM, Trupkiewicz JG. Reptile neoplasia at the Philadelphia Zoological Garden, 1901–2002. *J Zoo Wildl Med* 2006;37(1):11–19.

Author Kurt K. Sladky, MS, DVM, DACZM, DECZM (Zoo Health Management & Herpetology)

STOMATITIS

BASICS

DEFINITION/OVERVIEW

Stomatitis is inflammation of the soft tissues of the oral cavity, which may be caused by a local or a systemic process.

ETIOLOGY/PATHOPHYSIOLOGY

- Immunosuppression or trauma can lead to bacterial or fungal colonization of oral tissues. Normal bacterial flora secondarily infect damaged oral tissue, particularly Gram-negative rods.
- Fungi, particularly *Candida* spp., *Penicillium* spp., *Aspergillus* spp. and *Mucor* spp.
- Systemic infections
- Varanid herpesvirus 1
- Foreign objects, such as splinters, food debris, cactus spines, bedding material.
- Electric burns from, for example, biting electric cord.
- Lacerations
- Prey injuries: bite or claw wounds from live prey; injuries from sharp teeth or claws from previously frozen prey.
- Facial injuries from striking at enclosure or from rubbing against enclosure.
- Rough handling and damage of teeth and oral mucosa during physical examination.
- Trauma during tong-feeding
- Improper assisted feeding resulting in oral, pharyngeal or esophageal injuries.
- Vomiting and regurgitation may create mucosal defects in esophagus, pharynx or oral mucosa.
- Neoplasia
- NSHP can lead to mandibular swelling and exposure of oral mucosa.
- Hypovitaminosis A, particularly in chameleons.
- Exposure gingivitis secondary to metabolic bone disease is most common in lizards.

SIGNALMENT/HISTORY

- No specific age, breed, sex predisposition.
- Animals with a history of poor husbandry, specifically inappropriate temperatures and hygiene.

CLINICAL PRESENTATION

- Anorexia, dysphagia
- Periorbital swelling, exophthalmos
- Nasal discharge and secondary tracheitis or pneumonia.
- White plaques on mucous membranes, particularly with oral candidiasis.
- Rostral abrasions or callus from persistent facial rubbing or scratching.
- Hemorrhage, edema, swelling of lips and gingiva, ulceration, plaques, ptyalism, tongue dysfunction, halitosis, anorexia, or dysphagia.
- Dyspnea in some animals with choanal or periglottal lesions.
- Electrocution: vesicular and/or charred tissue often associated with a flared pattern; lesions usually associated with tongue, oral cavity, or front digits.
- Non-specific clinical signs associated with infiltrating bacteria causing lesions in liver, kidney, heart, or central nervous system, secondary to osteomyelitis

RISK FACTORS

Husbandry

- Chronic suboptimal temperature is considered one of the most important risk factors.
- Poor hygiene, overcrowding, improper light cycles, poor air quality, excess or insufficient humidity, toxin exposure, improper brumation, malnutrition.

Others

- Pathogen contaminated food or water: hay-based bedding is subject to molding.
- Bite wounds and facial injuries from territorial disputes.
- Feeding live prey

DIAGNOSIS

DIFFERENTIAL DIAGNOSIS

- Rule out septicemia as cause of oral petechiation. Usually ulceration and caseous lesions with stomatitis.
- Ulcerated neoplasms are usually focal whereas stomatitis is more typically diffuse.
- Consider neoplasia in cases unresponsive to supportive therapy and correction of improper husbandry.
- Abnormal maxilla and/or mandibles with NSHP.
- Tongue dysfunction from infection, trauma, electrocution, inflammatory masses, neoplasia, and NSHP.

DIAGNOSTICS

- Physical examination: pay particular attention to eyes, teeth, choana, and oral tissues.
- Use of a small otoscope or endoscope may be necessary for complete examination and to facilitate collection of samples. Anesthesia or sedation may be necessary.
- Cytology and culture: must target the deeper layers of affected tissue to minimize superficial contamination. The surface of the lesions can also be cleaned /disinfected prior to collection of samples. Aerobic, anaerobic and fungal cultures should be considered.
- Biopsy: particularly in recurring or persistent lesions; preclean the tissue to collect samples for culture. Histopathology is key to further understanding the results of cytology and culture. Herpesvirus is often associated with intranuclear inclusion bodies associated with necrotic epithelium.
- CBC and plasma biochemistry may be useful to detect systemic disease and severity of tissue damage. CBC may be normal or may show toxic changes within heterophils if bacterial or fungal infection.
- Advanced imaging: radiography, CT or MRI can be used to identify severity of bone or ocular involvement.

PATHOLOGICAL FINDINGS

Histopathologic finding will vary depending on the etiologic agent involved.

TREATMENT

APPROPRIATE HEALTH CARE

- Therapy will fail if underlying cause is not identified and corrected.
- Maintain sick reptiles, and those receiving medications, at high end of POTZ for the species, (80–90 degrees F for most reptiles; 100 degrees F for desert species). Some pathogens may be less pathogenic at higher temperatures and the reptile immune system may be more efficient; increases heart rate, improves circulation, improves fluid and antibiotic distribution, improves neural response, increases muscular activity, and stimulates enzyme activity.
- Mild and acute lesions: debride and clean lesions followed by application of topical antimicrobial and/or antifungal.
- Deep and severe lesions require topical treatment described above as well as broad-spectrum systemic antimicrobials for bacteria (aerobic or anaerobic) or fungi, based on results of cytology. Adjust therapy as needed based on results of culture.
- Antimicrobial therapy alone is unlikely to be successful if the infection is walled off; there is poor drug penetration into exudates. A combination of aggressive debridement, wound care, and antibiotic therapy is likely to yield better results.

NUTRITIONAL SUPPORT

- Correct dehydration and maintain normal hydration level (20–30 ml/kg q24h, IV, IO, ICe in divided dose) during treatment; reptiles that are sufficiently ill to require antimicrobial therapy should be considered dehydrated.
- After rehydration, supportive nutrition is needed to maintain positive nitrogen balance.
- Feed small amounts more frequently.
- Use high protein and fat diets for carnivores and complex carbohydrate diets for herbivores.
- Esophagostomy tube may be needed in severe cases.

CLIENT EDUCATION/HUSBANDRY RECOMMENDATIONS

- Quarantining new arrivals will minimize the risk of introducing a new pathogen to an established collection and will allow the new arrival time to acclimatize to its new environment.
- Follow proper husbandry guidelines for the species at hand.
- Environmental temperature, proper housing, and feeding regimen all play a crucial role in the wellbeing of reptilian species kept in captivity.

MEDICATIONS

DRUG(S) OF CHOICE

- Antibiotic selection is largely empiric based initially on in-clinic cytology and Gram staining, owing to the delay in return of culture results; disease-associated organisms may be noted on cytology that are not cultured.
- Bactericidal drugs are preferable to bacteriostatic drugs.

Antibiotics of Choice for Empirical Treatment

- Amikacin 5 mg/kg IM, then 2.5 mg/kg q72h.
- Azithromycin 10 mg/kg PO q3–7d.
- Carbenicillin 200 mg/kg IM q24h.
- Ceftazidime 20 mg/kg IM q72h.
- Enrofloxacin 5-10 mg/kg IM q48h.
- Metronidazole 20 mg/kg PO q48h.
- Topical antimicrobials/antifungals: iodine, chlorhexidine, and silver based products.
- Antimicrobials may be required for 4–8 weeks.

PRECAUTIONS/INTERACTIONS

Enrofloxacin given parentally can cause tissue necrosis, use with caution.

FOLLOW-UP

PATIENT MONITORING

- Evaluate hydration frequently after starting treatment.
- Make husbandry changes to provide proper environment and nutrition.

EXPECTED COURSE AND PROGNOSIS

- Varies with underlying cause, chronicity and condition of patient.
- Lesions can progress from petechial hemorrhage to overwhelming infection and septicemia within 2–3 days.
- Acute and uncomplicated lesions usually respond to appropriate therapy.
- Untreated infections frequently progress to osteomyelitis, septicemia and death.
- Prognosis is guarded to poor with osteomyelitis depending on chronicity and severity.
- Neoplasia has a poor prognosis unless completely resected and with no metastasis.

MISCELLANEOUS

COMMENTS

Associated Conditions

- Osteomyelitis, sinusitis, septicemia, pneumonia and/or gastroenteritis
- Ocular or periocular disease
- Permanent tongue damage resulting in dysphagia or anorexia
- Pharyngeal cellulitis
- Gout in chameleons

ZOONOTIC POTENTIAL

- Many bacteria and fungi that infect reptiles can also cause disease in humans.
- Any bites from reptiles should be treated as contaminated; immediately wash wounds with soap and water and seek medical attention; humans with open wounds on the hands should not handle reptiles or their secretions or excretions without gloves.

SYNONYMS

- Infectious stomatitis
- Mouth rot
- Ulcerative stomatitis

ABBREVIATIONS

- CBC = complete blood count
- CT = computed tomography
- NSHP = nutritional secondary hyperparathyroidism
- ICe = intracoelomic
- IM = intramuscular
- IO = intraosseous
- IV = intravenous
- MRI = magnetic resonance imaging
- POTZ = preferred optimal temperature zone

INTERNET RESOURCES

- Suedmeyer K, Pollock C, Tristan T. Presenting problem: stomatitis in reptiles. Lafeber Vet, November 11, 2013. https://lafeber.com/vet/presenting-problem-stomatitis-in-reptiles
- Divers SJ. Bacterial diseases of reptiles. MSD Manual Veterinary Manual, June 2020. https://www.merckvetmanual.com/exotic-and-laboratory-animals/reptiles/bacterial-diseases-of-reptiles

Suggested Reading

Jacobson ER, ed. *Infectious Diseases and Pathology of Reptiles: Color Atlas and Text.* Boca Raton, FL: CRC Press, 2007.

Mader DR, Divers SJ, eds. *Current Therapy in Reptile Medicine and Surgery.* St. Louis MO: Elsevier Saunders, 2014.

Author Sam Rivera, DVM, MS, DABVP (avian), DACZM, DECZM (Zoo Health Management)

THERMAL BURNS

BASICS

DEFINITION/OVERVIEW

Reptiles are classified as ectothermic, meaning that they actively seek appropriate environmental temperatures to satisfy metabolic requirements. Periods of increased metabolic activity, such as foraging and digestion, are usually preceded and followed by actively raising core body temperature. Traditionally, heat production has been categorized into three types: radiant heat such as solar energy; convective heat such as currents of warm air; conductive heat such as direct contact with a heat source. Reptiles usually use a combination of all three types of heat acquisition. Ventilation and humidity are also important components of thermodynamics. Most thermal burns are associated with excessive exposure to radiant and/or conductive heat.

ETIOLOGY/PATHOPHYSIOLOGY

- Thermal burns have assorted causes most of which fall into the following categories: close/direct contact with an unprotected focal heat or light source, faulty electrical equipment, or human error.
- Nociception is still poorly understood in reptiles and consequently the question remains unanswered as to why reptiles do not recognize when excessive heat is burning the integument.
- Heated-simulated rocks with faulty thermostats have been associated with ventral burns in lizards. Fortunately, these devices are used with decreasing frequency today.
- Reptiles that are placed outdoors for exposure to UVB light can overheat, particularly if they are not provided with areas of shade.
- Burns can occur when the heating elements are placed dangerously close to the reptile.
- Overhead lights should be outside of the tank entirely, with a tank lid between the lamp and the reptile or placed high enough in the enclosure that the reptile cannot reach it.
- Thermal burns can also occur when a reptile is weak or lethargic due to systemic disease.

SIGNALMENT/HISTORY

- Thermal burns may affect reptiles of all ages and may be more prevalent during the cooler seasons when additional heating devices are used.
- History usually involves exposure to heated-simulated rocks, adhesive heating elements used on the outside of the bottoms of aquariums, or bulbs placed inside the enclosures.

CLINICAL PRESENTATION

- A complete clinical examination should be performed to determine whether there is an underlying disease.
- Clinical signs depend primarily on the severity of lesions.
- Traditionally, thermal burns have been classified according to the depth of damaged tissue.
- First-degree burns cause damage confined to the epidermis and present as erythema and sloughing of damaged scales.
- Second-degree burns involve the epidermis and dermis. These burns present as erythema plus vesicles. The vesicles may rupture causing loss of tissue fluid and protein with a higher risk for secondary bacterial infections.
- Third-degree burns involve destruction of epidermis, dermis and underlying tissues.
- Secondary bacterial and/or fungal infections commonly occur.
- A more recent classification makes use of the terms "partial thickness" and "full thickness" when defining severity of burns.

RISK FACTORS

Husbandry

Exposure to inappropriate or malfunctioning heating sources is the most common cause of thermal burns.

Others

Debilitation secondary to internal disease can predispose a reptile to being too weak to move away from a heat source.

DIAGNOSIS

DIFFERENTIAL DIAGNOSIS

Other causes of dermatoses should be excluded, such as chronic dysecdysis, bacterial/fungal infections, ectoparasitism, trauma, and neoplasia.

DIAGNOSTICS

Diagnosis is based upon history, clinical signs and physical examination.

PATHOLOGICAL FINDINGS

- For a description of gross lesions see section on clinical presentation.
- Histopathologic findings of first-degree burns consist of dilatation of arterioles and venules, increased capillary permeability with filtration of plasma into tissue spaces and migration of erythrocytes and leukocytes.
- Second-degree burns consist of vesicles filled with an acellular transudate in addition to changes associated with first-degree burns.
- Third-degree burns are characterized by destruction of the entire integument followed by sloughing of necrotic tissue. Surrounding this zone are areas of lesser degree burns, as described above.

TREATMENT

APPROPRIATE HEALTH CARE

N/A

NUTRITIONAL SUPPORT

- Nutritional support and proper temperatures are important factors that influence tissue regeneration.
- A 5–10 degree F increase in the basking area may help improve healing but care must be taken that this does not cause additional evaporative losses.
- If the affected reptile was in a positive energy balance prior to the thermal injury and the wounds are not severe, most reptiles resume feeding as healing commences aided with the judicious use of analgesics.
- A weight loss of 10% acutely or 20% chronically should prompt nutritional intervention.
- Tube feeding with the use of an appropriate enteral, such as Oxbow Critical Care for Herbivores® (Oxbow Animal Health, Omaha, NE) or EmerAid Sustain Herbivore® (EmerAid, LLC, Cornell, IL) aid in promoting anabolism and healing.
- An esophagostomy tube should be considered for long-term feeding and medication, in anorectic, difficult to handle or stressed animals.

• CLIENT EDUCATION/HUSBANDRY RECOMMENDATIONS

- The owner should check the affected reptile's condition daily, implement suggested husbandry modifications and administer medications as directed.
- Follow-up veterinary visits at prescribed intervals should be adhered to.

MEDICATIONS

DRUG(S) OF CHOICE

- If the affected reptile presents acutely aftera burn (less than 30 minutes), skin cooling isrecommended, with application of coldcompresses for 15–20 minutes to furtherreduce inflammation and limit tissueswelling.
- Where blisters form, an effort should bemade to minimize trauma and resultantrupture to limit tissue fluid loss and preventsecondary infection.
- Topical therapy, such as dilute chlorhexidine (0.05%), and silver sulfadiazine cream, and non-adherent sterile dressings, is advised to limit secondary infection.

• Silver sulfadiazine is particularly useful due to its broad-spectrum activity and its efficacy against *Pseudomonas*—a common contaminant of burns—as well as its ability to reduce further fluid loss from evaporation.
• Ophthalmic ointments can also be used topically.
• Patients should be kept on non-adherent substrates to minimize further wound trauma and infection. An empty glass enclosure is the simplest to keep clean.
• IV, IO or ICe crystalloid fluid therapy is
• recommended for second- and third-degree burns.
• For extensive wounds, a semipermeable hydrophilic wound dressing (e.g., GranuflexR, ConvaTec Inc., Oklahoma City, OK), may be used to cover defects.
• The use of wet-to-dry sterile bandagesin-fused with sterile saline or even honey bandages also work well and initially should be changed every 24 hours.
• Other products that have been used widely include the porcine xenograft dressing VetBiosist™(Smiths Medical North America, Waukesha, WI), a sterile non-allergenic dressing that may be sutured over extensive wounds to provide a semi-permeable membrane, protecting the granulation bed and encouraging rapid epithelialization.
• Aquatic chelonians can be dry-docked during the day and kept on damp towels. In the evenings they can be placed in their aquatic environment with fresh, clean water.
• Narcotic analgesics (hydromorphone 0.5-1 mg/kg IM q12–24h, tramadol 5–10 mg/kg PO, SC q24h), NSAIDs (meloxicam 0.2–0.5 mg/kg IM, SC q24–48h), parenteral fluids (lactated Ringer's 10–25 ml/kg IV, IO, ICE, SC q24h) and antibiotics based upon microbiological culture and sensitivities are recommended.
• Depending on the severity of lesions, the author prefers the use of antibacterials such as piperacillin 100 mg/kg IM q24h, ceftazadime 20 mg/kg IM q72h or amikacin 5 mg/kg loading dose followed by 2.5 mg/kg q72h combined with metronidazole 20 mg/kg q24h.
• A complete blood count and biochemical analysis should also be done, especially in reptiles with third-degree burns.
• Treatment can last weeks to months depending on the severity and extent of the burns.
• Permanent scarring with abnormal pigmentation usually occurs in the burn area.

PRECAUTIONS/INTERACTIONS

• Adequate hydration should be addressed, particularly for those reptiles being treated with aminoglycosides.
• Soaking in sterile saline or water for 2-4 hours on the days that antibiotics are administered can help to provide additional hydration.
• Care must be taken when soaking reptiles in antiseptic solutions (dilute betadine, dilute chlorhexidine) due to the risk of ingestion.
• Direct application of these solutions to the wounds is recommended.

FOLLOW-UP

PATIENT MONITORING

• Affected animals should be re-evaluated every 1–2 weeks by a veterinarian.
• If this is not feasible, the owner can send pictures for appraisal until healing is progressing in a positive manner.

EXPECTED COURSE AND PROGNOSIS

• First-degree burns: damaged tissue heals in approximately 2–4 weeks.
• Second-degree burns: healing usually takes 6–8 weeks and eschar may form.
• Third-degree burns: healing can take from months to years and is accompanied with extensive scarring. The prognosis is guarded for third-degree burns due to the possibility of sepsis.

MISCELLANEOUS

COMMENTS

• Exposure to high-intensity and/or inappropriate wavelengths of UV radiation can cause signs of phototoxicity, such as photokeratoconjunctivitis and photodermatitis.
• Affected reptiles can present acutely with corneal and dermal opacities, excessive ecdysis, hyperkeratosis and epidermal erosions.
• Chronic cases may present with cataracts and cutaneous neoplasia. These cases must be differentiated from thermal burns.
• Figures 5 and 6 – see web image supplementary content for Section III (Lizards).

ZOONOTIC POTENTIAL

N/A

SYNONYMS

N/A

ABBREVIATIONS

• ICe = intracoelomic
• IM = intramuscular
• IO = intraosseus
• IV = intravenous
• NSAIDs = nonsteroidal anti-inflammatory drugs
• PO = by mouth
• SC = subcutaneously
• UVB = ultraviolet B

INTERNET RESOURCES

Divers SJ. Management and husbandry of reptiles. MSD Manual Veterinary Manual, June 2020. https://www.msdvetmanual.com/en-gb/exotic-and-laboratory-animals/reptiles/management-and-husbandry-of-reptiles

Suggested Reading

Girling SJ, Raiti P, eds. *BSAVA Manual of Reptiles*. 2nd ed. Gloucester, UK: BSAVA; 2004.
Mader DR, ed. *Reptile Medicine and Surgery*. 2nd ed. St. Louis, MO: Elsevier Saunders; 2006.

Author Paul Raiti, DVM DABVP (Reptile and Amphibian Practice)

LIZARDS

TICKS

BASICS

DEFINITION/OVERVIEW

Ticks are ectoparasites that feed on blood and can potentially transmit disease through their bite, together with causing local irritation, secondary infection, or rarely anemia. They are mainly seen in wild-caught animals, so any known wild-caught animals should be closely examined for their presence. They may also be found on animals that are otherwise weak or debilitated. Rarely, they may be seen in captive specimens that spend time outdoors.

ETIOLOGY/PATHOPHYSIOLOGY

- Ticks can parasitize reptiles, including hard ticks of the genera *Ixodes*, *Hyalomma*, *Haemaphysalis*, *Amblyomma*, and *Aponomma*, and the soft ticks *Argasidae* and *Ornithodoros*.
- Soft ticks live in nests and burrows while hard ticks live in fields or scrub areas and attach to a host as it passes by. Some are host specific.
- Ticks use their mouthparts to attach and feed on blood. Soft ticks become engorged and drop off within hours and may feed repeatedly while hard ticks remain attached for several days.
- Females lay eggs after a blood meal. Eggs hatch as a larval stage, which feed on blood from the host as well. They progress through two or more nymph stages before becoming adults, feeding on blood between each stage.
- Larvae, nymphs, and adults can live for months without a blood meal.

SIGNALMENT/HISTORY

- No age or sex predisposition
- Typically only seen in wild-caught animals, or those that spend significant time outdoors or are kept in unsanitary conditions with poor husbandry.

CLINICAL PRESENTATION

- Identification of tick attached to skin.
- Ticks often attach in skin folds, under scales, or around the ears, lips, cloaca.
- There may be swelling, erythema, or discharge at the site of attachment from local irritation or secondary bacterial infection.
- The monitor lizard ticks *Aponomma exornatium* and *A. flavimaculatum* attach inside nostrils, where heavy infestation can cause dyspnea and suffocation.
- In some cases, animals may be otherwise debilitated, weak, or have other underlying problems.
- Animals may also soak frequently in an attempt to dislodge the parasites, and if the infestation is severe there may be signs of dysecdysis, anemia, or disease possibly transmitted by the tick.
- Ticks can serve as vectors of hemogregarines.

RISK FACTORS

Husbandry

- Ticks are typically only seen in wild-caught animals, and rarely in captive animals that spend significant time outdoors.
- There is no specific way to avoid picking up ticks other than regular control measures such as mowing the lawn regularly, removing debris piles or refuse, avoid overwatering or standing water, limiting access by wildlife, and using tick control pesticides in the enclosure.
- Infestations can also occur in severe cases of poor husbandry and sanitation, stress, and other underlying medical conditions.

Others

N/A

DIAGNOSIS

DIFFERENTIAL DIAGNOSIS

- Diagnosis is pathognomonic
- Other ectoparasites such as mites, and chiggers are significantly smaller and not confused with ticks.

DIAGNOSTICS

- Diagnosis of ticks is based on physical exam alone.
- Additional tests to evaluate the animal's overall condition may be necessary if the animal is otherwise weak or debilitated.
- Tests may include a fecal exam, CBC and chemistry panel, and/or radiography.

PATHOLOGICAL FINDINGS

- Ticks are obvious on physical exam.
- There may be evidence of inflammation or secondary bacterial colonization at the attachment site.
- Anemia is possible, but because ticks are large, they are often removed before significant anemia can occur.
- Other pathologic findings could include those from a pathogen transmitted by the tick.

TREATMENT

APPROPRIATE HEALTH CARE

N/A

NUTRITIONAL SUPPORT

- Not needed for this condition unless animal is otherwise debilitated.
- Most lizards can be fed at 1–2% of body weight once or twice daily of an appropriate carnivore, omnivore, or herbivore feeding formula.

CLIENT EDUCATION/HUSBANDRY RECOMMENDATIONS

- Ticks must be removed from the patient and the environment for successful management.
- If ticks were acquired in an outdoor environment, that area should be cleaned of debris and measures taken to reduce the possibility that ticks will colonize the area.
- Routine monitoring of animals and enclosures is needed.
- If the animal is wild caught and otherwise weak and debilitated, husbandry needs to be ideal to reduce stress on the animal and aid in recovery.
- Strict quarantine is necessary to avoid introducing ticks to other animals in a collection.

MEDICATIONS

DRUG(S) OF CHOICE

- Physical removal is recommended
- The tick must be grasped under the head on the mouthparts for full extraction.
- Secondary infection of the attachment site can be treated with topical antibacterial ointment, such as silver sulfadiazine cream, and systemic antibiotics if needed.
- FRONTLINE® (Merial Inc., Duluth, GA) spray is effective for prevention and may aid in removal. It should never be sprayed directly on the animal; spray on a towel and wipe the animal head to tail.
- Ivermectin 0.2 mg/kg SC may aid in tick removal, mainly for sites that are not easily accessible such as the nostrils. Provent-A-Mite™ (Pro Products, Mahopac, NY) is an over the counter permethrin product that appears to be both safe and effective.
- It can be applied to the animal or sprayed in the environment.
- Additional treatments may be needed based on the animal's overall condition.
- If the animal is anemic due to blood loss, consider additional therapies such as B vitamins, iron dextran, or even a blood transfusion.

PRECAUTIONS/INTERACTIONS

- Use caution with any over the counter remedies, particularly organophosphates or permethrins, as toxicity is possible.
- Cyfluthrin, a component of products for treating the environment, is toxic to lizards, even in small amounts, and should not be used for those species.

FOLLOW-UP

PATIENT MONITORING

- None needed if ticks are physically removed.
- If secondary bacterial infection is present, resolution of clinical signs will indicate response to therapy.

EXPECTED COURSE AND PROGNOSIS

- The prognosis for animals with ticks themselves is excellent.
- Once the ticks are removed there should be no further complications.
- The prognosis for secondary infection of the skin is good.
- The main concern is if the animal is weak or debilitated overall, or if there is potential for disease transmission from the tick. Depending on the animal's overall condition, the prognosis may be fair to guarded.

MISCELLANEOUS

COMMENTS

- One concern with ticks on wild-caught animals is potential foreign animal disease transmission.
- Any tick on a wild-caught animal from another country, and the animal itself, should be treated with suspicion.

ZOONOTIC POTENTIAL

- Ticks affecting reptiles can potentially attach to humans and cause irritation and pruritis at the site of a bite.
- Many can also carry and transmit disease to humans such as tularemia, Lyme disease, and other encephalitis-causing viruses.
- Use caution during removal and kill the tick immediately.

SYNONYMS

N/A

ABBREVIATIONS

- CBC = complete blood count
- SC = subcutaneous

INTERNET RESOURCES

- Burridge, MJ. Controlling and Eradicating Tick Infestations on Reptiles. Veterinary Compendium, 2005. https://vetfoliovetstreet.s3.amazonaws.com/mmah/5d/12368b9df24fabb6fd86b1b65e51df/filePV_27_05_371.pdf
- PetCoach Editorial. Reptile Tick and Mite Infestation: Causes, Signs, Diagnosis, and Treatment. Petco Animal Supplies Stores, Inc. http://www.peteducation.com/article.cfm?c=17+1796&aid=2433
- Greek T. How to Recognize and Treat Reptile Ectoparasites. Reptiles, July 1, 2014. http://www.reptilesmagazine.com/Snake-Care/How-to-Recognize-and-Treat-Reptile-Ectoparasites

Suggested Reading

Burridge MJ, Simmons L. Control and eradication of exotic tick infestations on reptiles. *Proc ARAV* 2001:21–23.

Fitzgerald KT, Vera R. Acariasis. In: Mader DR, ed. *Reptile Medicine and Surgery*. 2nd ed. St. Louis, MO: Elsevier Saunders; 2006:720–738.

Jacobson ER. Parasites and parasitic disease of reptiles. In: Jacobson ER, ed. *Infectious Diseases and Pathology of Reptiles*. Boca Raton, FL: CRC Press; 2007:571–665.

Author Stacey Leonatti Wilkinson, DVM, DABVP (Reptile and Amphibian)

UPPER RESPIRATORY TRACT DISEASE

BASICS

DEFINITION/OVERVIEW

Lizards can suffer diseases of the respiratory tract but often less commonly so than snakes and chelonians. Signs of URTD in lizards can include nasal or oral discharge, respiratory sounds, and dyspnea. Primary infections of the oral cavity or esophagus can also lead to URTD. There is a wide range of pathogens and etiologies. URTD often occurs concurrently with LRTD; thus patients with signs of URTD must also be evaluated for LRTD. Respiratory diseases often take a long time to develop before clinical signs are evident. Lizards normally breathe with their mouths closed, with air entering the URT through the external nares. The air is passed from the external nares through the vestibulum nasi, the cavum nasi proprium, the conchae, the ductus nasopharyngeus, and the internal nares. The vomeronasal organ, which is well developed in lizards, is associated with the nose. Lizards lack a secondary palate. Some lizards (e.g., iguanas, uromastyx) possess salt glands in their nostrils (located lateronasally), which discharge their content into the nasal cavities. Thus, dry white discharge on the nostrils of these lizards is not a sign of disease, but rather a sign of physiologic electrolyte secretion.

ETIOLOGY/PATHOPHYSIOLOGY

There is a wide range of etiologies associated with URTD, but infectious causes are some of the most common. URTD may also be secondary to other diseases such as stomatitis.

Infectious

- Bacteria: *Mycobacterium chelonae*; Gram-negative such as *Pseudomonas* spp., *Aeromonas* spp., *Klebsiella* spp., *Salmonella* spp., *Proteus* spp. and anaerobic bacteria such as *Bacteroides* spp.
- Fungi
- Viruses: varanid or gerrhosaurid herpesvirus, shingleback nidovirus.
- Parasites may cause physical damage to epithelium and serve as vectors for other infections, sometimes a combination of parasitic and bacterial or viral: *Rhabdias* infecting the oral cavity or esophagus; pentastomids (in oral cavity, pharynx, trachea, bronchi, lung), which sometimes exit via the glottis and then through the mouth and nares.

Non-Infectious

- Foreign bodies within the choana, nasal or oral cavity.
- Physical trauma/injuries affecting the nasal or oral cavity or the choana.
- Neoplasia (e.g., cervical and pharyngeal lymphoma in a green iguana causing obstruction of the oropharynx; lymphoma in the maxilla of a green iguana causing severe lesions in the oral cavity; thyroid adenocarcinoma in a crocodile lizard causing stomatitis and rhinitis).
- Inhalation of dust, smoke, aerosols or disinfectants leading to rhinotracheitis.
- Improper husbandry

SIGNALMENT/HISTORY

No age, sex, or species predisposition.

CLINICAL PRESENTATION

- Depending on the underlying cause and lizard species.
- Nasal discharge/exudate (clear to mucopurulent) not to be confused with salt secretions.
- Stridor, wheezing or clicking respiratory sounds.
- Dyspnea, open mouth-breathing
- Excess salivation or mucous secretion in the oral cavity.
- Oculonasal discharge
- Stomatitis
- Ulceration of the nasal and buccal mucosa.
- Swelling of the face due to obstruction of the nasolacrimal duct (secondary to inflammation).
- Purulent material in the subspectacular space (provoked by bacterial infections of the spectaculocorneal space) or bullous spectaculopathy in species lacking eyelids.
- Obstruction of the nostrils by retained skin, mites, dried exudate, etc.
- Elevated head and straightened cranial part of the body due to forced breathing.
- Excessive air-filled digestive tract (aerophagia) due to increased and forced inspiration.
- Non-specific signs such as anorexia, lethargy, inactivity.

RISK FACTORS

Husbandry

- Stressors
- Poor hygiene
- Stagnant water, substrate with irritating compounds (e.g., cedar shavings), poor ventilation.
- Improper diet (including starvation) and endoparasitism may also be predisposing factors.
- Inappropriate temperatures and humidity; sudden changes in temperature or humidity.

Others

- Immunosuppression, which may be caused by stress, overcrowding, relocation, concurrent disease or inappropriate husbandry.

DIAGNOSIS

DIFFERENTIAL DIAGNOSIS

- Infectious diseases (bacterial, viral, fungal, parasitic)
- Traumata
- Neoplasia
- Abscess
- Foreign bodies
- Inhalation of irritating substances

DIAGNOSTICS

- Physical examination, including thorough exam of the oral cavity and choana. The use of magnification may aid in identifying subtle lesions.
- Bacterial culture and sensitivity (aerobic and anaerobic) and/or fungal culture of nasal discharge, nasal flush, or inflamed tissue in the upper alimentary or respiratory tract.
- Cytology of the nasal discharge or any gross lesions of the respiratory tract or oral cavity.
- Biopsy and histopathology of nasal or oral mucosa.
- For suspected mycoplasmosis: culture and PCR of oral mucosa.
- For suspected viral infections: culture and PCR of nasal flush or nasal, oral, or pharyngeal swab.
- Diagnostic imaging (radiography, CT, MRI) for detection of foreign bodies, osteolysis, osteomyelitis, or concurrent LRTD.
- Endoscopy of the URTD (and LRTD); possibly including nasal lavage and biopsy for further diagnostics such as cytology, histopathology, virology, and electron microscopy.
- Fecal exam

PATHOLOGICAL FINDINGS

- Depending on the underlying cause, signs of mild to severe inflammation, lesions and ulcerations of the nasal and oral mucosa and submucosa may be found.
- Bacteria, fungal hyphae, virus associated inclusion bodies, as well as parasites may be visible histologically.
- Inflammation of the mucosa and submucosa or lingual epithelium is mostly characterized by granulocytic and lymphocytic inflammation with epithelial erosion.
- In cases of herpesvirus infections, eosinophilic intranuclear inclusion bodies may be visible in the lingual epithelium.
- Osteomyelitis (with sometimes severe granulomatous inflammation of the bone marrow) and osteolysis (osteonecrosis) leading to necrotic bone tissue and bone remodeling in the adjacent structures of the skull may occur.

TREATMENT

APPROPRIATE HEALTH CARE

N/A

NUTRITIONAL SUPPORT

- Force-feeding with easily digestible proteins.
- Direct feeding by stomach tube can be performed in some species; placement of an esophagostomy tube should be considered for chronic management.
- Supportive fluid therapy should be provided, at a rate of 10–30 ml/kg/day as supportive care.

CLIENT EDUCATION/HUSBANDRY RECOMMENDATIONS

- Correct any husbandry deficiencies with special attention to temperature, humidity, and ventilation.
- Isolate animal from others in collection, especially when viral etiology is suspected.
- It is important to ensure a full course of treatment to avoid recurrence of disease.

SURGICAL CONSIDERATIONS

- Neoplasia: surgical removal if feasible.
- Parasites: in some cases, physical removal of the parasites via surgery or endoscopy may be necessary.

MEDICATIONS

DRUG(S) OF CHOICE

- Bacteria: systemic or nebulized antibiotics (e.g., amikacin, ceftazidime, enrofloxacin, tylosin), preferably according to sensitivity panel for at least 4–6 weeks. Local instillation of antibiotics (injectable or ophthalmic solutions) in the nasal passage may also be effective.
- Fungi: systemic, local, nebulized antifungals (e.g., terbinafine, voriconazole, amphotericin B).
- Systemic use of itraconazole may cause severe adverse effects in some lizards.
- Viral: separation, strict quarantine, and intensive supportive therapy. Antiviral therapy has had low success and euthanasia is often required, depending on the state of the animal and the disease.
- Parasites: antiparasitic treatment according the species. In some cases, parasites can be physically removed via surgery or endoscopy.
- Treatment depends on the underlying cause and the affected lizard species.
- In case of confirmed mycobacterial infection: no treatment, euthanasia.
- Foreign body within the choana, nasal/oral cavity: extraction.

PRECAUTIONS/INTERACTIONS

- Many systemic antibiotics (e.g. aminoglycosides, fluoroquinolones) are excreted through the kidney or show renal toxicity.
- Adequate hydration and regular monitoring of renal values is recommended.

FOLLOW-UP

PATIENT MONITORING

- Improvement of clinical signs should be expected within 1–2 weeks for bacterial and fungal infections when definitive diagnosis and treatment are employed.
- It is critical to continue treatment until clinical signs are fully resolved and repeating cultures to confirm resolution of infection if unsure.
- In cases that do not show any improvement or worsen during the first 1–2 weeks of treatment, it should be considered that the etiology and/or treatment are not accurate.
- Viral infections should also be considered in cases that do not respond to therapy or have chronic, intermittent recurrence of disease.
- Repeat diagnostics may be needed to assess resolution or progression of disease.

EXPECTED COURSE AND PROGNOSIS

- Bacterial: good prognosis depending on response to antibiotics.
- Fungal: guarded to poor prognosis
- Viral: poor to grave prognosis, especially when showing clinical signs.
- Parasitic: good prognosis
- Neoplastic: poor to grave prognosis
- Others: depend on severity and involvement of other tissues.

MISCELLANEOUS

COMMENTS

N/A

ZOONOTIC POTENTIAL

- Depending on the causative agent
- Mycobacteria, salmonella, and pentastomids have zoonotic potential.

SYNONYMS

- Upper respiratory tract infection (URTI)
- Upper respiratory disease syndrome
- Flu ("Bobtail flu" in cases of nidovirus infections in Australian shingleback lizards)

ABBREVIATIONS

- CT = computed tomography
- LRTD = lower respiratory tract disease
- MRI = magnetic resonance imaging
- PCR = polymerase chain reaction
- URT = upper respiratory tract
- URTD = upper respiratory tract disease

Suggested Reading

Hernandez-Divers SM = Garner MM. Neoplasia of reptiles with an emphasis on lizards. *Vet Clin North Am Exot Anim Pract* 2003;6(1):251–273.

Jacobson ER. Overview of reptile biology, anatomy, and histology. In: Jacobson ER, ed. *Infectious Diseases and Pathology of Reptiles: Color Atlas and Text.* Boca Raton, FL: CRC Press; 2007:1–130.

O'Dea MA, Jackson B, Jackson C, et al. Discovery and partial genomic characterisation of a novel nidovirus associated with respiratory disease in wild shingleback lizards (*Tiliqua rugosa*). *PloS One* 2016;11(11):e0165209.

Wellehan JF, Johnson AJ, Latimer KS, et al. Varanid herpesvirus 1: a novel herpesvirus associated with proliferative stomatitis in green tree monitors (*Varanus prasinus*). *Vet Microbiol* 2005;105(2):83–92.

Wellehan JF, Nichols DK, Li LL, Kapur V. Three novel herpesviruses associated with stomatitis in Sudan plated lizards (*Gerrhosaurus major*) and a black-lined plated lizard (*Gerrhosaurus nigrolineatus*). *J Zoo Wildl Med* 2004;35(1):50–54.

Wyneken J, Witherington D. Respiratory anatomy: Form and function in reptiles. *Exotic DVM* 2001;3:17–22.

Author Karina A. Mathes, DVM, Dr. med. vet., DECZM (Herpetology), European Veterinary Specialist in Zoological Medicine (Herpetology), Certified Specialist in Reptiles (Fachtieraerztin fuer Reptilien), Certified Specialist in Reptiles and Amphibians (ZB Reptilien und Amphibien)

UROLITHIASIS

BASICS

DEFINITION/OVERVIEW

Urolithiasis is the formation of calculi within the urinary tract. While most reptiles are uricotelic, some can be ureotelic, ammoniotelic, or a combination of these. Uric acid is actively secreted by the proximal tubules of the kidneys and excreted in the urine. It is the end product of nitrogen metabolism through a series of enzymatic reactions that involve xanthine oxidase. Endogenous uric acid production results from de novo purine synthesis and tissue catabolism. The form in which uric acid is excreted is dependent on urine pH. When urine pH is < 5, uric acid is present in the urine, whereas when urine pH is > 6.5, most of the uric acid is excreted as urate salts. The majority of uroliths are composed of salts of uric acid and ammonium, sodium, potassium, or calcium. In reptiles, urinary calculi have been identified in the kidneys, ureters, urinary bladder, urodeum and distal cloaca. Some lizards (i.e., bearded dragons, monitor lizards) do not possess urinary bladders; hence, cystic calculi do not occur in these reptiles. Inciting factors for calculus formation are chronic dehydration, renal insufficiency, high-protein diets, and lack of exercise.

ETIOLOGY/PATHOPHYSIOLOGY

- The formation of urinary calculi is initiated by the precipitation of excretory metabolites in supersaturated urine.
- Factors credited with stone nidation include dehydration, alterations in urinary pH, abnormalities of urinary tract structure and function, high levels of urolith mineral components in the diet, nutrient deficiencies such as hypovitaminosis A, atypical metabolism of calculus precursors, and the presence of bacteria and other foreign materials within the urinary tract.
- An additional characteristic of reptiles is that urine is not sterile, since the bladder communicates with the coprodeum (the opening of the GI tract into the cloaca).
- Once a nidus is formed that is too large to pass through the urethra, a bladder stone results.
- Cystic calculi are relatively common in green iguanas (*Iguana iguana*) and spiny-tailed lizards (*Uromastyx* spp.).
- Some owners of *Uromastyx* spp. neither provide standing water nor mist the enclosures since these lizards are from xeric habitats.
- The presumption is that water present in fresh vegetables provides adequate hydration, which has been shown not to be true.

SIGNALMENT/HISTORY

- Urolithiasis is usually a problem of adult herbivorous reptiles.
- Deficiencies in husbandry such as chronic dehydration, suboptimal ambient temperatures and inappropriately high-protein diets (usually mammalian based) are commonly identified during anamnesis.

CLINICAL PRESENTATION

- Many reptiles with small uroliths show no clinical signs.
- Small uroliths may be voided; however, larger calculi may pass from the urinary bladder into the cloaca and obstruct the vent.
- As calculi grow larger, hematuria, hindleg dysfunction, cloacal prolapse, dystocia, dysuria, or tenesmus may occur.

RISK FACTORS

Husbandry

- Urolith formation is commonly associated with chronic dehydration, high-protein diets, and lack of exercise.
- Exogenous uric acid production is dependent on diet and is particularly high when the diet is rich in animal protein; hence, the feeding of dog or cat food to herbivorous reptiles is contraindicated.
- Fresh water should always be present in the enclosure and supplemented with daily misting.
- Weekly soakings for most reptiles are also recommended.

Others

Underlying renal insufficiency

DIAGNOSIS

DIFFERENTIAL DIAGNOSIS

- Space-occupying lesions of the intestinal tract including cloaca.
- GI foreign bodies
- Ileus
- Dystocia
- Constipation

DIAGNOSTICS

- Palpation of the caudal coelom is relatively straightforward in lizards.
- Diagnosis can be confirmed with radiography.
- If a radiolucent calculus or soft tissue mass is suspected, ultrasound should be performed.
- Ultrasound is also useful to determine whether an ectopic egg is located in the urinary bladder.

PATHOLOGICAL FINDINGS

- Uroliths cause mucinosis, cystitis, and inflammatory hypertrophy of the bladder wall, while very large uroliths can cause pressure necrosis of the bladder wall, with subsequent rupture and septic coelomitis.
- Necropsies have revealed concurrent renal gout, membranous glomerulopathy, renal interstitial fibrosis, glomerulonephritis and interstitial fibrosis, and renal interstitial fibrosis with mineralization.

TREATMENT

APPROPRIATE HEALTH CARE

N/A

NUTRITIONAL SUPPORT

- Reptiles that are anorexic will benefit from placement of an esophagostomy tube for administering oral medications and feeding before and up to several months postoperatively.
- Subsequent to stone removal, recovery is usually quite rapid with appetite returning to normal within several days.
- Oxbow Critical Care for Herbivores® (Oxbow Animal Health, Omaha, NE) or EmerAid Sustain Herbivore® (EmerAid, LLC, Cornell, IL) is commonly used to provide proper nutrition during the recovery period.

CLIENT EDUCATION/HUSBANDRY RECOMMENDATIONS

- Husbandry parameters should be adhered to meticulously with special emphasis on ambient temperature ranges, diet, hydration, and hygiene during the immediate and long-term convalescent period.
- Follow-up visits with the veterinarian are also important for successful recovery.

MEDICATIONS

DRUG(S) OF CHOICE

- Currently, there are no drugs that have been used to successfully dissolve uroliths in reptiles; however allopurinol, a xanthine oxidase inhibitor, at 10-20 mg/kg PO q24hr is used to reduce uric acid levels in reptiles to discourage stone formation.
- Extraction of the urolith is required and can be done via an assortment of techniques.
- Sometimes, smaller calculi can be passed successfully by soaking affected animals.
- Calculi present in the cloaca can usually be removed with sedation and the use of forceps to fragment the calculi.
- Visualization is dramatically enhanced with the use of endoscopic guidance (cloacoscopy) and the use of a dental drill to fragment cloacoliths has been described.

- Coeliotomy and cystotomy are the procedures most commonly done to remove calculi located in the urinary bladder.
- Postsurgical broad spectrum antibiotics are recommended.

PRECAUTIONS/INTERACTIONS

N/A

FOLLOW-UP

PATIENT MONITORING

- Any reptile recovering from an invasive surgical procedure should be isolated so it may be carefully monitored.
- Appetite should be closely monitored
- It is essential to keep the cage warm.
- A basking light, typically a 60 -100-watt spotlight, should be set up at one end of the tank. The temperature underneath the spotlight should reach 95 -100°F. The other end of the cage should be about 15 -20°F cooler.
- It is recommended that the owner uses an infrared (laser) thermometer to directly measure the temperature of the reptile. If the animal spends all its time on the heated side, the cage may be too cool. If it spends all its time at the cool end of the cage, the basking spot may be too hot.
- Some source of floor heat, such as heat tape, is useful for night-time heat.
- A UVB light should be provided for proper vitamin D synthesis and to stimulate proper healing. The light should be set up to illuminate the area around the basking light.
- The reptile should have a shallow water bowl for drinking, but it should not be soaked until the incision has healed or the patch has been on long enough that there is good granulation tissue beneath. For other reptiles, a 2-week soak pause is adequate.
- Esophagostomy tubes can be removed once the patient begins feeding. It is also important to monitor urine and fecal output throughout recovery.

EXPECTED COURSE AND PROGNOSIS

- In the author's experience, reptiles that have been diagnosed concurrently with urinary calculi and gout (articular/visceral) carry a significantly more guarded prognosis than those that are not hyperuricemic.
- Cystotomy cases usually respond rapidly during convalescence particularly when analgesia is addressed with the use of NSAIDs (meloxicam 0.2 mg/kg IM or PO once daily) or opioids (morphine or hydromorphone at 0.5–1 mg/kg IM q12h).

MISCELLANEOUS

COMMENTS

N/A

ZOONOTIC POTENTIAL

N/A

SYNONYMS

- Bladder stones
- Cystic calculi
- Cystoliths
- Urinary concretions
- Urolithiasis
- Uroliths

ABBREVIATIONS

- GI = gastrointestinal
- IM = intramuscular
- NSAIDs = nonsteroidal anti-inflammatory drugs
- PO = per os
- UVB = ultraviolet B

INTERNET RESOURCES

Mader D. Tortoise bladder stones. Reptiles, December 1, 2011. https://www.reptilesmagazine.com/tortoise-bladder-stones

Suggested Reading

Jacobson ER. *Biology, Husbandry and Medicine of the Green Iguana*. Malabar, FL: Krieger; 2003.

Mader DR. Calculi: Urinary. In: Mader DR, ed. *Reptile Medicine and Surgery*. 2nd ed. St. Louis, MO: Elsevier Saunders; 2006:763–771.

Author Paul Raiti, DVM, DABVP (Reptile and Amphibian Practice)

VOMITING

BASICS

DEFINITION/OVERVIEW

Vomiting is the forcible ejection of partially or wholly digested contents from the stomach and small intestine through the mouth.

ETIOLOGY/PATHOPHYSIOLOGY

- Vomiting in reptiles is under active neural control from the autonomic and somatic nervous systems.
- Details of this process are not completely understood, but they are likely similar to that in mammals.
- The difference between vomiting and regurgitation may be difficult to discern.

SIGNALMENT/HISTORY

- All species, ages, sexes may be affected.
- Owner may report observing vomiting or only that vomited material was found.
- Lethargy, anorexia, weight loss, respiratory distress, or increased basking frequency.
- Ingestion of foreign material

CLINICAL PRESENTATION

- No clinical signs are specific to vomiting, and physical exam may be normal.
- Presentation varies depending on the underlying cause and chronicity.
- Dehydration and/or emaciation/cachexia
- Hard mass on palpation of the coelomic cavity due to an obstructive lesion or organomegaly.
- Skeletal abnormalities that may include pathological fractures or abnormal growth patterns.
- Lethargy and/or obtunded mentation.
- Ulceration and accumulation of caseous material in the oral cavity.
- Secondary respiratory disease (e.g., oral/ nasal discharge, abnormal respiratory sounds) or enteritis (e.g., diarrhea).

RISK FACTORS

Husbandry

- Too much disturbance or lack of hiding places (increases stress/anxiety).
- Poor sanitation, overcrowding, hyper- or hypothermia, lack of quarantine for new individuals (increases stress, possibility of secondary infections, and disease transmission).
- Toxin exposure (cleaning chemicals, pesticides, heavy metals).
- Excessive/inappropriate handling (especially soon after feeding).
- Inadequate diet (incorrect calcium/ phosphorus ratio, improper prey items, excessive feeding).
- Inappropriate substrate (may be accidentally ingested).

Others

Concomitant infectious or parasitic disease.

DIAGNOSIS

DIFFERENTIAL DIAGNOSIS

- Stomatitis
- Esophagitis
- Esophageal stricture
- Gastritis
- Handling/stress (e.g., excessive pressure to coelom)
- Obstructive lesions (e.g., GI foreign body, intussusception, neoplasia, abscess, granuloma)
- Metabolic disease (e.g., nutritional secondary hyperparathyroidism, renal or hepatic dysfunction)
- Toxicoses (e.g., zinc)
- Iatrogenic (e.g., enrofloxacin, xylazine, levamisole)
- Trauma to esophagus or stomach
- Parasites (e.g., *Cryptosporidium*, amoebiasis, ascaridiasis, cestodiasis)
- Viruses
- Bacteria/septicemia (e.g., *Chlamydophila*)
- Congenital GI defects

DIAGNOSTICS

- Husbandry review
- Physical examination
- Complete blood count and plasma biochemistries.
- Radiography with or without contrast
- Ultrasound
- Fecal parasite exam
- Bacterial cultures from oral lesions.
- GI endoscopy or coeliotomy (direct tissue evaluation and biopsy).
- Testing for cryptosporidiosis

PATHOLOGICAL FINDINGS

- Dependent on underlying cause
- Cryptosporidiosis in lizards primarily affects the intestinal tract but could also potentially affect the stomach.

TREATMENT

APPROPRIATE HEALTH CARE

- The primary goal is to identify and address the underlying cause.
- Institute quarantine procedures for new animals, including 30–60-day period, veterinary evaluation, and 1–3 weekly fecal exams for parasites.
- Animals affected by cryptosporidiosis should be isolated from all other reptiles.

NUTRITIONAL SUPPORT

- Correct fluid deficits and maintain hydration.
- Intracoelomic, subcutaneous, or intravenous routes for administration of a reptile Ringer's solution are most effective. Maintenance rate is 10–30 ml/kg/day.
- Tube or assist-feeding liquid or gel diets (e.g., Hill's® Prescription Diet® a/d®, Hills Pet Nutrition, Inc., Topeka, KS; Mazuri® Amphibian & Carnivorous Reptile Gel, Mazuri Exotic Animal Nutrition, St. Louis, MO; Oxbow Critical Care® formulas, Oxbow Animal Health, Omaha, NE) may be beneficial during initial treatment/recovery.
- Gradually add normal diet items as the animal improves.

CLIENT EDUCATION/HUSBANDRY RECOMMENDATIONS

- Review husbandry and correct any problems.
- Avoid overfeeding and disturbing carnivorous lizards 1–2 days after feeding.

MEDICATIONS

DRUG(S) OF CHOICE

- Cimetidine 4 mg/kg IM, PO q8–12h, or famotidine 0.25–0.5 mg/kg SC, PO q24–72h.
- Metoclopramide 0.06 mg/kg PO q24h for 7 days, or cisapride 0.5–2 mg/kg PO q24h.
- Sucralfate 500–1000 mg/kg PO q6–8h.

PRECAUTIONS/INTERACTIONS

N/A

FOLLOW-UP

PATIENT MONITORING

Monitor for continued signs of vomiting and possible complications.

EXPECTED COURSE AND PROGNOSIS

- Prognosis is dependent on the underlying cause.
- Prognosis for subclinical cryptosporidiosis is fair to good.
- Prognosis for clinical disease is poor to grave, and euthanasia is often indicated.

MISCELLANEOUS

COMMENTS

N/A

ZOONOTIC POTENTIAL

N/A

SYNONYMS

Emesis

ABBREVIATIONS

- GI = gastrointestinal
- IM = intramuscular
- PO = per os
- SC = subcutaneous

Suggested Reading

Funk RS. Vomiting and regurgitation. In: Mader DR, ed. *Reptile Medicine and Surgery*. 2nd ed. St. Louis, MO: Elsevier Saunders; 2006:939–940.

Gibbons PM, Klaphake E, Carpenter JW. Reptiles. In: Carpenter JW, Marion CJ, eds. *Exotic Animal Formulary*. 4th ed. St. Louis, MO: Elsevier Saunders; 2013:83–182.

Mitchell MA, Diaz-Figueroa O. Clinical reptile gastroenterology. *Vet Clin N Am Exot Anim Pract* 2005;8:277–298.

Author Tamara Kruse, DVM, MS, and Trevor T. Zachariah, DVM, MS, DACZM

WEIGHT LOSS

BASICS

DEFINITION/OVERVIEW

For reptiles, weight loss can take the form of body mass loss (i.e., cachexia) or fluid loss. In mammals, it is generally accepted that weight loss becomes clinically significant when the loss exceeds 10% of normal body weight (and when it is not completely due to fluid loss). From a clinical perspective, weight loss of more than 10–20% of a healthy, species-specific body weight is significant and must be systematically evaluated, with rapid weight loss being considered most urgent. Weight loss in reptiles may be a normal physiologic process (e.g., brumation/estivation, reproductive activity and behavior), and is not considered a primary disease, but, rather, a clinical manifestation of other disease processes.

ETIOLOGY/PATHOPHYSIOLOGY

- In reptiles, normal weight loss (fluid and body mass loss) will occur during times of torpor or brumation/estivation.
- Once post-torpor normal behavior returns, the reptile will replenish lost fluids and body mass under normal circumstances or given normal access to clean water and appropriate food and environmental conditions.
- Normal weight loss may be associated with reproductive behavior or gravidity.
- Pathologic weight loss may be associated with a variety of noninfectious and infectious disease processes.
- In pet reptiles, inappropriate husbandry is the most common underlying cause of pathologic weight loss.
- Poor husbandry may frequently lead to metabolic diseases of secondary infectious diseases due to immune system compromise of the animal.
- Infectious diseases, and debilitating non-infectious diseases, will commonly result in weight loss due to both body mass and fluid loss.
- In some cases, reptiles succumb to a nonspecific disease process referred to as "maladaptation or failure to thrive syndrome," which is characterized by the failure of a captive reptile to adapt to its current conditions, or a wild-caught reptile unable to adapt to the captive environment.
- Many of these animals will lose weight and die, and a specific disease process is not diagnosed.

SIGNALMENT/HISTORY

- Weight loss in reptiles has no specific signalment, and can affect males or females of any species and any age.
- A typical history suggests rapid weight loss of ≥ 10% acutely or ≥ 20% chronically.
- Weight loss in reptiles typically includes some degree of dehydration, in addition to loss of body mass and/or fat stores.
- If the individual or species normally brumates/estivates, weight loss can be expected as a normal physiologic process.
- With pathologic weight loss, the husbandry and environment must be evaluated thoroughly, and infectious and noninfectious diseases must be considered as underlying causes for the weight loss.

CLINICAL PRESENTATION

- Reptiles presenting with weight loss typically show observable loss of muscle mass.
- The vertebral column and pelvic bones become more readily apparent, and the hind limb muscles will decrease in mass.
- In some lizard species (e.g., geckos), the normally plump tail becomes thin and the coccygeal vertebrae are readily apparent.
- Externally, the coelomic cavity may appear sunken on both sides.
- Palpation of the coelomic cavity may reveal lack of fat bodies.
- With dehydration, the eyes may sink into the bony orbits, and the severe tenting of the skin may become distinct, depending on the species.

RISK FACTORS

Husbandry

- Poor husbandry is the most common contributing factor to pathologic process in reptiles, including weight loss.
- Inappropriate housing type or improper placement within a client's household or other facility.
- Ambient temperature and humidity
- Lack of access to clean water or dechlorinated water in aquatic species.
- Lack of presence and appropriate maintenance of an ultraviolet light source (position, distance from reptiles, appropriate duration between bulb changes).
- Inappropriate type, quality and quantity of food offered for the species.
- Intra- or inter-specific competition for food.
- Type of substrate, cage furniture, and frequency of cleaning/replacing substrate.
- Toxicity associated with environmental cleaning solutions.
- Common diseases associated with inappropriate husbandry include foreign body ingestion and gastrointestinal impaction; thermal burns; nutritional secondary hyperparathyroidism (metabolic bone disease); dental disease; chronic renal disease; starvation due to competition for food by other individuals; and exposure to toxic chemicals (e.g., ammonia, nitrites, or chloramines in aquatic species; heavy metals; cleaning solutions; toxic food items, such as fireflies etc.).
- In some cases, maladaptation syndrome or failure to thrive syndrome should also be considered as an underlying cause of weight loss.

Others

N/A

DIAGNOSIS

DIFFERENTIAL DIAGNOSIS

Normal Behavior

- Periods of torpor, brumation and estivation are normal for some species and may be associated with weight loss (loss of body mass and fluids).
- In some species, fluid loss during brumation/estivation can contribute to > 10% of total weight loss.
- Reproductive activity, behavior and gravidity may contribute to normal seasonal weight loss.

Non-Infectious Diseases

Exposure to toxic substances, especially in aquatic species, or developing disease processes secondary to poor husbandry or nutrition, will commonly lead to weight loss.

Neoplasia

- A number of neoplastic diseases have been identified in reptile species, with many different organ systems affected.
- Most of these neoplastic diseases have an expected clinical sequela of hyporexia, dehydration, and weight loss.

Infectious Diseases

- Reptiles are susceptible to many infectious diseases, all of which can contribute to hyporexia, dehydration, and weight loss.
- Simply attempting to list all infectious diseases of reptiles that may contribute to weight loss is beyond the scope of this chapter.
- Common reptile diseases observed in clinical practice, include endoparasites (gastrointestinal protozoa, nematodes, amoebae, and hemoparasites); ectoparasites (mites, ticks); Gram-negative bacterial infections and septicemia; *Chrysosporium* species and other fungal infections; and viruses (e.g., adenoviruses, paramyxoviruses, herpesviruses, retroviruses).

DIAGNOSTICS

- Since weight loss is not a specific disease, a significant clinical diagnostic workup will be necessary.
- A thorough history, including the following will be useful: housing; feeding practices; maintenance temperature and humidity; presence of other animals; access to UVB light spectrum; ad libitum access to water and water quality.

- Comparison to conspecifics housed in the same environment may confirm individual or group disease.
- A complete physical examination is critical to identify obvious lesions on the skin, within the oral cavity, on the extremities, or associated with the eyes.
- A fecal sample should be evaluated by direct smear and fecal float, if possible.
- A complete blood count and biochemical profile, along with imaging modalities (radiography, ultrasound, and/or CT), should be considered.
- Aerobic and anaerobic bacterial cultures of blood samples can be useful in debilitated reptiles due to the possibility of sepsis.
- Intracoelomic or gastrointestinal endoscopy, with or without biopsy and histopathology, may help with the diagnosis.
- In cases of obvious skin disease, a biopsy with histopathologic examination is important.

PATHOLOGICAL FINDINGS

- Pathologic findings are non-specific for weight loss, but the underlying cause may be associated with obvious gross pathologic or histopathologic lesions.
- Gross pathology of nonspecific weight loss might include loss of intracoelomic fat bodies, lack of intracoelomic organ-associated fat, and generalized muscle wasting.

TREATMENT

APPROPRIATE HEALTH CARE

N/A

NUTRITIONAL SUPPORT

- Nonspecific nutritional support may include regular force-feeding of an appropriate commercial diet and/or placement of a pharyngostomy tube to facilitate administering nutritional supplements.
- The directions on the label of the commercial diet can be followed for appropriate volume per feeding and frequency.
- Alternatively, force-feeding whole prey items (e.g., gut-loaded invertebrates, pinkie mice or small fish) may be useful.

CLIENT EDUCATION/HUSBANDRY RECOMMENDATIONS

N/A

MEDICATIONS

DRUG(S) OF CHOICE

- Based on the diagnosis of the underlying cause of weight loss, treatment should be focused on the primary disease process.
- Correct hydration status by soaking or administering appropriate fluid therapy due to fluid loss (typically an isotonic solution), as any debilitated reptile will likely be moderately to severely dehydrated.
- Based on the primary disease process underlying the weight loss, antimicrobial and anti-inflammatory drugs may be warranted.
- In addition, vitamin and mineral supplements (e.g., calcium in the form of parenteral calcium gluconate or oral calcium glubionate) may be beneficial if nutritional deficiencies underlie the weight loss; or oversupplementation of vitamins and minerals may need to be discontinued if this appears to be causing primary disease.

PRECAUTIONS/INTERACTIONS

N/A

FOLLOW-UP

PATIENT MONITORING

- Correction of inappropriate husbandry and/or feeding practices will significantly benefit the reptile patient.
- If medical treatment is necessary, the body weight can be measured, and the body condition assessed daily.
- If appropriate, medical therapy can be initiated and the patient monitored for improving condition.

EXPECTED COURSE AND PROGNOSIS

- Replenishing lost fluids from normal physiologic processes, such as brumation/estivation, may be warranted and should improve the reptiles' condition and provide a good prognosis.
- Depending on the primary underlying disease process and duration, the prognosis will range from poor to good for re-establishing normal body weight and condition.
- If husbandry problems can be corrected in a relatively short amount of time, the prognosis may be good.
- If the underlying disease process is progressive and debilitating, the prognosis will be poor.
- In cases of some infectious diseases, antimicrobials can be administered for bacterial or fungal diseases using topical, parenteral, or oral solutions.

MISCELLANEOUS

COMMENTS

N/A

ZOONOTIC POTENTIAL

N/A

SYNONYMS

- Cachexia
- Wasting

ABBREVIATIONS

- CT = computed tomography
- UVB = ultraviolet B

Suggested Reading

Mader DR, ed. *Reptile Medicine and Surgery, Reptile Medicine and Surgery*. 2nd ed. St. Louis, MO: Elsevier Saunders; 2006.

Author Kurt K. Sladky, MS, DVM, DACZM, DECZM (Zoo Health Management & Herpetology)

YEAST INFECTIONS

BASICS

DEFINITION/OVERVIEW

Infection with *Candida* spp., *Cryptococcus* spp., or, exceptionally, other yeasts. Rare in reptiles in comparison with mammals and birds.

ETIOLOGY/PATHOPHYSIOLOGY

- Many yeasts, especially *Candida* spp., are normal constituents of reptile GI and even respiratory tracts.
- Typically found secondary to concurrent condition or infection.

SIGNALMENT/HISTORY

Any reptile species, any sex, any age.

CLINICAL PRESENTATION

- Anorexia, diarrhea, weight loss, debilitation
- Signs may be non-specific or depend on affected organ system.
- Cryptococcosis has manifested as a granulomatous pneumonia and meningoencephalitis in an anaconda, but as a cutaneous swelling in at least two skinks.

RISK FACTORS

Husbandry

Poor husbandry likely a factor with these often-opportunistic pathogens.

Others

- Breaches in mucosal epithelia from concurrent issues/infections may allow deep tissue access to yeasts.
- Prolonged antibiotic treatment may also favor yeast proliferation.
- Cold stunning in sea turtles
- Hibernation under suboptimal conditions may also predispose to disease.

DIAGNOSIS

DIFFERENTIAL DIAGNOSIS

- Viral and/or bacterial stomatitides and enteritides, or even protozoal GI infections
- Viral/bacterial/parasitic or other respiratory infections

DIAGNOSTICS

- Cytology of swabs or washes that demonstrate budding yeast, and ideally inflammatory cells.
- Culture of swabs, exudates, and biopsies are needed, but the isolation of *Candida* is insufficient to confirm causality.
- Cytology of fine-needle aspirates from cutaneous lesions may identify yeast clusters with morphology consistent with *Cryptococcus* spp.
- Histopathological evidence of yeast infection in biopsy/tissue sections is essential to establish causality.

PATHOLOGICAL FINDINGS

Necrosis, inflammation, and budding yeast with pseudohyphae.

TREATMENT

APPROPRIATE HEALTH CARE

- Systemic antifungals, fluid therapy, thermal and nutritional support.
- Debridement or resection of skin lesions when needed.
- Isolation of sick animals
- Review of captive husbandry

NUTRITIONAL SUPPORT

Assist-feeding if needed

CLIENT EDUCATION/HUSBANDRY RECOMMENDATIONS

- Isolation of sick animals and thorough hygiene.
- Critical review of husbandry

MEDICATIONS

DRUG(S) OF CHOICE

- Fluconazole may be efficient in treating yeast infections, but some *Candida* spp. are inherently fluconazole resistant.
- Superficial gastric or intestinal mucosal infections may respond to nystatin. Probably better to use wider-spectrum, systemically absorbed triazoles like itraconazole.

PRECAUTIONS/INTERACTIONS

N/A

FOLLOW-UP

PATIENT MONITORING

- Might require intensive care
- Monitor response to antifungal therapy and supportive measures.

EXPECTED COURSE AND PROGNOSIS

- Variable, depending on duration and severity of disease, affected organ systems, and extent of lesions.
- As these infections are often diagnosed late in the disease process, prognosis should be guarded.

MISCELLANEOUS

COMMENTS

- A presumptive diagnosis of candidiasis or other yeast infection may be possible cytologically from clinical samples, but every effort should be made to pursue identification of these yeast to species. Yeast identification may carry treatment implications, as sensitivity panels can be determined.
- Cryptococcal species infecting reptiles may differ from those infecting other vertebrates. Only with proper identification can we understand which yeast carry pathogenic potential for reptiles.

ZOONOTIC POTENTIAL

- Cryptococcosis, a zoonotic disease, has been documented in reptiles.
- Candidiasis is rare in reptiles, but also is a potential zoonosis.

SYNONYMS

N/A

ABBREVIATIONS

GI = gastrointestinal

Suggested Reading

Paré JA, Jacobson ER. Mycotic diseases of reptiles. In: Jacobson ER, ed. *Infectious Disease and Pathology of Reptiles, Color Atlas and Text.* Boca Raton, FL: CRC Press; 2007:527–570.

Author Jean A. Paré, DMV, DVSc, DACZM, DECZM (Zoo Health Management)

SECTION IV

SNAKES

ADENOVIRUS

BASICS

DEFINITION/OVERVIEW

AdVs have been found to infect all classes of bony vertebrates and most appear to have co-evolved with their hosts. Adenoviral infections in reptiles have ranged from clinically inapparent to enteritis, necrotizing hepatitis, esophagitis, splenitis, and encephalopathy.

ETIOLOGY/PATHOPHYSIOLOGY

- Adenoviruses are double-stranded non-enveloped DNA viruses.
- The family Adenoviridae is further classified into five currently accepted genera: *Mastadenovirus* isolated from mammals; *Aviadenovirus* in birds; *Atadenovirus* isolated from squamates; *Siadenovirus* found in some chelonians, amphibians, and birds; and *Ichtadenovirus* isolated from a sturgeon. A sixth genus, *Testadenovirus*, isolated from tortoises, has been proposed.
- AdV infections have been identified in wild-caught and captive lizards, snakes, chelonians, and crocodiles.
- Disease is often a combination of other disease agents and/or stress and the viral infection.

SIGNALMENT/HISTORY

- Species reported with an adenovirus isolate are the Colubridae: corn snake, milk snake, bull snake, kingsnake, California mountain kingsnake, coastal mountain kingsnake; Pythonidae: royal python; Boidae: boa constrictor, rosy boas; Viperidae: European asp, and an Indonesian pit viper.
- With molecular diagnostics, more affected species are expected to be identified.
- There is no sex predilection.
- Juvenile and/or stressed animals are more frequently reported with disease.

CLINICAL PRESENTATION

- The clinical presentation is non-specific and often the animal is found dead.
- Chronic enteritis is the most common presentation in snakes.
- Other clinical signs include inappetence, regurgitation, coelomic distention, disequilibrium and unresponsiveness to stimuli, weight loss, and dehydration.

RISK FACTORS

Husbandry

- Adenoviruses are very stable in the environment and commonly spread through fecal–oral transmission.
- Poor biosecurity can help to disseminate the virus throughout a collection.

Others

- Stressors such as capture, substandard housing, nutritional inadequacies or underlying disease play a role in the development of clinical infection.
- Concurrent disease and/or immunosuppression increases the likelihood of severe systemic disease.
- California mountain kingsnakes have had co-infection with *Dependovirus*-like agent.
- Corn snakes have been reported as co-infected with cryptosporidia.

DIAGNOSIS

DIFFERENTIAL DIAGNOSIS

- Septicemia, gastroenteritis from any cause
- Inclusion body disease of boids (arenavirus), herpesvirus.

DIAGNOSTICS

- PCR may be diagnostic if the test is specific for the adenovirus commonly isolated from the reptile species.
- Necropsy and histopathology: the appropriate tissues need to be evaluated and, in some cases, additional tests such as TEM and/or PCR molecular diagnostics need to be performed.

PATHOLOGICAL FINDINGS

- Gross lesions: coelomic cavity fluid, enlarged, mottled liver, dilated small intestines.
- Histology: large basophilic or amphophilic inclusions in mucosal epithelial cells of the stomach, intestines, esophagus and liver. Specifically, there is enteritis, hepatic necrosis, secondary bacterial septicemias, foci of gliosis primarily within the caudal cerebrum, brainstem, and cervical spinal cord.

TREATMENT

APPROPRIATE HEALTH CARE

N/A

NUTRITIONAL SUPPORT

Nutritional support should be provided as needed only when the reptile is well hydrated and at an ideal environmental temperature for the species.

CLIENT EDUCATION/HUSBANDRY RECOMMENDATIONS

- Quarantine: the current recommendation is for approximately six months' isolation for most reptiles, with PCR testing at various intervals.
- Post-outbreak: after diagnosis of an adenovirus infection in a collection, cages and hard surfaces must be thoroughly cleaned with a detergent followed by disinfection with a 10% bleach solution. A minimum of 10-minute contact time with the bleach is recommended. All bleached supplies and cages should be thoroughly rinsed afterward and dried. Bleach can be corrosive and can cause respiratory irritation in enclosed spaces. Direct unfiltered sunlight or other intense ultraviolet sources may also aid disinfection. Proper contact time must be followed if using other disinfectants.
- All reptiles should be kept at the appropriate temperature and humidity, and offered food consistent with their dietary requirements.

MEDICATIONS

DRUG(S) OF CHOICE

N/A

PRECAUTIONS/INTERACTIONS

N/A

FOLLOW-UP

PATIENT MONITORING

- Reptiles showing clinical signs should be isolated and provided supportive care.
- Any co-infections should be treated, if possible.
- Monitoring weight, appetite, and fecal production will help assess response to therapy and progression of infection.
- Utensils and cage furniture should not be transferred from room to room or animal to animal.

EXPECTED COURSE AND PROGNOSIS

- There is no specific treatment.
- The disease progression is unknown as antemortem diagnosis is seldom determined.
- Cases have ranged from acute to chronic protracted presentation of clinical signs.
- Identifying adenovirus from a healthy animal is not diagnostic for a disease caused by the virus.
- Reptiles can be inapparent hosts for adenoviruses.

MISCELLANEOUS

COMMENTS

N/A

ZOONOTIC POTENTIAL

N/A

SYNONYMS

N/A

ABBREVIATIONS

- AdV = adenovirus
- PCR = polymerase chain reaction
- TEM = transmission electron microscopy

INTERNET RESOURCES

- Kik MJL. Adenovirus Infection in Reptiles. EAZWV Transmissible Disease Fact Sheet, sheet no. 2, April 2009. http://c.ymcdn.com/sites/www.eazwv.org/resource/resmgr/Files/Transmissible_Diseases_Handbook/Fact_Sheets/002_Adenovirus_Infection_In_.pdf
- Jacobson E, Wellehan J, Stacy B. Reptile Adenovirus PCR and Sequencing at the University of Florida CVM. http://www.dachiu.com/beardeddragons/Adenovirus.pdf

Suggested Reading

Ball I, Ofner S, Funk RS, et al. Prevalence of neutralising antibodies against adenoviruses in lizards and snakes. *Vet J* 2014;202(1):176–181.

Farkas SL, Harrach B, Benkö M. Completion of the genome analysis of snake adenovirus type 1, a representative of the reptilian lineage within the novel genus *Atadenovirus*. *Virus Res* 2008;132(1–2):132–139.

Papp T, Fledelius B, Schmidt V, et al. PCR-sequence characterization of new adenoviruses found in reptiles and the first successful isolation of a lizard adenovirus. *Vet Microbiol* 2009;134(3–4):233–240.

Author Drury R. Reavill, DVM, DABVP (Avian and Reptile & Amphibian Practice), DACVP

ANEMIA

BASICS

DEFINITION/OVERVIEW

Anemia is a sign of disease and is characterized by a decreased number of erythrocytes, hemoglobin deficiency, or both. Anemia can occur due to one of four main categories: decreased erythropoietic activity, hemorrhage, destruction of red blood cells, or sequestration.

ETIOLOGY/PATHOPHYSIOLOGY

The etiology of anemia in reptiles includes:

- Traumatic
- Hemorrhagic
- Maladaptation syndrome associated anemia: reported in stressed reptiles, associated with captivity or with capture of wild reptiles.
- Blood parasites
- Virus-associated anemia
- Autoimmune hemolytic anemia: rare in reptiles.

SIGNALMENT/HISTORY

Wild-caught reptiles or those housed under poor husbandry conditions may be more predisposed.

CLINICAL PRESENTATION

- Anemic reptiles often present with nonspecific clinical signs including lethargy, anorexia, and behavioral changes.
- Pallor of skin and mucus membrane color may be observed.

RISK FACTORS

Husbandry

- Inadequate husbandry, including diet, is often a predisposing factor for many diseases of captive reptiles.
- Any reptile maintained under poor husbandry conditions should be considered susceptible to disease.
- Wild-caught reptiles are more likely to have underlying diseases, especially endoparasites and hemoparasites, which may be the underlying cause of chronic anemia.

Others

Any reptile with a chronic illness may be predisposed to anemia.

DIAGNOSIS

DIFFERENTIAL DIAGNOSIS

- Trauma leading to external or internal hemorrhage.
- Maladaptation syndrome associated anemia (reported in stressed reptiles, associated with captivity or trapping of wild reptiles).
- Hemoparasites
- Malnutrition
- Toxicity
- Viral infection

DIAGNOSTICS

Blood sampling

- Blood sampling is essential for diagnosis and monitoring of anemic reptiles. Patient's size, condition, and venous access all must be considered.
- Venipuncture sites with minimal lymphatic contamination are preferred to obtain a more representative sample of the peripheral blood.
- In snakes, the two most common sampling sites are cardiac puncture and the ventral coccygeal vein. The palatine vessel and jugular may also be accessible in some species.
- In critically ill, possibly anemic, reptiles, aim to collect a blood volume of no more than 0.5% of the body weight (0.5 ml/100 g body weight) so as to not exacerbate the anemic condition.
- The use of EDTA or lithium heparin is widely debated in reptile medicine and is largely based on experience and few scientific studies. In general, EDTA is recommended unless artifacts are documented for a particular species.

Physical Exam

- Examination of mucous membranes and general pallor.
- Compared with mammals, reptiles' mucous membranes are lighter in color but should still appear pink.
- Among reptiles, snakes tend normally have rather pale mucus membranes, making it more difficult to make a proper assessment.

Hematology

Although there is limited ability to assess all the same hematologic parameters as in mammals, some basic guidelines can be found for certain values.

Hematocrit/PCV

- The normal values range from 20% to 45%. Values below 20% suggest anemia in most cases.
- A blood transfusion should be considered in animals with values below 10%, although there is little research in reptilian blood transfusions.
- Seasonal variations in this parameter should also be considered before making clinical decisions.
- A low hematocrit with an increased polychromasia index is a normal physiologic change during brumation, but pathologic during the active season.

Hemoglobin

- Normal values are 5–12 g/dl according to the species. Lower values should suggest anemia.
- Mean corpuscular hemoglobin concentration is calculated according to hematocrit and hemoglobin; parameters show variation in anemia. Individual variations should also be considered, as reptiles have different types of hemoglobin, which may influence the expression of clinical signs.

Polychromasia and Erythroblasts

- An increased polychromasia and erythroblasts in general suggests an increased need for erythrocytes in peripheral blood and can be interpreted as evidence of a regenerative anemia.
- Occasionally, a high number of erythroblasts may be found in the microhematocrit tube, forming an intermediate layer between the buffy coat and the red blood concentrate.
- This activity is usually accompanied by the presence of erythrocyte precursors in peripheral blood (erythroblasts, occasionally polychromatophils).
- Hemoparasites may also lead to increased erythroblast and polychromasia.
- Polychromasia may also occur in the absence of anemia, and has been reported in shedding reptiles.

Erythrocytic Mitoses

- When detected in peripheral blood as an anecdotal finding, erythrocyte mitoses are not a manifestation of anemia.
- Anemia should only be considered when mitoses appear in erythrocytes together with the presence of abundant erythroblasts and other markers described, such as altered hematocrit and irregular erythrocytic nucleus.

Erythrocyte Counts

- Total erythrocyte counts are lower than in mammals and birds.
- Erythrocytes in snakes are medium sized compared with other reptiles; they tend to have erythrocyte counts between 400,000 and 1.5 million erythrocytes/microliter.

Fecal Occult Blood Test and Urinalysis

- Fecal occult blood test and urinalysis may allow for the detection of small amounts of blood in an animal's urine or feces.
- Fecal occult test may produce false positives in carnivorous species.

PATHOLOGICAL FINDINGS

Pathologic findings will be specific to the underlying cause of anemia.

TREATMENT

APPROPRIATE HEALTH CARE

- Anemia is often a chronic presentation in most reptiles.
- A slower metabolism and physiologic adaptation mechanisms allow them to compensate better than birds or mammals.
- Treatment is often not needed on an emergency basis, but is rather focused on addressing the underlying diseases and providing supportive therapy.

NUTRITIONAL SUPPORT

- Proper nutrition is key for the prevention and treatment of anemia.
- The diet should be as varied as possible and adapted to each species.
- Diet should be balanced and contain natural sources of vitamin B12 and iron.
- Nutritional support via gavage feeding should be implemented in very ill and/or anorectic animals.

CLIENT EDUCATION/HUSBANDRY RECOMMENDATIONS

- It is recommended to perform annual health evaluations of the animals at risk. These evaluations should include blood tests and fecal exams.
- Any treatments must be performed based on the results of the exams and the historical data for the collection.
- These tests should also be done on newly acquired and quarantined animals.
- A proper nutritional plan is also essential for good health.

MEDICATIONS

DRUG(S) OF CHOICE

- Hemorrhagic anemia: control bleeding by applying pressure.
- Maladaptation syndrome: treatment consists of fluid therapy and stimulation of blood regeneration.
- The use of hemostatic agents such as D-aminocaproic acid or ethamsylate has not been reported in reptiles, so doses are empirical (0.1 ml/kg). The efficacy of blood replacers or transfusions has not been well studied at this time.
- Fluid therapy: isotonic fluids should be administered at a rate of 20–30 ml/kg IV or SC for maintenance.
- Fluid losses can be replaced, being careful not to overhydrate the patient. Close monitoring is necessary when treating hypoproteinemic patients to avoid overhydration.
- Colloids may also be used at a rate 10–20 ml/kg with a bolus of 3–5 ml/kg IV as needed. The main challenge in snakes is placement of an intravenous catheter, which often requires a cutdown technique.
- Blood replacers: availability varies across the world. If available, products like Oxyglobin® (bovine hemoglobin glutamer; 1 ml/100 g IV for 5 minutes by means of perfusion; repeat 4 hours later) may improve the success of such cases of severe anemia.
- Blood transfusion: homologous transfusions are preferred over heterologous. A blood volume of up to 1% body weight is extracted from the donor by means of syringes and needles filled with anticoagulant at a ratio of 1 : 6 to 1 : 9 anticoagulant to blood. The blood is administered to the recipient by means of an infusion pump at 5 ml/hour flow rate. True efficacy is not well documented but clinical experience suggests some short-term benefits.
- Maladaptation syndrome: iron dextran 12 mg/kg, IM every 7 days and cyanocobalamin (vitamin B12) 0.5 mg/kg or 10–2000 iu, according to the animal's weight,, as single IM or SC dose.

PRECAUTIONS/INTERACTIONS

N/A

FOLLOW-UP

PATIENT MONITORING

- Because of the small size of some snakes and difficulty in obtaining blood, monitoring should rely on assessment of the behavior and clinical signs of the affected animal, not just on blood sampling.
- If the treatment is appropriate, the snake should become progressively more active and alert, with interest in hunting, seeking shelter or mating behaviors.
- Normal attitude and shedding are two common aspects that can be monitored in reptiles after the start of treatment, because they are related to the overall health of the animal.
- In addition, signs of healing of the other diseases that have contributed to the animal's anemia should be observed.

EXPECTED COURSE AND PROGNOSIS

- Repeat blood sampling after 1 week and 1 month may show early signs of regeneration.
- Repeat blood sampling may be contraindicated, especially in cases of non-regenerative anemia, when working with small patients, or if the underlying etiology is not being treated.
- If the underlying cause of anemia is properly diagnosed and can be effectively treated, prognosis is good.

MISCELLANEOUS

COMMENTS

Figure 1 – see web image supplementary content for Section II (Snakes)

ZOONOTIC POTENTIAL

N/A

SYNONYMS

- Inadaptation syndrome
- Maladaptation syndrome

ABBREVIATIONS

- EDTA = ethylenediaminetetraacetic acid
- IM = intramuscular
- IV = intravenous
- PCV = packed cell volume
- SC = subcutaneous

INTERNET RESOURCES

Cital S. Exotic animal blood transfusions: An overview. VetBloom. http://blog.vetbloom.com/exotics/exotic-animal-blood-transfusions-an-overview

Suggested Reading

Boyer TH. Autoimmune hemolytic anemia in a parson's chameleon, *Calumna parsonii parsonii*. *Proc ARAV.* 2002;9: 81-84.

Martínez-Silvestre A. How do I treat anemia in reptiles. *Proc SEVC-AVEPA* 2013;48:1–5.

Saggese MD. Clinical approach to the anemic reptile. *J Exot Pet Med* 2009;18(2):98–111.

Wu C, Chie CHH. Case study: Successful treatment of acute anaemia with whole blood transfusion and supportive care in two turtles. *Proc UPAV/AAVAC/ARAV* 2014:13–20.

Author Albert Martínez-Silvestre, DVM, MSc, PhD, DECZM (Herpetology), EBVS European Veterinary Specialist in Herpetological Medicine and Surgery, Acred. AVEPA (Exotic Animals)

ANOREXIA

BASICS

DEFINITION/OVERVIEW

Anorexia is the lack of appetite or intake of food; it does not define an underlying cause. Many pathological and even physiological conditions can result in decreased food intake. Anorexia is distinct from decreased appetite, which is also known as hypophagia. Anorexia in some snakes (e.g., *Python regius*) is thought to be physiologic and has a seasonal influence.

ETIOLOGY/PATHOPHYSIOLOGY

- Anorexia may be a normal physiologic/behavioral occurrence during certain times of the year (e.g., brumation, estivation, reproductive season).
- Pathologic causes of anorexia may stem from either GI or extra-GI disease (e.g., any painful condition or systemic illness).
- Improper husbandry and offering the wrong type and size of food may also lead to anorexia.
- Anorexia may also result in dehydration.
- Prolonged anorexia may lead to hepatic lipidosis, which may result in nausea, leading to continued lack of food intake.
- Nutritional imbalances and metabolic derangements can occur with chronic anorexia and cachexia may ensue.
- Primarily, the gastrointestinal and musculoskeletal systems are affected with anorexia.
- Animals that are not consuming food for prolonged periods of time may not defecate significant amounts.
- As the body begins to break down adipose tissue stores and muscle, bony prominences become more obvious as body condition decreases.

SIGNALMENT/HISTORY

- Anorexia has no age or sex predilection.
- It is important to differentiate physiologic/behavioral anorexia from that caused by an underlying pathology or disease process.
- Lack of appetite is a normal finding in estivating or hibernating animals.

CLINICAL PRESENTATION

- An isolated incident or occasional episodes of anorexia in otherwise healthy animals may be inconsequential, especially in an animal presenting in good body condition.
- Decreased food intake over an extended period.
- Clients may report repeated attempts at feeding.
- Clinical signs of chronic anorexia include a decreased body condition score with prominent bony protuberances, dehydration, and muscle wasting.

RISK FACTORS

- Different types of stress may result in decreased food intake.
- Any disease process could result in anorexia.

Husbandry

- Adjusting to captivity: often seen in newly acquired animals. A period of acclimation may be necessary prior to an animal feeling secure enough to start eating on its own. While a snake is adapting to its new environment over the first few days to weeks in its new enclosure, handling should be minimized to limit stress. Prey should be offered only after the snake has become more comfortable in its new habitat.
- Improper husbandry: inappropriate environmental temperature or humidity, inappropriate food items (type and/or size), malnutrition, poor water quality, overcrowding, rapid change of diet, lack of provision of hiding areas.
- Stress: social or environmental

Others

- Physiologic: often seen in adult ball pythons (*Python regius*) that fast for weeks to months without overt negative effects; snakes just prior to or undergoing ecdysis may not eat.
- Cardiovascular disease: cardiomyopathy, congestive heart failure.
- Reproductive activity: gravid females, breeding males.
- Reproductive disease: pre- or postovulatory dystocia.
- Respiratory tract pathology: bacterial pneumonia; tracheal ring granulomas.
- Viral infections
- Fungal infections: Fungal pneumonia; *Ophidiomyces ophiodiicola, Paranannizziopsis* spp. infections.
- Systemic illness: septicemia
- GI disease: stomatitis, damage to tongue, foreign bodies, neoplasia, constipation, gastroenteritis, prolapses.
- Parasitic disease: ectoparasites and endoparasites; infestation with *Ophionyssus natricis* often results in anorexia in captive snakes.
- Neurologic disease: inclusion body disease.
- Toxic diseases
- Urogenital: renal disease
- Metabolic: nutritional secondary hyperparathyroidism
- Any potentially painful condition: ophthalmic disease, orthopedic conditions, cellulitis, trauma.

DIAGNOSIS

DIFFERENTIAL DIAGNOSIS

- Conditions that result in failed food prehension (disorders of the oral cavity) or processing (regurgitation with gastric hyperplasia from cryptosporidiosis) may result in animals that attempt to eat (have an appetite) but are unable to do so successfully.
- Hypophagia may be mistaken for anorexia in certain circumstances.

DIAGNOSTICS

- Diagnostic procedures should be tailored towards identifying the underlying cause of the anorexia and identifying potential negative sequelae (e.g., hepatic lipidosis).

Baseline Blood Work

- CBC, PCV, total solids, biochemistry
- Findings on CBC and biochemistry panels are usually non-specific but may be suggestive of underlying disease process(es) resulting in the observed anorexia.
- Bile acids and liver leakage enzymes (AST) may be increased if hepatic lipidosis is present secondary to prolonged anorexia.

Imaging

Radiography can help to identify abnormalities of the GI tract such as foreign bodies and masses. Ultrasound and CT can provide more detailed information about possible hepatic lipidosis, ileus, and coelomic masses.

Other Tests

- Additional diagnostics, including infectious or parasitic disease testing, may be warranted based on patient history and physical examination findings.
- The presumed underlying causes should be thoroughly investigated.

PATHOLOGICAL FINDINGS

- Findings depend on underlying cause of the anorexia.
- Hepatic lipidosis may be suspected based on the findings of advanced imaging or biochemistry evaluation.

TREATMENT

APPROPRIATE HEALTH CARE

N/A

NUTRITIONAL SUPPORT

- Nutritional support should be started in anorectic animals that have lost 10% of their body weight acutely (≤ 7 days or less) or 20% chronically (> 7 days).
- This weight loss must also be monitored together with an assessment of BCS.
- Anorectic animals with a BCS of 2/5 or lower may be immediate candidates for nutritional support.
- Animals should be housed in appropriate environments and maintained at their preferred optimum temperature zones, to facilitate proper takeup of the provided nourishment.
- Liquid diets may be provided via syringe or gavage in smaller animals.
- In otherwise stable patients in which the mouth can be teased open, assist-feeding may be attempted by gently placing killed prey items in the back of the oral cavity to promote swallowing.

• Although poorly understood in veterinary medicine, the potential exists for refeeding syndrome in chronically anorectic patients, necessitating careful planning of nutritional support in these animals.
• Recommendations include feeding chronically anorectic animals half of their calculated energy requirements initially, then slowly increasing up to the full energy requirement over 7–10 days.

CLIENT EDUCATION/HUSBANDRY RECOMMENDATIONS

• The clinician should perform a thorough review of the patient's current husbandry including feeding.
• It is important to ensure that a proper diet of an appropriate size is being offered.
• The diet must be presented to the animal appropriately (e.g., feeding diurnal animals during daylight hours, offering prey on land vs. in the water or vice versa).
• Any husbandry or dietary deficiencies should be corrected.
• Clients should be notified that offering live food items to anorectic animals could result in rapid, serious injury secondary to prey attacks.
• For most cases, live prey (especially rodents and crickets) should not be offered to snakes without direct supervision.

MEDICATIONS

DRUG(S) OF CHOICE

Commercial, high calorie formulations designed for nutritional support in reptiles are recommended when feeding anorectic snakes.

PRECAUTIONS/INTERACTIONS

• Exercise caution when force-feeding to prevent dental trauma.
• Be careful not to administer too large a volume of nutritional formula in small patients.
• Feed 1–3% f body weight initially to ensure the animal will tolerate the feedings.

FOLLOW-UP

PATIENT MONITORING

• Individuals should be monitored for resolution of anorexia following correction of any husbandry and dietary deficiencies.
• Serial imaging and blood chemistry evaluation may be considered to monitor for development or resolution of secondary liver diseases such as hepatic lipidosis.

EXPECTED COURSE AND PROGNOSIS

• Anorexia may continue until the underlying reason is identified and treated, if applicable.
• Prognosis for resolution of anorexia depends on the severity of the underlying cause.

MISCELLANEOUS

COMMENTS

• Simply providing appropriate husbandry will help to prevent many causes of anorexia in snakes.
• Prompt diagnosis of true anorexia enables initiation of proper nutritional support and may prevent formation of hepatic lipidosis, which can perpetuate the lack of appetite.
• Supportive care should be continued while an underlying cause for the anorexia is identified and corrected.
• Gravid individuals may decrease their amount of food consumption from lack of coelomic space for GI distension.
• Animals that are anorectic from an underlying pathologic condition may cease or abort reproductive activity due to preferential allotment of energy for other physiologic functions.
• Male snakes may drop substantial body weight during the active breeding season.

ZOONOTIC POTENTIAL

N/A

SYNONYMS

• Aphagia
• Anophagia
• Inappetence

ABBREVIATIONS

• AST = aspartate aminotransferase
• BCS = body condition score
• CBC = complete blood count
• CT = computed tomography
• GI = gastrointestinal
• PCV = packed cell volume

Suggested Reading

De Voe RS. Nutritional support of reptile patients. *Vet Clin North Am Exot Anim Pract* 2014;17:249–261.
Divers SJ, Stahl S, eds. *Mader's Reptile and Amphibian Medicine and Surgery*. 3rd ed. St. Louis, MO: Elsevier; 2019.

Author Grayson Doss, DVM, DACZM

BALANTIDIUM

BASICS

DEFINITION/OVERVIEW

Balantidium is a large ciliated protozoal organism that resides within the gastrointestinal tract. The trophozoite is elliptical in shape and ranges in size from 30 × 25 μm to 300 × 120 μm. It is densely covered with cilia along its surface. At the tapered front end lies the cystostome (mouth). Cysts have a thick wall, spherical in shape, and have a kidney bean-shaped macronucleus. *Balantidium* is typically found in herbivorous reptiles and its pathogenicity is often debated. There is a report of concurrent *Balantidium coli* and *Escherichia coli* in a group of snakes.

ETIOLOGY/PATHOPHYSIOLOGY

- Transmission is through fecal–oral route.
- Cysts are ingested and then undergo excystation in the intestinal tract.
- Trophozoites inhabit the large colon and replicate by binary fission.
- Trophozoites undergo encystation in which infective cysts are formed and then excreted in feces.
- *Balantidium* spp. are facultative parasites and only become pathogenic when other virulence factors such as hyaluronidase are present. This then allows them to penetrate the intestinal mucosa and cause extensive hemorrhage and necrosis.
- The parasites are generally limited to the large intestinal tract.
- In severe infections, the protozoal organisms migrate to the liver and cause abscessation.

SIGNALMENT/HISTORY

No age or sex predisposition

CLINICAL PRESENTATION

Vomiting, weight loss, diarrhea

RISK FACTORS

Husbandry

- Improper husbandry
- Imported
- Wild-caught animals

Others

Immunocompromised animals with active parasitic/bacterial infections are more predisposed for the protozoan to become pathogenic.

DIAGNOSIS

DIFFERENTIAL DIAGNOSIS

Nyctotherus sp.

DIAGNOSTICS

- Microscopic evaluation of fresh fecal material to visualize trophozoites and cysts. In a single case report in snakes, the parasite was also observed in the vomit.
- SAF technique can be used for better visualization.
- The addition of iodine will stain the contents of the cysts, making them more visible.

PATHOLOGICAL FINDINGS

Hemorrhagic necrotizing enteritis

TREATMENT

APPROPRIATE HEALTH CARE

N/A

NUTRITIONAL SUPPORT

N/A

CLIENT EDUCATION/HUSBANDRY RECOMMENDATIONS

Practice proper hygiene

MEDICATIONS

DRUG(S) OF CHOICE

- Metronidazole 50 mg/kg PO q24h for 7 days
- Nimorazole 125 mg/kg PO q24 for 4 days
- Tetracyclines 5–10 mg/kg PO q24h for 5–8 days

PRECAUTIONS/INTERACTIONS

N/A

FOLLOW-UP

PATIENT MONITORING

Recheck feces on a routine basis.

EXPECTED COURSE AND PROGNOSIS

- Since most cases do not require therapy, prognosis is usually good as long as the disease does not have effects beyond the intestines.
- Treatment should be started only if clinical disease is observed.
- Snakes in the case report responded to treatment with metronidazole.

MISCELLANEOUS

COMMENTS

N/A

ZOONOTIC POTENTIAL

N/A

SYNONYMS

N/A

ABBREVIATIONS

- PO = per os
- SAF = sodium acetate-acetic acid formalin

INTERNET RESOURCES

- De Bosschere H, Roels S. *Balantidium* sp. and *Nyctotherus* sp: Two common members of the digestive-tract flora in Mediterranean tortoises. Tortoise Trust. https://www.tortoisetrust.org/articles/balantidium.htm
- Divers SJ. Parasitic Diseases of Reptiles. MSD Manual Veterinary Manual, June 2020. http://www.merckvetmanual.com/exotic-and-laboratory-animals/reptiles/parasitic-diseases-of-reptiles

Suggested Reading

Adaszek L, Winiarczyk S, Tomczuk K, et al. Balantidiosis in snakes. *Medycyna Weterynaryjna* 2005;61:583–584.

Hnizdo J, Pantchev N. Protozoa (digestive tract). In: Medical Care of Turtles and Tortoises. Diagnosis. Surgery. Pathology. Parasitology. Frankfurt, Germany: Edition Chimaira; 2011: 194–195.

Jacobson ER. Parasites and parasitic diseases of reptiles. In: Jacobson ER, ed. *Infectious Diseases and Pathology of Reptiles: Color Atlas and Text.* Boca Raton, FL: CRC Press; 2007:571–665.

Rataj AV, Lindtner-Knific R, Vlahovic K,et al. Parasites in pet reptiles. *Acta Vet Scand* 2011;53(1):33.

Author Elsburgh O. Clarke III, DVM, DACZM

BUPHTHALMOS

BASICS

DEFINITION/OVERVIEW

Buphthalmos is an enlarged globe that is positioned normally in the socket.

ETIOLOGY/PATHOPHYSIOLOGY

An increase in IOP causing enlargement and distention of the globe secondary to chronic glaucoma.

SIGNALMENT/HISTORY

- There is no standard signalment for this disease.
- Common findings in the history may include asymmetry of the globes and loss of vision on the affected side(s).

CLINICAL PRESENTATION

- While it can be bilateral, most cases in snakes are unilateral.
- The corneal diameter of the affected eye is increased due to globe stretching.
- Unlike exophthalmia, the conjunctiva is usually normal.
- There may be a red ciliary flush (red ring around the cornea) and congested episcleral vessels.
- There may be lens luxation and/or cataracts in the affected eye(s).
- Retropulsion of the globe is normal but the globe itself may feel more firm than normal.

RISK FACTORS

Husbandry

- Diet and environmental factors are likely to have an effect on the development of cataracts.
- Cataract development in brumating snakes has been associated with damage from freezing temperatures.

Others

- Trauma, especially if there is corneal penetration can induce uveitis and cataract formation.
- The presence of a cataract may increase the chance of lens luxation and/or lens induced uveitis, both of which can lead to glaucoma.

DIAGNOSIS

DIFFERENTIAL DIAGNOSIS

- It is important to first differentiate between exophthalmia, buphthalmos, and pesudobuphthalmos, which occurs when fluid builds up between the spectacle and cornea.
- Glaucoma in snakes is usually secondary to outflow obstruction of the aqueous humor, which is most often caused by uveitis, lens luxation, or intraocular neoplasia.

DIAGNOSTICS

- Physical examination findings should raise suspicion of buphthalmos, which is confirmed by finding elevated IOP.
- Normal IOP has not been reported in any snake species, but in other reptiles where it has been measured, it generally ranges from 5 mmHg to 15 mmHg.
- Since most cases are unilateral, a significant difference in IOP between the eyes may be most indicative of a problem.
- Ocular examination and ultrasound are helpful in further evaluating the root cause.

PATHOLOGICAL FINDINGS

Chronically elevated IOP will lead to pain and blindness.

TREATMENT

APPROPRIATE HEALTH CARE

N/A

NUTRITIONAL SUPPORT

- Additional nutritional support is not necessary in most cases if the IOP can be brought down.
- If needed, tube feeding can be used to provide nutritional support.

CLIENT EDUCATION/HUSBANDRY RECOMMENDATIONS

- While buphthalmos can occur in any animal, those with husbandry deficiencies may be at increased risk.
- In addition to medical and surgical therapy, maximizing the husbandry of the animal will improve the chance for a successful outcome.

SURGICAL CONSIDERATIONS

Enucleation as a salvage procedure is usually indicated.

MEDICATIONS

DRUG(S) OF CHOICE

- Most cases present in a chronic state.
- Vision is often already lost.
- Medications are used to control pain and slow the disease process during diagnostic evaluation.
- If acute glaucoma is suspected, it is important to start treatment immediately with mannitol 1–2 g/kg IV slowly over 20–30 minutes, to reduce the IOP and preserve vision.
- If uveitis is suspected, systemic antibiotics such as ceftazidime 20 mg/kg IM or SC q48–72h and steroids (prednisolone: 0.25–0.5 mg/kg daily or dexamethasone SP: 0.04–0.08 mg/kg daily) should also be instituted.

PRECAUTIONS/INTERACTIONS

N/A

FOLLOW-UP

PATIENT MONITORING

Serial IOP measurements are useful to determine the response to therapy.

EXPECTED COURSE AND PROGNOSIS

- Prognosis is related to the underlying cause of the glaucoma, which is not always readily identifiable.
- Enucleation of the diseased globe will resolve the issue in most cases.

MISCELLANEOUS

COMMENTS

N/A

ZOONOTIC POTENTIAL

Depends on the cause of the buphthalmos but low to most often no zoonotic potential.

SYNONYMS

N/A

ABBREVIATIONS

- IM = intramuscular
- IOP = intraocular pressure
- IV = intravenous
- SC = subcutaneous

Suggested Reading

Hochleithner C, Holland M. Ultrasonography. In: Mader, DR, Divers SJ, eds. *Current Therapy in Reptile Medicine and Surgery*. Saint Louis, MO: Elsevier Saunders; 2014:93–106.

Lawton, MPC. Reptilian Ophthalmology. In: Mader DR, ed. *Reptile Medicine and Surgery*. 2nd ed. St. Louis, MO: Elsevier Saunders; 2006:323–342.

Author Christopher S. Hanley, DVM, DACZM

CARDIAC DISEASE

BASICS

DEFINITION/OVERVIEW

Cardiovascular disease encompasses a group of disorders of the heart and blood vessels including:

- Cardiomyopathy
- Septic endocarditis
- Valvular insufficiency (with no current evidence of primary degenerative endocardiosis)
- Myocarditis
- Pericardial effusion
- Infarct
- Atherosclerosis
- Aneurysm (rupture of aortic or carotid aneurysms)
- Gout
- Arterial calcification
- Thrombus
- Parasitic infestations
- Congenital heart defects
- Tumors

ETIOLOGY/PATHOPHYSIOLOGY

Infectious

- Often secondary to systemic infections in captive reptiles.
- Bacterial: aerobic Gram-negative bacteria: *Salmonella* spp., *Corynebacterium* spp., *Pseudomonas* spp. (endocarditis). *Chlamydophila* spp. (granulomatous pericarditis and myocarditis, necrotizing myocarditis and histiocytic granulomas in the heart).
- Viral: *Arenavirus*—large eosinophilic intracytoplasmic inclusion bodies in many different organs including the heart in snakes. *Adenovirus*—hepatitis and endocarditis in rosy boas (*Lichanura trivirgata*).
- Parasitic: filarial nematodes (*Macdonaldius oschei*) within the cardiovascular system can cause edema, thrombosis and necrosis. Besnoitiosis and sarcosporidiosis have also been observed in histological sections of ophidian hearts.

Non-Infectious

- Neoplastic (primary neoplasia is uncommon in reptiles): hemangioma, hemangiosarcoma, cardiac rhabdomyosarcoma, fibrosarcoma. Metastasis to the heart: metastatic chondrosarcoma, metastasis of oviductal adenocarcinoma, disseminated mast cell, multicentric lymphoblastic lymphoma, and lymphoblastic malignant lymphoma.
- Metabolic: visceral gout can cause urate crystals deposition in the pericardium. Cardiomyopathy is of undetermined origin in snakes.
- Traumatic hemopericardium with the formation of hematomas and myocardial fibrosis can occur as a result of cardiac blood sampling.
- Pericardial effusion was reported in many species but a small amount of fluid within the pericardial sac may also be normal. The etiology of pathologic pericardial effusion is unknown.

SIGNALMENT/HISTORY

- There are no known species, sex, or age predilections.
- Weakness and dyspnea
- Swelling in the area of the heart and/or peripheral edema.

CLINICAL PRESENTATION

- Presentation is similar to that seen in mammals.
- Certain differences exist due to differing cardiovascular physiology and anatomy.
- Non-specific clinical signs such as lethargy, depression, anorexia, weight loss, weakness, dyspnea, and sudden death.
- Swelling around the cardiac region (cardiomegaly).
- Cyanosis
- Peripheral edema (e.g., in gular region).
- Pulmonary edema, ascites
- Neurological signs such as ataxia and head tilt in case of brain anoxia.
- Peripheral thrombosis and necrosis in case of filarial infestation of the cardiovascular system.
- Coughing is not a feature of congestive heart failure as observed in mammals.

RISK FACTORS

Husbandry

Inadequate husbandry, resulting in chronic stress, immune suppression and malnutrition, is the most likely common predisposing factor for the development of cardiovascular conditions in captive reptiles.

Others

Atherosclerosis and viral diseases can also be predisposing factors.

DIAGNOSIS

DIFFERENTIAL DIAGNOSIS

All other diseases that induce lethargy and/or respiratory distress.

DIAGNOSTICS

- Ambient temperature can influence cardiopulmonary parameters in reptiles so must be considered during examination.

Auscultation

- Use a pressure sensitive acoustic stethoscope.
- A continuous Doppler ultrasonic probe (8 MHz) can also be used for cardiac "auscultation." It allows determination of heart rate and rhythm but only indicates blood flow (not valve closure).

Ultrasound

- The most practical diagnostic tool for antemortem evaluation of reptilian heart diseases.
- Allows visualization of blood flow within the heart. In snakes, the heart can be easily accessed via a ventral and intercostal approach.

Hematology and Biochemistry

Blood pressure measurement and pulse oximetry are not reliable in reptiles.

Clinical Pathology

- CK and LDH may increase with conditions affecting the cardiac muscle in reptiles such as myocarditis or infarct. However, these are non-specific measurements and may also increase with skeletal muscle damage from traumatic injuries, loss of body condition, and intramuscular injections.
- Cardiac troponins have been assessed in snakes.
- Leukocytosis, lymphocytosis, and heterophilia may be present, and are suggestive of underlying infections or hematopoietic neoplasia with secondary cardiac effects.

Electrocardiography

- Low electric amplitudes (usually < 1.0 mV) and standard parameters not established for many species.
- Common findings in the normal reptilian ECG include P-wave pleomorphism, very small Q and S deflections and prolonged Q-T intervals compared with similar sized mammals.
- Correct electrode placement (challenging in reptiles) is essential to avoid erroneous ECG readings.

Radiography

Can be used to evaluate the size of the cardiac silhouette in snakes.

CT and MRI

- Apart from obvious cardiomyopathy, neither CT nor MRI (unless using a very high magnetic field strengths) are of use for visualizing intracardiac structures and large vessels.
- Evaluate for concurrent disease to determine whether cardiac issue is primary or secondary (neoplastic, infectious).

PATHOLOGICAL FINDINGS

Gross and histopathologic findings depend on the type of heart disease.

TREATMENT

APPROPRIATE HEALTH CARE

- Little information
- Actions of cardiac drugs in reptiles are poorly understood and few data are available in the literature (pharmacokinetics, toxicity, etc.).

NUTRITIONAL SUPPORT

No specific nutritional support considerations and/or recommendations.

CLIENT EDUCATION/HUSBANDRY RECOMMENDATIONS

Reduce stress by minimizing handling, separating from cage mates, and maintaining the reptile at its preferred optimum temperature.

MEDICATIONS

DRUG(S) OF CHOICE

- Beta-blockers: unknown effectiveness in reptile patients.
- Methylatropine: administration results in an increase in resting heart rate of iguanas. No data available for snakes.
- Pimobendan and digoxin: unknown effects in reptiles.
- Enalapril: inhibited angiotensin I conversion in alligators at 0.5–0.7 mg/kg once every 24 hours (combined with spironolactone and furosemide). No data available for snakes.
- Furosemide: possible diuretic effect in chelonians and ophidians despite lacking the loop of Henle.
- Hydrochlorothiazide has been used as a diuretic in lizards with renal disease. No data available for snakes.
- Methylated xanthines (aminophylline and theophylline) have successfully induced diuresis.
- Nothing is known about the potential use of spironolactone in reptiles.

PRECAUTIONS/INTERACTIONS

N/A

FOLLOW-UP

PATIENT MONITORING

Repeated echocardiographic examinations

EXPECTED COURSE AND PROGNOSIS

As no specific treatment is available, fast deterioration can be expected.

MISCELLANEOUS

COMMENTS

N/A

ZOONOTIC POTENTIAL

Can be zoonotic in case of salmonellosis and other Gram-negative bacteria.

SYNONYMS

- Cardiovascular disease
- Heart disease

ABBREVIATIONS

- CK = creatine kinase
- CT = computed tomography
- ECG = electrocardiogram
- LDH = lactate dehydrogenase
- MRI = magnetic resonance imaging

Suggested Reading

Beaufrère H, Schilliger L, Pariaut R. Cardiovascular system In: Mitchell MA, Tully TN, eds. *Current therapy of exotic animal practice*. St. Louis, MO: Elsevier; 2016:151–220.

Mitchell MA. Reptile cardiology. *Vet Clin North Am Exot Anim Pract* 2009;12:65–79.

Schilliger L, Girling S. Cardiology. In: Divers S, Stahl S, eds. *Mader's Reptile and Amphibian Medicine and Surgery*. St. Louis, MO: Elsevier; 2019:669–698.

Author Lionel Schilliger, DVM, DECZM (Herpetology), DABVP (Reptile & Amphibian Practice)

CHLAMYDIOSIS

BASICS

DEFINITION/OVERVIEW

Chlamydia sp. are obligate intracellular bacteria that infect both animals and humans. Besides crocodilians, snakes are the only other reptile group with well-documented cases of chlamydiosis.

ETIOLOGY/PATHOPHYSIOLOGY

- *Chlamydia pneumoniae* is the most commonly diagnosed chlamydial pathogen in snakes.
- The source of exposure to snakes in unknown.
- Other novel species (*C. serpentis* and *C. poikilothermis sp. nov.*) from snakes have also been reported.

SIGNALMENT/HISTORY

- Chlamydiosis has been reported form a wide range of snake species.
- There is no age or sex predilection.
- Animals may come from a stable collection or one with a recent history of additions.
- Chronic regurgitation may be reported as part of the history for the collection.

CLINICAL PRESENTATION

- Affected animals regurgitate food a few days after feeding.
- This is followed by a loss of body condition, emaciation, and death.

RISK FACTORS

- Addition of new snakes without quarantine, wild-caught snakes, and snakes from infected collections.
- Stress from transport and brumation may precipitate disease expression in subclinical carriers.

Husbandry

- A lack of quarantine and biosecurity can lead to spread of the disease within a facility.
- Inadequate husbandry, specifically temperature and humidity causing stress, may also precipitate clinical signs.

Others

N/A

DIAGNOSIS

- Diagnosis is based on histopathology and PCR.
- The liver, spleen, heart, lungs, and intestines are some of the tissues that should be tested by PCR.
- Choana and cloacal swabs can be collected for antemortem diagnosis.

DIFFERENTIAL DIAGNOSIS

- Cryptosporidiosis
- Inclusion body disease
- Parasitic enteritis

DIAGNOSTICS

- Real-time quantitative PCR is the most commonly reported diagnostic tool. Liver and spleen are the ideal tissues to be tested.
- Histopathology helps to confirm and characterize the infection.
- Electron microscopy can help to confirm the presence of a chlamydial organism within tissues.

PATHOLOGICAL FINDINGS

Granulomatous inflammation of the liver, spleen, heart, lungs, and intestines.

TREATMENT

APPROPRIATE HEALTH CARE

N/A

NUTRITIONAL SUPPORT

Force-feeding once weekly with a critical care formula may help to facilitate nutrient absorption if the snake does not regurgitate the formula.

CLIENT EDUCATION/HUSBANDRY RECOMMENDATIONS

- Antemortem PCR can help to identify subclinical carriers in the collection, to aid in designing management protocols for feeding order and biosecurity.
- It is critical to implement quarantine and biosecurity protocols to prevent spread of the disease during an outbreak.
- It is important to keep good records of feeding events, regurgitation, and body weights.
- Consider testing new animals during quarantine or prior to purchasing.
- An infected collection should be closed to any movement of snakes in or out of the collection.

MEDICATIONS

DRUG(S) OF CHOICE

- Oxytetracycline 10 mg/kg PO, IM, IV q24h
- Fluoroquinolones: marbofloxacin 10 mg/kg PO q48h; 5 mg/kg IM q24h; ciprofloxacin 10 mg/kg PO q48h; enrofloxacin 10 mg/kg PO, SC q24h

PRECAUTIONS/INTERACTIONS

N/A

FOLLOW-UP

PATIENT MONITORING

Once regurgitation steady weight loss begins despite nutritional support, the snake is unlikely to recover, and euthanasia should be considered.

EXPECTED COURSE AND PROGNOSIS

- Prognosis for clinically ill snakes is grave, as most will die from the disease.
- Those with subclinical infections have a good to guarded prognosis.

MISCELLANEOUS

COMMENTS

N/A

ZOONOTIC POTENTIAL

C. pneumoniae is a human pathogen; zoonosis and reverse zoonosis must be considered.

SYNONYMS

Emerald regurgitation syndrome

ABBREVIATIONS

- IM = intramuscular
- IV = intravenous
- PCR = polymerase chin reaction
- PO = per os

Suggested Reading

Lock B, Heard D, Detrisac C, Jacobson E. An epizootic of chronic regurgitation associated with chlamydophilosis in recently imported emerald tree boas (*Corallus caninus*). *J Z Wildl Med* 2003;34(4):385–393.

Ruegg SR, Regenscheit N, Origgi FC, et al. Detection of *Chlamydia pneumoniae* in a collection of captive snakes and response to treatment with marbofloxacin. *Vet J* 2015;205(3):424–426.

Taylor-Brown A, Ruegg S, Polkinghorne A, Borel N. Characterisation of *Chlamydia pneumoniae* and other novel chlamydial infections in captive snakes. *Vet Microbiol* 2015;178(1–2):88–93.

Author Javier G. Nevarez, DVM, PhD, DACZM, DECZM (Herpetology)

CLOACAL PROLAPSE

BASICS

DEFINITION/OVERVIEW

A prolapse is the moving or slipping of a body part from its usual position or anatomic relation. In the reptile, a prolapse from the vent may be of cloacal, rectal, hemipenal, oviductal, or bladder in origin.

ETIOLOGY/PATHOPHYSIOLOGY

- The underlying causes for prolapse is often unknown.
- See Differential Diagnosis for a list of possible etiologies.

SIGNALMENT/HISTORY

- There appears to be no specific signalment or predilections noted for the various reptilian prolapses.
- Female reptilians may be overrepresented due to occurrences of dystocia.

CLINICAL PRESENTATION

- A prolapse is easy to visualize as abnormal tissue protruding from the cloacal/vent region.
- In reptiles housed outdoors and in case of small prolapses, the owners may not notice a problem until days after it has occurred.
- For this reason, a prolapse should be considered an emergency and evaluated promptly.
- The tissue should be kept moist either through gentle washing the area with water and loosely wrapped in a damp cloth or paper towel until the animal can be evaluated a veterinarian.
- The extruded material should be identified to the tissue(s) involved, such as cloacal with/without bladder, oviduct, proctodeum, colon, hemipenis.
- Once the issues are identified, the clinician may be able to narrow the diagnosis to determine the course of diagnostics and therapeutics.

RISK FACTORS

- In cases of NSHP, the muscle tone around the cloacal opening is decreased, leading to potential tissue exposure.
- Any generalized physical straining of the patient can lead to tissue exposure through the cloaca, such as dyspnea, obstipation, parasites, infection.
- Space-occupying lesions located in the coelomic cavity, such as uroliths, neoplasia, hepto- or renomegaly, eggs, may also cause increase straining and cloacal prolapse.

Husbandry

- Several factors of husbandry may lead to one of the differential diagnoses.
- Corrections of the deficient aspects of the husbandry can lead to reversal of some conditions.

Others

- Some cloacal tissue may prolapse during normal oviposition.
- Iatrogenic prolapses may occur when owners attempt to manually manipulate ova in suspected cases of dystocia or feces in constipated animals.

DIAGNOSIS

DIFFERENTIAL DIAGNOSIS

- Parasites
- Hypocalcemia
- Dehydration
- Metabolic disease
- Neoplasia
- Impaction
- Obstruction
- Trauma
- Coelomic space-occupying lesion
- Obesity
- Bacterial infection
- Intoxication

DIAGNOSTICS

- Radiography and ultrasound may be useful in determining internal abnormalities (e.g., impactions, masses, obstructions).
- The small size of some reptiles may lead to reduced imaging detail, which makes interpretation challenging.
- Dental radiography may be a better alternative in smaller species (< 100 g).
- A fecal examination should be performed in all cases. This can be directly from the feces, a saline cloacal wash, or direct impression smear of the prolapsed tissue may reveal the presence of parasites such as nematode larvae or eggs.
- A complete blood count and chemistry panel may assist in the determination of underlying physiologic abnormalities.

PATHOLOGICAL FINDINGS

- Protozoal infections affecting the gastrointestinal tract may be diagnosed on histopathology.
- Other findings will be consistent with the underlying cause but often no specific cause or pathology can be identified.

TREATMENT

APPROPRIATE HEALTH CARE

- Treatment often involves direct replacement of the tissue back into normal anatomic position, by either manual or surgical means, in combination with correction of the underlying etiology.
- The patient should be fully evaluated for general health status and treated accordingly.
- The prolapsed tissue should be evaluated for presence of devitalization, which must be surgically or medically addressed prior to prolapse reduction.
- In some cases, the internal reproductive structures may be medically or surgically repaired, although further reproductive events could result in dystocia.
- The prolapse may be reduced in size by coating with a hyperosmotic solution such as 2–5% ophthalmic saline or concentrated sugar solution.
- Direct application of dry salt or sugar may be attempted, but the extreme osmolar difference could lead to direct tissue damage and should be closely monitored.
- After several minutes of application, the prolapsed tissue should become less edematous and capable of reduction back into the body cavity.
- A moistened and lubricated (water soluble) cotton tip applicator or metal probe is used to gently push the tissue back inside the body cavity, aligning the lumen.
- A purse-string suture around the cloaca or lateral sutures across the cloacal margin may be placed for 10–14 days to allow for the tissue swelling to resolve in place.

NUTRITIONAL SUPPORT

The reptilian patient may need weight and body condition monitoring to determine whether additional caloric supplementation is needed.

CLIENT EDUCATION/HUSBANDRY RECOMMENDATIONS

- If surgical correction of the prolapse is undertaken, the client should be directed on postoperative care of any surgical sites, suture, etc.
- A detailed log of activity, as well as food intake/defecations, should be maintained and related back to the veterinarian.
- If any changes to the husbandry were determined, such as changes to temperature and/or humidity, exposure to ultraviolet lighting, the owner should correct them prior to the patient returning home.
- Surgical options such as resection of the diseased tissue and double-layer closure can be performed prior to tissue replacement.
- In more extensive cases, a coeliotomy may be performed, with the tissue resection performed within the coelomic cavity where the tissue is in approximate "normal" anatomic position.
- Colonic prolapses may require a colopexy where sutures are placed to facilitate the "tacking" of the colon to the dorsolateral body wall.
- In cases of reproductive system prolapse (i.e., oviduct), the tissue may be replaced but damage to the suspensory ligaments and internal vasculature may be present.

CLOACAL PROLAPSE (CONTINUED)

- In severe oviductal prolapses, discussion with the owner about desired reproductive status should take place with a potential for coeliotomy and ovariosalpingectomy.

MEDICATIONS

DRUG(S) OF CHOICE

- NSAIDs or opioids may be used in management of the inflammation and pain associated with the physical discomfort of the prolapse or surgery.
- Depending on the determined etiology, antibiotics or anti-parasiticides may be indicated.

PRECAUTIONS/INTERACTIONS

- When replacing the prolapse, extreme care must be taken not to tear or perforate the delicate, inflamed tissue.
- After the sutures are removed, the tissue may re-prolapse if swelling/inflammation are still present or the underlying etiology has not been corrected.
- Placement of additional sutures may be required.
- Hydration status of the patent must be considered before use of NSAIDs.

FOLLOW-UP

PATIENT MONITORING

- The patient should be followed up daily after clinical repair of the prolapse for reoccurrence.
- The owner should monitor and record all food intake and defecations during this time.
- Any abnormal changes should be related back to the veterinarian to determine any further changes to the therapy.

EXPECTED COURSE AND PROGNOSIS

- Prolapses of the oviduct and bladder tend to have a guarded to grave prognosis due to the degree of underlying physical damage to the affected tissues and cloaca.
- Rectal and cloacal prolapses tend to have a fair prognosis if treated promptly.
- Hemipenal prolapses have excellent to good prognosis, as these are purely copulatory organs.
- The length of time the prolapse presents has an inverse effect on the prognosis.
- When treated early in the disease process and the tissue appears viable, cloacal prolapse replacement may lead to clinical resolution if the underlying etiology is addressed.
- Once the tissue begins to desiccate and become devitalized, there is a guarded to grave prognosis.

MISCELLANEOUS

COMMENTS

N/A

ZOONOTIC POTENTIAL

N/A

SYNONYMS

N/A

ABBREVIATIONS

- NSAIDs = nonsteroidal anti-inflammatory drugs
- NSHP = nutritional secondary hyperparathyroidism

Suggested Reading

Barten, SL. Penile prolapse. In: Mader DR, ed. *Reptile Medicine and Surgery*. 2nd ed. St. Louis, MO: Elsevier Saunders; 2006:862–864.

Bennett, RA. Cloacal prolapse. In: Mader DR, ed. *Reptile Medicine and Surgery*. 2nd ed. St. Louis, MO: Elsevier Saunders; 2006:751–755.

Author Rob L. Coke, DVM, DACZM, DABVP (Reptile & Amphibian), CVA

CRYPTOSPORIDIUM

BASICS

DEFINITION/OVERVIEW

Cryptosporidia are apicomplexan parasites typified by possessing an apical complex, and with four naked sporozoites within each oocyte. *Cryptosporidium* spp. can be distinguished from other coccidian parasites by the location that they occupy within the host cell membrane, their capacity for autoinfection, and their resistance to anti-parasitic medication. Possessing a durable oocyst wall consisting of a double layer of a protein–lipid–carbohydrate matrix, cryptosporidia are highly resistant to environmental degradation and chemical disinfection. Historically, oocyst morphology has been used for species identification, but this is considered unreliable and species assignment is now determined by molecular characteristics. *Cryptosporidium* spp. are ubiquitous in the environment and are globally distributed.

ETIOLOGY/PATHOPHYSIOLOGY

- *Cryptosporidium* infections are common in reptiles and have been reported in at least 57 different species.
- *C. serpentis* is the species predominately seen snakes and is typically found within the gastric mucosa.
- *Cryptosporidium* oocysts from chelonians can cause severe infections in snakes when experimentally transferred.
- Transmission is direct, with reptiles becoming infected after ingesting oocysts that have been shed in feces.
- Autoinfection may also occur with some oocysts releasing their sporozoites within the host's body.
- No prepatent period has been determined.

SIGNALMENT/HISTORY

Snakes are typically presented due to mid-body swelling and regurgitation.

CLINICAL PRESENTATION

- Two common clinical manifestations exist in snakes:
  - In the subclinical (carrier state), animals may appear healthy and are able to shed oocysts intermittently for years.
  - In the clinical state, gastric hyperplasia manifests as a large, palpable swelling in the gastric region with a history of postprandial regurgitation.

RISK FACTORS

The greatest risk factor for developing infection is poor quarantine of new animals entering a collection.

Husbandry

N/A

Others

N/A

DIAGNOSIS

DIFFERENTIAL DIAGNOSIS

Gastric hyperplasia: neoplasia or abscess/granulomatous disease.

DIAGNOSTICS

- Examination of mucus from regurgitated food items: unstained smears are useful but sensitivity of detection increases with an acid-fast stain and is greatest with an IFA stain.
- Sensitivity may be increased if performed postprandially.
- An important limitation of these tests is their lack of specificity to differentiate *Cryptosporidium* spp.
- False positive results can occur in animals that have ingested food items (e.g., mice) infected with other *Cryptosporidium* spp. that are not pathogenic to reptiles.
- Gastric lavage is a highly sensitive test performed by inserting a feeding tube into the stomach and infusing 2% of body weight of NaCl followed by gentle aspiration. The resultant fluid is then centrifuged for 15 minutes at 7,500 g and stained with acid-fast or IFA. Sensitivity increased if performed 3 days after feeding.
- Serum antibody titers take 6 weeks for antibodies to develop, and can be assessed using ELISA. Best if combined with fecal or gastric lavage.
- ELISA positive, fecal positive—animal infected and shedding.
- ELISA negative, fecal negative—not infected.
- ELISA negative, fecal positive—recent infection (< 6 weeks) or passing non-reptilian *Cryptosporidium* spp.
- ELISA positive, fecal negative—has been infected at some point but not shedding or shedding at undetectable levels.
- PCR is a highly sensitive test that can be used for lavage samples. Can also differentiate between *Cryptosporidium* spp.
- Barium studies can be used to differentiate non-gastrointestinal masses from gastric hyperplasia.
- Gastric biopsy: organisms may have a patchy distribution within the stomach and so false negatives may occur.

PATHOLOGICAL FINDINGS

- Gross: gastric lesions may range from normal in appearance to a marked increase in gastric mucosa and subsequent decrease in gastric lumen. The mucosa may appear edematous and thickened with copious amounts of stringy mucus.
- Histopathology: gastric tissue may have widely dilated tubules and increased interstitial connective tissue.

TREATMENT

APPROPRIATE HEALTH CARE

Elimination of *Cryptosporidium* spp. from reptiles is difficult and rarely rewarding.

NUTRITIONAL SUPPORT

- Force-feeding with easily digestible proteins by stomach tubing can be performed in most species.
- This approach should be re-evaluated when dealing with venomous species.
- Supportive fluid therapy should be provided.

CLIENT EDUCATION/HUSBANDRY RECOMMENDATIONS

- Clients should be made aware of the insidious nature of infection, the unlikelihood of successful treatment, and the risks that affected animals pose to the remaining collection.
- Owners should be reminded that while *C. serpentis* has no zoonotic potential, prey items fed to reptiles might harbor *Cryptosporidium* that can pose a risk to immunocompromised individuals.

MEDICATIONS

DRUG(S) OF CHOICE

- Trimethoprim sulfonamide 30 mg/kg PO once a day for 14 days, then 1–3 times weekly for 3 months may reduce oocyst shedding but does not eliminate *Cryptosporidium* organisms from the gastrointestinal mucosa.
- Paromomycin 100 mg/kg PO once a day for 7 days; then twice weekly for 6 weeks; and 360 mg/kg q48h for 10 days resulted in complete resolution in experimentally infected bearded dragons (*Pogona vitticeps*).
- Hyperimmune bovine colostrum 1% body weight by volume PO once weekly for 6 weeks. Currently not available commercially.

PRECAUTIONS/INTERACTIONS

- Euthanasia should be strongly considered for affected animals to limit spread.
- If this is not an option, then diseased reptiles should be separated from the remaining collection and strict barrier nursing protocols enacted to prevent spread.

FOLLOW-UP

Regular fecal examination and ELISA assays for suspected at risk animals.

PATIENT MONITORING

Monitor for signs of disease (i.e., wasting, diarrhea, persistent regurgitation).

CRYPTOSPORIDIUM (CONTINUED)

EXPECTED COURSE AND PROGNOSIS

Grave prognosis, likely chronic wasting and death.

MISCELLANEOUS

COMMENTS

N/A

ZOONOTIC POTENTIAL

- *C. serpentis* has no zoonotic potential.
- It should be remembered that prey items fed to reptiles may harbor *Cryptosporidium* spp. that can pose a risk to immunocompromised individuals.

SYNONYMS

N/A

ABBREVIATIONS

- ELISA = enzyme-linked immunosorbent assay
- IFA = immunofluorescent antibody
- NaCl = sodium chloride
- PCR = polymerase chain reaction
- PO = per os

Suggested Reading

Cranfield MR, Graczyk TK. Cryptosporidiosis. In: Mader DR, ed. *Reptile Medicine and Surgery*. 2nd ed. St. Louis, MO: Elsevier Saunders; 2006:756–762.

Fayer R, Graczyk TK, Cranfield MR. Multiple heterogenous isolates of *Cryptosporidium serpentis* from captive snakes are not transmissible to neonatal BALB/c mice (*Mus musculus*). *J Parasitol* 1995;81(3):482–484.

Graczyk TK, Owens R, Cranfield MR. Diagnosis of subclinical cryptosporidiosis in captive snakes based on stomach lavage and cloacal sampling. *Vet Parasitol* 1996;67:143–151.

Grosset C, Villeneuve A, Brieger A, Lair S. Cryptosporidiosis in juvenile bearded dragons (*Pogona vitticeps*) effects of treatment with paromomycin. *J Herp Med Surg* 2011;21:10–15.

Pedraza-Diaz S, Ortega-Mora LM, Carrion BA, et al. Molecular characterisation of *Cryptosporidium* isolates from pet reptiles. *Vet Parasitol* 2009;160(3–4):204–210.

Plutzer J, Karanis P. Genetic polymorphism in *Cryptosporidium* species: an update. *Vet Parasitol* 2009;165(3–4):187–199.

Scullion FT, Scullion MG. Gastrointestinal protozoal diseases in reptiles. *J Exot Pet Med* 2009;18(4):266–278.

Shahiduzzaman M, Daugschies A. Therapy and prevention of cryptosporidiosis in animals. *Vet Parasitol* 2012;188(3–4):203–214.

Traversa D, Iorio R, Otranto D, et al. *Cryptosporidium* from tortoises: Genetic characterisation, phylogeny and zoonotic implications. *Mol Cell Probes* 2008;22(2):122–128.

Author T. Franciscus Scheelings, BVSc, MVSc, PhD, MANCVSc (Wildlife Health), DECZM (Herpetology)

DIARRHEA

BASICS

DEFINITION/OVERVIEW

Diarrhea is the production of unformed or liquid fecal matter. It is often associated with increased fecal volume and frequency of defection.

ETIOLOGY/PATHOPHYSIOLOGY

- Diarrhea is usually associated with enteritis due to primary infectious (e.g., endoparasites) or non-infectious (e.g., dietary) causes.
- Sudden diet changes
- Environmental factors, such as low temperatures, lead to decreased gastrointestinal motility, dysbacteriosis and diarrhea due overgrowth of opportunistic pathogens.
- Endoparasites causing diarrhea in snakes include coccidia, *Cryptosporidia serpentis*, strongylids (*Kalicephalus* spp.—hookworms), ascarids—most important nematode pathogen in snakes.
- Other less common infectious causes, include viral, fungal, and bacterial organisms.

SIGNALMENT/HISTORY

- Inappropriate husbandry: low environmental temperatures and overcrowding (stress) can lead to enteritis and diarrhea.
- Owners report liquid feces, frequently malodorous, and increased frequency of defecation.
- Possible straining to defecate, weight loss, anorexia, and cloacal prolapse.

CLINICAL PRESENTATION

- Depending on duration (acute vs. chronic), severity and etiology of diarrhea.
- Fecal staining around cloaca
- Presence of abnormally soft or liquid fecal matter in transport container.
- Dehydration
- Chronic diarrhea can lead to weight loss and cachexia due to malabsorption of nutrients.
- Cloacal prolapse

RISK FACTORS

Husbandry

- Change in diet
- Poor sanitation
- Inappropriate (too low or to high) environmental temperatures
- Young age—endoparasites cause higher morbidity and mortality in young snakes.
- Lack of fecal parasitology screening after acquisition of the snake.

Others

N/A

DIAGNOSIS

DIFFERENTIAL DIAGNOSIS

- Enteritis - bacterial, parasitic, dietary

DIAGNOSTICS

- Fecal direct wet mount to evaluate for motile protozoa.
- Fecal flotation to evaluate for helminths and protozoa (coccidian, amoeba cysts).
- Diagnostic imaging (radiography, CT, ultrasound) as needed.

PATHOLOGICAL FINDINGS

- Enteritis
- Malodorous and liquid intestinal content.
- Emaciation

TREATMENT

APPROPRIATE HEALTH CARE

N/A

NUTRITIONAL SUPPORT

- Provide nutritional support to emaciated and/or anorexic animals.
- Provide fluid therapy to dehydrated animals.

CLIENT EDUCATION/HUSBANDRY RECOMMENDATIONS

N/A

MEDICATIONS

DRUG(S) OF CHOICE

- Coccidiosis: Toltrazuril 10 mg/kg PO once or q7d for 2–3 treatments; sulfonamides: e.g., trimethoprim/sulfa 30 mg/kg PO q24h.
- Metronidazole 25 mg/kg PO q24h for 5–10 days effective against motile protozoal organism.
- Fenbendazole 10–20 mg/kg PO q24h for 3–5 days effective against nematodes and flagellates.
- Ivermectin 0.2 mg/kg PO, SC, IM effective against nematodes.
- Emodepside/praziquantel 1 ml/kg topical on skin, repeat after 14 days effective against nematodes, trematodes, and cestodes.
- Prevention of reinfection is critically important during and following antiparasitic treatments against parasites with a direct life cycle.
- Keep the animal on newspaper until treatment is completed and recheck fecal samples.
- Immediate removal of feces to prevent ingestion.
- Bathing the lizard and cleaning of the pericloacal region to remove feces and eggs or cysts are recommended.

PRECAUTIONS/INTERACTIONS

N/A

FOLLOW-UP

PATIENT MONITORING

- Return to normal fecal consistency
- Weight gain and maintenance of hydration.
- Repeat fecal parasitology to ensure that treatment is effective.

EXPECTED COURSE AND PROGNOSIS

- If dietary causes are responsible for the diarrhea, prognosis is excellent to good.
- Animals in good body condition and no concurrent morbidities have an excellent to good prognosis.
- Animals in poor body condition with signs of systemic illness (dehydration, lethargy, etc.) have a guarded to poor prognosis.
- There is currently no effective treatment against *Cryptosporidium* spp.

MISCELLANEOUS

COMMENTS

- Diarrhea is a clinical sign associated with an underlying diseases, improper husbandry or nutrition.
- Identification of the underlying cause is necessary to improve outcome and reduce the risk of recurrence.
- Correction of husbandry is always recommended to in help to improve the outcome.

ZOONOTIC POTENTIAL

Salmonella spp. are commonly shed by snakes with and without diarrhea.

SYNONYMS

N/A

ABBREVIATIONS

- CT = computed tomography
- IM = intramuscular
- PO = per os
- SC = subcutaneous

INTERNET RESOURCES

Divers SJ. Parasitic Diseases of Reptiles. MSD Manual Veterinary Manual, June 2020. http://www.merckvetmanual.com/exotic-and-laboratory-animals/reptiles/parasitic-diseases-of-reptiles

Suggested Reading

Funk RS. Diarrhea. In: Mader DR, ed. *Reptile Medicine and Surgery*. 2nd ed. St. Louis, MO: Elsevier Saunders; 2006:772–773.

Greiner EC, Mader DR. Parasitology. In: Mader DR, ed. *Reptile Medicine and Surgery*. 2nd ed. St. Louis, MO: Elsevier Saunders; 2006:343–364.

Author Christoph Mans, Dr. med. vet., DACZM

DYSECDYSIS

BASICS

DEFINITION/OVERVIEW

Dysecdysis is difficult or abnormal shedding, and is a common presentation for reptile species. True dysecdysis implies that the snake has retained shed that requires assistance for removal or that the shed has come off in an abnormal pattern that could lead to further problems.

ETIOLOGY/PATHOPHYSIOLOGY

- In snakes, shedding is a discontinuous process through a well-described ecdysis cycle.
- For simplicity, the ecdysis cycle can be split into a resting phase and a renewal phase, which has up to five stages.
- During the beginning of the renewal phase, the skin begins to appear duller as regeneration of cells and enzymatic separation of the skin layers becomes activated. This period lasts approximately 5 ± 2 days. Afterwards, the skin becomes even duller and the spectacles turn opaque in what is commonly described as snakes being in "blue".
- This appearance is in large part due to lymphatic fluid accumulation that helps to separate the old and new skin layers. This lymphatic fluid accumulation is in large part what causes the opacity observed on the spectacles.
- This second period lasts 5 ± 2 days, and is followed by the last stage, during which lymphatic fluid resorption occurs leading to a clearing of the skin and spectacle. At this time, the skin regains some of its sheen.
- Shedding typically occurs 5 ± 2 days later.
- Ecdysis in snakes should occur as a single piece of skin, starting at the head and progressing to the tip of the tail.
- The snake usually uses a rough surface to help break the skin at the snout and aid in its removal.
- The shed skin should be inspected to ensure that both spectacles have been shed appropriately.

SIGNALMENT/HISTORY

- There is no typical signalment for dysecdysis.
- Snakes presenting with dysecdysis typically have a history of piecemeal shedding or simply appearing to have delayed shedding stages.

CLINICAL PRESENTATION

- Snakes with dysecdysis can present with patches of retained skin through the body or segmental dysecdysis in a specific region.
- Others may present with the skin falling off in segments as opposed to one continuous piece.
- Even if the skin comes off easily, it should not come off in fragments.
- The eyes and tip of the tail must be examined carefully, as dysecdysis at these two sites can lead to further complications such as subspectacular abscess and tail necrosis.
- It is also possible to see focal dysecdysis in areas of previous injuries or surgical incisions that have scarred over.
- In some instances, there will always be an abnormal shed observed over these areas, even in well-hydrated patients.

RISK FACTORS

Husbandry

- Inappropriate humidity, temperature, and access to water are common husbandry deficiencies.
- A lack of a rough surface within the enclosure may also be the cause of dysecdysis, as the snake will have difficulty making the initial tear of the skin.
- Dehydration is a key contributor to dysecdysis because dehydrated animals may not be able to mobilize enough lymphatic fluid, which is an essential part of the renewal phase.

Others

- Ecdysis is under pituitary–thyroid control.
- In snakes, it is reported that thyroid hormones help to downregulate the ecdysis process.
- Hypophysectomy or thyroidectomy of snakes results in repeated shedding.
- Skin disease (bacterial or fungal) may also lead to dysecdysis or even increased shedding frequency.

DIAGNOSIS

DIFFERENTIAL DIAGNOSIS

Bacterial or fungal dermatitis

DIAGNOSTICS

- Dysecdysis is easily diagnosed at physical examination.
- Any snake presenting with retained, incomplete, or abnormal shedding is suffering from dysecdysis.
- The spectacle should be carefully examined with an ophthalmoscope to diagnose retained spectacles.
- While most snake species have smooth and clear spectacles, it is important to recognize that some snake species such as ball pythons (*Python regius*) can normally have wrinkled spectacles that should not be confused with a retained spectacle.
- Retained spectacles tend to have more dull appearance and irregular pieces of skin may be observed in the periocular/perispectacular area.
- Fluid accumulation may also be present in the subspectacular space unilaterally or bilaterally.

PATHOLOGICAL FINDINGS

- The different stages of ecdysis can be identified microscopically.
- It may be possible to obtain a histologic diagnosis, although this is seldom required.
- Histological examination would be beneficial in cases where an underlying bacterial or fungal infection is suspected.
- Microscopic examination can help identify organisms that are present in between skin layers or deep within the dermis, which would be more indicative of true pathology, as opposed to organisms on the epidermis layer alone, which may be suggestive of superficial contamination.
- In cases of retained spectacles, grossly there will be opacity of the spectacle.
- Microscopically, layering of retained skin with bacterial and or fungal contamination may be observed.

TREATMENT

APPROPRIATE HEALTH CARE

N/A

NUTRITIONAL SUPPORT

There are no specific nutritional requirements other than ensuing proper hydration.

CLIENT EDUCATION/HUSBANDRY RECOMMENDATIONS

- Ensuring access to water and proper temperature and humidity is essential for preventing dehydration.
- In snake species that do not originate from habitats with high environmental humidity, a humidity box consisting of a plastic container with sphagnum moss or moist paper towels should be provided so the animal can seek additional humidity as needed.
- Water bowls must also be large enough for the snakes to soak in if they chose to do so.
- Prey items can also be soaked in water prior to feeding to provide additional moisture.
- Every shed should be inspected to ensure that the spectacles and tip of the tail were shed properly.

MEDICATIONS

DRUG(S) OF CHOICE

- Because dysecdysis is often associated with poor husbandry, any deficiencies must be corrected.
- Retained skin must not be removed if still firmly adhered to the animal.
- The treatment approach should consist of subcutaneous fluid therapy 20–30 ml/kg SC, since dehydration is a significant contributor to dysecdysis.

- In addition, the snake should be misted and/or soaked in water, or covered with a wet towel to increase the moisture of the skin and aid in the shedding process.
- In snakes with firmly adhered skin, it may take up to a week of daily soaking before the retained shed can be peeled off easily.
- In cases of retained spectacles, the spectacle must not be forcibly removed unless it is loosely adhered.
- In addition, topical treatment with artificial tears q6–8h can help to soften the spectacle. This can be done until it can either be removed or until the next shed occurs.
- If waiting until the next shed, the frequency of applying artificial tears can be decreased once the husbandry is corrected and the animal is properly hydrated.

PRECAUTIONS/INTERACTIONS

N/A

FOLLOW-UP

PATIENT MONITORING

- The character of future sheds should be recorded to determine if the issue has been resolved.
- It may take 1–2 shed cycles for the animals to shed properly again.
- Remember that retained shed over scars and old incisions may occur despite appropriate husbandry.

EXPECTED COURSE AND PROGNOSIS

- Dysecdysis has a good to excellent prognosis as long as husbandry is corrected, and snakes are provided enough access to water.
- Even snakes with retained spectacles have a good prognosis due to the eye's ability to heal.

MISCELLANEOUS

COMMENTS

Subspectacular abscesses may occur as a result of retained spectacles but also have other etiologies.

ZOONOTIC POTENTIAL

N/A

SYNONYMS

Retained shed

ABBREVIATIONS

SC = subcutaneous

Suggested Reading

Cooper, JE. Dermatology. In: Mader DR, ed. *Reptile Medicine and Surgery*. 2nd ed. St. Louis, MO: Elsevier Saunders; 2006:196–199.

Jacobson ER. Overview of reptile biology, anatomy, and histology. In: Jacobson ER, ed. *Infectious Diseases and Pathology of Reptiles: Color Atlas and Text*. Boca Raton, FL: CRC Press; 2007:4–6.

Author Javier G. Nevarez, DVM, PhD, DACZM, DECZM (Herpetology)

DYSTOCIA

BASICS

DEFINITION/OVERVIEW

Dystocia is difficulty laying eggs or giving birth.

ETIOLOGY/PATHOPHYSIOLOGY

- The reproductive hormone mechanism in reptiles is not as well understood as it is in mammals.
- It is suspected that a multitude of environmental and behavioral factors, as well as underlying diseases, contribute to an abnormal function of the endocrine system, which in turn leads to dystocia.
- It is also possible that a lack of breeding and exposure to males may be contributing factors.
- In addition to basic husbandry aspects such as temperature, humidity, and a proper diet, female reptiles also have a need for appropriate substrate and environment that is conductive for egg laying or birthing in the case of viviparous species.
- Dystocia is less commonly reported in viviparous species.
- It is also less common in snakes compared with other reptile groups.

SIGNALMENT/HISTORY

- Dystocia occurs in female snakes of reproductive age or size.
- Most animals have a history of inadequate nutrition and husbandry.

CLINICAL PRESENTATION

- Signs of dystocia may include coelomic distention, straining, decreased fecal production, cloacal prolapse, lethargy, and anorexia.
- In some instances, the eggs may be grossly visible during physical exam.
- Palpation of the coelomic cavity must be done gently to avoid rupturing the eggs.
- In the majority of cases, the owners are not aware of the fact that their snake is in dystocia.
- Other abnormalities identified in physical exam may include dehydration and poor body condition score.

RISK FACTORS

Husbandry

- Inappropriate husbandry is likely a significant contributing factor to the occurrence of dystocia.
- Inappropriate temperature and humidity are key deficiencies that may contribute to dystocia in snakes.
- The provision of an adequate substrate for nesting/oviposition and parturition is not as critical in snakes as in other species.
- Stress is likely a significant contributing factor in snakes.
- Reptiles that may not perceive the environmental conditions are adequate for successful oviposition may not have the proper stimuli to lay their eggs.

Others

- A less discussed topic is the effect that lack of exposure to males may have on the reproductive cycle of reptiles.
- Many reptiles display courtship and breeding behaviors that likely influence the proper hormonal stimulation of prospective females.
- Many female snakes in captivity are kept alone without the benefit of behavioral cues from a male counterpart.
- This possibility of a behavioral effect must be considered, especially when animals are maintained in proper husbandry and are otherwise healthy.

DIAGNOSIS

DIFFERENTIAL DIAGNOSIS

- Follicular stasis
- Neoplasia
- Egg yolk coelomitis
- Ovarian cysts
- GI obstruction

DIAGNOSTICS

Radiography

- Eggs can appear as minimally calcified to calcified, round to ovoid, depending on the species of snakes. In viviparous species, the skeletons of the offspring may be observed.

Ultrasound

- The calcification of the egg varies widely across snake species; the ultrasonographic appearance varies from a well-delineated hyperechogenic eggshell membrane to significant acoustic shadowing.
- In those with poorly calcified eggshell, ultrasound may be more sensitive than radiography at diagnosing broken eggs, which may be associated with egg yolk coelomitis.
- In viviparous species, ultrasound can help to determine viability of the fetuses by documenting heart rate and blood flow.

CT and MRI

- Both these modalities are extremely sensitive at identifying eggs and can better assess their structure, integrity, and location.

Coelioscopy

Coelioscopic examination allows for confirmation of the presence of eggs and ruling out egg yolk coelomitis. The presence of eggs makes coelioscopy more difficult due to their space-occupying nature. It can also be used to assess the viability of the oviduct based on appearance and coloration.

Hematology and Biochemistry

- A chemistry panel is essential to help identify other possible underlying disease processes such as dehydration and NSHP. In addition to Ca and P, Mg levels should be documented as Mg also plays an important role in Ca homeostasis. Levels of Mg below 1 mg/dl and/or ionized Ca below 1 mmol/l should be considered deficient. Hypercalcemia and hyperphosphatemia are common findings in reproductively active female snakes.
- CBC: a leukocytosis indicates a significant inflammatory response that may suggest an additional underlying disease like egg yolk coelomitis.

PATHOLOGICAL FINDINGS

- Grossly, dystocia can be identified by the presence of eggs or fetuses within the oviduct.
- Pathologic findings may include variation in eggs size, calcification, malformations, broken eggshells, and oviduct torsions.
- Healthy eggs should be smooth, uniform in shape and white in color.
- A deviation from this appearance (i.e., dark, shriveled) is indicative of pathology.

TREATMENT

APPROPRIATE HEALTH CARE

- The treatment approach to dystocia is based on the species of snakes, clinical condition at presentation, amount and appearance of the eggs/fetuses based on imaging or coelioscopy and ability to provide a suitable environment for egg laying/parturition.
- All snakes will benefit from medical treatment even if surgery is ultimately required.
- Medical therapy consists of correcting the husbandry, providing a quiet area for nesting/birthing, and supportive therapy with emphasis on correcting calcium deficiencies.
- Oxytocin or arginine vasotocin can be administered, as long as an obstructive process is not suspected.
- Some recommend the use of beta-adrenergic blockers such as propranolol or atenolol before administration of oxytocin, as these have been shown to potentiate the effects of oxytocin in humans due to their ability to increase uterine activity.
- If the snake appears to be stable, medical therapy alone can be attempted and the animal monitored for evidence of egg laying/parturition.
- There are no specific timelines as to how quickly egg laying/parturition should occur once medical therapy is initiated.

- Many snakes will ultimately require surgical intervention if there is no response to medical therapy.
- Manual manipulation of eggs within the coelomic cavity (i.e., stripping) in an attempt to push them out of the cloaca is controversial as it can lead to rupture of the oviduct, ectopic eggs, and or egg yolk coelomitis.
- Surgery is best performed before dystocia progresses while the animal is metabolically stable.
- Surgery should be an immediate consideration for snakes with documented chronic dystocia, metabolic derangements, and when egg yolk coelomitis is suspected.
- The goal of surgery is to remove the eggs and to perform an ovariosalpingectomy to avoid reoccurrence.
- Extreme care must be taken to not rupture the eggs in the coelomic cavity, as the yolk is extremely antigenic and will cause a severe inflammatory response.
- If leakage occurs, the coelomic cavity should be thoroughly lavaged before closure.

NUTRITIONAL SUPPORT

Any dietary deficiencies must be corrected with special emphasis on Ca supplementation.

CLIENT EDUCATION/HUSBANDRY RECOMMENDATIONS

- Clients should be encouraged to seek veterinary care of snakes early on to establish individual baseline values and confirm the sex of the animal.
- Dystocia likely has a multifactorial cause, so all husbandry deficiencies must be corrected with emphasis on nutrition, temperature, humidity, and provision of adequate nesting/birthing area.
- Snakes should be weighed at least weekly to document any sudden weight increases that may be indicative of egg development.

MEDICATIONS

DRUG(S) OF CHOICE

- Propranolol 1 mg/kg PO once at least 3 hours prior to oxytocin administration.
- Atenolol 7 mg/kg PO once at least 3 hours prior to administration of oxytocin or arginine vasotocin.
- Arginine vasotocin 0.5–1 µg/kg IV, IO, IM, ICe q12–24h should be administered 30–60 minutes after IM or SC injection of calcium gluconate.
- Oxytocin 5–10 iu/kg IM, IV, IO q4–8h IV administration may be more efficacious but most be done slowly.
- Calcium: start with calcium gluconate 100 mg/kg IM, SC q12–24h followed by calcium glubionate 10–100 mg/kg PO q4–24h long term.
- Magnesium sulfate 20 mg/kg IM, SC q24–72h, or magnesium lactate (Rescue Cal+, Repashy Ventures, Saskatoon, SK) 20 mg/kg PO q24h.
- Crystalloid fluids 20–30 ml/kg SC, IV, IO q24h
- Meloxicam 0.5 mg/kg PO, IM, SC q24–48h

PRECAUTIONS/INTERACTIONS

- There is scant information about the safety and efficacy of oxytocin and arginine vasotocin when used for prolonged periods over 2–3 days.
- IV administration of oxytocin and arginine vasotocin should be done slowly as they can cause life-threatening hypotension.
- Beta-adrenergic blockers also may cause bradycardia and hypotension.

FOLLOW-UP

PATIENT MONITORING

- If performing medical therapy alone, especially with oxytocin or arginine vasotocin, the snake should be monitored closely to identify any signs of distress, although this is a rare occurrence.
- If an underlying disease process was diagnosed, appropriate follow-up diagnostics should be done to determine improvement of that condition or the need to alter therapy.
- For those undergoing surgery, a re-evaluation within 1–2 weeks is recommended to evaluate the surgical site and overall recovery.

EXPECTED COURSE AND PROGNOSIS

- Ultimately the prognosis will depend on the underlying cause of dystocia and the response to therapy.
- Cases with underlying infectious or metabolic disease that respond to medical therapy have a good prognosis.
- Many cases requiring surgical therapy have a good to guarded prognosis.

MISCELLANEOUS

COMMENTS

- The ultimate diagnosis of dystocia is based on interpretation of clinical signs, history, and results of physical exam and diagnostics.
- In all cases, it is essential to have at least one confirmatory test that there are indeed eggs present in the coelomic cavity.
- It must be mentioned that the sex of the animals must be confirmed as female before surgery is performed.
- While this may seem obvious, sex determination of snakes can be quite challenging for untrained individuals and males may present with coelomic neoplasias or GI obstructions that clinically appear very similar to dystocia.

ZOONOTIC POTENTIAL

N/A

SYNONYMS

- Egg bound
- Postovulatory follicular stasis

ABBREVIATIONS

- Ca = calcium
- CBC = complete blood count
- CT = computed tomography
- GI = gastrointestinal
- ICe = intracoelemic
- IM = intramuscular
- IO = intraosseous
- IV = intravenous
- Mg = magnesium
- MRI = magnetic resonance imaging
- NSHP = nutritional secondary hyperparathyroidism
- P = phosphorus
- PO = per os
- SC = subcutaneous

Suggested Reading

Hochleithner C, Holland M. Ultrasonography. In: Mader DR, Divers SJ, eds. *Current Therapy in Reptile Medicine and Surgery*. St. Louis, MO: Elsevier Saunders; 2014:107–127.

Jacobson ER. Overview of reptile biology, anatomy, and histology. In: Jacobson ER, ed. *Infectious Diseases and Pathology of Reptiles: Color Atlas and Text*. Boca Raton, FL: CRC Press; 2007:14–17.

Author Javier G. Nevarez, DVM, PhD, DACZM, DECZM (Herpetology)

EGG YOLK COELOMITIS

BASICS

DEFINITION/OVERVIEW

Egg yolk coelomitis occurs when yolk material is released into the coelomic cavity as a result of a ruptured follicle or egg due to oophoritis, follicular stasis, dystocia, salpingitis, or aggressive palpation. Egg yolk coelomitis is rarely reported in snakes.

ETIOLOGY/PATHOPHYSIOLOGY

- In all cases, yolk coelomitis is a result of yolk material free within the coelomic cavity overwhelming the body's activity to resorb the material.
- This leads to an intense inflammatory response that is often sterile but can also be associated with secondary bacterial infection.
- It can progress to adhesions throughout the coelomic cavity, septicemia, and death.

SIGNALMENT/HISTORY

- Egg yolk coelomitis occurs in female snakes of reproductive age or size, usually older than 1 year.
- Most animals have a history of inadequate husbandry, being housed alone without access to a male, and lacking an appropriate area for laying eggs or giving birth.

CLINICAL PRESENTATION

- Snakes with yolk coelomitis often present for non-specific clinical signs like anorexia, lethargy, and coloration changes.
- Some animals may present with coelomic distention.
- Other abnormalities identified in physical exam may include dehydration and poor body condition score.
- Some animals may present obtunded due to rapid progression of the disease.

RISK FACTORS

Husbandry

- Any factors that may results in follicular stasis or dystocia are also contributing factors to yolk coelomitis.
- These include inadequate husbandry, nutrition, brumation, and nesting/birthing environment.

Others

- A less discussed topic is the effect that lack of exposure to males may have on the reproductive cycle of reptiles.
- Many reptiles display courtship and breeding behaviors that likely influence the proper hormonal stimulation of prospective females.
- Many female snakes in captivity are kept alone without the benefit of behavioral cues from a male counterpart.
- This possibility of a behavioral effect must be considered, especially when animals are maintained in proper husbandry and are otherwise healthy.

DIAGNOSIS

DIFFERENTIAL DIAGNOSIS

- Follicular stasis
- Dystocia
- Neoplasia
- Ovarian cysts
- GI obstruction
- Septicemia

DIAGNOSTICS

Cytology

- Evaluation of free fluid in the coelomic cavity will be a confirmatory test of yolk coelomitis.
- In acute cases, the fluid is yellow to white with a high amount of proteinaceous material and inflammatory cells.
- In chronic cases, the fluid may appear cloudier. Blood and bacteria may also be observed with either presentation.

Imaging

- Radiographic findings may include free fluid, follicles, or ruptured eggs.
- Ultrasound: aspiration of any free fluid can be used to diagnose egg yolk coelomitis.
- CT and MRI: both these modalities are extremely sensitive for evaluation of the reproductive tract. They can also help assess damage to other organs.

Coelioscopy

- Coelioscopic examination allows for confirmation of yolk coelomitis.
- It may be confounded by changes in anatomy due to adhesions.

Hematology and Biochemistry

- A chemistry panel is essential to help in identifying other possible underlying disease processes such as dehydration.
- In addition to Ca and P, Mg levels should be documented, as Mg also plays an important role in Ca homeostasis.
- Levels of Mg below 1 mg/dl and/or ionized Ca below 1 mmol/l should be considered deficient.
- Hypercalcemia and hyperphosphatemia may be observed in reproductively active female snakes. Hyperproteinemia, anemia, and hypoglycemia may also be identified.
- CBC: a leukocytosis may be observed but does not always occur, especially in chronic cases. Leukopenia may be present if sepsis has ensued.

PATHOLOGICAL FINDINGS

- During the acute stages, egg yolk coelomitis presents as yellow to white, viscous, free fluid within the cavity.
- Fragments of more solid yolk may also be free floating within the cavity.
- Chronically, more adhesions develop and form a white fibrinous to fibrotic membrane on the serosal surfaces of the organs.
- The lesions are often severe enough that surgical repair is not possible.
- Many cases are diagnosed postmortem.

TREATMENT

APPROPRIATE HEALTH CARE

- Animals with yolk coelomitis must undergo surgery in an attempt to correct the condition, but it is often fatal.
- The goal of exploratory coeliotomy is to determine the severity of the diseases and whether successful lavage and cleaning of the cavity can be performed.
- Any free-floating material must be removed and the cavity lavaged copiously to remove the protein.
- If this can be accomplished, an ovariosalpingectomy is performed.
- Any underlying abnormalities (e.g., dehydration, anemia, septicemia) must be treated accordingly.
- These animals must also receive anti-inflammatories and analgesics, as the reaction to the yolk and subsequent adhesions is extremely painful.

NUTRITIONAL SUPPORT

- A proper diet for the species must be provided.
- Weekly nutritional support with carnivore critical care diets can be provided as needed in anorectic animals.

CLIENT EDUCATION/HUSBANDRY RECOMMENDATIONS

- Clients should be encouraged to seek veterinary care of snakes early on to establish individual baseline values and confirm the sex of the animal.
- Egg yolk coelomitis occurs as a sequel to multifactorial causes, so all husbandry deficiencies must be corrected.
- Snakes should be weighed at least weekly to document any sudden weight increases that may be indicative of follicular development that may lead to yolk coelomitis.

MEDICATIONS

DRUG(S) OF CHOICE

Meloxicam 0.5 mg/kg PO, IM, SC q24–48h

PRECAUTIONS/INTERACTIONS

N/A

FOLLOW-UP

PATIENT MONITORING

- If an underlying disease process was diagnosed, appropriate follow-up diagnostics should be done to determine improvement of that condition or the need to alter therapy.
- A re-evaluation within 1–2 weeks of surgery is recommended to evaluate the surgical site and overall recovery.

EXPECTED COURSE AND PROGNOSIS

- The overall prognosis will depend on the speed with which the diseases is recognized by the owners and diagnosed and treated by the veterinarian.
- Peracute to acute cases have a fair prognosis.
- Chronic cases have a grave prognosis.

MISCELLANEOUS

COMMENTS

N/A

ZOONOTIC POTENTIAL

N/A

SYNONYMS

- Egg coelomitis/peritonitis
- Yolk coelomitis/peritonitis

ABBREVIATIONS

- Ca = calcium
- CBC = complete blood count
- CT = computed tomography
- GI = gastrointestinal
- IM = intramuscular
- Mg = magnesium
- MRI = magnetic resonance imaging
- P = phosphorus
- PO = per os
- SC = subcutaneous

INTERNET RESOURCES

Pollock C. Reproductive disease in reptiles: twelve key facts. LafeberVet, September 23, 2012. https://lafeber.com/vet/reproductive-disease-in-reptiles-twelve-key-facts

Author Javier G. Nevarez, DVM, PhD, DACZM, DECZM (Herpetology)

EIMERIA

BASICS

DEFINITION/OVERVIEW

Eimeria are apicomplexan parasites characterized by oocytes having four sporocysts that each contain two sporozoites. *Eimeria* spp. are typically intracytoplasmic parasites, although some have been described as having intranuclear development. They rarely cause disease and commonly form a normal component of the gastrointestinal flora of reptiles.

ETIOLOGY/PATHOPHYSIOLOGY

- Over 200 species of *Eimeria* have been described in reptiles, and with the advent of molecular techniques, the rate of species discovery is increasing exponentially.
- *Eimeria* spp. have a direct life cycle with infective stages passed in the feces of the host.
- *Eimeria* spp. can be found in the gallbladder, bile ducts, and intestinal epithelium of snakes, lizards and crocodilians.
- Most reports of illness associated with *Eimeria* infection are from captive animals that have been housed under suboptimal conditions.
- Virulence may be exacerbated by a range of intrinsic and extrinsic factors such as concurrent disease and infective dose.
- *Eimeria cascabeli* infection has been associated with epithelial erosion and connective tissue proliferation in the gall bladder and extra hepatic ducts in rattlesnakes (*Crotalus* spp.).
- *E. bitis* infection resulting in pathology was reported in a range of ophidian species but this diagnosis has been questioned by some authors.

SIGNALMENT/HISTORY

Disease usually occurs under circumstances of high stocking density, unsanitary conditions, and maladaptation of wild animals entering captive situations.

CLINICAL PRESENTATION

- Most animals are asymptomatic carriers but when disease occurs then clinical signs are reflective of host cell destruction and are dependent on site of infection.
- Typically, signs are related to GI disorder and may include anorexia, weight loss, dehydration, diarrhea, and in severe cases death.

RISK FACTORS

Husbandry

New (captive or wild) animals entering a collection with poor hygiene and high stocking densities.

Others

Concurrent disease or excessive stress may cause immunosuppression thus increasing risks of disease expression.

DIAGNOSIS

DIFFERENTIAL DIAGNOSIS

Other GI disease such as bacterial or protozoal infections (i.e., *Isospora*).

DIAGNOSTICS

- Examination of feces for presence of oocysts using light microscopy is the most reliable test.
- Molecular techniques such as PCR may aid in species delineation but are unlikely to improve treatment efficacy or prognosis.
- Protozoa may also be seen in biopsy or necropsy samples.
- For preservation of coccidia for future diagnostics, fecal samples should be stored in 2–3% aqueous (w/v) potassium dichromate ($K_2Cr_2O_7$).

PATHOLOGICAL FINDINGS

- Lesions may include proliferation of connective tissue and erosions of epithelial cells lining the intestines, gallbladder, and extra hepatic ducts.
- There may also be an accompanying catarrhal or diphtheroid inflammatory response in the small and large intestines of affected animals.

TREATMENT

APPROPRIATE HEALTH CARE

N/A

NUTRITIONAL SUPPORT

- Ensure animals are well hydrated, especially if medicating with sulfa drugs.
- Force-feeding with easily digestible proteins by stomach tubing can be performed in most species.
- This approach should be re-evaluated when dealing with venomous species.
- Supportive fluid therapy should be provided.

CLIENT EDUCATION/HUSBANDRY RECOMMENDATIONS

- Remove and isolate sick individuals and reduce stress by providing optimal living conditions, and hygiene.
- Thorough cleaning of cage to reduce environmental contamination of oocysts.
- Ensure that quarantine protocols have been adopted for all new arrivals and during quarantine all animals should be subjected to repeated clinical and fecal examinations.

MEDICATIONS

DRUG(S) OF CHOICE

- Ponazuril 30 mg/kg PO q48h for 2 treatments, or 30 mg/kg PO q24h for 4 treatments, then repeat for 2–4 treatments 2 weeks apart.
- Toltrazuril 15 mg/kg PO q48h for 30 days
- Sulfadimethoxine 50 mg/kg q24h for 21 days
- Trimethoprim-sulfa 30 mg/kg daily for 5 days, then q48h until the coccidia are eliminated.
- Because *Eimeria spp.* are often non-pathogenic, prophylactic therapy or treatment based on the identification of *Eimeria spp.* alone should not be performed in order to avoid development of resistance.
- Treatment should only be performed after *Eimeria* spp. has been confirmed to be causing clinical signs.

PRECAUTIONS/INTERACTIONS

Sulfa drugs are known to be nephrotoxic and care should be taken with their use particularly in dehydrated or severely compromised individuals.

FOLLOW-UP

PATIENT MONITORING

Repeat fecal examination at monthly intervals.

EXPECTED COURSE AND PROGNOSIS

- Treatment may have variable efficacy as many protozoa are resistant to a range of anticoccidial medication.
- Prognosis is good to guarded and is determined primarily by the state of the animal at initial presentation and the presence or absence of concurrent disease.

MISCELLANEOUS

COMMENTS

N/A

ZOONOTIC POTENTIAL

Due to their high host-specificity there is no known zoonotic risk with any *Eimeria* species.

SYNONYMS

N/A

ABBREVIATIONS

- GI = gastrointestinal
- PCR = polymerase chain reaction
- PO = per os

Suggested Reading

Gibbons PM. Advances in reptile clinical therapeutics. *J Exot Pet Med* 2014;23(1):21–38.

Helke KL, Cooper TK, Mankowski JL, Poynton SL. Disseminated visceral coccidiosis in Indo-gangetic flap-shelled turtles, *Lissemys punctata andersonii*. *J Wildl Dis* 2006;42(4):788–796.

Jacobson ER. Parasites and parasitic diseases of reptiles. In: Jacobson ER, ed. *Infectious Diseases and Pathology of Reptiles: Color Atlas and Text*. Boca Raton, FL: CRC Press; 2007:571–665.

Scullion FT, Scullion MG. Gastrointestinal protozoal diseases in reptiles. *J Exot Pet Med* 2009;18(4):266–278.

Vetterling JM, Widmer EA. *Eimeria cascabeli* sp. n. (Eimeriidae, Sporozoa) from rattlesnakes, with a review of the species of *Eimeria* from snakes. *J Parasitol* 1968;54(3):569–576.

Author T. Franciscus Scheelings, BVSc, MVSc, PhD, MANCVSc (Wildlife Health), DECZM (Herpetology)

ENTAMOEBA

BASICS

DEFINITION/OVERVIEW

Entamoeba is considered to be one of the most significant parasites of reptilian species. They are capable of forming pseudopodia. *Entamoeba* species are characterized into two groupings based on morphology and the number of nuclei present. *Entamoeba* species in the group containing four nuclei are considered to be pathogenic and are the main concern for reptilian species. *Entamoeba* species in the group containing eight nuclei are considered to be non-invasive. *Entamoeba invadens* is the most common pathogenic species seen in reptiles and has been known to cause significant mortality. Virulence can differ between strains of E. *invadens*. Infectious cysts are 11–20.2 μm with four nuclei and a small central karyosome. Trophozoites are 17.5–50 μm in length (average 36.18 μm), 10–25 μm in width (average 12 μm), with an average diameter of 24.1 μm. Trophozoites also possess a single nucleus with a large central karyosome that is 5–7.5 μm in diameter (average 5.65 μm).

ETIOLOGY/PATHOPHYSIOLOGY

- *E. invadens* has a direct life cycle and transmission is the through fecal–oral route.
- Cysts are ingested and then undergo excystation in the intestinal tract.
- In snakes, *E. invadens* will start within the colon, causing mucosal necrosis.
- The parasite will then move to the small intestine and stomach, and trophozoites shower the liver.
- Once in systemic circulation, trophozoites can spread to virtually all other organs within the body including the lungs, kidneys, pancreas, and brain.
- The parasite can migrate to the brain causing abscessation and meningoencephalitis.
- The motile feeding trophozoite can also encyst and then be passed through the host's GI tract and out in the feces.
- Trophozoites undergo encystation in which infective cysts are formed and then excreted in feces.
- Cysts can remain infective for 14+ days at temperatures of 8 degrees C and for several days at 37 degrees C.
- Secondary bacterial infections with *Salmonella* sp. are common occurrences with the infection.

SIGNALMENT/HISTORY

All ages and species can be affected. Animals consistently kept in temperatures 25–33 degrees C.

CLINICAL PRESENTATION

- Anorexia, diarrhea, dehydration, weight loss, bloody and mucoid stools, hardening of the large intestinal tract that can be palpated, intussusception, vomiting, convulsions, listlessness, and sudden death.
- Diffuse necrotizing enterohepatitis is the most common clinical presentation in afflicted snakes.

RISK FACTORS

Husbandry

- Improper husbandry, improper hygiene, diarrhea, housed with infected animals, decreased immune status, temperatures held at 25–33 degrees C.
- Snakes housed with chelonians may be at higher risk of exposure. Invertebrates (i.e., roaches and flies) act as mechanical vectors.

Others

N/A

DIAGNOSIS

DIFFERENTIAL DIAGNOSIS

- Salmonellosis
- GI helminths

DIAGNOSTICS

- Microscopic evaluation of fresh fecal material to visualize trophozoites and cysts.
- Trophozoites may be seen in fresh fecal but die within 20–30 minutes once outside the host.
- SAF technique can be used for better visualization.
- Fecal/cysts can be placed within a petri dish with water and trophozoites will emerge from the dissolved envelope within several hours.
- Immunohistochemistry with *E. invadens* poly clonal antibody is developed for snakes.
- PCR assays can be used to distinguish species of *Entamoeba*.

PATHOLOGICAL FINDINGS

- Diarrhea
- Dehydration
- Weight loss

TREATMENT

APPROPRIATE HEALTH CARE

Medical therapy as appropriate

NUTRITIONAL SUPPORT

Nutritional supplementation may be indicated if diarrhea, dehydration is severe.

CLIENT EDUCATION/HUSBANDRY RECOMMENDATIONS

- Practice proper hygiene
- Refrain from housing chelonians and squamates within the same enclosure/exhibit or sharing the same water system.

MEDICATIONS

DRUG(S) OF CHOICE

Metronidazole 25 mg/kg PO q24h for 5–7 days

PRECAUTIONS/INTERACTIONS

N/A

FOLLOW-UP

PATIENT MONITORING

- Monitor for weight gain
- Take fecal samples

EXPECTED COURSE AND PROGNOSIS

- High morbidity and mortality is observed in snakes.
- Animals may survive if diagnosed and treated early in disease process, but prognosis is poor once clinical signs progress and grave if neurologic signs are present.

MISCELLANEOUS

- *Entamoeba invadens* in culture, dies at 37°C, so can raise the temperature to 37°C if it is within the animal's preferred optimum temperature range.
- *E. histolytica* and *E. dispar* which are found in humans GI tracts are morphologically similar to *E. invadens* but considered to be non-pathogenic.

COMMENTS

N/A

ZOONOTIC POTENTIAL

E. histolytica and *E. dispar*, species found in humans, are morphologically similar to *E. invadens* but are considered to be non-pathogenic.

SYNONYMS

Amebiasis

ABBREVIATIONS

- GI = gastrointestinal
- PCR = polymerase chain reaction
- PO = per os
- SAF = sodium acetate acetic acid formalin

INTERNET RESOURCES

- PetMD Editorial. Amebiasis in reptiles. October 1, 2008. https://www.petmd.com/reptile/conditions/digestive/c_rp_amebiasis
- Amebiasis in snakes. Wag! https://wagwalking.com/reptile/condition/amebiasis-in-snakes
- Divers SJ. Parasitic Diseases of Reptiles. MSD Manual Veterinary Manual, June 2020. http://www.merckvetmanual.com/exotic-and-laboratory-animals/reptiles/parasitic-diseases-of-reptiles

Suggested Reading

Denver MC. Reptile Protozoa. In: Fowler M, Miller E, eds. *Zoo and Wildlife Medicine: Current Therapy 6*. St. Louis, MO: Elsevier Saunders; 2008:154–159.

Hnizdo J, Pantchev N. Protozoa (digestive tract). In: *Medical Care of Turtles and Tortoises*. Diagnosis. Surgery. Pathology. Parasitology. Frankfurt, Germany: Edition Chimaira; 2011: 194–195.

Jacobson ER. Parasites and parasitic diseases of reptiles. In: Jacobson ER, ed. *Infectious Diseases and Pathology of Reptiles: Color Atlas and Text*. Boca Raton, FL: CRC Press; 2007:571–665.

Author Elsburgh O. Clarke III, DVM, DACZM

FOLLICULAR STASIS

BASICS

DEFINITION/OVERVIEW

Follicular stasis is the retention of ovarian follicles. Normally, follicles ovulate into the oviduct or undergo atresia. If neither happens, then the reptile is considered to be in follicular stasis. Identifying whether the presence of follicles is pathologic or physiologic is difficult given the fact that, most of the time, the stage of the reproductive cycle in an individual animal is unknown. A diagnosis of follicular stasis is often made once the animal starts showing clinical signs of illness or follicles are present for a longer period than expected for the species. Follicular stasis can occur in either oviparous or viviparous species and is an uncommon presentation in snakes.

ETIOLOGY/PATHOPHYSIOLOGY

- Follicles can fail to ovulate and undergo atresia for a number of reasons but in most cases an abnormal hormonal status can be assumed.
- The reproductive hormone mechanism in reptiles is not as well understood as it is in mammals.
- It is suspected that a multitude of environmental and behavioral factors, as well as underlying disease, contribute to an abnormal function of the endocrine system, which in turn leads to follicular stasis.
- It is also possible that a lack of breeding and exposure to males may have a negative impact on the reptiles' ability to properly ovulate.
- In addition to basic husbandry aspects such as temperature, humidity, and a proper diet, female reptiles also have a need for appropriate substrate and environment that is conductive for egg laying or birthing in the case of viviparous species.

SIGNALMENT/HISTORY

- Follicular stasis occurs in female snakes of reproductive age or size.
- A history of inadequate husbandry, being housed alone without access to a male, and lacking an appropriate area for laying eggs or giving birth may be part of the presenting history.
- There may also be snakes with appropriate husbandry that still suffer from follicular stasis for unknown reasons.

CLINICAL PRESENTATION

- Snakes with follicular stasis often present with non-specific clinical signs such as anorexia and lethargy. These could be due to the pathologic effects of the retained follicles, an underlying disease, or both.
- Some animals may present with coelomic distention, but follicles are not as easily palpable as in lizards.
- Palpation of the coelomic cavity must be done gently to avoid rupturing the follicles.
- In the majority of cases, the owners are not aware of the fact that their snake is in follicular stasis.
- Other abnormalities identified in physical exam may include dehydration, poor body condition score, and significant weight gain that does not match the growth of the animal.

RISK FACTORS

Husbandry

- Inappropriate husbandry is likely a significant contributing factor to the occurrence of follicular stasis.
- Beyond temperature and humidity, and inadequate nutrition can have a significant impact in calcium availability and follicular development.
- An often-forgotten aspect of the husbandry of reproductive female snakes is the provision of an adequate substrate for oviposition or an area deemed safe for parturition.
- It is often accepted that reptiles that may not perceive the environmental conditions are adequate for successful reproduction will resorb the follicles through atresia.
- In captivity, there may be a combination of factors that do not allow for normal follicular atresia.

Others

- A less discussed topic is the effect that lack of exposure to males may have on the reproductive cycle of reptiles.
- Many reptiles display courtship and breeding behaviors that likely influence the proper hormonal stimulation of prospective females.
- Many female snakes in captivity are kept alone without the benefit of behavioral cues from a male counterpart.
- This possibility of a behavioral effect must be considered, especially when animals are maintained in proper husbandry and are otherwise healthy.

DIAGNOSIS

DIFFERENTIAL DIAGNOSIS

- Dystocia
- Neoplasia
- Egg yolk coelomitis
- Ovarian cysts
- GI obstruction
- Constipation

DIAGNOSTICS

Imaging

- Radiography: follicles appear as non-calcified, round to ovoid, variably sized soft-tissue opacities in the caudal coelom. At times, the follicles may either be large enough or of large enough numbers to encompass the majority of the caudal coelomic cavity.
- Ultrasound: early follicles appear as anechoic and progress to have more echogenicity as they mature or fail to ovulate. Follicles with a more heterogeneous distribution within the lumen should be highly suspicious of being retained follicles, as the material within becomes firmer and inspissated. Ultrasound examination and aspiration of any free fluid can also be used to rule out egg yolk coelomitis.
- CT and MRI: both modalities are extremely sensitive at identifying follicles and can better assess the differences in size, shape and content of the follicles.
- Coelioscopic examination allows for confirmation of the presence of follicles and evaluation of their color and size to help in making a determination of whether the presentation may be pathologic.

Hematology and Biochemistry

- A chemistry panel is essential to help to identify other possible underlying disease processes such as dehydration and renal disease. In addition to Ca and P, Mg levels should be documented as Mg also plays an important role in Ca homeostasis. Levels of Mg below 1 mg/dl should be considered deficient. Hypercalcemia and hyperphosphatemia are common findings in reproductively active female snakes.
- CBC: a leukocytosis indicates a significant inflammatory response, which may suggest an additional underlying disease like egg yolk coelomitis.

PATHOLOGICAL FINDINGS

- Grossly, follicular stasis can be differentiated from dystocia by the presence of follicles outside of the oviduct.
- At times, the follicles may be large enough to appear to be in chains but are surrounded by the ovarian membrane rather than the oviduct.
- Healthy follicles should be smooth and white to yellow in color.
- A deviation from this appearance (i.e., dark, shriveled, or cystic follicles) is indicative of pathology.

TREATMENT

APPROPRIATE HEALTH CARE

- The treatment approach to follicular stasis is based on diagnosis and treatment of contributing factors leading to the stasis and treatment of the stasis itself.
- The species of snake, clinical condition at presentation, amount and appearance of the follicles based on imaging or coelioscopy, and ability to provide a suitable environment all contribute to the decision-making process.

• All snakes will benefit from medical treatment even if surgery is ultimately required.
• Medical therapy consists of correcting the husbandry, providing an appropriate nesting/birthing area, and supportive therapy with emphasis on calcium supplementation.
• If the snake appears to be stable, medical therapy alone can be attempted and the animal monitored for evidence of follicular atresia.
• There are no timelines as to how quickly atresia can be expected.
• Many snakes will ultimately require surgical intervention.
• Surgery is best performed before stasis progresses, while the animal is metabolically stable.
• Surgery should be an immediate consideration for snakes with documented chronic stasis, metabolic derangements, and when egg yolk coelomitis is suspected.
• The goal of surgery is to remove the follicles and perform an ovariectomy to avoid reoccurrence.
• Follicular stasis is commonly associated with follicles on both ovaries but even if only one is affected, bilateral ovariectomy is recommended.
• Extreme care must be taken to not rupture the follicles in the coelomic cavity, as the yolk is extremely antigenic and will cause a severe inflammatory response.
• If leakage occurs, the coelomic cavity should be thoroughly lavaged before closure.

NUTRITIONAL SUPPORT

Dietary deficiencies must be corrected, with special emphasis on proper nutrition.

CLIENT EDUCATION/HUSBANDRY RECOMMENDATIONS

• Clients should be encouraged to seek veterinary care of snakes early on to establish individual baseline values and confirm the sex of the animal.
• Follicular stasis likely has a multifactorial cause, so all husbandry deficiencies must be corrected, including the provision of adequate nesting substrate for oviparous species or birthing areas for viviparous.
• It is also important to avoid disturbing snakes that are known to be reproductively active.
• Snakes should be weighed at least weekly to document any sudden weight increases that may be indicative of follicular development.

MEDICATIONS

DRUG(S) OF CHOICE

• Calcium: start with calcium gluconate 100 mg/kg IM, SC q12–24h followed by calcium glubionate 10–100 mg/kg PO q4–24h long term.
• Magnesium sulfate 20 mg/kg IM, SC q24–72h, or magnesium lactate (Rescue Cal+, Repashy Ventures, CA, USA Saskatoon, SK) 20 mg/kg PO q24h.
• Crystalloid fluids 20–30 ml/kg SC, IV q24h
• Meloxicam 0.5–1 mg/kg PO, IM, SC q24–48h

PRECAUTIONS/INTERACTIONS

N/A

FOLLOW-UP

PATIENT MONITORING

• If performing medical therapy alone, the weight of the snake should be recorded weekly to provide an early indication that follicle atresia may be occurring.
• Any acute weight losses beyond 10% of the body weight should prompt re-evaluation by a veterinarian.
• If an underlying disease process was diagnosed, appropriate follow-up diagnostics should be performed to determine improvement of that condition or the need to alter therapy.
• For those undergoing surgery, a re-evaluation within 1–2 weeks is recommended to evaluate the surgical site and overall recovery.

EXPECTED COURSE AND PROGNOSIS

• Ultimately, the prognosis will depend on the underlying cause of follicular stasis and the required therapy.
• Cases with underlying infectious or metabolic disease that respond to medical therapy have a good prognosis.
• Many cases requiring surgical therapy have a good to guarded prognosis.

MISCELLANEOUS

COMMENTS

• The ultimate diagnosis of follicular stasis is based on interpretation of clinical signs, history, results of the physical exam, and diagnostics.
• Before ovariectomy is performed, it is essential to have at least one confirmatory test that there are indeed follicles present in the coelomic cavity.
• The sex of the animals must be confirmed as female before surgery is performed. While this may seem obvious, sex determination in some snakes, especially at a young age, can be quite challenging and males may present with coelomic neoplasias or GI obstructions that clinically appear very similar to follicular stasis.

ZOONOTIC POTENTIAL

N/A

SYNONYMS

Preovulatory follicular stasis

ABBREVIATIONS

• Ca = calcium
• CBC = complete blood count
• CT scan = computed tomography
• GI = gastrointestinal
• IM = intramuscular
• Mg = magnesium
• MRI = magnetic resonance imaging
• P = phosphorus
• PO = per os
• SC = subcutaneous

Suggested Reading

Jacobson ER. Overview of reptile biology, anatomy, and histology. In: Jacobson ER, ed. *Infectious Diseases and Pathology of Reptiles: Color Atlas and Text.* Boca Raton, FL: CRC Press; 2007:14–17.

Author Javier G. Nevarez, DVM, PhD, DACZM, DECZM (Herpetology)

Gout

BASICS

DEFINITION/OVERVIEW

Gout is a common disease seen in reptiles. It occurs due to the buildup of uric acid crystals deposited in or around the joints or throughout visceral organs.

ETIOLOGY/PATHOPHYSIOLOGY

- Increased production of uric acid may occur due to excessive levels of dietary proteins or potentially due to an inherited enzyme defect, as occurs in humans.
- Alternatively, excretion may be compromised, for example by dehydration, starvation, nephrotoxic drugs, or renal pathology.
- Uric acid is a relatively insoluble substance so when levels are elevated in the blood or in other body fluids, crystallization will occur and deposits will form.
- In snakes, these uric acid crystals usually deposit throughout internal organs such as the kidneys, liver, spleen, pericardial sac, lungs, and subcutaneous tissue.

SIGNALMENT/HISTORY

- Often seen in snakes with a history of husbandry deficits.
- Sometimes the animal may have been previously treated with potentially nephrotoxic drugs.

CLINICAL PRESENTATION

- Snakes may be asymptomatic or may have non-specific signs such as lethargy and reduced appetite.
- Sometimes white nodules may be visualized on examination of the oral cavity.

RISK FACTORS

Husbandry

- Inappropriate environmental temperatures
- Inappropriate water provision (e.g., low humidity or lack of fresh water).

Others

Administration of potentially nephrotoxic drugs (e.g., aminoglycosides), especially to dehydrated patients.

DIAGNOSIS

Gout may be suspected on history and clinical examination, but diagnostic testing will be necessary for definitive diagnosis.

DIFFERENTIAL DIAGNOSIS

- Pseudogout
- Metastatic or dystrophic calcification
- Bacterial abscess
- Fungal granuloma

DIAGNOSTICS

- Demonstration of uric acid (usually monosodium urate) crystals within diseased tissue is necessary for definitive diagnosis. Surgical biopsies should be submitted for histopathological analysis.
- Blood uric acid levels may be elevated, but this is not always a consistent finding as this depends on the stage in the disease process.
- Ultrasound of the coelomic organs may reveal echodense areas of precipitates within internal organs in cases of visceral gout.

PATHOLOGICAL FINDINGS

- On gross postmortem examination, small white nodules (tophi) can be seen scattered throughout visceral organs.
- On histopathological examination, tophi are often surrounded by granulomatous inflammation.

TREATMENT

APPROPRIATE HEALTH CARE

- Treatment aims to lower blood uric acid levels and promote uric acid excretion.
- Supportive treatment should always include appropriate analgesia, as in other species this is known to be a painful condition.
- Euthanasia may be considered in severe cases.

CLIENT EDUCATION/HUSBANDRY RECOMMENDATIONS

- Husbandry should be reviewed to identify any predisposing factors, such as inappropriate temperatures or low humidity, and these should be corrected.
- Clean fresh water should always be available in a recognizable form for the species.
- Clients should be advised that this is a condition that will require long-term management.

NUTRITIONAL SUPPORT

- Some patients may be anorexic and severely dehydrated on presentation.
- Fluid deficits should always be corrected and nutritional support provided.

MEDICATIONS

DRUG(S) OF CHOICE

- Allopurinol is the most common choice for treating gout. It is a xanthine oxidase-inhibiting drug that works by inhibiting the conversion of hypoxanthine and xanthine to uric acid in the liver, consequently reducing blood uric acid levels. If blood uric acid levels remain consistently low, then existing deposits may potentially dissolve. Doses of 10–20 mg/kg PO q24h are recommended for most species.
- Other drugs to promote uric acid excretion, such as probenecid, can theoretically be used, but are contraindicated in dehydrated patients.
- In cases of visceral gout, probenecid should be avoided as it increases uric acid excretion by the kidneys and could theoretically make the condition worse.

PRECAUTIONS/INTERACTIONS

Allopurinol and probenecid may potentially interact, although the clinical significance of this in reptiles is unknown.

FOLLOW-UP

PATIENT MONITORING

- Response to therapy may be based on clinical signs (e.g., increase in activity levels).
- Repeat blood samples can also be taken to recheck uric acid levels which would be expected to start reducing within 7 days of treatment.

EXPECTED COURSE AND PROGNOSIS

- The prognosis for patients with severe widespread signs is poor, but if diagnosed early the condition can often be managed successfully.
- If left untreated, the disease will progress with widespread uric acid deposition, ultimately resulting in organ failure and death.

MISCELLANEOUS

COMMENTS

N/A

ZOONOTIC POTENTIAL

N/A

SYNONYMS

N/A

ABBREVIATIONS

PO = per os

INTERNET RESOURCES

Veterinary Information Network: www.vin.com

Suggested Reading

Dallwig R. Allopurinol. *J Exot Pet Med* 2010;19(3):255–257.

Mader DR. Gout. In: Mader DR, ed. *Reptile Medicine and Surgery*. 2nd ed. St. Louis, MO: Elsevier Saunders; 2006:374–379.

Montali RJ, Bush M, Smeller JM. The pathology of nephrotoxicity of gentamicin in snakes: *A model for reptilian gout. Vet Path* 1979;16(1):108–115.

Author Joanna Hedley BVM&S, DZooMed (Reptilian), DECZM (Herpetology), MRCVS

HEMIPENE PROLAPSE

BASICS

DEFINITION/OVERVIEW

A prolapse is the moving or slipping of a body part from its usual position or anatomic relation. A prolapse of one or both paired hemipenes may occur in snakes.

ETIOLOGY/PATHOPHYSIOLOGY

- The underlying causes for prolapse is often unknown.
- See Differential Diagnosis for a list of possible etiologies.

SIGNALMENT/HISTORY

- There appears to be no specific signalment or predilections noted.
- Prolapse may occur more commonly in breeding animals.

CLINICAL PRESENTATION

- A prolapse is easy to visualize as abnormal tissue protruding from the vent region. Sometimes the owners may not notice a problem until days after it has occurred.
- A prolapse should be considered an emergency and evaluated promptly.
- The tissue should be kept moist either through gentle washing the area with water and loosely wrapped in a damp cloth or paper towel until the animal can be evaluated by a veterinarian.
- The extruded tissue should be identified to the tissue(s) involved.
- In the case of the hemipenis, the tissue may be pink to purple, although some species have black pigmentation normally.
- Some species of snakes may have "ornate" hemipenes with a flower-like end and/or small spike-shaped papilla.
- Exposure of the prolapsed tissue may result in further damage due to desiccation and trauma.
- The act of crawling and walking exposes the prolapsed organ to mechanical damage from the ground, branches, etc.

RISK FACTORS

- Any generalized physical straining by the patient such as dyspnea, obstipation, parasites, infection, can lead to tissue exposure through the vent.
- Space-occupying lesions located in the coelomic cavity, such as uroliths, neoplasia, hepato/renomegaly, may also cause increase straining and hemipenal prolapse.
- Seminal plugs are not frequently produced in male snakes. The plugs are white to brown structures emerging from the cloacal area and may be mistaken for parasites.
- Seminal plugs are waxy discharges mixed with semen that form a "plug" inside the inverted hemipenes.
- Manual rubbing or pressure often removes these structures. In some cases, the plug enlarges to a point where it is not able to be expressed without causing damage.
- The patient may continue to rub the area and inadvertently prolapse the hemipenes in the process. On occasion, attempting to remove these plugs may also lead to a prolapse.

Husbandry

- Several factors of husbandry may lead to one of the clinical conditions listed in the Differential Diagnosis section.
- Corrections of the deficient aspects of the husbandry can lead to reversal of some of those listed conditions.
- The act of copulation may result in trauma to the hemipenis resulting in swelling and the inability to invert the organ.
- Any eversion of the organ may result in direct trauma with the environment (i.e., ground, dirt, etc.) or bite wounds from a cage mate.

Others

- A prolapse of the hemipenes may be iatrogenic through sex determination, where a probe is placed inside the inverted hemipenis and it is torn.
- The act of "popping" the hemipenes through digital pressure to evert the tissue to determine sex may cause direct damage.

DIAGNOSIS

DIFFERENTIAL DIAGNOSIS

- Trauma
- Sexual activity
- Constipation
- Cloacal impaction (urates, cystic calculi, cage substrate)
- Neurological deficits
- Coelomic masses
- Parasites
- Hypocalcemia
- Metabolic disease
- Bacterial infection

DIAGNOSTICS

- Radiography and ultrasound may be useful in determining internal abnormalities (e.g., impactions, masses, obstructions).
- The small size of some reptiles may lead to reduced imaging detail, which makes interpretation challenging.
- Dental radiography may be a better alternative in smaller species (< 100 g).
- A fecal examination should be performed in all cases. This can be directly from the feces, from a saline cloacal wash, or a direct impression smear of the prolapsed tissue may reveal the presence of parasites such as nematode larvae or eggs.
- A complete blood count and chemistry panel may assist in determining underlying physiologic abnormalities.

PATHOLOGICAL FINDINGS

- The length of time the prolapse presents has an inverse effect on the prognosis.
- The longer an internal mucosal tissue is exposed to the outside environment, the higher the risk for the tissue to desiccate and potentially devitalize.
- Any devitalized tissue must be removed.
- The greater the amount of tissue devitalized, the lower the prognosis to save the organ.

TREATMENT

APPROPRIATE HEALTH CARE

- Treatment often involves direct replacement of the tissue back into normal anatomic position, by either manual or surgical means, in combination with correction of the underlying etiology. The patient should be fully evaluated for general health status and treated accordingly.
- The prolapsed tissue should be evaluated for presence of devitalization, which must be surgically or medically addressed prior to prolapse reduction.
- The prolapsed hemipenis may be reduced in size by coating it with a hyperosmotic solution such as 2–5% ophthalmic saline or concentrated sugar solution.
- Direct application of dry salt or sugar may be attempted, but the extreme osmolar difference could lead to direct tissue damage and should be closely monitored.
- After several minutes of application, the prolapsed tissue should become less edematous and capable of reduction back into the body cavity.
- A moistened and lubricated (water soluble) cotton tip applicator or metal probe is used to gently push the tissue by inversion back inside the body cavity aligning the lumen.
- Lateral sutures across the cloacal margin may be placed for 10–14 days to allow for the tissue swelling to resolve in place.
- If the tissue is devitalized or traumatized, or the prolapsed tissue cannot be easily replaced, the best option may be amputation.
- Since the hemipenis is not associated with the urinary system, the tissue can be amputated with no long-term effects.
- To perform amputation the exteriorized tissue should be further removed to identify and isolate the base of the organ.
- The base should be ligated with a transfixation and/or mattress suture.
- A double ligation is warranted due to the well-developed vascular system, as well as the vascular stimulation secondary to the prolapse.

HEMIPENE PROLAPSE (CONTINUED)

• The remaining surgical stump should be replaced back into the hemipenal pocket at the base of the tail.
• When replacing the prolapse, extreme care must be taken not to tear or perforate the delicate, inflamed tissue.
• After the sutures are removed, the tissue may re-prolapse if swelling/inflammation is still present or the underlying etiology has not been corrected.
• Placement of additional sutures may be required.
• Amputation may be considered at this time.

NUTRITIONAL SUPPORT

The patient may need weight and body condition monitoring to determine whether additional caloric supplementation is needed.

CLIENT EDUCATION/HUSBANDRY RECOMMENDATIONS

• If surgical correction of the prolapse was undertaken, the client should be directed on postoperative care of any surgical sites, suture, etc.
• A detailed log of activity and food intake/defecations should be maintained and related back to the veterinarian.
• If any changes to the husbandry were determined (e.g., changes to temperature and/or humidity, exposure to ultraviolet lighting), the owner should make corrections prior to the patient returning home.

MEDICATIONS

DRUG(S) OF CHOICE

• NSAIDs or opioids may be used in management of the pain and inflammation associated with the physical discomfort of the prolapse or surgery.
• Depending on the underlying etiology, antibiotics or anti-parasiticides may be indicated.

PRECAUTIONS/INTERACTIONS

• When replacing the prolapse, extreme care must be taken not to tear or perforate the delicate, inflamed tissue.
• After the sutures are removed, the tissue may re-prolapse if swelling/inflammation is still present or the underlying etiology has not been corrected.
• Placement of additional sutures may be required.
• Amputation may be considered at this time.
• Hydration status of the patent must be considered before use of NSAIDs.

FOLLOW-UP

PATIENT MONITORING

• The patient should be followed up daily after clinical repair of the prolapse for reoccurrence.
• The owner should monitor and record all food intake and defecations during this time.
• Any abnormal changes from the routine should be related back to the veterinarian to determine any further changes to the therapy.

EXPECTED COURSE AND PROGNOSIS

• Hemipenal prolapses have excellent to good prognosis, as these are purely copulatory organs.
• Even in if amputation is required, there are rarely any ill effects on the patient.
• Even if one hemipene is amputated, the animal could still breed with the contralateral organ.

MISCELLANEOUS

COMMENTS

N/A

ZOONOTIC POTENTIAL

N/A

SYNONYMS

N/A

ABBREVIATIONS

NSAIDs = nonsteroidal anti-inflammatory drugs

Suggested Reading

Barten, SL. Penile prolapse. In: Mader DR, ed. *Reptile Medicine and Surgery*. 2nd ed. St. Louis, MO: Elsevier Saunders; 2006:862–864.
Bennett, RA. Cloacal prolapse. In: Mader DR, ed. *Reptile Medicine and Surgery*. 2nd ed. St. Louis, MO: Elsevier Saunders; 2006:751–755.

Author Rob L. Coke, DVM, DACZM, DABVP (Reptile & Amphibian), CVA

HEPATIC LIPIDOSIS

BASICS

DEFINITION/OVERVIEW

Hepatic lipidosis is the excessive accumulation of triglycerides in the hepatocytes. It can result in altered hepatic function. It is expected to be a reversible lesion if the underlying cause is corrected. It is a common lesion diagnosed in reptiles.

ETIOLOGY/PATHOPHYSIOLOGY

- Triglyceride accumulation in hepatocytes can occur due to disturbances of lipid metabolism from primary metabolic liver disease, toxins, protein malnutrition, diabetes mellitus, obesity, anorexia (increased fatty acid mobilization from peripheral stores), extrahepatic visceral inflammation, and anoxia (inhibits fatty acid oxidation).
- In female reptiles, the change can be associated with folliculogenesis.
- The common factor for each of these possible etiologies is a negative balance between the rates of deposition and dispersal of fat from the liver, resulting in an accumulation of triglycerides in the liver.
- Obesity from rich diets can result in hepatic lipidosis and enlargement of the coelomic fat bodies.
- Reduced activity may also contribute to increased fat deposits.

SIGNALMENT/HISTORY

Hepatic lipidosis is reported to be less common in snakes. Data from one lab (D Reavill, unpublished) found the percentages of hepatic lipidosis in the reptile groups with the liver submitted for evaluation to be: chelonians (turtles and tortoises) 14% (97/676); lizards 20% (304/1485); snakes 5.4% (91/1672).

CLINICAL PRESENTATION

- Clinical signs are generally non-specific, including weakness, depression, pale oral mucous membranes, and non-specific neurologic signs.
- Green to blue urates are reported, and clay-like, tan, or watery feces may also be noted.

RISK FACTORS

Husbandry

- Inappropriate diet, overfeeding, and feeding fatty prey.
- Chronic stress: inappropriate captive husbandry conditions (temperature, cage size, feeding strategies).
- Inactivity: restricted physical activity due to space or adequate stimulation.
- Inappropriate support for reproduction
- Inappropriate hibernation conditions
- Anorexia/hyporexia

Others

N/A

DIAGNOSIS

- Although the presumptive diagnosis is based on history, clinical signs, laboratory data, and imaging, the definitive diagnosis is made by microscopic evaluation of a liver biopsy or necropsy examination.

DIFFERENTIAL DIAGNOSIS

- Vascular congestion: underlying cardiovascular disease.
- Toxins: mycotoxins, pesticides, heavy metals.
- Infectious diseases: herpesvirus, adenovirus, salmonella, mycobacteria, Gram-negative bacterial infections, abscesses/granulomas, protozoa.
- Tumor: lymphoma, hepatoma

DIAGNOSTICS

Imaging

- Radiographs ± contrast, ultrasound, CT, and MRI.
- There may an enlarged hepatic silhouette on radiography.
- Ultrasound may reveal a brightly reflective, enlarged, rounded liver.
- CT provides measurements of radiodensity of the liver.

Hematology and Biochemistry

- Serum biochemistry: lack of species-specific reference ranges make interpretation challenging.
- In general, decreased plasma proteins; increased triglycerides, cholesterol, AST, and LDH; glucose and bile acid levels vary; blood is often noticeably lipemic.

PATHOLOGICAL FINDINGS

- The gross appearance is of an enlarged, friable liver, pale tan to yellow, which typically has a greasy feel.
- Biopsy and/or necropsy histopathology: the hepatocytes will be variably enlarged, and supporting cytoplasmic vacuolization with H&E stains.
- Additional stains will demonstrate the prominent, oil red O-positive lipid droplets in all the hepatocytes.

TREATMENT

APPROPRIATE HEALTH CARE

Antibiotics if needed

NUTRITIONAL SUPPORT

- Caloric reduction with a nutritionally complete, low-fat, high-quality protein, liquid diet (Lafeber's Emeraid®, or Oxbow Carnivore Care®).
- Ensure adequate hydration

CLIENT EDUCATION/HUSBANDRY RECOMMENDATIONS

Advise client to maintain the animal at an appropriate temperature and humidity, and to provide exercise.

MEDICATIONS

DRUG(S) OF CHOICE

- Antibiotic of choice: ceftazidime
- Nutraceuticals such as silymarin, milk thistle (reported to be an anti-inflammatory and antioxidant, although there are no studies to support its claim for hepatic benefits).

PRECAUTIONS/INTERACTIONS

Avoid hepatotoxic agents use in reptiles:

- Antibiotics: doxycycline, clindamycin, erythromycin
- Antivirals: acyclovir
- Antifungals: itraconazole, ketoconazole
- Antiparasitic: metronidazole, dichlorvos, tiabendazole, ivermectin.

FOLLOW-UP

PATIENT MONITORING

Regular checkups to assess body weight, change in serum biochemistries, and possibly repeat biopsy.

EXPECTED COURSE AND PROGNOSIS

After support through any acute crisis, the long-term prognosis depends on associated conditions and whether they can be changed.

MISCELLANEOUS

COMMENTS

N/A

ZOONOTIC POTENTIAL

N/A

SYNONYMS

- Fatty liver
- Vacuolar hepatopathy

ABBREVIATIONS

- AST = aspartate aminotransferase
- CT = Computed tomography
- H&E = hematoxylin and eosin
- LDH = lactate dehydrogenase
- MRI = magnetic resonance imaging

Suggested Reading

Divers SJ, Cooper JE. Reptile hepatic lipidosis. *Semin Avian Exot Pet* 2000;9(3):153–164.

HEPATIC LIPIDOSIS (CONTINUED)

Knotková Z, Dorrestein GM, Jekl V, et al. Fasting and postprandial serum bile acid concentrations in 10 healthy female red-eared terrapins (*Trachemys scripta elegans*). *Vet Rec* 2008;163(17):510–514.

Marchiori A, da Silva ICC, de Albuquerque Bonelli M, et al. Use of computed tomography for investigation of hepatic lipidosis in captive *Chelonoidis carbonaria* (spix, 1824). *J Zoo Wildl Med* 2015;46(2):320–324.

Martínez-Silvestre, A. *Hepatic lipidosis in reptiles*. Proc SEVC, October 2013, Barcelona, Spain.

West G. Endoscopic hepatic biopsy in Coahuilan box turtles, *Terrapene coahuila*. *J Herpetol Med Surg* 2001;11(2):28–29.

Author Drury R. Reavill, DVM, DABVP (Avian and Reptile & Amphibian Practice), DACVP

HYPERGLYCEMIA

BASICS

DEFINITION/OVERVIEW
Hyperglycemia is abnormally high blood glucose concentration. In most species, glucose concentrations fluctuate. Normal glucose concentration ranges from 10 mg/dl to 80 mg/dl (0.55–4.4 mmol/l).

ETIOLOGY/PATHOPHYSIOLOGY
- The etiology is largely unknown.
- Transient hyperglycemia may be postprandial or stress induced.
- Elevated glucose may be seen during ovulation/gestation, and with certain neoplastic processes.
- Iatrogenic from prior glucose or glucocorticosteroid administration.
- It is speculated that endocrine pancreas disease may lead to insulin deficiency resulting in a diabetes mellitus-like syndrome, but this has not been documented.

SIGNALMENT/HISTORY
N/A

CLINICAL PRESENTATION
- Unspecific
- Possibly increased water consumption, increased urine (urate) production, and weight loss.

RISK FACTORS

Husbandry
Stress from handling or improper housing may predispose.

Others
Largely unknown

DIAGNOSIS
Blood glucose levels above 100 mg/dl (5.5 mmol/l) indicate hyperglycemia.

DIFFERENTIAL DIAGNOSIS
N/A

DIAGNOSTICS
- Blood glucose measurements should be repeated, as a single elevated value is likely insignificant.
- Persistent hyperglycemia is a more relevant finding.
- Glucosuria should be evaluated to identify chronic hyperglycemia.
- Underlying causes should be investigated: ovarian activity, neoplasia, metabolic disease.

PATHOLOGICAL FINDINGS
The etiology for persistent hyperglycemia is unknown, but endocrine pancreas should be thoroughly evaluated.

TREATMENT

APPROPRIATE HEALTH CARE
- In cases with persistent hyperglycemia, where systemic disease has been ruled out, experimental insulin treatment may be attempted.
- Suggested starting dose: 1–5 iu/kg q24–48h.

NUTRITIONAL SUPPORT
N/A

CLIENT EDUCATION/HUSBANDRY RECOMMENDATIONS
- Correct any improper husbandry
- Avoid stress from handling

MEDICATIONS

DRUG(S) OF CHOICE
N/A

PRECAUTIONS/INTERACTIONS
N/A

FOLLOW-UP

PATIENT MONITORING
- Follow up with repeated glucose measurements.
- Monitor general health of patient.

EXPECTED COURSE AND PROGNOSIS
Transient hyperglycemia is likely insignificant, while chronically elevated levels carry a poor prognosis.

MISCELLANEOUS

COMMENTS
N/A

ZOONOTIC POTENTIAL
N/A

SYNONYMS
N/A

ABBREVIATIONS
N/A

INTERNET RESOURCES
Kaplan M. Hypoglycemia and Hyperglycemia in Reptiles. Melissa 's Herp Care Collection, January 1, 2014. http://www.anapsid.org/diabetes.html

Suggested Reading
Campbell TW. Clinical pathology. In: Mader DR, Divers SJ, eds. *Current Therapy in Reptile Medicine and Surgery*. St. Louis, MO: Elsevier; 2014: 70–92.

Stahl SJ. Hyperglycemia in reptiles. In: Mader DR, ed. *Reptile Medicine and Surgery*. 2nd ed. St. Louis, MO: Elsevier Saunders; 2006:822–830.

Author Mads F. Bertelsen, DVM, DVSc, DACZM, DECZM (Zoo Health Management)

HYPOGLYCEMIA

BASICS

DEFINITION/OVERVIEW

Hypoglycemia is abnormally low blood glucose concentration. In most species, glucose concentrations fluctuate, and normal concentrations range from 10 mg/dl to 80 mg/dl (0.55–4.4 mmol/l). Values approaching zero may be physiological.

ETIOLOGY/PATHOPHYSIOLOGY

- Exhaustion, starvation, malnutrition
- Septicemia
- Hepatobiliary disease
- Pancreatic disease

SIGNALMENT/HISTORY

- Animals with severe systemic disease may be predisposed.
- Long-lasting anorexia

CLINICAL PRESENTATION

- Weakness
- Tremors
- Loss of righting reflex
- Torpor
- Unresponsiveness

RISK FACTORS

Husbandry

N/A

Others

- Systemic disease
- Poor nutritional status

DIAGNOSIS

Blood glucose levels below 10 mg/dl (0.55 mmol/l) indicate hypoglycemia.

DIFFERENTIAL DIAGNOSIS

N/A

DIAGNOSTICS

- Detection of hypoglycemia in a clinically healthy animal should not cause concern.
- In animals with clinical signs and hypoglycemia, attempts should be made to rule out septicemia, hepatobiliary disease and pancreatic neoplasia.
- Glucose may be artificially low in blood samples stored for too long prior to separation of plasma/serum.

PATHOLOGICAL FINDINGS

- Depends on underlying etiology
- Pancreas should be thoroughly evaluated.

TREATMENT

APPROPRIATE HEALTH CARE

N/A

NUTRITIONAL SUPPORT

Consider energy-rich nutritional support by stomach tube in anorectic animals.

CLIENT EDUCATION/HUSBANDRY RECOMMENDATIONS

If related to poor nutrition and management, educate clients on appropriate feeding practices.

MEDICATIONS

DRUG(S) OF CHOICE

- Treat underlying disease
- Supportive administration of glucose or dextrose parenterally (e.g., 2.5% in 0.45% saline, 20–40 ml/kg SC) or orally (3 g/kg PO) may be indicated.

PRECAUTIONS/INTERACTIONS

N/A

FOLLOW-UP

PATIENT MONITORING

Monitor glucose levels and clinical signs.

EXPECTED COURSE AND PROGNOSIS

- If related to nutritional status, prognosis is good.
- If secondary to severe systemic disease, prognosis is poor.

MISCELLANEOUS

COMMENTS

N/A

ZOONOTIC POTENTIAL

N/A

SYNONYMS

N/A

ABBREVIATIONS

- PO = per os
- SC = subcutaneous

INTERNET RESOURCES

Kaplan M. Hypoglycemia and Hyperglycemia in Reptiles. Melissa Kaplan's Herp Care Collection, January 1, 2014). http://www.anapsid.org/diabetes.html .

Suggested Reading

Campbell TW. Clinical pathology. In: Mader DR, Divers SJ, eds. *Current Therapy in Reptile Medicine and Surgery*. St. Louis, MO: Elsevier; 2014:70–92.

Stahl SJ. Hyperglycemia in reptiles. In: Mader DR, ed. *Reptile Medicine and Surgery*. 2nd ed. St. Louis, MO: Elsevier Saunders; 2006:822–830.

Author Mads F. Bertelsen, DVM, DVSc, DACZM, DECZM (Zoo Health Management)

INCLUSION BODY DISEASE

BASICS

DEFINITION/OVERVIEW

IBD is a progressive degenerative disease affecting boas and pythons. It is characterized by the presence of intracytoplasmic inclusions in neurons and epithelial cells of various organs. The inclusions are made up of a unique protein, IBDP. The disease is caused by viruses in the family *Arenaviridae*, genus *Reptarenavirus*. Arenaviruses are enveloped, pleomorphic single-stranded RNA viruses that are easily disinfected. Many arenaviruses have rodents as reservoir hosts, while reptarenaviruses have only been found in snakes so far.

ETIOLOGY/PATHOPHYSIOLOGY

- Reptarenaviruses have been detected in various boa and python species, detections in other snake species are extremely rare.
- Transmission is not fully understood, but seems to require close contact; transmission via blood appears to be likely.
- Snake mites (*Ophionyssus natricis*) have been suggested as a possible vector.
- Vertical transmission is possible, and offspring from infected parents are often (but not always) infected and develop disease.
- Studies of viruses in affected snakes have shown that the reptarenaviruses are genetically highly variable, and it has been hypothesized that this genetic variability may influence the development of clinical disease.
- IBD causes immune suppression in affected animals; clinical disease may therefore also depend on a wide variety of other opportunistic pathogens and have very varied clinical signs.
- The CNS is most often affected.

SIGNALMENT/HISTORY

- Boas and pythons of various species can be affected by IBD.
- In recent years, it has most commonly been detected in the boa constrictor.
- Similar disease processes have been reported in viperid and colubrid snakes, but it is not known whether these were caused by the same agents.
- Juvenile animals infected in utero or at birth may develop disease more quickly, although not all offspring will be affected.
- In boas, typical inclusion bodies can often be found in a wide range of cells throughout the body.
- In pythons, inclusions are rare and may only be found in a few neurons within the brain.
- Clinical disease appears to develop much faster in pythons, while boas can live for extended periods of time with no apparent clinical signs.
- A large number of captive boas may be carriers.
- There is evidence that some boas may live for years with IBD.

CLINICAL PRESENTATION

- The development of IBD-associated disease often depends on the affected snake species, and pythons appear to develop severe signs more quickly than boas.
- In general, IBD is considered a progressive debilitating disease with fatal outcome.
- IBD is immunosuppressive and can be associated with a variety of clinical signs.
- CNS signs may include anisocoria, opisthotonus, disorientation, inability of the animal to right itself, head tremors, and flaccid paralysis.
- Some snakes may react to stimuli with thrashing or uncontrolled lunging.
- In many cases, especially in boas, the first signs noted may be associated with the digestive tract and can include inappetence, regurgitation, and stomatitis.
- Pneumonia has also frequently been observed in affected animals.
- Lymphoproliferative disease and round cell tumors appear to occur more frequently in IBD-positive snakes.
- Skin disorders may also be observed.
- IBD should always be considered in cases in which disease is chronic and therapy resistant and in cases of CNS disease in boas and pythons.

RISK FACTORS

Husbandry

- Mixing of infected animals, particularly boas and pythons, may provoke disease development.
- Inadequate hygiene practices can lead to spread of IBD and other secondary pathogens.

Others

Snake mites may transmit infection and may be a factor in the spread of disease within a collection.

DIAGNOSIS

DIFFERENTIAL DIAGNOSIS

Depending on the clinical presentation, many other infectious and noninfectious causes of disease may need to be considered.

DIAGNOSTICS

- Virus detection: PCR detection of reptarenavirus RNA in esophageal swabs, whole blood, esophageal tonsils, liver, kidney, pancreas, brain, and other tissues.
- In boas, esophageal swabs may be the most sensitive minimally invasive sample, but biopsies of a variety of other tissues can be helpful for diagnosis, if they can be obtained.
- In pythons, whole blood may sometimes be arenavirus positive.
- In most pythons and in some cases in boas, virus is found only in the brain, and detection in live animals may therefore not be possible in these cases.

PATHOLOGICAL FINDINGS

- IBD was originally defined by the presence of eosinophilic to amphophilic intracytoplasmic inclusions in various tissues, particularly neurons and epithelial cells of various organs.
- Inclusions are sometimes, but not always, associated with inflammation.
- Inclusions are made up of a unique protein, IBDP, and appear as granular, electron dense material by electron microscopy.
- In pythons, inclusions are frequently found only in neurons, while in boas, inclusions are much more common and can often be found in large numbers in various tissues (e.g., in the liver, pancreas, kidney, esophageal tonsils) in addition to neurons.

TREATMENT

APPROPRIATE HEALTH CARE

- IBD is a progressive degenerative disease.
- Supportive therapy can help extend the life of affected snakes, but no curative therapy is available.
- Euthanasia should be considered for positive snakes with clinical disease.

NUTRITIONAL SUPPORT

N/A

CLIENT EDUCATION/HUSBANDRY RECOMMENDATIONS

- IBD is currently present in many collections of boas and possibly pythons.
- Preventing the introduction of IBD into a collection must include various strategies, including quarantine, ectoparasite control, and a preventive medicine program.
- Managing a collection in which IBD has been detected should include similar programs and ridding a collection of IBD can be challenging and take an extended period.
- An effective quarantine regimen should include testing for both virus and inclusion bodies.
- Since IBD can develop very slowly, an extended quarantine is necessary to increase the chances of preventing the introduction of this disease into a collection.

INCLUSION BODY DISEASE (CONTINUED)

- Any animals that test positive should be permanently removed from a collection and either euthanized or kept separate from other snakes.
- Ectoparasite control should be implemented to control spread of disease.
- Offspring from IBD or arenavirus positive animals may also be positive, so positive parents should not be bred and offspring from such animals should not be mixed with other snakes, sold, or given away.
- Thorough necropsy with histopathology and virological testing should be carried out on all animals that die within a collection.
- Animals should be purchased from breeders in which the history is known and who are known to have a preventive medicine program in place.

MEDICATIONS

DRUG(S) OF CHOICE

N/A

PRECAUTIONS/INTERACTIONS

- Affected animals should be placed in quarantine and should not have contact with negative animals.
- Ectoparasites, particularly snake mites, should be treated as these may transmit infection.
- Optimization of husbandry and prevention of secondary infections may help to prolong the life of infected animals.

FOLLOW-UP

PATIENT MONITORING

Development of disease in contact animals may take weeks, months, or even years, depending on the host species, the virus involved, as well as husbandry conditions and the presence of secondary pathogens, so monitoring of a collection should remain active at all times.

EXPECTED COURSE AND PROGNOSIS

- Morbidity is generally low, although the slow course of disease can make the establishment of IBD-free large collections difficult to impossible.
- Mortality is considered to be high, although duration of the disease varies depending mostly on the host species, with pythons developing severe neurological disease and succumbing faster than boas.
- Virus specific factors may also play a role in the course of disease, although these are not yet fully understood.

MISCELLANEOUS

COMMENTS

N/A

ZOONOTIC POTENTIAL

Although reptarenaviruses are related to several zoonotic viruses, including mammalian arenaviruses and filoviruses, currently there is no indication that they are zoonotic.

SYNONYMS

Boid inclusion body disease (BIBD)

ABBREVIATIONS

- BIBD = boid inclusion body disease
- CNS = central nervous system
- IBD = inclusion body disease
- IBDP = inclusion body disease protein
- PCR = polymerase chain reaction

INTERNET RESOURCES

- Stenglein MD, Jacobson ER, Chang W, et al. Widespread recombination, reassortment, and transmission of unbalanced compound viral genotypes in natural arenavirus infections. *PLoS Pathog* 2015;11:e1004900.
- Stenglein MD, Sanders C, Kistler AL, et al. Identification, characterization, and in vitro culture of highly divergent arenaviruses from boa constrictors and annulated tree boas: candidate etiological agents for snake inclusion body disease. *MBio* 2012;3:e00180-12.

Suggested Reading

Chang LW, Jacobson ER. Inclusion body disease, a worldwide infectious disease of boid snakes: A review. *J Exot Pet Med* 2010;19:216–225.

Marschang RE. Virology. In: Divers SJ, Stahl SJ, eds. *Mader's Reptile and Amphibian Medicine and Surgery*. St. Louis, MO: Elsevier; 2019:247–269.

Author Rachel E. Marschang, PD, Dr. med. vet., DECZM (Herpetology), FTÄ Mikrobiologie

BASICS

DEFINITION/OVERVIEW

Viruses in the family *Iridoviridae* are large, double-stranded DNA viruses that contain a lipid component and can be enveloped. Iridoviruses that have been described in reptiles include ranaviruses, erythrocytic viruses (named hemocytiviruses) and invertebrate iridoviruses. The ranaviruses are the most commonly described with the greatest clinical importance. They can infect a wide range of ectothermic vertebrates including reptiles, amphibians, and bony fish. In reptiles, they are most commonly described in chelonians, but have also been found in a wide range of squamate species. Hemocytiviruses have also been described in a wide range of species, while invertebrate iridoviruses have been described mostly in insectivorous squamates.

ETIOLOGY/PATHOPHYSIOLOGY

- Ranaviruses have been described in a few snake cases. Numerous ranavirus strains can be transmitted between different animal classes.
- In North America, the ranaviruses described in reptiles have all been closely related to *Frog virus 3*, the type species of the genus, while ranaviruses found in reptiles in other parts of the world (particularly Europe) have been more genetically diverse. In infected reptiles, ranaviruses can cause severe disease, often associated with lesions in the mouth, liver, and blood vessels.
- Hemocytiviruses have mostly been described in wild-caught reptiles, as well as amphibians and fish. They lead to the development of intracytoplasmic inclusions in blood cells, mostly erythrocytes, and can cause anemia and systemic disease in infected animals.

SIGNALMENT/HISTORY

- Ranavirus infections in snakes are rare. They have been associated with the movement of groups of animals, generally through the pet trade. Affected species have included *Morelia viridis*, *Python* spp., and *Eunectes* spp.
- Erythrocytic viruses have been detected in lizards, snakes, and turtles from various parts of the world, often in blood smears from wild-caught animals.

CLINICAL PRESENTATION

- Ranaviruses: in snakes, anorexia, oral and nasal ulcers, skin lesions, and increased erythema of the skin and mucous membranes have been reported.
- Erythrocytic viruses have been found in animals with no apparent signs of disease, in animals with anemia and in animals with systemic fatal disease. Affected animals may become lethargic and lose weight. In some cases, infection has been associated with oral lesions and hepatic necrosis. The temperature appears to play a role in the course of infection.

RISK FACTORS

- Inappropriate management, stress, temperature variation, species mixing, contact with infected amphibians, fish or other reptiles may all play significant role in promoting ranavirus infection and eventually in the occurrence of the disease.
- Contaminated water can also lead to transmission.
- Ranaviruses do not replicate at high temperatures, so keeping animals at low temperatures may increase the risk of infection.
- Hemocytiviruses are likely transmitted by hematophagous invertebrates, so keeping biting insects away from animals is important.

Husbandry

N/A

Others

N/A

DIAGNOSIS

DIFFERENTIAL DIAGNOSIS

Bacterial and/or fungal infections

DIAGNOSTICS

Ranaviruses

- In the United States, all the ranaviruses described in reptiles to date have been genetically closely related, and highly sensitive real-time PCRs are available for their detection.
- In other parts of the world, ranaviruses found in reptiles have been more genetically diverse, and PCRs capable of detecting these should be used.
- Ranaviruses can be relatively easily isolated in cell culture.
- Skin has been used for virus detection in lizards with skin lesions.
- Liver and kidney should also be tested if possible.

Hemocytiviruses

- Infections with erythrocytic viruses have most often been initially diagnosed by cytological examination of blood smears, with confirmation of etiology carried out by electron microscopy.
- Genomic information is now available from several members of this proposed genus, and PCRs for virus detection are likely to become more available.
- Virus detection is generally carried out from blood samples, but liver can also be used.

PATHOLOGICAL FINDINGS

- Gross findings in snakes consist of oral mucosa chronic ulcerations and pharyngeal necrosis.
- On histology necrosis of the pharyngeal submucosa, ulceration of the nasal mucosa, hepatic degeneration, and necrosis (*M. viridis*) have been reported.
- Subclinical infections might not be associated with histological changes, or at least not specific.

TREATMENT

APPROPRIATE HEALTH CARE

- There is no specific treatment available for iridovirus infections in reptiles.
- All viruses in this family replicate at temperatures below 32 degrees C (89.6 degrees F); environmental temperature has been shown to influence the pathogenicity of ranaviruses in turtles.
- It is, however, important to keep the POTZ of the affected species in mind when adjusting environmental temperature.
- Antibiotic therapy to prevent secondary bacterial infections should be evaluated case by case.

NUTRITIONAL SUPPORT

N/A

CLIENT EDUCATION/HUSBANDRY RECOMMENDATIONS

- All newly introduced animals into an established collection must undergo appropriate quarantine period (at least 6 months).
- Appropriate hygiene measures should be maintained.
- Routinely carry out diagnostic tests (at least once a year).
- Do not introduce individuals from collections that have experienced a ranavirus outbreak or general multiple deaths within a short period of time.
- Avoid species mixing and overcrowding, and separate animals showing abnormal behavior.
- Pre- and post-brumation are particularly critical times to monitor because of the more likely occurrence or recurrence of infection.
- Clean and disinfect terraria regularly and replace bedding and water frequently.

IRIDOVIRUS (CONTINUED)

• Disinfection of gear, footwear, and potential fomites is an important precaution.
• Carcasses from dead animals should be disposed of appropriately and must not come in contact with other animals.
• Since ectoparasites may play a role in the transmission of various iridoviruses, effective measures for parasite control should be implemented.

MEDICATIONS

DRUG(S) OF CHOICE

N/A

PRECAUTIONS/INTERACTIONS

• Affected animals should be barrier nursed.
• Viruses can cross species and class barriers, so contact with any other ectothermic vertebrates should be avoided.
• It has been suggested that ranaviruses and hemocytiviruses may be transmitted by hematophagus invertebrates, so control of mosquito populations may be helpful.

FOLLOW-UP

PATIENT MONITORING

• Molecular testing for virus shedding over time is suggested.
• Molecular testing is also suggested after the end of the outbreak, in case of incomplete clearance of the virus by the survivors.
• The time to development of disease in contact animals can vary, depending on the route of infection, amount of infectious material, virus strain, and host species, so monitoring should be continued for several months in an affected collection.
• Surviving infected animals can become carriers.

EXPECTED COURSE AND PROGNOSIS

Animals that survive infection may remain carriers and should be kept separate from susceptible animals, including reptiles, amphibians, and fish.

MISCELLANEOUS

COMMENTS

N/A

ZOONOTIC POTENTIAL

• Viruses in the family *Iridoviridae* are generally temperature restricted and can only replicate at temperatures below 32 degrees C (89.6 degrees F).
• Iridoviruses are unable to infect mammals or birds.

SYNONYMS

• Erythrocytic necrosis virus
• Ranavirus

ABBREVIATIONS

• PCR = polymerase chain reaction
• POTZ = preferred optimal temperature zone

INTERNET RESOURCES

Gray MJ, Chinchar VG. Ranaviruses: Lethal pathogens of ectothermic vertebrates. Heidelberg: Springer Open; 2015. http://link.springer.com/book/10.1007%2F978-3-319-13755-1

Suggested Reading

Alves de Matos AP, Paperna I, Crespo E. Experimental infection of lacertids with lizard erythrocytic viruses. *Intervirology* 2002;45:150–159.

Marschang RE. Virology. In: Divers SJ, Stahl SJ, eds. *Mader's Reptile and Amphibian Medicine and Surgery*. St. Louis, MO: Elsevier; 2019:247–269.

Stöhr AC, Blahak S, Heckers KO, et al. Ranavirus infections associated with skin lesions in lizards. *Vet Res* 2013;44:84.

Wellehan JF Jr, Strik NI, Stacy BA, et al. Characterization of an erythrocytic virus in the family Iridoviridae from a peninsula ribbon snake (*Thamnophis sauritus sackenii*). *Vet Microbiol* 2008;131:115–122.

Author Rachel E. Marschang, PD, Dr. med. vet., DECZM (Herpetology), FTÄ Mikrobiologie, and Francesco C. Origgi, DVM, PhD, DACVM (Virology), DACVP, DECZM (Herpetology)

ISOSPORA

BASICS

DEFINITION/OVERVIEW

Isospora is a genus of apicomplexan parasites with two sporocysts containing four sporozoites. *Isospora* is typically an intracytoplasmic parasite, but some species may have intranuclear development.

ETIOLOGY/PATHOPHYSIOLOGY

- *Isospora* spp. have a direct life cycle, with infective stages passed in the feces of the host. Infections are confined to the intestines.
- Most reports of illness associated with *Isospora* infection are from captive animals that have been housed under suboptimal conditions, with infection often further complicated by concurrent disease.
- There are no reports of infection with *Isospora* resulting in disease in snakes.

SIGNALMENT/HISTORY

- High stocking density
- Unsanitary conditions
- Maladaptation of wild animals entering captivity

CLINICAL PRESENTATION

None reported but may relate to GI upset.

RISK FACTORS

Husbandry

- Breeding colonies at high stocking density are at greatest risk.
- Poor hygiene and stress are likely to predispose to infection and disease.

Others

Concurrent disease or excessive stress may cause immunosuppression, thus increasing risks of disease expression.

DIAGNOSIS

DIFFERENTIAL DIAGNOSIS

Other GI disease such as bacterial or protozoal infections (i.e., *Eimeria*).

DIAGNOSTICS

- Examination of feces for presence of oocysts using light microscopy.
- Molecular techniques such as PCR may aid in species delineation but are unlikely to improve treatment efficacy or prognosis.
- Protozoa may also be seen in biopsy or necropsy samples.
- Fecal samples should be stored in 2–3% aqueous (w/v) potassium dichromate ($K_2Cr_2O_7$).

PATHOLOGICAL FINDINGS

- Gross lesions may be mild and unapparent in many cases.
- Histologically, there may be small intestinal villous atrophy with intracytoplasmic coccidia within enterocytes.

TREATMENT

APPROPRIATE HEALTH CARE

N/A

NUTRITIONAL SUPPORT

- Ensure animals are well hydrated, especially if medicating with sulfa drugs.
- Force-feeding with easily digestible proteins by stomach tubing can be done in most species.
- This approach should be re-evaluated when dealing with venomous species.
- Supportive fluid therapy should be provided.

CLIENT EDUCATION/HUSBANDRY RECOMMENDATIONS

- Remove and isolate sick individuals and reduce stress by providing optimal living conditions and hygiene.
- Thoroughly clean the cage to reduce environmental contamination of oocysts.
- Ensure that quarantine protocols have been adopted for all new arrivals.
- During quarantine, all animals should be subjected to repeated clinical and fecal examinations.
- Keep stocking densities as low as possible, especially in stressful conditions such as breeding colonies.

MEDICATIONS

DRUG(S) OF CHOICE

- Because *Isospora* spp. are not known to be pathogenic in snakes, prophylactic therapy or treatment should not be based on the identification of *Isospora* spp. alone, to avoid developing resistance.
- Treatment should only be performed after an *Isospora* sp. has been confirmed to be causing clinical signs.
- Ponazuril 30 mg/kg PO q48h for 2 treatments, or 30 mg/kg PO q24h for 4 treatments, then repeat for 2–4 treatments 2 weeks apart.
- Toltrazuril 15 mg/kg PO q48h for 30 days
- Sulfadimethoxine 50 mg/kg PO q24h for 21 days
- Trimethoprim-sulfa 30 mg/kg daily for 5 days, then q48h until the coccidia are eliminated.

PRECAUTIONS/INTERACTIONS

Sulfa drugs are known to be nephrotoxic.

FOLLOW-UP

PATIENT MONITORING

Repeat fecal examination at monthly intervals.

EXPECTED COURSE AND PROGNOSIS

- Treatment may have variable efficacy as many protozoa are resistant to a range of anticoccidial medication.
- Prognosis is good to guarded and is determined primarily by the state of the animal at initial presentation and the presence or absence of concurrent disease.

MISCELLANEOUS

COMMENTS

N/A

ZOONOTIC POTENTIAL

N/A

SYNONYMS

N/A

ABBREVIATIONS

- GI = gastrointestinal
- PCR = polymerase chain reaction
- PO = per os

Suggested Reading

Gibbons PM. Advances in reptile clinical therapeutics. *J Exot Pet Med* 2014;23(1):21–38.

Jacobson ER. Parasites and parasitic diseases of reptiles. In: Jacobson ER, ed. *Infectious Diseases and Pathology of Reptiles: Color Atlas and Text.* Boca Raton, FL: CRC Press; 2007:571–665.

Kim DY, Mitchell MA, Bauer RW, et al. An outbreak of adenoviral infection in inland bearded dragons (*Pogona vitticeps*) coinfected with dependovirus and coccidial protozoa (*Isospora* sp.). *J Vet Diagn Invest* 2002;14:332–334.

Scullion FT, Scullion MG. Gastrointestinal protozoal diseases in reptiles. *J Exot Pet Med* 2009;18(4):266–278.

Walden M, Mitchell MA. Evaluation of three treatment modalities against *Isospora amphiboluri* in inland bearded dragons (*Pogona vitticeps*). *J Exot Pet Med* 2012;21(3):213–218.

Wolf D, Vrhovec MG, Failing K, et al. Diagnosis of gastrointestinal parasites in reptiles: comparison of two coprological methods. *Acta Vet Scand* 2014;56:1–13.

Author T. Franciscus Scheelings, BVSc, MVSc, PhD, MANCVSc (Wildlife Health), DECZM (Herpetology)

LEUKEMIA

BASICS

DEFINITION/OVERVIEW

Leukemia is a neoplasia of the white blood cells, which starts in the bone marrow.

ETIOLOGY/PATHOPHYSIOLOGY

- No confirmed etiology has been proved for any of the leukemia cases described in snakes, including viral etiology.
- Leukemias are classified as myeloid or lymphoid, depending upon the neoplastic blood cell.
- It is generally accepted, based on previously reported cytochemical staining characteristics, that reptilian granulocytes, monocytes, and azurophils are from the myeloid cell lineage, whereas reptilian lymphocytes are from the lymphoid cell lineage.
- Leukemias are commonly graded as acute or chronic, depending on the number of blast cells in peripheral circulation.
- Blast cells predominate in acute leukemia, whereas mature forms predominate in chronic onset leukemia with less than 30% of the peripheral leukocytes being blast cells.
- Acute leukemias are rapidly fatal in untreated patients.

SIGNALMENT/HISTORY

- Leukemia has been reported in both adult and immature snakes.
- Lymphoid leukemia is reported more frequently than myeloid leukemia.

CLINICAL PRESENTATION

- Anorexia and lethargy are frequently reported.
- Weight loss is common in chronic leukemia.

RISK FACTORS

Husbandry

N/A

Others

N/A

DIAGNOSIS

DIFFERENTIAL DIAGNOSIS

- Multiple myeloma or plasma cell myeloma.
- Monoclonal gammopathy

DIAGNOSTICS

- Hemogram: a marked leukocytosis characterized by lymphocytosis/monocytosis (depending upon the type of leukemia) is observed in many cases.
- Cytological evaluation of blood smears and/or bone marrow aspirates.
- Necropsy and subsequent histopathology
- Cytochemical and immunocytochemical stains to confirm cell lineage.
- Peroxidase activity, chloroacetate esterase activity, and α-naphthyl butyrate esterase activity can be used as markers to distinguish myeloid or lymphoid origin; it is important to study comparison samples from both clinically healthy and affected animals of the same species because of the paucity of cytochemical characterization of blood cells for most reptiles.
- CD3 antibody identifies T-cell lymphocytes and CD79 antibody identifies B-cell lymphocytes.
- L1-calprotectin antibody has been used to identify myeloid cells in lizards.
- Transmission electron microscopy can be attempted to determine histogenesis and to identify viral particles.

PATHOLOGICAL FINDINGS

- Cytological evaluation of blood smears and/or bone marrow aspirates can reveal abnormal cell morphology of the neoplastic cells, abnormal nuclear to cytoplasm ratio, and anisokaryosis; mitotic figures are frequently detected.
- Histopathologic examination of tissue samples can reveal infiltration of neoplastic cells in several organs and occasional mitotic figures.

TREATMENT

APPROPRIATE HEALTH CARE

N/A

NUTRITIONAL SUPPORT

As needed

CLIENT EDUCATION/HUSBANDRY RECOMMENDATIONS

An early diagnosis can maximize the success of therapy.

MEDICATIONS

DRUG(S) OF CHOICE

- No successful specific treatment protocol has been reported in snakes (see Leukemia in Section II: Lizards for a treatment protocol which can be used as a reference point).
- Cytosine arabinoside is the most frequently used treatment for small mammals with chronic monocytic leukemia, whereas prednisone therapy is widely used and accepted for small mammals with lymphoid leukemia and lymphoma, not being effective for myeloid leukemias.

PRECAUTIONS/INTERACTIONS

Suspected cytosine arabinoside toxicity characterized by renal failure has been reported in a rhinoceros viper.

FOLLOW-UP

PATIENT MONITORING

Complete blood count must be done for monitoring the overall white blood cell count and different leukocyte counts to gauge response to the drugs.

EXPECTED COURSE AND PROGNOSIS

The prognosis of the disease, especially in acute leukemia, is poor.

MISCELLANEOUS

COMMENTS

N/A

ZOONOTIC POTENTIAL

N/A

SYNONYMS

N/A

ABBREVIATIONS

N/A

Suggested Reading

Frye FL. Diagnosis and surgical treatment of reptilian neoplasms with a compilation of cases 1966–1993. *In Vivo* 1994;8:885–892.

Hruban Z, Vardiman J, Meehan T, et al. Haematopoietic malignancies in zoo animals. *J Comp Pathol* 1992;106:15–24.

János G, Mihály A, Mihály DK. Myeloid leukaemia in black head python (*Aspidites melanocephalus*). *Magyar Allatorvosok Lapja* 2002;124:491–495.

Mauldin GN, Done LB. Oncology. In: Mader DR, ed. *Reptile Medicine and Surgery*. 2nd ed. St. Louis, MO: Elsevier Saunders; 2006:299–322.

Author Jorge Orós, DVM, PhD, DECZM

LOWER RESPIRATORY TRACT DISEASE

BASICS

DEFINITION/OVERVIEW

Diseases of the respiratory tract are common and are often responsible for considerable morbidity and mortality in reptiles. LRTD is a common presentation in snakes. Often, the URT is affected concurrently. In snakes, the LRT consists of the glottis, larynx, trachea, paired bronchi, and, depending on the species, single or multichambered lungs. The forward-lying glottis is situated in the front part of the oral cavity and lies against the choana dorsally when the mouth is closed. The glottis is very mobile and can be pulled forward or extended laterally by special muscles to allow breathing while ingesting prey. The trachea, which is composed of incomplete cartilaginous rings, runs down the neck and, in the majority of snakes, continues as a single bronchus. In some snakes, a tracheal lung arises from the dorsal surface of the trachea. The lung in snakes is oblong according to their elongated total body plan. In general, the right lung is always larger in snakes while the left lung is reduced or absent. Some snakes completely lack a left lung; some, such as colubrids, have a vestigial one; and some snakes, such as boas, have a fairly developed left lung. In general, only the first third to the first half of the lung consists of a highly vascular portion and contains functional respiratory tissue, the remainder consisting of an avascular air sac-like portion. The transition from lung to air sac happens at the level of the liver, with the air sac extending up to the cloaca in some species. Inspiration is achieved by expansion of the ribs, while expiration is a passive process through relaxation of the muscles. Snakes are unable to cough. Ciliary action is disrupted at the glottis, and snakes lack a diaphragm.

ETIOLOGY/PATHOPHYSIOLOGY

- There is a wide range of etiologies associated with LRTD; infectious causes are some of the most common.
- LRTD may also be secondary to other diseases such as stomatitis.

Infectious

- Bacteria (*Mycobacterium genavense*; *Chlamydia* spp.; Gram-negatives such as *Bordetella* spp., *Pseudomonas* spp., *Salmonella* spp., *Morganella morganii*, *Acinetobacter* spp., *Klebsiella* spp., *Serratia marcescens*, *Proteus* spp., *Alcaligenes faecalis*, *Providencia rettgeri*; Gram-positive alpha-hemolytic *Streptococcus* spp.).
- *Mycoplasma* spp. (sp. *novum*)
- Fungi (*Rhizopus arrhizus*, *Paecilomyces variotii*)
- Viruses (ferlavirus, arenaviruses, adenoviruses, nidovirus, ranaviruses).
- Parasites may cause physical damage to epithelium and serve as vectors for other infections, sometimes a combination of parasitic and bacterial or viral.
- The mite *Ophionyssus natricis* has been linked to transmission of *Aeromonas hydrophila*, one of the agents associated with stomatitis in snakes and a possible cause of respiratory tract infections.
- *Kalicephalus* spp. in the nasal cavity.
- *Rhabdias*, *Kalicephalus*, *Renifers* infecting the oral cavity or esophagus.
- Pentastomids (in oral cavity, pharynx, trachea, bronchi, lung) sometimes exit via the glottis and then through the mouth and nares.
- Adult flukes (in oral cavity, pharynx, trachea, bronchi, lungs).
- Cartilaginous hyperplasia of the trachea (ball pythons).

Non-Infectious

- Neoplasia (intratracheal chondromas in ball pythons, bronchogenic adenocarcinoma in a cobra).
- Cartilaginous hyperplasia of the trachea (ball pythons).
- Foreign bodies within the choana, nasal or oral cavity.
- Physical trauma/injuries
- Inhalation of dust, smoke, aerosols, or disinfectants leading to rhinotracheitis.
- Improper husbandry

SIGNALMENT/HISTORY

No age, sex, or species predisposition.

CLINICAL PRESENTATION

- Dependent on the underlying cause and snake species.
- Tachypnea or dyspnea
- Respiratory distress (intermittent or persistent)
- Elevated head and straightened cranial part of the body (vertical positioning of the head and neck) due to forced breathing.
- Stridor, gurgling, or wheezing
- Glottal discharge/exudate (clear to mucopurulent)
- Excess salivation/oral exudate
- Sometimes nasal discharge/exudate and obstructed external nares.
- Sometimes glottal discharge, reddening and/or edema of the glottis.
- Cyanosis in severe cases
- Simultaneous occurrence of stomatitis (sometimes necrotizing)
- Excessive air-filled digestive tract (aerophagia) due to increased and forced inspiration.
- Acute death due to blockage with plug (sometimes mucopurulent) or tissue (hyperplasia or neoplasia).
- Nonspecific signs, such as anorexia, lethargy, inactivity.
- Sometimes purulent material in the subspectacular space (provoked by bacterial infections of the spectaculocorneal space) or bullous spectaculopathy.

RISK FACTORS

- Inadequate husbandry
- Stressors
- Poor hygiene

Husbandry

Improper husbandry, including inappropriate temperatures and humidity, stagnant water, substrate with irritating compounds (e.g., cedar shavings), poor ventilation.

Others

- Immunosuppression
- Sudden changes in temperature or humidity.
- Improper diet (including starvation)
- Endoparasitism may also be a predisposing factor.

DIAGNOSIS

DIFFERENTIAL DIAGNOSIS

- Infectious diseases (bacterial, viral, fungal, parasitic)
- Trauma
- Neoplasia
- Foreign bodies
- Inhalation of irritating substances

DIAGNOSTICS

- Physical exam, including thorough exam of the oral cavity and choana. The use of magnification may aid in identifying subtle lesions.
- Bacterial culture and sensitivity (aerobic and anaerobic) and/or fungal culture of tracheal or lung lavage are critical for proper diagnosis.
- Cytology of oral mucus and tracheal or lung lavage.
- Diagnostic imaging (radiography, CT, MRI)
- Endoscopy, including nasal lavage and biopsy for further diagnostics such as cytology, histopathology, virology, and electron microscopy.
- Biopsy, cytology, and histopathology of the affected lung(s) may be beneficial in refractory cases.
- In cases of virus infection, virus isolation and/or PCR using tracheal or lung lavage, nasal flush or nasal swab, choanal, oral, esophageal swabs, or lung tissue; detection of antibodies in blood samples (serology), biopsies of liver and/or esophageal tonsils for arenaviruses.
- In case of suspected mycobacteria infection: immunohistochemistry and PCR.
- Fecal exam

LOWER RESPIRATORY TRACT DISEASE (CONTINUED)

PATHOLOGICAL FINDINGS

- Pathologic findings will vary according to the underlying cause and may range from mild to severe.
- Histopathology of intratracheal chondroma in ball pythons has revealed an intratracheal mass occluding the lumen. Calcium deposits were observed within the tissue as eosinophilic cytoplasmic inclusions.
- In another study in ball pythons, the benign chondromas were composed of variably disorganized chondroid matrix populated by quiescent, chondrocytes within lacunae.
- Space-occupying masses in the trachea have been seen in ball pythons with cartilaginous hyperplasia of the trachea.
- Pneumonia usually affects the well-developed right lung but can also affect the left lung, if present, as in the case of a green tree python (*Morelia viridis*) with fibrinopurulent pneumonia of the rudimentary left lung.
- Snakes with a *Mycobacterium genavense* infection had white nodules in the trachea, lung and liver. Microscopic examination revealed pneumonia characterized by inflammatory interstitial infiltration and necrotic areas surrounded by heterophils, macrophages, and giant cells. Similar lesions were found in the esophagus, trachea, and liver.
- Various forms of pneumonias have been described in a study detecting pathogens in boas and pythons.
- Pneumonias were characterized by an inflammatory reaction of different stages and, in most cases, by detectable bacterial foci and one case had intralesional mycotic hyphae. Variations of pneumonia included catarrhal, fibrinous, chronic, and granulomatous.
- During a ferlavirus epizootic in snakes, major microscopic findings included proliferative interstitial pneumonia with or without infiltrates of mononuclear inflammatory cells and heterophils.
- Nidovirus infections in pythons are associated with pneumonia, tracheitis, and esophagitis. The lungs of infected snakes were characterized by marked pneumocyte hyperplasia and mixed mononuclear and granulocytic inflammation and epithelial necrosis.
- Inflammatory and hyperplastic changes were also present in the trachea.
- In another study, histopathology of nidovirus infected ball pythons revealed proliferative interstitial pneumonia, as well as thickened and edematous lung tissue with mucoid to caseous material in the airways.

TREATMENT

APPROPRIATE HEALTH CARE

- Dependent on the underlying cause and the affected snake species.
- Viral: separation, strict quarantine, and intensive supportive therapy.
- In case of confirmed mycobacterial infection, no treatment: euthanasia.
- In some cases, physical removal of the parasites via surgery or endoscopy may be necessary.
- Intratracheal chondromas: removal via endoscopy or partial tracheal resection and anastomosis.
- Cartilaginous hyperplasia of the trachea: surgical removal of the affected area.

NUTRITIONAL SUPPORT

Nutritional supplementation for anorexic animals is essential for recovery. Carnivore critical care diets can be fed once weekly until the snake starts eating on its own.

CLIENT EDUCATION/HUSBANDRY RECOMMENDATIONS

- Correct any husbandry deficiencies with special attention to temperature, humidity, and ventilation.
- Isolate animal from others in collection, especially when viral etiology is suspected.
- It is important to ensure a full course of treatment to avoid recurrence of disease.

MEDICATIONS

DRUG(S) OF CHOICE

- Systemic use of itraconazole may cause severe adverse effects in some snakes.
- Bacteria: systemic or nebulized antibiotics (amikacin, ceftazidime, enrofloxacin, tylosin), preferably according to sensitivity panel for at least 4–6 weeks. Local instillation of antibiotics (injectable or ophthalmic solutions) in the nasal passage may also be effective.
- Fungi: systemic, local, nebulized antifungals (e.g., terbinafine, voriconazole, amphotericin B).
- Antiviral therapy has had low success and euthanasia is often required, depending on the state of the animal and the disease.
- Parasites: antiparasitic treatment according the species.
- In case of tracheal obstruction, saccular lung cannulation via air sac tube and suction from material from the lung and trachea.
- Oxygen cage therapy in severe cases.
- Fluid therapy at a fluid rate of 10–30 ml/kg/day as supportive care.

PRECAUTIONS/INTERACTIONS

- Many systemic antibiotics (e.g., gentamycin or enrofloxacin) are excreted through the kidney or show renal toxicity, thus adequate hydration and regular monitoring of renal values is recommended.

FOLLOW-UP

PATIENT MONITORING

- Improvement of clinical signs should be expected within 1–2 weeks for bacterial and fungal infections when definitive diagnosis and treatment are employed.
- It is critical to continue treatment until clinical signs are fully resolved and to repeat cultures to confirm resolution of the infection if unsure.
- In cases that do not show any improvement or worsen during the first 1–2 weeks of treatment, it should be considered that the etiology and/or treatment are not accurate.
- Viral infections should be considered in cases that do not respond to therapy or have chronic, intermittent recurrence of disease.
- Repeat diagnostics may be needed to assess resolution or progression of disease.

EXPECTED COURSE AND PROGNOSIS

- Bacterial: good prognosis depending on response to antibiotics.
- Fungal: guarded to poor prognosis.
- Viral: poor to grave prognosis especially when showing clinical signs.
- Parasitic: good prognosis
- Neoplastic: poor to grave prognosis
- Others: depend on severity and involvement of other tissues.

MISCELLANEOUS

COMMENTS

N/A

ZOONOTIC POTENTIAL

- Dependent on the causative agent
- Mycobacteria, *Salmonella* spp., pentastomids, and other etiologies have zoonotic potential.

SYNONYMS

Pneumonia

ABBREVIATIONS

- CT = computed tomography
- LRT = lower respiratory tract
- LRTD = lower respiratory tract disease
- MRI = magnetic resonance imaging
- PCR = polymerase chain reaction
- URT = upper respiratory tract

Suggested Reading

Chang LW, Jacobson ER. Inclusion body disease, a worldwide infectious disease of boid snakes: A review. *J Exot Pet Med* 2010;19(3):216–225.

Drew ML, Phalen DN, Berridge BR, et al. Partial tracheal obstruction due to chondromas in ball pythons (*Python regius*). *J Zoo Wildl Med* 1999;30(1):151–157.

Greenacre CB, Ritchie BW, Latimer KS. Treatment of cartilaginous hyperplasia in ball pythons. *Comp Cont Educ Pract* 1999;21(7):633–637.

Hyndman TH, Shilton CM, Doneley RJT, Nicholls PK. Sunshine virus in Australian pythons. *Vet Microbiol* 2012;161(1–2):77–87.

Jacobson E. Diseases of the respiratory system in reptiles. *Vet Med Small Anim Clin* 1978;73(9):1169–1175.

Junge RE, Miller RE. Reptile respiratory diseases. In: Kirk RW, Bonagura JD, eds. *Kirk's Current Veterinary Therapy XI. Small Animal Practice.* 11th ed. Philadelphia, PA: WB Saunders; 1992:1204–1210.

Myers DA, Wellehan JF Jr, Isaza R. Saccular lung cannulation in a ball python (*Python regius*) to treat a tracheal obstruction. *J Zoo Wildl Med* 2009;40(1):214–216.

O'Malley B. Snakes In: O'Malley B, ed. *Clinical Anatomy and Physiology of Exotic Species.* Edinburgh: WB Saunders; 2005:77–93.

Schmidt V, Marschang RE, Abbas MD, et al. Detection of pathogens in Boidae and Pythonidae with and without respiratory disease. *Vet Rec* 2013;172(9):236.

Stenglein MD, Jacobson ER, Wozniak EJ, et al. Ball python nidovirus: a candidate etiologic agent for severe respiratory disease in *Python regius. mBio* 2014;5(5):e01484-14.

Ullmann LS, das Neves Dias-Neto R, Cagnini DQ, et al. Mycobacterium genavense infection in two species of captive snakes. *J Venom Anim Toxins incl Trop Dis* 2016;22(1):27.

Wyneken J, Witherington D. Respiratory anatomy: Form and function in reptiles. *Exotic DVM* 2001;3:17–22.

Author Karina A. Mathes, DVM, Dr. med. vet., DECZM (Herpetology), European Veterinary Specialist in Zoological Medicine (Herpetology), Certified Specialist in Reptiles (Fachtieraerztin fuer Reptilien), Certified Specialist in Reptiles and Amphibians (ZB Reptilien und Amphibien)

LYMPHOMA

BASICS

DEFINITION/OVERVIEW

Lymphoma is a lymphoid neoplasia that originates in the lymphocyte cells.

ETIOLOGY/PATHOPHYSIOLOGY

- Although a lymphosarcoma associated with virus-like intranuclear inclusions in a California king snake (*Lampropeltis getula californiae*) has been reported, no viral etiology has been identified in most cases of lymphoid neoplasias in reptiles.
- The first description of a neoplasm of the reptilian hematopoietic system was a metastatic lymphosarcoma in an anaconda (*Eunectes murinus*). Since then, lymphoid neoplasias have been more frequently reported in snakes and lizards than in other reptiles, and they most commonly have a multicentric distribution.
- There is insufficient information about lymphoma in reptiles to be able to stage this entity meaningfully.
- In some of the reptile lymphomas, immunohistochemistry has been attempted to determine the cellular origin, but no correlation to the biological behavior of the tumor was made.

SIGNALMENT/HISTORY

Most cases of lymphoma/lymphosarcoma reported in snakes have affected adults.

CLINICAL PRESENTATION

- Anorexia, chronic weight loss, and lethargy are frequently reported.
- A complete blood count can reveal marked lymphocytosis.
- Physical examination can reveal single or multiple tumor nodules.

RISK FACTORS

Unknown

DIAGNOSIS

DIFFERENTIAL DIAGNOSIS

- Other tumors
- Inflammatory reactions (abscesses, granulomas, etc.)

DIAGNOSTICS

- Hemogram: a marked leukocytosis characterized by lymphocytosis can be observed. In advanced stages of the disease, it is unclear whether the neoplasia originates within the bone marrow or whether leukemia is a feature of disseminated, end-stage lymphoma.
- Histological examination of direct smears from a fine-needle aspirate of the nodular masses and/or of the biopsy specimen can reveal the presence of neoplastic lymphoid cells.
- Necropsy and subsequent histopathology
- Transmission electron microscopy can be attempted to identify viral particles.

PATHOLOGICAL FINDINGS

- Gross lesions include white and firm nodules in several organs, not limited to lymphoid organs.
- Splenomegaly is also frequently observed.
- Histologically, unencapsulated masses or monotonous sheets composed of hyperchromatic neoplastic lymphoid cells are observed.
- Mitotic figures are variable.

TREATMENT

APPROPRIATE HEALTH CARE

N/A

NUTRITIONAL SUPPORT

An esophagostomy tube should be considered in anorexic animals or for long-term administration of medications.

CLIENT EDUCATION/HUSBANDRY RECOMMENDATIONS

N/A

MEDICATIONS

DRUG(S) OF CHOICE

- No successful specific treatment protocol has been reported in snakes.
- See Lymphoma in Section III: Lizards for a treatment protocol that can be used as a reference point.
- A king cobra (*Ophiophagus hannah*) has been treated with subcutaneous L-asparagine amidohydrolase, intravenous vincristine, and oral prednisone over a three-week period, but the tumors metastasized.
- The protocol was modified using oral prednisone and chlorambucil but the snake showed a gradual decline in condition.

PRECAUTIONS/INTERACTIONS

A heterophil count threshold may be used as an indicator of drug toxicity.

FOLLOW-UP

PATIENT MONITORING

It can be adequate to monitor the overall WBC count and lymphocyte count to gauge response to the drugs, together with reduction in tumor size, weight gain, and quality of life.

EXPECTED COURSE AND PROGNOSIS

- Because little is known about most chemotherapeutic agents in snakes, the prognosis of the disease is poor.
- Most cases are diagnosed postmortem.

MISCELLANEOUS

COMMENTS

N/A

ZOONOTIC POTENTIAL

N/A

SYNONYMS

- Lymphoid neoplasm
- Lymphosarcoma

ABBREVIATIONS

WBC = white blood cell

Suggested Reading

Jacobson ER. Neoplastic diseases. In: Cooper JE, Jackson OF, eds. *Diseases of the Reptilia*. New York, NY: Academic Press; 1981:429–468.

Jacobson ER, Calderwood MB, French TW, et al. Lymphosarcoma in an Eastern king snake and a rhinoceros viper. *J Am Vet Med Assoc* 1981;179:1231–1235.

Mauldin GN, Done LB. Oncology. In: Mader DR, ed. *Reptile Medicine and Surgery*. 2nd ed. St. Louis, MO: Elsevier Saunders; 2006:299–322.

Schilliger L, Selleri P, Frye FL. Lymphoblastic lymphoma and leukemic blood profile in a red-tail boa (*Boa constrictor constrictor*) with concurrent inclusion body disease. *J Vet Diagn Invest* 2011;23:159–162.

Willette MM, Garner MM, Drew M. Chemotherapeutic treatment of lymphoma in a king cobra. *Proceedings of the American Association of Zoo Veterinarians*; 2001:20.

Author Jorge Orós, DVM, PhD, DECZM

MITES

BASICS

DEFINITION/OVERVIEW

Wild and captive snakes can be affected by external parasites (e.g., ticks and mites). The most commonly encountered ectoparasite of captive snakes is the hematophagous snake mite (*Ophionyssus natricis*). *Ophioptid* mites (*Ophioptes* spp.) live under the scales in a few species of snakes from widely scattered geographic areas of the world.

ETIOLOGY/PATHOPHYSIOLOGY

- *O. natricis* belongs to the sub-order Mesostigmata of the Macronyssidae family.
- Only protonymphs and adults are parasitic.
- *Ophionyssus* has a life span of about 40 days, irrespective of feeding. The life cycle is 7–16 days.
- The female (up to 1.5 mm in length) is larger than the male and takes 2–3 blood meals lasting 4–8 days at an interval of 1–2 weeks.
- A clutch of about 20 eggs is laid on the inner surfaces of the terrarium.
- When the humidity rises above 85% and the temperature ranges between 20–30 degrees C (68 degrees F to 86 degrees F), larvae hatch in 1–4 days.
- The free-living larvae measure about 400 µm, are whitish in color, and possess three pairs of legs.
- When the temperature reaches between 25–30 degrees C (77 degrees F and 86 degrees F) with a humidity above 75%, the larvae molt into protonymphs within 24 hours.
- The protonymphs, which possess four pairs of legs, take a single blood meal, which enables them to survive 3–7 days at 25 degrees C (77 degrees F).
- 12–48 hours following their meal, 90% molt into deutonymphs. Like larvae, the deutonymph stage is a free-living non-parasitic stage.
- At 25 degrees C (77 degrees F), the deutonymphs molt into adults, a process that takes approximately 24 hours.
- Adults are highly mobile, and following mating, females lay eggs that hatch into females only.
- If the eggs are not fertilized, they hatch into males only by arrhenotokous parthogenesis.
- *Ophioptes* spp. has been found only in a few species of snakes in Bolivia (*Erythrolamprus aesculapii*), Australia (*Simoselaps fasciolatus*), and central Africa (colubrid snakes).

SIGNALMENT/HISTORY

- Infected snakes often exhibit lethargy, dysecdysis, pruritus, crusting dermatitis (sometimes progressing to abscesses), and behavioral changes (increased bathing time, rubbing against objects).
- Owners may also notice infestation when they find mites on their own skin after handling infested snakes.

CLINICAL PRESENTATION

- The presence of small black granules between scales or on the hand after handling snakes should lead to a thorough examination of the entire skin of the snake.
- The snake mite can most commonly be found around the eyes, where they cause a characteristic annular swelling on the rims of the spectacle.
- Mites can also be found on the thinner part of the skin between the mandibles.

RISK FACTORS

Husbandry

The snake mite is a nest parasite, and is well adapted to reptile collections, with cages and other enclosures providing an ideal nesting environment.

Others

- Mites are usually introduced into a collection with substrate, pieces of wood, plants, and prey in a cage.
- A newly acquired infested snake can transmit parasites to a whole collection.

DIAGNOSIS

DIFFERENTIAL DIAGNOSIS

- Other ectoparasites such as ticks (*Amblyomma* spp., *Hyalomma* spp., *Ornithodoros* spp.) can be encountered.
- They differ markedly from *Ophionyssus* in size and shape.

DIAGNOSTICS

- Snake mites are easily identified with the naked eye or with a magnifying glass.
- Water bowls can be examined for drowned parasites.
- Definitive diagnosis is made by microscopic identification.

PATHOLOGICAL FINDINGS

N/A

TREATMENT

APPROPRIATE HEALTH CARE

The predatory mite *Cheyletus eruditus* (Taurrus®, APPI Biological Control, Haverhill, UK) is a good candidate for the biological control of *O. natricis*. It has strong predatory potential, good environmental survival, and a temperature range adapted to captive snake conditions. It can only be used only if substrate is present in the enclosure.

NUTRITIONAL SUPPORT

N/A

CLIENT EDUCATION/HUSBANDRY RECOMMENDATIONS

- Environmental treatment involves removal of all objects in the terrarium.
- The terrarium should be washed and scrubbed with hot water (> 122 degrees F; 50 degrees C) and then thoroughly sprayed with an acaricide.
- Decorations such as stones and bowls can be treated in the same manner, but substrate should be disposed.
- All stages are killed if the temperature in the terrarium rises above 50–55 degrees C (122–131 degrees F), and development is arrested if the humidity remains below 50%.
- Quarantine new individuals

MEDICATIONS

DRUG(S) OF CHOICE

- Many insecticidal and acaricidal compounds used in dogs, cats, and other mammals can be used.
- Pyrethrins, pyrethroids (0.5% spray) and fipronil can be applied on the animal and used for environmental treatment.
- Enclosures, bowls, and other inanimate objects should be thoroughly rinsed after using these compounds.
- Ivermectin 0.2 mg/kg IM, SC, or PO q14d
- Ivermectin: prepare a diluted topical spray of 5–10 mg/l of water applied q3–5d weekly or every other week for 6 to 8 weeks.
- Fipronil: apply directly to the animal and wipe off within 5 minutes q7d as needed; alternatively, spray on gauze or cloth and then wipe the snake with it to spread over the skin.

PRECAUTIONS/INTERACTIONS

- Snakes may present neurological disorders when they soak or drink from a water bowl that has not been carefully rinsed after application of an acaricide.
- Ivermectin should not be used in indigo snakes as toxicity has been reported.

FOLLOW-UP

Repeated and thorough examination of the entire skin of the snake.

PATIENT MONITORING

N/A

EXPECTED COURSE AND PROGNOSIS

- Eliminating snake mites from a collection is notoriously frustrating, as they are expensive and time consuming to kill and have a high rate of recurrence.

MITES (CONTINUED)

- Total elimination is only successful if coupled with rigorous environmental control.

MISCELLANEOUS

COMMENTS

- Anemia and septicemia are occasional complications.
- *Ophionyssus* spp. may serve as vector for hemogregarines (e.g., *Karyolyssus* spp.) and *Aeromonas hydrophila.*
- They may be implicated in the transmission of the agent of inclusion body disease in snakes (*Arenavirus*), but this has not been scientifically proven.
- Figure 1 – see web image supplementary content for section IV: Snakes.

ZOONOTIC POTENTIAL

Snake mites typically do not infest humans, but anecdotal cases of dermatitis induced by *O. natricis* in humans have been reported.

SYNONYMS

N/A

ABBREVIATIONS

- IM = intramuscular
- PO = per os
- SC = subcutaneous

INTERNET RESOURCES

http://www.taurrus.fr

Suggested Reading

Amanatfard E, Youssefi MR, Barimani A. Human dermatitis caused by *Ophionyssus natricis, a snake mite. Iran J Parasitol* 2014;9(4):594–596.

Fitzgerald K. Acariasis. In: Divers S, Stahl S, eds. *Mader's Reptile and Amphibian Medicine and Surgery.* St. Louis, MO: Elsevier; 2019:1290–1291.

Jacobson ER. Parasites and parasitic diseases of reptiles. In: Jacobson ER, ed. *Infectious Diseases and Pathology of Reptiles.* Boca Raton, FL: CRC Press; 2007:571–665.

Schilliger LH, Morel D, Bonwitt J. Marquis O. *Cheleytus eruditus* (Taurrus®): an effective candidate for the biological control of the snake mite (*Ophionyssus natricis*). *J Zoo Wildl Med* 2013;44(3):654–659.

Author Lionel Schilliger, DVM, DECZM (Herpetology), DABVP (Reptile & Amphibian Practice)

SNAKES

MYCOBACTEROSIS

BASICS

DEFINITION/OVERVIEW

Mycobacteriosis is a cosmopolitan disease that affects all classes of vertebrates. In reptiles, atypical or non-tuberculosis *Mycobacterium* spp. are most common. *Mycobacterium* spp. are more fastidious in ectothermic animals, and thus can appear as latent or chronic infections. While the apparent prevalence of mycobacteriosis in reptiles is low, it is likely underdiagnosed. Systemic and localized infections of *Mycobacterium* spp. have been documented in snakes. Infections are more commonly reported in aquatic reptiles.

ETIOLOGY/PATHOPHYSIOLOGY

- Aerobic, Acid-fast+, Gram-positive rod bacteria.
- *Mycobacterium chelonae, M. szulgai, M. marinum, M. fortuitum, M. ulcerans, M. leprae, M. haemophilum, M. avium, M. lepraemurium, M. kansasii, M. terrae, M. intracellulare M. genavense, M. kumamotonense, M. fuscus, M. nonchromogenium, M. smegmatis, M. confluentis, M. hiberniae.*
- The epidemiology of mycobacteriosis in reptiles is not well documented.
- Transmission of *Mycobacterium* spp. in reptiles is most likely through direct and indirect contact with infected animals and materials in the captive environment.
- Infected animals can shed the organisms through various body excretions (e.g., respiratory, skin, gastrointestinal), contaminating the environment and directly exposing conspecifics.
- Non-tuberculosis mycobacterial species are ubiquitous within the environment; thus, water, soil, dust, and plants can all serve as sources of exposure.
- Stress likely plays a role in the dissemination of this disease, as animals with compromised immune systems are more susceptible to infection.

SIGNALMENT/HISTORY

- No species, age, or sex predilection.
- Aquatic species more commonly affected then terrestrial species.
- Animals are typically housed under poor husbandry conditions: inappropriate environmental temperature, high organic loads, and poor water quality.

CLINICAL PRESENTATION

- Affected animals may be clinically inapparent or show clinical signs that include emaciation and weight loss with or without anorexia.
- Skin lesions may be present that are draining or nodular.
- Animals with systemic mycobacteriosis may show no apparent signs.
- Documented cases of *Mycobacterium* in snakes include, disseminated infection, pulmonary disease, biliary disease, subcutaneous, muscle, and gastrointestinal lesions.
- Fecal production and consistency may vary in animals with lesions in their gastrointestinal tract.

RISK FACTORS

Husbandry

- Inappropriate husbandry, such as a low environmental temperature, can lead to immunosuppression, making individuals more susceptible to infection.
- An absence of a quarantine program can lead to the introduction of an infected animal to a collection.
- High stocking densities in a production system may lead to an increased risk of exposure in a closed system.
- Mycobacterial infections are more common in aquatic species.
- High organic load and poor water quality likely contribute to the buildup and dissemination of the bacteria in these systems.

Others

- Stress
- Inappropriate nutrition
- Chronic disease
- Captive wild animals, wild-caught or imported animals.

DIAGNOSIS

DIFFERENTIAL DIAGNOSIS

- Any chronic disease process
- Tachypnea: pulmonary disease
- Organ dysfunction: liver failure, renal failure.
- Cholecystitis
- Salpingitis
- Malabsorptive gastrointestinal disease
- Infectious: parasitism, viral disease, other bacterial disease.
- Neoplasia

DIAGNOSTICS

Polymerase Chain Reaction

- PCR testing for *Mycobacterium* spp. does exist and is a more sensitive test than historical methodologies.
- The most common PCR primer used to diagnose *Mycobacterium* spp. in most laboratories is the 16s ribosomal RNA primer; however, a nested PCR assay targeting a 65 kDA heat shock protein (hsp65) has also been used as a diagnostic tool.
- Sensitives and specificities for these diagnostics have yet to be evaluated in reptiles. Sequencing is important to confirm the species of *Mycobacterium.*

Cytology

- Cytologic examination of skin lesions can be a useful first line diagnostic tool for diagnosing a *Mycobacterium* sp. infection. Cytology can be used to provide direct evidence of chronic inflammation in the lesions and demonstrate the presence of bacteria. Gram stain and acid-fast staining can be used to further characterize the presence of the bacteria, directing the clinician to other more sensitive diagnostics such as PCR and histopathology.
- Tissue biopsy and histopathology are considered the gold standard for diagnosing a *Mycobacterium* sp. infection.
- In addition to granulomatous lesions being present in the microscopic tissue architecture, acid-fast stains, including Ziehl–Nelsen and the Fite method, can be used to confirm the presence of acid-fast bacteria within the lesions.
- The sensitivity of these stains is considered low for *Mycobacterium* spp.

Microbiological Culture

- Microbiological culture has fallen out of favor for clinical samples because of the special media required to culture *Mycobacterium* spp. and the long culture times associated with growing these organisms.
- Speciation can be performed on cultured samples.
- Antibacterial sensitivities can also be performed on cultured *Mycobacterium* spp. if therapy is elected.

Hematology and Biochemistry

- Hematology and biochemistry testing can be used to characterize the physiologic status of the reptile patient.
- A chronic inflammatory leukogram characterized by a heterophilia and monocytosis may be observed.
- Anemia of chronic disease is also common.
- Biochemistry testing typically reveals dehydration (hyperproteinemia, hyperuricemia, hypernatremia, hyperchloremia).
- If the liver is involved, elevated bile acids may be identified.

PATHOLOGICAL FINDINGS

- Gross necropsy findings can range from a single white to gray focal lesion/nodule to multifocal to coalescing white lesions/nodules within any organ system.
- Granulomatous inflammation is the most common histopathological finding in reptile mycobacteriosis cases.
- Granulomas can range from compact nests of macrophages containing intracellular acid-fast bacilli to complex granulomas containing caseated centers.

MYCOBACTEROSIS (CONTINUED)

• Acute mycobacteriosis can have extracellular proliferation of acid-fast organisms with associated caseous necrosis and infiltrative heterophils and macrophages.

TREATMENT

APPROPRIATE HEALTH CARE

N/A

NUTRITIONAL SUPPORT

• If treatment is pursued, nutritional support should be considered.
• Mycobacteriosis in reptiles often leads to weight loss because of the negative energy balance that develops in these patients.

CLIENT EDUCATION/HUSBANDRY RECOMMENDATIONS

• Disease exposure and dissemination can be limited by quarantine and testing (PCR) new arrivals.
• Implementing husbandry practices that reduce organic loads in both aquatic and terrestrial vivariums is highly recommended.
• Regular water changes can minimize pathogen build up in a closed system.
• Husbandry recommendations should be species specific to minimize stress and the potential for compromising the immune system of a reptile.
• Clients and veterinary staff should follow standard hygiene practices to minimize zoonotic potential.

MEDICATIONS

DRUG(S) OF CHOICE

• No proven or approved treatments exist for mycobacteriosis in reptiles.
• Treatment is controversial due to the lack of clinical data on appropriate therapy, poor response to therapy, and the implications that treating reptiles may have in the increase of multidrug-resistant *Mycobacterium* spp., which may have implications for human health.
• Euthanasia should be considered to mitigate zoonotic potential and further dissemination of the organism within a collection.
• In human medicine, *Mycobacterium* infections are treated based on culture and sensitivity results, with a multidrug treatment protocol including macrolides, aminoglycosides, ethambutol, and/or rifamycins.
• Treatment is long term until there is no evidence of disease for at least 12 months.

PRECAUTIONS/INTERACTIONS

If treatment is elected, owner compliance is critical to minimize the development of multidrug resistance.

FOLLOW-UP

PATIENT MONITORING

Humane euthanasia is recommended for these cases; however, if treatment is pursued, regular examinations and blood work (hematology and biochemistry testing) should be done to evaluate the patient's quality of life and physiologic status.

EXPECTED COURSE AND PROGNOSIS

• Reptiles diagnosed with *Mycobacterium* spp. have a grave prognosis.
• The likelihood for mycobacterial transmission to other reptiles and the zoonotic potential of these organisms present a challenge.
• Therapeutic options, if pursued, are long term and are not commonly reported to be successful in reptiles.
• Animals that do not undergo therapy often develop disseminated mycobacteriosis, which includes chronic weight loss, cachexia, and emaciation.
• Because of these challenges, euthanasia is recommended.

MISCELLANEOUS

COMMENTS

N/A

ZOONOTIC POTENTIAL

• *Mycobacterium* spp. can be zoonotic
• Atypical mycobacteria are most commonly isolated from reptiles, and while not the most common forms found in humans, they are known to infect humans.
• Atypical *Mycobacterium* spp. are classified as the Runyon group IV and are characterized as antibiotic resistant.
• Preventive measures that should be followed to reduce the zoonotic potential of these organisms include minimizing direct contact with infected animals, wearing appropriate personal protective equipment (e.g., gloves, face mask) when handling infected animals, and following strict personal hygiene practices such as hand washing and not using human wash basins to clean these animals or materials from their environment.
• Immunocompromised individuals and children should avoid contact with infected animals and their environment.

SYNONYMS

• Atypical mycobacterium
• Granulomatous disease
• Vivarium granuloma

ABBREVIATIONS

PCR = polymerase chain reaction

Suggested Reading

Ebani VV, Fratini F, Bertelloni F, et al. Isolation and identification of mycobacteria from captive reptiles. *Res Vet Sci* 2012;93:1136–1138.
Jacobson ER. Bacterial diseases of reptiles. In: Jacobson ER, ed. *Infectious Diseases and Pathology of Reptiles: Color Atlas and Text.* Boca Raton, FL: CRC Press; 2007:461–526.
Mitchell MA. Mycobacterial infections in reptiles. *Vet Clin North Am Exot Anim Pract* 2012;15(1):101–111.

Authors Sean M. Perry, DVM, PhD, and Mark A. Mitchell, DVM, MS, PhD, DECZM (Herpetology)

NYCTOTHERUS

BASICS

DEFINITION/OVERVIEW

Nyctotherus is a large ciliated protozoal organism that resides within the GI tract. The trophozoite is dorsoventrally flattened like a bean and ranges in size from 60 µm to 200 µm. It has peristomal cilia that is characteristic for the organism. The cystostome (mouth) is long and curved. Cysts are brown, have a thick wall, ovoid in shape and have a polar cap. *Nyctotherus* spp. have been observed in snakes including *Platyceps karelini*.

ETIOLOGY/PATHOPHYSIOLOGY

- Transmission is through fecal–oral route.
- Cysts are ingested and then undergo excystation in the GI tract.
- Trophozoites hatch and emerge in the small intestine.
- They then migrate and manifest in the large colon and replicate by cell division.
- They feed on the chyme, bacteria, fiber, and other ingesta within the intestinal tract.
- Trophozoites undergo encystation in which infective cysts are formed and then excreted in feces.
- If in a moist environment, cysts remain infective for several weeks.
- *Nyctotherus* spp. are generally not considered pathogens.
- Animals with diarrhea have been observed to large amounts of trophozoites within fecals, but this is believed to be secondary due to the more liquid environment within the large intestine.

SIGNALMENT/HISTORY

All ages can be affected.

CLINICAL PRESENTATION

- Diarrhea, dehydration, weight loss
- Clinical signs are only likely to occur in severely immunocompromised individuals.

RISK FACTORS

Husbandry

Improper husbandry

Others

Diarrhea

DIAGNOSIS

DIFFERENTIAL DIAGNOSIS

- Oxyurid nematodiasis
- Trematodes

DIAGNOSTICS

- Microscopic evaluation of fresh fecal material to visualize trophozoites and cysts.
- SAF technique can be used for better visualization.
- Fecal samples or cysts can be placed within a petri dish with water; trophozoites will emerge from the dissolved envelope within several hours.

PATHOLOGICAL FINDINGS

- Diarrhea
- Dehydration
- Weight loss

TREATMENT

APPROPRIATE HEALTH CARE

Treatment is rarely required because they are mostly non-pathogenic.

NUTRITIONAL SUPPORT

Nutritional supplementation may be indicated if diarrhea and dehydration is severe.

CLIENT EDUCATION/HUSBANDRY RECOMMENDATIONS

- Practice proper hygiene
- House infected animals separately

MEDICATIONS

DRUG(S) OF CHOICE

Metronidazole 25 mg/kg PO q24h for 5–7 days.

PRECAUTIONS/INTERACTIONS

N/A

FOLLOW-UP

PATIENT MONITORING

- Weight gain
- Fecal samples

EXPECTED COURSE AND PROGNOSIS

Good

MISCELLANEOUS

COMMENTS

N/A

ZOONOTIC POTENTIAL

Unknown

SYNONYMS

N/A

ABBREVIATIONS

- GI = gastrointestinal
- PO = per os
- SAF = sodium acetate acetic acid formalin

INTERNET RESOURCES

- De Bosschere H, Roels S. *Balantidium* sp. and *Nyctotherus* sp: Two common members of the digestive-tract flora in Mediterranean tortoises. Tortoise Trust. https://www.tortoisetrust.org/articles/balantidium.htm
- Divers SJ. Parasitic diseases of reptiles. MSD Manual Veterinary Manual, June 2020. http://www.merckvetmanual.com/exotic-and-laboratory-animals/reptiles/parasitic-diseases-of-reptiles

Suggested Reading

Hnizdo J, Pantchev N. Protozoa (digestive tract). In: Medical Care of Turtles and Tortoises. Diagnosis. Surgery. Pathology. Parasitology. Frankfurt, Germany: Edition Chimaira; 2011: 194–195.

Jacobson ER. Parasites and parasitic diseases of reptiles. In: Jacobson ER, ed. *Infectious Diseases and Pathology of Reptiles: Color Atlas and Text.* Boca Raton, FL: CRC Press; 2007:571–665.

Author Elsburgh O. Clarke III, DVM, DACZM

OPHIDIOMYCOSIS

BASICS

DEFINITION/OVERVIEW

Ophidiomycosis is a fungal infection of mostly wild snakes in North America and of captive snakes worldwide, caused by *Ophidiomyces ophiodiicola* (formerly *Chrysosporium ophiodiicola*), an onygenalean fungus related to the Nannizziopsiaceae. The fungus has been recently identified in free-ranging snakes in Europe. It is the most common fungal disease of snakes by far, manifesting as mild to severe dermatomycosis.

ETIOLOGY/PATHOPHYSIOLOGY

- Contagious disease
- Spores/conidia on the skin invade the epidermal corneum, deeper strata and then dermis, sometimes underlying muscles and bones.
- Can rarely disseminate to liver and elsewhere internally.

SIGNALMENT/HISTORY

- Causes disease in snakes only, thus far.
- Some crotalids (massasaugas, timber and pygmy rattlesnakes, copperhead) and colubrids (corn snake, rat snakes, water snakes) seem particularly vulnerable, but all snakes are probably susceptible.
- No age or sex predilection

CLINICAL PRESENTATION

- Dermatomycosis with focal/multifocal, often extensive, necrotic lesions.
- Discolored and/or thickened scales, coalescing necrotic and/or crusty scales, ulcers.
- Most often over the head/face/rostrum, but also over the body.
- Facial features may be distorted from dermal and deeper infection.
- Some snakes, particularly rat snakes, present with scattered subcutaneous granulomas/mycetomas.
- Often significant scarring in snakes with prior or ongoing chronic infection.

RISK FACTORS

Husbandry

- Occurs in wild and captive snakes.
- Breaches in the skin may facilitate infection, but it can occur in seemingly healthy snakes in well-managed operations.
- Any inadequacies in husbandry will contribute to disease and contagion.

Others

- The fungus does not grow well at 35 degrees C (95 degrees F) or higher, as it prefers cooler temperatures.
- Heat, sunlight and successive shedding may help to clear infection in some snakes.

DIAGNOSIS

DIFFERENTIAL DIAGNOSIS

- Trauma
- Thermal injuries/burns
- Prey-inflicted skin trauma
- Bacterial dermatitides
- Abscesses, parasites, and tumors when presenting with subcutaneous mycetomas.

DIAGNOSTICS

- When present, arthroconidia on stained impression smears of skin lesions are highly suggestive.
- Both histopathology and culture of skin biopsies are essential for definitive diagnosis.
- Morphologically similar to *Nannizziopsis* and *Paranannizziopsis* spp.
- PCR on fungal isolate or on tissue sections or skin is required.

PATHOLOGICAL FINDINGS

- Epidermal/dermal hyalohyphomycosis with epidermal necrosis, heterophilic, and then mixed inflammatory cell infiltration, with or without dermal or deeper granulomas.
- PAS or silver stains may be required to identify fungal elements.
- Rarely evolves to systemic involvement.

TREATMENT

APPROPRIATE HEALTH CARE

- Review and improvement of captive husbandry.
- Supportive measures
- Topical antiseptic or antifungal
- Systemic antifungal drugs are often indicated.

NUTRITIONAL SUPPORT

- Assist-feeding if needed
- Fluids

CLIENT EDUCATION/HUSBANDRY RECOMMENDATIONS

- Isolation of sick snakes, hygiene.
- Thorough review of husbandry

SURGICAL CONSIDERATIONS

Surgical debridement of necrotic/crusty lesions is indicated to decrease fungal load.

MEDICATIONS

DRUG(S) OF CHOICE

- Often susceptible in vitro to itraconazole, terbinafine, voriconazole.
- Oral delivery in prey items if snake eats, or via stomach tube if anorectic.
- Injectable voriconazole is possibly linked with adverse reactions.
- Itraconazole and terbinafine accumulate and persist in the epidermis.
- Terbinafine nebulization and implants can be considered.

PRECAUTIONS/INTERACTIONS

- Triazole antifungal and terbinafine are possibly synergistic.
- Interactions with other drugs are possible.

FOLLOW-UP

PATIENT MONITORING

- Monitor appetite, demeanor, and skin improvement with treatment, and post-ecdysis.
- Blood work to monitor liver enzymes while on antifungals and/or immune status indicated.

EXPECTED COURSE AND PROGNOSIS

- Good if lesions mild and/or superficial and snake provided with thermal support and/or systemic antifungals. Successive sheds often result in marked improvement.
- Prognosis is reserved to poor when multiple and/or deeper lesions are present, or when more chronic.

MISCELLANEOUS

COMMENTS

N/A

ZOONOTIC POTENTIAL

None identified to date

SYNONYMS

- *Chrysosporium* anamorph of *Nannizziopsis vriesii* (all complex snake isolates deposited in fungal collections were *O. ophiodiicola* when molecular probes were used).
- Snake fungal disease.

ABBREVIATIONS

- PAS = periodic acid–Schiff
- PCR = polymerase chain reaction

Suggested Reading

Allender MC, Raudabaugh DB, Gleason FH, Miller AN. The natural history, ecology, and epidemiology of *Ophidiomyces ophiodiicola* and its potential impact on free-ranging snake populations. *Fungal Ecol* 2015;17:187–196.

Paré JA, Sigler L. An overview of reptile fungal pathogens in the genera *Nannizziopsis*, *Paranannizziopsis*, and *Ophidiomyces*. *J Herp Med Surg* 2016;26:46–53.

Sigler L, Hambleton S, Paré JA. Molecular characterization of reptile pathogens currently known as members of the *Chrysosporium* anamorph of *Nannizziopsis vriesii* complex and relationship with some human-associated isolates. *J Clin Microbiol* 2013;51:3338–3357.

Author Jean A. Paré, DMV, DVSc, DACZM, DECZM (Zoo Health Management)

OXYURIDS

BASICS

DEFINITION/OVERVIEW

Oxyurids (pinworms) have a direct life cycle and are host specific. Oxyurid infection is rare in snakes. It is considered non-pathogenic in animals without clinical signs.

ETIOLOGY/PATHOPHYSIOLOGY

- Animals are usually asymptomatic
- Parasites inhabit the lower intestinal tract.
- Severe infestations may cause secondary problems, especially in debilitated and dehydrated animals.

SIGNALMENT/HISTORY

Oxyurid ova found in snake feces often originate from prey items.

CLINICAL PRESENTATION

- Disease caused by oxyurids is usually a secondary complication due to an underlying disease.
- Anorexia
- Lethargy
- Diarrhea
- Dehydration

RISK FACTORS

Husbandry

- Inadequate husbandry may lead to stress, immunosuppression, and a myriad of secondary conditions.
- Poor hygiene, high fecal loads, and overcrowding may contribute to higher infection rates.

Others

N/A

DIAGNOSIS

DIFFERENTIAL DIAGNOSIS

- Rule out prey items as the source of oxyurid ova.
- Commensals of the rodent cecum.

DIAGNOSTICS

- Eggs vary in shape, can be ovoid, elongate, or D-shaped, and lack the thick wall of ascarid eggs.
- The eggs measure approximately 130 × 40 μm.
- Some eggs can be larvated.
- Adult worms are visible in fecal material.

PATHOLOGICAL FINDINGS

- Intestinal impaction of the intestinal tract may be observed in sick animals with severe pinworm infection.
- This is rare in snakes

TREATMENT

APPROPRIATE HEALTH CARE

Excessive numbers of these organisms in sick animals may require medical treatment.

NUTRITIONAL SUPPORT

In ill animals, nutritional support after rehydration is needed to maintain positive nitrogen balance.

CLIENT EDUCATION/HUSBANDRY RECOMMENDATIONS

- Follow proper husbandry guidelines for the species at hand.
- Environmental temperature, proper housing, and feeding regimen all play a crucial role in the wellbeing of reptilian species kept in captivity.

MEDICATIONS

DRUG(S) OF CHOICE

- Fenbendazole 25–50 mg/kg PO q24h for 5 days, 50–100 mg/kg PO q14d
- Oxfendazole 66 mg/kg PO once, may repeat in 14 days as needed.
- Pyrantel pamoate 25 mg/kg PO once a day for 3 days, repeat in 3 weeks.
- Ivermectin 0.2 mg/kg IM, SC, PO, once, then repeat in 14 days.

PRECAUTIONS/INTERACTIONS

- Avoid fenbendazole and oxfendazole in severely debilitated and dehydrated animals to minimize the risk of the potential adverse effects (bone marrow suppression, intestinal cell damage) associated with these drugs.
- Lower doses of these drugs should also be considered in species of critical conservation status if previous, safe use of these drugs is unknown.

FOLLOW-UP

PATIENT MONITORING

- Evaluate hydration frequently after starting treatment.
- Make husbandry changes to provide proper environment and nutrition.

EXPECTED COURSE AND PROGNOSIS

- Oxyurids are non-pathogenic in healthy, immunocompetent animals.
- In sick animals, treatment is aimed at decreasing the parasite load in the gut to minimize the chances of impaction.
- Prognosis is excellent to good, as long as the underlying source of illness is identified and treated effectively (husbandry mismanagement, primary disease process).

MISCELLANEOUS

COMMENTS

N/A

ZOONOTIC POTENTIAL

N/A

SYNONYMS

N/A

ABBREVIATIONS

- IM = intramuscular
- PO = per os
- SC = subcutaneous

Suggested Reading

Mader DR, ed. *Reptile Medicine and Surgery*. 2nd ed. Saint Louis, MO: Elsevier; 2006.

Rataj AV, Lindtner-Knific R, Vlahovic K, et al. Parasites in pet reptiles. *Acta Vet Scand* 2011;53(1):33.

Author Sam Rivera, DVM, MS, DABVP (Avian), DACZM, DECZM (Zoo Health Management)

PAPILLOMAVIRUS

BASICS

DEFINITION/OVERVIEW

Papillomaviruses cause mucocutaneous and cutaneous epithelial proliferative lesions in several vertebrate hosts, including reptiles.

ETIOLOGY/PATHOPHYSIOLOGY

- The members of the family Papillomaviridae are non-enveloped, icosahedral viral particles with a diameter of 50–55 nm and a small (7–8 kb), circular, double-stranded DNA.
- Recently, genomic characterization of a novel snake papillomavirus from papilloma-like lesions of an Australian diamond python (*Morelia spilota spilota*) has been described, which represents the first complete papillomavirus genome discovered in a Squamata host.
- According to phylogenetic analysis, this snake papillomavirus clusters with papillomaviruses of mammalians rather than sauropsid hosts.

SIGNALMENT/HISTORY

Among snakes, the only species in which confirmed papillomavirus infection associated with cutaneous proliferative lesions has been reported is the Australian diamond python (*Morelia spilota spilota*).

CLINICAL PRESENTATION

The only documented case of confirmed papillomavirus infection in a snake showed small black papillated and pedunculated exophytic skin proliferations.

RISK FACTORS

Husbandry

Because transmission is likely by direct contact, absence of quarantine for new admitted snakes can contribute to widespread the disease.

Others

In mammals, the presence of papillomaviral lesions may be an indication of immunosuppression.

DIAGNOSIS

DIFFERENTIAL DIAGNOSIS

Other tumor types affecting the integumentary system: histopathological study must be done to achieve an accurate diagnosis of papilloma.

DIAGNOSTICS

Although TEM can be used for detecting intranuclear aggregates of virions consistent in morphology with papillomavirus, a definitive diagnosis of papillomavirus in suspected samples must be done by PCR.

PATHOLOGICAL FINDINGS

- Gross lesions resemble papillomavirus lesions in mammals.
- Histologically, the lesions are benign in appearance and consist of epidermal hyperplasia with prominent anisocytosis and anisokaryosis of keratinocytes and severe parakeratotic hyperkeratosis.

TREATMENT

APPROPRIATE HEALTH CARE

N/A

NUTRITIONAL SUPPORT

N/A

CLIENT EDUCATION/HUSBANDRY RECOMMENDATIONS

Affected snakes should be isolated, and their cages should be cleaned and disinfected to minimize virus transmission and secondary infections.

MEDICATIONS

DRUG(S) OF CHOICE

- Surgical removal may be performed when lesions affect quality of life or normal function of the animal.
- No drug therapy has been reported in reptiles.
- Several antiviral drugs (cidofovir and imiquimod) have been effective in mammalian papillomavirus infections.

PRECAUTIONS/INTERACTIONS

N/A

FOLLOW-UP

PATIENT MONITORING

N/A

EXPECTED COURSE AND PROGNOSIS

- In most cases, the lesions in reptiles are benign and regression of lesions is expected.
- Secondary bacterial infections can be observed.

MISCELLANEOUS

COMMENTS

N/A

ZOONOTIC POTENTIAL

- Papillomaviruses are highly species-specific pathogens.
- There is no evidence for zoonosis from papillomaviruses affecting reptiles.

SYNONYMS

N/A

ABBREVIATIONS

- PCR = polymerase chain reaction
- TEM = transmission electron microscopy

Suggested Reading

Lange CE, Favrot C, Ackermann M, et al. Novel snake papillomavirus does not cluster with other non-mammalian papillomaviruses. *Virol J* 2011;8:436.

Author Jorge Orós, DVM, PhD, DECZM

PARAMYXOVIRUS

BASICS

DEFINITION/OVERVIEW

Reptilian paramyxoviruses are among the most relevant viral infectious agents of reptiles infecting mainly snakes, but also lizards and chelonians. They have been associated with outbreaks causing significant mortality. Paramyxovirus infections have been mostly reported in captive reptiles, but the presence of antibodies directed against paramyxoviruses has been reported in free-ranging individuals.

ETIOLOGY/PATHOPHYSIOLOGY

- Paramyxoviruses are enveloped, negative-stranded, RNA virus members of the family Paramyxoviridae. All the paramyxoviruses infecting reptiles are in the genus *Ferlavirus*. The first *Ferlavirus* was detected in the 70s in Switzerland. Since then it has been reported in the United States, other European countries, Brazil, and Asia.
- A recently discovered virus in Australian snakes, named *Reptile sunshinevirus 1*, originally believed to be a paramyxovirus, is now classified into a new family named *Suniviridae*.
- Within the genus *Ferlavirus* are three distinct genogroups named A, B, and C, and a separate chelonian lineage. There are no studies carried out on large numbers of individuals, although reptilian paramyxoviruses appear to be relatively common, especially in snake collections.
- Koch's postulates have been fulfilled for *Ferlavirus* in snakes. The natural route of infection is unknown; however, experimentally intratracheal inoculation of the virus is associated with the development of disease. Similar to other paramyxoviruses, inhalation of aerosolized viral particles might be a route of infection for *Ferlavirus*. Possible vertical transmission has been suggested for the Sunshine virus and vectors (mites) have been proposed for *Ferlavirus* infections.
- Infection with paramyxovirus is more likely to cause clinical disease in snakes, whereas in lizards, overt disease has been reported only in two cases.
- The respiratory system is the organ more commonly affected but CNS disease has also been reported in snakes infected with the *Ferlavirus* or *Reptile sunshinevirus 1*. The virus can also be detected in other tissues.

SIGNALMENT/HISTORY

- Reptilian paramyxoviruses have been detected in a variety of snakes including Colubridae, Elapidae, Viperidae, Crotalidae, Boidae and Pythonidae.
- *Reptile sunshinevirus 1* has been detected in *Antaresia* sp., *Aspidites* sp., and *Morelia* sp., all Australian snakes.

CLINICAL PRESENTATION

- Classic signs are not specific and may impact more commonly the respiratory and neurological systems.
- Reptiles infected with *Ferlavirus* have been reported to show brown to hemorrhagic discharge from the nostrils and/or trachea or from the oral cavity, stridor and/or respiratory noise, clear mucus in mouth, clear nasal discharge, mouth gaping, complete flaccid paralysis, decreased cutaneous sensation, head tremors, abnormal posturing/disequilibrium (i.e., opisthotonus: star gazing) or inability to right itself, anorexia, occasional regurgitation, lethargy, and sudden death.
- Occasional mucoid diarrhea or malodorous stools have also been reported.
- Neurorespiratory signs have also been reported in snakes infected with *Reptile sunshinevirus 1*, along with tracheal exudate.

RISK FACTORS

- Any type of stress-associated mismanagement, including but not limited to temperature variation, species mixing, contact with infected reptiles, may be critical in promoting the infection and eventually in priming the development of disease.
- It is not clear if a species predisposition to develop the disease following the infection does exist; however, the infection is more commonly followed by overt disease in snakes.

Husbandry

N/A

Others

N/A

DIAGNOSIS

DIFFERENTIAL DIAGNOSIS

- No pathognomonic clinical signs of paramyxovirus infection in reptiles exist.
- Nidovirus
- *Orthoreovirus* infections
- *Mycoplasma* sp. infection
- Inclusion body disease
- Mixed infections may also occur.
- Secondary bacterial and/or fungal infections have been reported in *Ferlavirus*-positive reptiles.

DIAGNOSTICS

- Molecular and serological tests are commonly performed; virus isolation is also available, but in fewer laboratories.
- Molecular tests are able to detect the presence of the viral nucleic acids into the tissues of the affected animals, whereas serological tests allow the detection of the exposure of reptiles to paramyxoviruses.
- Molecular test include RT-PCR and sequencing. They can be qualitative or quantitative in nature.
- RT-PCR can be performed on a number of tissues and can be carried out on samples collected from the live animal or from necropsied individuals.
- Intravitam samples include tracheal wash and cloacal swabs, whereas ideal postmortem samples include lung, pancreas, small intestine, and brain tissues.
- RT-PCR allows the detection of the viral RNA as early as 4 days post-infection and it can be detected at least up to 49 days post-infection.
- Viral detection can be as early as at 16 days post-infection when the tracheal wash is tested, whereas cloacal swabs allows the detection of the virus not before 28 days post-infection.
- Serological tests include hemagglutination inhibition or, more rarely, ELISA.
- The actual length of time necessary for seroconversion following paramyxovirus infection in reptiles is not known, but it is supposed to take more than 22 days and likely between 4 and 8 weeks post-infection.
- Serological tests need to be interpreted cautiously because they might provide conflicting results when antigens belonging to distinct genogroups are used.
- Molecular tests are generally more indicated during the acute stage of the disease, whereas serological tests allow the detection of the exposure to the pathogen also when viral shedding is not occurring anymore or is inconsistent, which might be the case in the subacute chronic stage of the disease or in case of asymptomatic infections.
- Molecular and serological tests are complementary in paramyxovirus diagnostics.
- Viral isolation is the most conclusive diagnostic test concerning reptile paramyxovirus infection and ideally should be carried out together with the molecular and serological tests.
- Electron microscopy is also a valuable diagnostic resource.
- Histology complemented by immunohistochemistry and/or in situ hybridization is also an important diagnostic test that may also help in clarify the etiology of the disease when the other tests would be inconclusive.

PATHOLOGICAL FINDINGS

- Gross findings can range from pneumonia with accumulation of variable amount of exudate to frank hemorrhages in hyperacute infections.
- The most significant histological change observed in reptiles infected with paramyxovirus is the occurrence of proliferative interstitial pneumonia.
- Although these lesions are not pathognomonic, they are very characteristic.

PARAMYXOVIRUS (CONTINUED)

- The presence of intracytoplasmic eosinophilic inclusions is also an important finding, but they are not always detectable in the infected tissues.
- Syncytial cells can be detected in the lungs.
- Inclusions have also been reported in liver and pancreas, along with pancreatitis and necrosis.
- Neurological disease has been associated with perivascular cuffing, demyelination, axonal degeneration and multifocal gliosis.
- In Australian snakes infected with *Reptile sunshinevirus 1*, gross findings might not be present.
- Histologically, spongiosis of the white matter of the hindbrain has been reported.
- More recently, multisystemic necrotizing inflammation with most severe lesions in the kidney (pan-nephritis) was reported in snakes.

TREATMENT

APPROPRIATE HEALTH CARE

N/A

NUTRITIONAL SUPPORT

Supportive feeding in case of prolonged anorexia is suggested.

CLIENT EDUCATION/HUSBANDRY RECOMMENDATIONS

- It is highly recommended to quarantine for not less than 2–3 months. Longer periods (6 months) have been proposed.
- Repeated molecular and serological testing is highly recommended during the quarantine period.
- Avoiding species mixing and overcrowding, along with separating animals showing abnormal behavior is also important.
- Paramyxoviruses can cross species and, consequently, it is critical to avoid mixing of susceptible taxa (snakes, lizards and chelonians) or handling different individuals without having first changes disposable gloves or disinfected hands.
- Avoiding introducing individuals from collections that experienced paramyxovirus outbreaks or of questionable source is critical.
- The virus has an envelope and consequently is not supposed to survive for long in the environment; however, it is of paramount importance to clean and disinfect terraria regularly and replace bedding and water frequently.
- Disinfection of gear, footwear, and potential fomites is also important.

MEDICATIONS

DRUG(S) OF CHOICE

- No specific therapy is available for reptiles infected with reptilian paramyxoviruses.
- Supportive care consistent in fluid administration together with antibiotics has been proposed.
- Treatment of secondary bacterial and protozoal infection has been reported to improve the survival time of the infected animals.
- Experimental vaccination protocols have been attempted in the past but no current vaccines are available for the prevention of paramyxovirus infections in reptiles.

PRECAUTIONS/INTERACTIONS

N/A

EXPECTED COURSE AND PROGNOSIS

- Some experimentally infected snakes might overcome the disease.
- Fatal outcome is common among snakes.

FOLLOW-UP

PATIENT MONITORING

- Molecular testing should be regularly carried out during the supportive therapy to assess the reduction and, ideally, the resolution of the viral shedding.
- Testing should also be performed on animals that eventually recovered from the disease to determine if they still shed virus (RT-PCR) and to monitor their antibody titer (serology).
- Diseased and molecular/serologically positive reptiles should be separated from the rest of the collection and undergo long-term monitoring.

MISCELLANEOUS

COMMENTS

N/A

ZOONOTIC POTENTIAL

There is no evidence zoonotic potential of *Ferlavirus* or any other reptilian paramyxoviruses currently.

SYNONYMS

Previously, the paramyxoviruses infecting reptiles were also indicated as "ophidian paramyxoviruses". This term is not currently used and has been replaced by the term *Ferlavirus* or by the broader "reptilian paramyxoviruses."

ABBREVIATIONS

- ELISA = enzyme-linked immunosorbent assay
- PCR = polymerase chain reaction
- RT-PCR = reverse transcription polymerase chain reaction

Suggested Reading

Hyndman TH, Shilton CM, Marschang RE. Paramyxoviruses in reptiles: A review. *Vet Microbiol* 2013;165:200–213.

Jacobson ER. Viruses and viral diseases of reptiles. In: Jacobson ER, ed. *Infectious Diseases and Pathology of Reptiles: Color Atlas and Text*. Boca Raton, FL: CRC Press; 2007:395–460.

Author Francesco C. Origgi, DVM, PhD, DACVM (Virology), DACVP, DECZM (Herpetology)

PARANANNIZZIOPSIS MYCOSES

BASICS

DEFINITION/OVERVIEW

Parananannizziopsis mycoses is an infection caused by any of five fungal species in the genus *Paranannizziopsis*. It is an important disease of captive tentacled snakes, and of tuataras in New Zealand.

ETIOLOGY/PATHOPHYSIOLOGY

- *Paranannizziopsis crustacea*, *P. californiensis*, *P. longispora*, and *P. tardicrescens* cause severe dermatitis in captive tentacled snakes, with focal to extensive epidermal necrosis and sloughing.
- *P. australasiensis* causes fungal skin disease in captive tuataras and may be linked with multifocal punctate dermatomycosis in acrochordid snakes.
- *P. tardicrescens* has caused dermatitis in captive tentacled snakes, but also in captive arboreal snakes housed in proximity to infected tentacled snakes.

SIGNALMENT/HISTORY

- *P. crustacea*, *P. californiensis*, and *P. longispora* are only known to infect captive tentacled snakes.
- No age or sex predilection is reported.
- It is contagious and often affects all snakes in a captive setting.
- Case fatality rate is high
- *P. tardicrescens* has also infected rhinoceros snakes and Wagler's pit vipers.
- *P. australasiensis* can infect acrochordid snakes, tuataras, coastal bearded dragons, and probably other lizards but, up until recently, was only reported from Australia and New Zealand.

CLINICAL PRESENTATION

- Very typical in tentacled snakes.
- Sick snakes present with swollen, discolored, edematous to necrotic epidermis that sloughs off the body.
- In acrochordid snakes and arboreal snakes, punctate, raised, white lesions are seen.
- In tuataras, dermatitis with raised, yellow to brown crusts can progress to necrosis and ulcers. Similar disease was seen in one coastal bearded dragon housed near diseased tuataras.

RISK FACTORS

Husbandry

- Substandard husbandry
- Inadequate water parameters, especially pH, may predispose tentacled snakes to infection.
- Housing of arboreal or terrestrial snake species in proximity to infected tentacled snakes probably underlies infection in these non-aquatic species.

Others

N/A

DIAGNOSIS

DIFFERENTIAL DIAGNOSIS

- Fairly characteristic presentation in tentacled snakes.
- Caustic, thermal, bacterial, viral, or even parasitic dermatitides or dermatoses should be ruled out.

DIAGNOSTICS

- Presentation in tentacled snakes is highly suggestive of infection with *P. crustacea*, *P. californiensis*, and *P. longispora*.
- Arthroconidia may be seen on stained impression smears of lesions.
- Culture of clinical samples (crusts, sloughed skin or shed skin, lesion biopsies) is required, and PCR is necessary to identify *Paranannizziopsis* isolates to genus and species.
- Histopathology should always be performed to support causality.

PATHOLOGICAL FINDINGS

Hyphae or other fungal elements within inflamed and/or necrotic epidermis and in the underlying dermis.

TREATMENT

APPROPRIATE HEALTH CARE

- Correct perceived husbandry deficiencies
- Assess water quality parameters, especially pH.
- Fluids, antibiotics, thermal and nutritional support as needed.
- *P. crustacea* is susceptible in vitro to itraconazole, voriconazole, and terbinafine.

NUTRITIONAL SUPPORT

Assist-feeding if needed

CLIENT EDUCATION/HUSBANDRY RECOMMENDATIONS

- Quarantine of incoming animals
- Thorough and meticulous review of captive husbandry.
- Close monitoring of water quality parameters.

SURGICAL CONSIDERATIONS

Debulking of lesions and/or sloughed skin, when possible.

MEDICATIONS

DRUG(S) OF CHOICE

Wide-spectrum antifungals (itraconazole, voriconazole, terbinafine) are indicated pending culture and sensitivity results.

PRECAUTIONS/INTERACTIONS

- Triazole antifungal and terbinafine are possibly synergistic.
- Interactions with other drugs possible.

FOLLOW-UP

PATIENT MONITORING

- Monitor appetite, demeanor, and skin improvement with treatment.
- Blood work to monitor liver enzymes and other parameters while on antifungals.

EXPECTED COURSE AND PROGNOSIS

- Often diagnosed late in the course of disease.
- Progression of lesions may be rapid, and disease may spread.
- Systemic antifungals and water pH adjustments may result in improvement in tentacled snakes.
- Outcome is often fatal

MISCELLANEOUS

COMMENTS

The most important infectious disease of tentacled snakes.

ZOONOTIC POTENTIAL

None identified to date

SYNONYMS

Used to be referred to as *Chrysosporium* anamorph of *Nannizziopsis vriesii* (CANV) complex before reassignment based on molecular studies to the genus *Paranannizziopsis*.

ABBREVIATIONS

PCR = polymerase chain reaction

Suggested Reading

Bertelsen MF, Crawshaw GJ, Sigler L, Smith DA. Fatal cutaneous mycosis in tentacled snakes (*Erpeton tentaculatum*) caused by the *Chrysosporium* anamorph of *Nannizziopsis vriesii*. *J Zoo Wildl Med* 2005;36:82–87.

Paré JA, Sigler L. An overview of reptile fungal pathogens in the genera *Nannizziopsis*, *Paranannizziopsis*, and *Ophidiomyces*. *J Herp Med Surg* 2016;26:46–53.

Sigler L, Hambleton S, Paré JA. Molecular characterization of reptile pathogens currently known as members of the *Chrysosporium* anamorph of *Nannizziopsis vriesii* complex and relationship with some human-associated isolates. *J Clin Microbiol* 2013;51:3338–3357.

Author Jean A. Paré, DMV, DVSc, DACZM, DECZM (Zoo Health Management)

PENTASTOMIDS

BASICS

DEFINITION/OVERVIEW

Pentastomids are crustacean endoparasites of the respiratory system of snakes. Approximately 90% of pentastomids use carnivorous reptiles as their definitive hosts, with 70% being found in snakes. Pentastomiasis occurs on all continents except Antarctica.

ETIOLOGY/PATHOPHYSIOLOGY

- Adult pentastomids live in the lungs or air sacs of snakes, where they breed and feed.
- Females are larger and longer lived than males.
- Copulation takes place 3–4 months after infection of the definitive host.
- Approximately 4–8 months later, fertilized females begin to deposit millions of embryonated eggs into the environment.
- Eggs are coughed up from the lungs or ingested and passed in feces.
- Intermediate hosts, such as insects, fish, anurans, squamates, birds, or mammals (especially rodents), ingest pentastomid eggs, which hatch, and go through two instars (growth periods between molts), before becoming encysted somewhere in the intermediate host's body.
- When the intermediate host is eaten by the definitive host, third-stage larvae emerge from the cyst and migrate to the host's lungs, where they feed on blood through the lung wall (hematophagous).
- Pentastomids damage the lungs which may lead to secondary bacterial or fungal colonization, pneumonia, septicemia, pericarditis, or death.
- Heavy infestations can occlude the lungs or trachea.
- Numerous pentastomid genera parasitize snakes, including *Kiricephalus*, *Porocephalus*, *Armillifer*, *Raillietiella*, *Waddycephalus*, *Cubirea*, *Gigliolella*, *Parasambonia*, and *Cephalobaena* spp.

SIGNALMENT/HISTORY

Wild-caught large tropical to subtropical viperids, crotalids, elapids, boids, and colubrids, especially African and Australasian species.

CLINICAL PRESENTATION

- Can be subclinical or have subcutaneous swellings, respiratory tract disease, pneumonia, dyspnea, weight loss, or poor growth.
- One Australian study found almost 60% of 81 road-killed snakes, 7/10 species, to be infected with at least one pentastomid species.

RISK FACTORS

Wild-caught snakes

Husbandry

Yet another compelling reason for quarantine and fecal examinations.

Others

N/A

DIAGNOSIS

- Detection of pentastomid eggs on fecal flotation, lung or colonic washes, or tracheal discharge.
- Adult pentastomids are sometimes visible on radiography, or by pulmonoscopy or ultrasound.
- Adults may also be found during exploratory surgery, necropsy, or histopathology.

DIFFERENTIAL DIAGNOSIS

- Respiratory signs may also be caused by other parasites, viruses, bacterial, fungi, neoplasia, trauma, or foreign bodies.
- In tissue sections, pentastomes can be mistaken for parasitic metazoan, especially cysticerci, spargana, nematodes, and fly larvae.

DIAGNOSTICS

- Fecal examination revealing thin-walled, sometimes double-walled, large (up to 130 μm in diameter), distinct ova, containing larvae with four claw-like hooklets.
- A complete blood count may reveal anemia or eosinophilia.

PATHOLOGICAL FINDINGS

- Pentastomids are medium to large (0.25–15 cm), superficially segmented, wormlike parasites, with two compound pairs of hooks surrounding the mouth.
- Adults may be recovered from the mouth, trachea, lungs, and air sacs, while encysted instars may be found throughout the body.
- In tissues, pentastomids are identified histologically by the presence of acidophilic glands adjacent to the intestine, and black sclerotized openings in the body wall.
- Inflammatory response in the lung may be mild with pentastomids because all life stages secrete surfactant very similar to host surfactant, which is thought to help them evade the host's immune system.
- Degrading molted pentastomid cuticles shed into the lung lumen may induce putrid pneumonia.
- Feed attachment sites on the lung surface can cause multiple crateriform ulcers.
- Pentastomids can be identified by morphological and molecular techniques.

TREATMENT

APPROPRIATE HEALTH CARE

- Stabilize patient first with antibiotics, fluids and nutritional support, if indicated.
- If medical therapy fails consider transcutaneous pulmonary laparoscopic removal.

NUTRITIONAL SUPPORT

Emeraid™ Sustain Carnivore (EmerAid, LLC, Cornell, IL), or Oxbow Critical Care Carnivore® (Oxbow Animal Health, Omaha, NE) via stomach tube only if indicated.

CLIENT EDUCATION/HUSBANDRY RECOMMENDATIONS

- Pentastomids are zoonotic, although typically through eating raw snakes.
- Wash hands after handling snakes or wear gloves.

MEDICATIONS

DRUG(S) OF CHOICE

Four Boelen's pythons (*Morelia boeleni*) stopped shedding pentastomid ova and adult parasites could no longer be visualized radiographically in the lungs after treatment with fenbendazole (100 mg/kg) and ivermectin (0.2 mg/kg) PO once a day for 3 days.

PRECAUTIONS/INTERACTIONS

Living pentastomids secrete surfactant that helps them evade the host's immune system but on their death in tissue or lungs, a severe antigenic release, or putrefaction, with serious and potential lethal complications can occur.

FOLLOW-UP

PATIENT MONITORING

Monitor fecals post-treatment to determine therapeutic effectiveness.

EXPECTED COURSE AND PROGNOSIS

- Highly variable depending on parasitic burden (one road-killed lesser black whipsnake, *Demansia vestigiata*, had 77 *Raillietiella orientalis* present in its lungs, the largest up to 6.5 cm long), chronicity, condition of patient, and therapeutic options.
- Medical therapy alone may not eliminate infection.

MISCELLANEOUS

COMMENTS

N/A

ZOONOTIC POTENTIAL

• In intermediate hosts, pentastome larvae often hatch and bore through the stomach wall and encyst in nearby mesentery, peritoneum, and viscera.
• Species infecting humans belong to the families Linguatulidae, Armilliferidae, Porocephalidae, and Raillietiellidae, and have different geographic distributions.
• More than 90% of human cases are caused by two species, *Armillifer armillatus* (most prevalent in West and Central Africa and Malaysia, where raw snakes are eaten; 40–45% prevalence rate in humans) and *Linguatula serrata*, which uses dogs as definitive host, and spreads by fecal–oral contamination (most prevalent in the Middle East, with sporadic cases in Central and South America).
• *Porocephalus taiwana* infects humans in China.
• *Sebekia* spp. can cause a parasitic dermatitis in humans.
• All pentastomids should be considered potentially zoonotic.

SYNONYMS

• Colloquial human disease called golf caddy's disease (Democratic Republic of the Congo), halzoun (Middle East), and marrara (Sudan, Southwest Asia).
• Pentastomiasis
• Tongue worms

ABBREVIATIONS

PO = per os

Suggested Reading

Greiner EC, Mader DR. Parasitology. In Reptile Medicine and Surgery, 2nd ed. Mader DR, ed. Elsevier Saunders: St. Louis, MO; 2006:360–363.

Jacobson ER. Parasites and parasitic diseases of reptiles. In: Jacobson ER, ed. *Infectious Disease and Pathology of Reptiles*. Boca Raton, FL: CRC Press; 2007:571–665.

Kelehear C, Spratt DM, O'Meally D, Shine, R. Pentastomids of wild snakes in the Australian tropics. *Int J Parasitol Parasites Wildl* 2014;3:20–31.

Pare JA. An overview of pentastomiasis in reptiles and other vertebrates. *J Exot Pet Med* 2008;17:285–294.

Stahl SJ, Hernandez-Divers SJ, Cooper TL, Blas-Machado U. Evaluation of transcutaneous pulmonoscopy for examination and biopsy of the lungs of ball pythons and determination of preferred biopsy specimen handling and fixation procedures. *J Am Vet Med Assoc* 2008;233(3):440–445.

Author Thomas H. Boyer, DVM, DABVP (Reptile and Amphibian Practice)

PHAEOHYPHOMYCOSES

BASICS

DEFINITION/OVERVIEW

Phaeohyphomycosis refers to any infection with dematiaceous (pigmented) fungi: *Exophiala*, *Cladosporium*, *Ochroconis*, *Ulocladium*, *Trichoderma*, and many others. The cell walls of these fungi contain variable amounts of melanin, and hyphae are therefore easily seen on routine H&E histological sections. They are relatively uncommon in reptiles.

ETIOLOGY/PATHOPHYSIOLOGY

- All dematiaceous fungi are environmental, often found in soil and/or water; they usually infect cutaneous wounds, or less often infect sick or debilitated animals.
- These opportunistic pathogens typically cause deep granulomatous infections of the feet, especially in tortoises, and rarely disseminate.
- Exophiala species have been isolated with some regularity from reptiles with phaeohyphomycosis.

SIGNALMENT/HISTORY

Any reptile, any age, or sex.

CLINICAL PRESENTATION

- Swellings, nodules, wounds, often on the feet or ventrum (body parts in contact with soil).
- Slow progression
- Tends to not disseminate

RISK FACTORS

Husbandry

- Substandard or otherwise deficient husbandry.
- Soil substrate
- Poor water quality

Others

Open wounds or other cutaneous breaches may facilitate invasion by these opportunistic fungi.

DIAGNOSIS

DIFFERENTIAL DIAGNOSIS

- Other fungal infections
- Mycobacteriosis
- Abscesses
- Neoplasia

DIAGNOSTICS

- Biopsy and histopathology
- Culture of biopsy tissue or PCR.
- Pigmented fungi associated with inflammation/necrosis in histological section, and morphology of fungi in tissues consistent with morphology of putative isolate cultured from biopsy.

PATHOLOGICAL FINDINGS

Pigmented hyphae or other fungal elements within inflamed and/or necrotic tissue or within granulomas, consistent in morphology (e.g., pigmentation, diameter, septation, branching) to those of fungal isolates from the lesion.

TREATMENT

APPROPRIATE HEALTH CARE

- Fluids, antibiotic coverage, thermal and nutritional support.
- Correct perceived husbandry deficiencies
- Debulking of lesions, when possible.
- Amputation may be indicated when lesion located on/in feet.

NUTRITIONAL SUPPORT

Assist-feeding if needed

CLIENT EDUCATION/HUSBANDRY RECOMMENDATIONS

- Quarantine of incoming animals
- Thorough and meticulous captive husbandry.

MEDICATIONS

DRUG(S) OF CHOICE

- Ideally based on fungal identification and known susceptibility of the causative fungus to the various antifungal drugs.
- In vitro assays might be available.
- Many, if not most, pigmented fungi display resistance to triazoles and allylamines.

PRECAUTIONS/INTERACTIONS

N/A

FOLLOW-UP

PATIENT MONITORING

- Monitor appetite, demeanor, and skin improvement with treatment.
- Blood work to monitor liver enzymes and other parameters while on antifungals.
- Assessment of immune status is indicated.

EXPECTED COURSE AND PROGNOSIS

- Often diagnosed late in the course of disease, when lesions are chronic and/or extensive.
- Prognosis is usually guarded, but may vary depending on duration, severity, and extent of lesions, and on the sensitivity pattern of the offending fungus.

MISCELLANEOUS

COMMENTS

N/A

ZOONOTIC POTENTIAL

- Minimal
- Some pigmented fungi can cause local infections and onychomycosis in humans, and rarely fungemia and disseminated disease.

SYNONYMS

N/A

ABBREVIATIONS

H&E = hematoxylin and eosin

Suggested Reading

Paré JA, Jacobson ER. Mycotic diseases of reptiles. In: Jacobson ER, ed. *Infectious Disease and Pathology of Reptiles, Color Atlas and Text*. Boca Raton, FL: CRC Press; 2007:527–570.

Author Jean A. Paré, DMV, DVSc, DACZM, DECZM (Zoo Health Management)

REGURGITATION

BASICS

DEFINITION/OVERVIEW

Regurgitation is passive discharge through the mouth of undigested food or other contents within a short time after eating.

ETIOLOGY/PATHOPHYSIOLOGY

- Regurgitation usually originates as an esophageal or pharyngeal problem.
- May be gastric if gastroesophageal sphincter is incompetent or stomach is markedly diseased.

SIGNALMENT/HISTORY

- All species, ages, sexes may be affected.
- Owner may report observing regurgitation or only that regurgitated material was found.
- Lethargy, anorexia, weight loss, respiratory distress, or increased basking frequency.
- Ingestion of foreign material
- Neurologic signs (e.g., tremors, disorientation)

CLINICAL PRESENTATION

- No clinical signs are specific to regurgitation, and physical exam may be normal.
- Presentation varies depending on the underlying cause and chronicity.
- Dehydration and/or emaciation/cachexia.
- Hard mass on palpation of the coelomic cavity due to an obstructive lesion or organomegaly.
- Skeletal abnormalities that may include pathological fractures or abnormal growth patterns.
- Lethargy and/or obtunded mentation.
- Ulceration and accumulation of caseous material in the oral cavity.
- Secondary respiratory disease (e.g., oral/nasal discharge, abnormal respiratory sounds) or enteritis (e.g., diarrhea).
- In boids, loss of righting reflex, tremors, and disorientation may occur with suspected IBD.

RISK FACTORS

Husbandry

- Too much disturbance or lack of hiding places (increases stress/anxiety).
- Poor sanitation, overcrowding, hyper- or hypothermia, lack of quarantine for new individuals (increases stress, possibility of secondary infections, and disease transmission).
- Toxin exposure (cleaning chemicals, pesticides, heavy metals).
- Excessive/inappropriate handling (especially soon after feeding).
- Inadequate diet (incorrect calcium/phosphorus ratio, improper prey items, excessive feeding).
- Inappropriate substrate (may be accidentally or inappropriately ingested).

Others

- Concomitant infectious or parasitic disease.
- Snake mites (*Ophionyssus natricis*) are a potential vector for IBD.

DIAGNOSIS

DIFFERENTIAL DIAGNOSIS

- Stomatitis
- Esophagitis
- Esophageal stricture
- Gastritis
- Handling/stress (e.g., excessive pressure to coelom)
- Obstructive lesions (e.g., GI foreign body, intussusception, neoplasia, abscess, granuloma).
- Metabolic disease (e.g., nutritional secondary hyperparathyroidism, renal or hepatic dysfunction).
- Toxicoses (e.g., zinc)
- Iatrogenic (e.g., miticides, xylazine, levamisole)
- Trauma to esophagus or stomach.
- Parasites (e.g., *Cryptosporidium*, amoebiasis, ascaridiasis, cestodiasis)
- Viruses (e.g., IBD in boids)
- Bacteria/septicemia (e.g., *Chlamydophila*)
- Congenital GI defects

DIAGNOSTICS

- Husbandry review
- Physical examination
- Complete blood count and plasma biochemistries.
- Radiography with or without contrast.
- Ultrasound
- Fecal parasite exam
- Bacterial cultures from oral lesions.
- GI endoscopy or coeliotomy (direct tissue evaluation and biopsy).

Suspected Cryptosporidiosis

- Acid-fast staining and/or IFA of feces, regurgitated material, or gastric wash (best collected 3 days after feeding); PCR of feces, regurgitated material, gastric wash, or biopsy from affected tissues (e.g., stomach).
- In boids with suspected IBD: buffy coat evaluation for cytoplasmic inclusion bodies; PCR of whole blood or biopsy from affected tissues (e.g., liver, stomach, esophageal tonsils).
- Histopathology of biopsy from affected tissues.

PATHOLOGICAL FINDINGS

- Dependent on underlying cause
- In cryptosporidiosis, no gross pathology may be present, especially in chronic, subclinical cases. In clinical cases, there usually is gastromegaly due to mucosal edema and thickening, excessive mucus production, and reduction of the luminal diameter. Enlargement of gastric rugae, mucosal petechiae, and focal necrosis may also be present.
- For IBD, the lack of inclusion bodies does not rule out infection.

TREATMENT

APPROPRIATE HEALTH CARE

The primary goal is to identify and address the underlying cause.

NUTRITIONAL SUPPORT

- Correct fluid deficits and maintain hydration.
- Intracoelomic, subcutaneous, or intravenous routes for administration of a reptile Ringer's solution are most effective. Maintenance rate is 10–30 ml/kg/day.
- Tube or assist-feeding liquid or gel diets, e.g., Hill's® Prescription Diet® a/d® (Hills Pet Nutrition, Inc., Topeka, KS); Mazuri® Amphibian & Carnivorous Reptile Gel (Mazuri Exotic Animal Nutrition, St. Louis, MO); Oxbow Critical Care Carnivore® (Oxbow Animal Health, Omaha, NE) may be beneficial during initial treatment/recovery.
- Gradually add normal prey items to diet as animal improves.

CLIENT EDUCATION/HUSBANDRY RECOMMENDATIONS

- Review husbandry and correct any problems.
- Avoid overfeeding and disturbing snakes 1–2 days after feeding.
- Institute quarantine procedures for new animals, including 30–60-day period, veterinary evaluation, and 1–3-weekly fecal exams for parasites.
- Animals affected by IBD or cryptosporidiosis should be isolated from all other reptiles.

MEDICATIONS

DRUG(S) OF CHOICE

- Cimetidine 4 mg/kg IM, PO q8–12h, or famotidine 0.25–0.5 mg/kg SC, PO q24–72h
- Metoclopramide 0.06 mg/kg PO q24h for 7 days, or cisapride 0.5–2 mg/kg PO q24h
- Sucralfate 500–1000 mg/kg PO q6–8h

PRECAUTIONS/INTERACTIONS

N/A

FOLLOW-UP

PATIENT MONITORING

Monitor for continued signs of regurgitation and possible complications.

REGURGITATION (CONTINUED)

EXPECTED COURSE AND PROGNOSIS

- Dependent on underlying cause
- Prognosis for IBD is poor, as there is no treatment.
- Prognosis for subclinical cryptosporidiosis is fair to good.
- Prognosis for clinical disease is poor to grave, and euthanasia is often indicated.

MISCELLANEOUS

COMMENTS

N/A

ZOONOTIC POTENTIAL

N/A

SYNONYMS

Reflux

ABBREVIATIONS

- GI = gastrointestinal
- IBD = inclusion body disease
- IFA = immunofluorescence antibody assay
- IM = intramuscular
- PCR = polymerase chain reaction
- PO = per os
- SC = subcutaneous

Suggested Reading

Cranfield MR, Graczyk TK. Cryptosporidiosis. In: Mader DR, ed. *Reptile Medicine and Surgery*. 2nd ed. St. Louis: Elsevier Saunders, 2006: 756–762.

Mitchell MA, Diaz-Figueroa O. Clinical reptile gastroenterology. *Vet Clin N Am Exot Anim Pract* 2005;8:277–298.

Schumacher, J. Inclusion body disease virus. In: Mader DR, ed. *Reptile Medicine and Surgery*. 2nd ed. St. Louis: Elsevier Saunders, 2006: 836–840.

Authors Tamara Kruse, DVM, MS, and Trevor T. Zachariah, DVM, MS, DACZM

SALMONELLOSIS

BASICS

DEFINITION/OVERVIEW

Salmonellosis is a cosmopolitan disease; it is an important reptile zoonosis. While much of the focus on reptile-associated salmonellosis has been on chelonians and lizards because of pet popularity, snakes can also serve as latent carriers or reservoirs and should be considered to harbor this pathogen in their indigenous microflora. Of the three major groups of reptiles, snakes are the most likely to present with salmonellosis. Affected animals can develop systemic disease, including vertebral osteomyelitis. Feeder rodents being fed to snakes can also serve as a source of *Salmonella* spp. to pet owners and captive snakes, so care should be taken when handling frozen/thawed mice and rats.

ETIOLOGY/PATHOPHYSIOLOGY

- Anaerobic, Gram-negative, straight rods, flagellated.
- Species: *Salmonella enterica* and *S. bongori*, subsp. *S. enterica* [1], *S. salamae* [II], *S. arizonae* [IIIa], *S. diarizonae* [IIIb], *S. houtenae* [IV], and *S. indica* [VI].
- Reptile patients often are infected with *S. arizonae* [IIIa] and *S. diarizonae* [IIIb].
- There are over 2,637 extant serovars of *Salmonella*. These organisms are characterized by the phenotype of their O (somatic) and H (flagellar) antigens. All serotypes should be considered pathogenic.
- The prevalence of *Salmonella* spp. in wild and captive snakes can be highly variable. Captive-raised animals have a higher prevalence because stocking densities lead to increased exposure, poor hygiene practices, and positive food sources. The low prevalence reported in wild snakes may be associated with the sampling method; single samples are typically collected for prevalence studies and may misclassify animals due to intermittent shedding.
- The epidemiology of *Salmonella* infection in snakes is not as well understood as in chelonians and lizards, but is expected to be similar, with both vertical and horizontal routes of transmission possible.

SIGNALMENT/HISTORY

Because many of the cases of snake-associated salmonellosis are from latent carriers, all animals should be considered *Salmonella* spp. positive.

CLINICAL PRESENTATION

- Of the three major groups of reptiles outlined here, snakes are the most likely group of reptiles to present with salmonellosis.
- Snakes presenting with primary salmonellosis may present with lethargy, anorexia, hyporexia, and diarrhea.
- Because *Salmonella* spp. can enter systemic circulation by ascending through the bile duct system, multisystemic disease, such as abscesses and osteomyelitis, can develop.
- Affected animals may have abnormal locomotion or palpable firm masses in the spine.

RISK FACTORS

Husbandry

- Inappropriate husbandry conditions can potentiate the likelihood of infection for conspecifics and the human caretakers of snakes.
- Environmental temperatures should be appropriate for the species, as low or high temperatures can lead to stress and the potential for increased shedding of the organism.
- In aquatic snake habitats, water should be changed regularly, as high organic loads can increase the potential growth of *Salmonella* spp.
- For terrestrial or arboreal snakes, substrate should also be replaced regularly to minimize organic buildup.
- Animal density and mixing of snakes can increase stress levels and *Salmonella* spp. shedding.
- Routine cleaning and disinfection of the enclosure is necessary to prevent dissemination of *Salmonella* spp.

Others

- Source of animals: confiscated or imported animals have an increased risk associated with clinical illness and zoonotic potential because of the increased likelihood of shedding *Salmonella* spp.
- Stress: shipping, overcrowding, and suboptimal husbandry conditions can lead to infection or increased shedding of *Salmonella* spp.

DIAGNOSIS

DIFFERENTIAL DIAGNOSIS

- Enteritis (other species of Enterobacteriaceae)
- Renal disease
- Liver disease
- Primary and secondary bacterial infections.
- Fungal infections
- Neoplasia
- Spondylosis
- Osteomyelitis (non-*Salmonella* spp.)

DIAGNOSTICS

- Microbiological culture of a gastrointestinal sample or abscess can be used to confirm the presence of *Salmonella* spp.
- Positive fecal cultures in clinically normal animals are not uncommon. These animals should not be treated for *Salmonella* spp., as this can lead to the development of antimicrobial resistance in the *Salmonella* spp.
- Culture of *Salmonella* spp. requires special consideration, as the organism can be outcompeted by other Enterobacteriaceae under standard culture methods. Thus, it is important to specifically request a *Salmonella* spp. culture from the diagnostic laboratory if the organism is suspected. Enrichment with selenite or tetrathionate is required. Samples are then plated on to specific agars such as XLD, Salmonella–Shigella, or XLT-4. XLD and XLT-4 agars have a hydrogen sulfide indicator system to detect lactose fermenting *Salmonella* spp.
- Factors that influence the reliability of culture include the collection method, quantity and/or type of sample collected, temporal variation in shedding, and culture methods. Time to perform culture can delay appropriate antimicrobial therapy and control/mitigation procedures.
- PCR testing can be used to confirm the presence of *Salmonella* spp. in a sample. This test is considered more sensitive than culture and provides faster turnaround times. One limitation of PCR is that it cannot provide an antibiotic sensitivity profile to guide treatment.
- Parallel testing with PCR and culture is recommended to increase the sensitivity of the testing methods.
- Complete blood counts can be used to confirm an inflammatory leukogram or toxic changes that might occur with salmonellosis.
- Radiography can be used to examine the coelomic cavity for organomegaly and bony structures for osteomyelitis.
- Ultrasound can be used to improve visualization of the coelomic organs.
- Fine-needle aspiration of coelomic fluid or osteomyelitis and cytologic review of the sample can be used to confirm the presence of Gram-negative bacteria and inflammatory cells.

PATHOLOGICAL FINDINGS

- *Salmonella* spp.is commonly isolated from the GI tract of snakes on postmortem examinations as an incidental finding.
- Snakes that have clinical salmonellosis will have typical inflammatory signs associated with the pathogen causing an enteritis, osteomyelitis, or systemic infection.

TREATMENT

APPROPRIATE HEALTH CARE

- Snakes that are clinically normal and not showing signs of disease should never be treated for *Salmonella* infection.

SALMONELLOSIS (CONTINUED)

- Treating animals that are latent carriers could potentiate antimicrobial resistance.
- Animals that are clinically affected by *Salmonella* should only be treated if an antibiotic sensitivity profile is available. This will help to minimize the likelihood of resistance.
- Some clinicians elect to not treat affected animals with antibiotics but instead provide supportive care and allow the infection to run its course.
- As with any bacterial disease, therapy should be driven by culture and sensitivity testing in addition to MIC, target plasma concentration, and volume of distribution of the medication.

NUTRITIONAL SUPPORT

- Nutritional support should be implemented in patients that have concurrent weight loss, hyporexia, or anorexia.
- Fluid support should be provided first to ensure that the GI tract is functioning properly.
- In animals with diarrhea, nutritional support can exacerbate the diarrhea.
- Assist-feeding can support the daily nutritional requirements of these patients with a highly digestible diet, which should be based on the species life history and nutritional requirements of the species.

CLIENT EDUCATION/HUSBANDRY RECOMMENDATIONS

- Clients should be educated on the risks of keeping snakes and provided information on the most appropriate husbandry and sanitation procedures.
- Owners should be made aware that it is not recommended to allow their snake to free roam in their household. This can serve as a source of indirect exposure for children.
- To minimize the zoonotic potential of snakes, it is important to practice strict hygiene and biosecurity.
- Hand washing with soap and warm water is one of the simplest and most effective methods of eliminating exposure to *Salmonella* spp.
- Individuals handling these animals or any part of their captive habitat should wash their hands thoroughly after working with them.
- The water removed from the enclosures of these animals should be discarded outside or down a toilet. It should never be discarded down a sink used for cooking or cleaning food or where water is obtained for drinking or a bathtub.
- The enclosure and its contents should be cleaned outside, if at all possible, and never in an area where food or drink is prepared.
- Separate washing receptacles, such as a plastic container, are recommended.
- Dilute bleach solution can be used to clean the environment and food and water bowls; however, it is important that the client rinse these thoroughly to minimize the potential for bleach toxicity.

MEDICATIONS

DRUG(S) OF CHOICE

- Ceftazidime 22 mg/kg IM q72h
- Amikacin 5 mg/kg IM q48h
- Enrofloxacin 5–10 mg/kg IM, PO q24–48h
- Oxytetracycline 42 mg/kg IM q6d

PRECAUTIONS/INTERACTIONS

N/A

FOLLOW-UP

PATIENT MONITORING

- Serial culture and PCR testing can be done to monitor the *Salmonella* spp. status and antimicrobial sensitivity profile of a patient or captive population of snakes.
- Complete blood counts to monitor responses to treatment.
- Repeat radiography to monitor for progression or resolution of osseous lesions.

EXPECTED COURSE AND PROGNOSIS

- Snakes diagnosed with *Salmonella* spp. from culture or PCR and without clinical signs may not require any intervention.
- Many snakes test positive for *Salmonella*; however, these animals are often latent carriers and do not show signs of disease.
- Animals that test negative for *Salmonella* on a single test may still be positive because intermittent shedding is common.
- Animals that test positive and have clinical signs, such as osteomyelitis, can require long-term treatment (e.g., weeks to months).
- The prognosis in these cases is fair to guarded, depending on the severity of disease at presentation.

MISCELLANEOUS

COMMENTS

N/A

ZOONOTIC POTENTIAL

- Snake-associated salmonellosis is not as commonly reported as for chelonians or lizards; however, it remains a concern and a reason for educating clients as to the risks of snake ownership.
- A recent case of meningitis in a child associated with exposure to a corn snake should reinforce the importance of pet owners following strict hygiene and biosecurity practices.

SYNONYMS

- Typhoid fever
- Salmonellosis

ABBREVIATIONS

- GI = gastrointestinal
- IM = intramuscular
- MIC = mean inhibitory concentration
- PCR = polymerase chain reaction
- PO = per os
- XLD = xylose lysine deoxycholate
- XLT-4 = xylose-lysine Tergitol 4

INTERNET RESOURCES

- Center for Food Security and Public Health. Reptile Associated Salmonellosis. January 2013. http://www.cfsph.iastate.edu/Factsheets/pdfs/reptile_associated_salmonellosis.pdf
- Association of Reptile and Amphibian Veterinarians http://www.ARAV.org

Suggested Reading

Briard E, Retornaz K, Miramont S, et. al. *Salmonella enterica* subsp. *arizonae* meningitis in a neonate exposed to a corn snake. *Pediatr Infect Dis J* 2015;34(10):1143–1144.

Clancy MM, Davis M, Valitutto MT, et. al. Salmonella infection and carriage in reptiles in a zoological collection. *J Am Vet Med Assoc* 2016;248(9):1050–1059.

Gray TZ. Update: Reptiles and Salmonella. *J Exot Pet Med* 2011;20(1):14–17.

Authors Sean M. Perry, DVM, PhD, and Mark A. Mitchell, DVM, MS, PhD, DECZM (Herpetology)

SQUAMOUS CELL CARCINOMA

BASICS

DEFINITION/OVERVIEW

SCCs are malignant epithelial cell tumors, most commonly associated with cutaneous or mucocutaneous regions of the body. SCCs are most commonly found on the skin or associated with oropharyngeal tissues. They tend to be well differentiated with some evidence of local infiltration of adjacent tissues, and limited evidence of metastatic behavior. SCCs are not uncommon in reptile species, and have been identified in a variety of snakes.

ETIOLOGY/PATHOPHYSIOLOGY

- An underlying cause of SCCs in reptiles is unknown.
- Published hypotheses with respect to risk factors and etiology include those based on mammalian or avian examples: overexposure to ultraviolet radiation, including exposure at higher altitudes, light skin color, chronic hypovitaminosis A, and possibly chronic viral infections.
- There is no evidence that any of these risk factors are associated with reptile SCCs.
- No viruses have been associated with SCCs in reptiles.
- Most reptile SCCs are locally invasive, but metastasis has yet to be reported in snakes.

SIGNALMENT/HISTORY

- In the reptile neoplasia literature, there is no clear predisposition with respect to species or sex.
- There may be an association between the presence of SCCs and increasing age of the reptile, but this has not been evaluated systematically.
- Historically, reptiles diagnosed with SCC are observed to have a focal mass or masses anywhere on the skin, within the oral cavity or at other mucocutaneous junctions.
- The raised tissue may become hemorrhagic, ulcerative and/or necrotic.
- With chronicity, bacterial abscessation may develop within or in close association with the tumor.
- Most commonly, the neoplastic cells invade adjacent tissues.
- Depending on the site of the tumor, the animal may become hyporexic/anorexic, exhibit a depressed attitude, and/or favor other anatomical sites that may be involved.
- If the eyes are involved, vision may become impaired and the animal may, uncharacteristically, fall from cage furniture or not be able to find food.

CLINICAL PRESENTATION

- The clinical signs may be somewhat variable depending on the anatomic locations of the mass.
- Discrete skin lesions tend to appear raised, with erythema, hemorrhage, and/or ulceration, or appear as chronic nonhealing wounds.
- With SCCs of the oropharynx, hyporexia or anorexia may be present, in addition to masticatory dysfunction and mild oral hemorrhage.

RISK FACTORS

Husbandry

- Purely hypothetical risk factors in reptiles are based on mammalian or avian risk factors.
- Hypovitaminosis A or excessive ultraviolet light exposure could be predisposing risk factors but there is no evidence documenting a link between these factors and SCCs.

Others

N/A

DIAGNOSIS

DIFFERENTIAL DIAGNOSIS

- Bacterial abscesses
- Fungal granulomas (especially *Chrysosporium* species)
- Viral papillomatous lesions
- Chronic traumatic wounds with fibrosis.
- Cloacal prolapse
- Other neoplastic diseases (e.g., melanoma, fibrosarcoma, cutaneous papilloma, fibropapilloma, lipoma, spindle cell sarcoma, chromatophorma).

DIAGNOSTICS

- Histopathology of the lesion is the gold standard for diagnosis, through complete surgical excision or biopsy of the mass.
- A fine-needle aspirate with cytologic evaluation may or may not be diagnostic.
- Imaging modalities, such as radiography or CT may be helpful in detecting local soft tissue or bone involvement.
- Contrast CT may be useful when trying to evaluate for metastases.

PATHOLOGICAL FINDINGS

- In domestic mammals, histologic subtypes of SCCs are typically described as poorly differentiated, moderately differentiated, or well differentiated.
- In general, SCCs are histopathologically characterized as round to polygonal cells with varying amounts of basophilic cytoplasm, and keratinization.
- The nuclei tend to be round, with significant variation in size and chromatin pattern; from coarsely stippled to pyknotic, and commonly with perinuclear vacuoles.
- Frequently, there is marked variation in nucleus to cytoplasmic ratio because the cells vary in degree of differentiation.
- In reptiles, the histologic description of SCC is similar.
- Typically, there are anastomosing cords and nests of polygonal cells with abundant eosinophilic cytoplasm, distinct intercellular bridges, and round to oval nuclei with finely stippled chromatin and multiple nucleoli, with occasional mitotic figures.
- Neoplastic cells are described as having differing levels of anisokaryosis, and frequently form circular keratinized foci consistent with keratin pearls and usually invade and/or replace adjacent tissues.

TREATMENT

APPROPRIATE HEALTH CARE

N/A

NUTRITIONAL SUPPORT

- Nonspecific nutritional support may include regular force-feeding of an appropriate commercial diet to facilitate administering nutritional supplements.
- The directions on the label of the commercial diet can be followed for appropriate volume per feeding and frequency.

CLIENT EDUCATION/HUSBANDRY RECOMMENDATIONS

N/A

MEDICATIONS

DRUG(S) OF CHOICE

- Surgical excision with histopathologic evidence of clean margins is the treatment of choice.
- In birds and mammals, focal SCCs have been treated with surgical debulking and intralesional platinum-based chemotherapeutic agents (e.g., cisplatin or carboplatin-impregnated beads).
- There is one report of a ground boa with a pharyngeal SCC treated with radiation therapy, but the mass continued to grow, and the snake was euthanized after two radiation treatments.
- Antimicrobial drugs may be used as needed for secondary bacterial infections.
- NSAIDs may help with any discomfort, but there are no systematically derived data with respect to efficacy of NSAIDs in any reptile species.
- There are no data demonstrating adverse effects of NSAIDs, such as renal impairment and/or gastrointestinal bleeding.
- Depending on the species, meloxicam may be administered orally or subcutaneously (0.2–0.5 mg/kg).

SQUAMOUS CELL CARCINOMA (CONTINUED)

PRECAUTIONS/INTERACTIONS

- With surgical excision of a SCC, recurrence should be considered and discussed with the owner.
- Should the owner elect intralesional chemotherapy, the possible outcomes include lack of therapeutic response, systemic absorption of the chemotherapeutic agent causing hyporexia/anorexia, depressed attitude, anemia or other blood cell changes, and necrosis of surrounding healthy tissues.

FOLLOW-UP

PATIENT MONITORING

- SCCs are likely to recur with incomplete surgical excision and may recur regardless of complete surgical excision.
- There are a few documented cases of local tissue invasion and/or metastasis.
- The patient should be monitored for recurrence of the tumor, and contrast CT may be of some use in monitoring for local invasion or metastatic disease.
- If treatment is recommended and accepted by the owner (partial excision and intralesional chemotherapy or electrochemotherapy), the treatment site should be monitored for secondary microbial infection or self-trauma.
- The owner should be instructed to report any signs of skin discoloration, discharge, or dysfunction of the anatomical region of the original tumor.
- Because of possible systemic absorption of locally administered chemotherapeutic agents, a complete blood count and biochemical profile should be evaluated prior to the start of chemotherapy, and serially evaluated during and after the course of chemotherapy.

EXPECTED COURSE AND PROGNOSIS

- With complete surgical excision and clean tissue margins, as evidenced by histopathology, the prognosis is good to guarded, with the possibility of recurrence.
- With recent published cases documenting metastatic disease in some reptiles, a guarded prognosis is wise until we know more about the behavior of SCCs across multiple species.
- There may be some promising new intralesional chemotherapeutic techniques or refined radiation therapy techniques applied to future cases of SCCs in reptiles, which may improve prognostic factors.

MISCELLANEOUS

COMMENTS

N/A

ZOONOTIC POTENTIAL

N/A

SYNONYMS

N/A

ABBREVIATIONS

- CT = computed tomography
- NSAIDs = Nonsteroidal anti-inflammatory drugs
- SCC = squamous cell carcinoma

Suggested Reading

Christman J, Devau M, Wilson-Robles H, et. al. Oncology of reptiles: Diseases, diagnosis, and treatment. *Vet Clin North Am Exot Anim Pract* 2017;20(1):87–110.

Sykes JM, Trupkiewicz JG. Reptile neoplasia at the Philadelphia Zoological Garden, 1901–2002. *J Zoo and Wildl Med* 2006;37(1):11–19.

Author Kurt K. Sladky, MS, DVM, DACZM, DECZM (Zoo Health Management & Herpetology)

STOMATITIS

BASICS

DEFINITION/OVERVIEW

Stomatitis is inflammation of the soft tissues of the oral cavity, which may be caused by a local or systemic process.

ETIOLOGY/PATHOPHYSIOLOGY

- Immunosuppression or trauma can lead to bacterial or fungal colonization of oral tissues.
- Normal bacterial flora secondarily infect damaged oral tissue, particularly Gram-negative rods.
- Fungi, particularly *Candida* spp., *Penicillium* spp., *Aspergillus* spp. and *Mucor* spp.
- Systemic infections
- Inclusion body disease/arenavirus
- Foreign objects: splinters, food debris, cactus spines, bedding material.
- Lacerations
- Facial injuries from striking at enclosure or from rubbing against enclosure.
- Prey injuries: bite or claw wounds from live prey; injuries from sharp teeth or claws from previously frozen prey.
- Rough handling and damage of teeth and oral mucosa during physical examination.
- Trauma during tong feeding
- Improper assisted feeding resulting in oral, pharyngeal or esophageal injuries.
- Vomiting and regurgitation may create mucosal defects in esophagus, pharynx or oral mucosa.
- Neoplasia

SIGNALMENT/HISTORY

- No specific age, breed, sex predisposition.
- Animals with a history of poor husbandry, specifically inappropriate temperatures and hygiene.

CLINICAL PRESENTATION

- Anorexia, dysphagia
- Sub spectacular swelling, buphthalmos
- Nasal discharge and secondary tracheitis or pneumonia.
- White plaques on mucous membranes, particularly with oral candidiasis.
- Rostral abrasions or callus from persistent facial rubbing or scratching.
- Hemorrhage, edema of lips and gingiva, ulceration, plaques, ptyalism, tongue dysfunction, halitosis, anorexia or dysphagia.
- Dyspnea in some animals with choanal or periglottal lesions.
- Non-specific clinical signs associated with infiltrating bacteria causing lesions in liver, kidney, heart or CNS secondary to osteomyelitis.

RISK FACTORS

Husbandry

- Chronic suboptimal temperatures considered one of the most important risk factors.
- Poor hygiene, overcrowding, improper light cycles, poor air quality, excess or insufficient humidity, toxin exposure, improper brumation, malnutrition.

Others

- Pathogen contaminated food or water
- Feeding live prey
- Secondary infection of the CNS may occur rapidly in snakes due to the short distance between the oral cavity and the thin bone encasing the brain.

DIAGNOSIS

DIFFERENTIAL DIAGNOSIS

- Rule out septicemia as cause of oral petechiation. Usually ulceration and caseous lesions with stomatitis.
- Ulcerated neoplasms are usually focal whereas stomatitis more typically diffuse.
- Consider neoplasia in cases unresponsive to supportive therapy and correction of improper husbandry.
- Abnormal maxilla and/or mandibles secondary to trauma.
- Tongue dysfunction from infection, trauma, inflammatory masses, neoplasia.

DIAGNOSTICS

- Physical examination: particular attention to eyes, teeth, choana and oral tissues.
- Use of a small otoscope or endoscope may be necessary for complete examination and to facilitate collection of samples. Anesthesia or sedation may be necessary.
- Cytology and culture: must target the deeper layers of affected tissue to minimize superficial contamination. The surface of the lesions can also be cleaned and disinfected prior to collection of samples. Aerobic, anaerobic and fungal cultures should be considered.
- Biopsy: particularly in recurring or persistent lesions; pre-clean tissue to collect samples for culture. Histopathology is key to further understanding the results of cytology and culture.
- CBC and plasma biochemistry: may be useful to detect systemic disease and severity of tissue damage. CBC may be normal or may see toxic changes within heterophils if bacterial or fungal infection.
- Advanced imaging: radiography, CT or MRI to identify severity of bone or ocular involvement.

PATHOLOGICAL FINDINGS

Histopathologic finding will vary depending on the etiologic agent involved.

TREATMENT

APPROPRIATE HEALTH CARE

- Therapy will fail if underlying cause is not identified and corrected.
- Maintain sick reptiles, and those receiving medications, at high end of POTZ for the specie.
- Some pathogens may be less pathogenic at higher temperatures and the reptile immune system may be more efficient; increases heart rate, improves circulation, improves fluid and antibiotic distribution, improves neural response, increases muscular activity, and stimulates enzyme activity.
- Oral lesions and rostral abrasions: debride, clean, and treat with appropriate antimicrobial.
- Mild and acute lesions: debride and clean lesions followed by application of topical antimicrobial and/or antifungal.
- Deep and severe lesions: require topical treatment described above as well as broad-spectrum systemic antimicrobials for bacteria (aerobic or anaerobic) or fungi, based on results of cytology. Adjust therapy as needed based on results of culture.

NUTRITIONAL SUPPORT

- After rehydration, supportive nutrition is needed to maintain positive nitrogen balance.
- Feed small amounts more frequently.
- Use high protein and fat diets.

CLIENT EDUCATION/HUSBANDRY RECOMMENDATIONS

- Quarantining new arrivals will minimize the risk of introducing a new pathogen to an established collection and will allow the new arrival time to acclimatize to its new environment.
- Follow proper husbandry guidelines for the species at hand.
- Environmental temperature, proper housing, and feeding regimen all play a crucial role in the wellbeing of reptilian species kept in captivity.

MEDICATIONS

DRUG(S) OF CHOICE

- Correct dehydration and maintain normal hydration level (15–25 ml/kg/24 hours, IV, IO, ICe in divided dose) during treatment.
- Reptiles that are sufficiently ill to require antimicrobial therapy should be considered to be dehydrated.
- Antimicrobial therapy alone is unlikely to be successful if the infection is walled off as there is poor drug penetration into exudates. A combination of aggressive debridement, wound care, and antibiotic therapy is likely to yield better results.
- Antibiotic selection is largely empiric based initially on in-clinic cytology and Gram staining, owing to the delay in return of culture results; disease-associated organisms

STOMATITIS (CONTINUED)

may be noted on cytology that are not cultured.

Antibiotics of Choice for Empirical Treatment

- Amikacin 5 mg/kg IM, then 2.5 mg/kg every 72 hours
- Azithromycin 10 mg/kg PO every 3–7 days
- Carbenicillin 200 mg/kg IM every 24 hours
- Ceftazidime 20 mg/kg IM every 72 hours
- Enrofloxacin 5–10 mg/kg IM every 48 hours
- Metronidazole 20 mg/kg PO every 48 hours
- Bactericidal drugs are preferable to bacteriostatic drugs.
- Topical antimicrobials/antifungals: iodine, chlorhexidine, and silver-based products.
- Antimicrobials may be required for 4–8 weeks.

PRECAUTIONS/INTERACTIONS

Enrofloxacin given parentally can cause tissue necrosis, use with caution.

FOLLOW-UP

PATIENT MONITORING

- Evaluate hydration frequently after starting treatment.
- Make husbandry changes to provide proper environment and nutrition.

EXPECTED COURSE AND PROGNOSIS

- Varies with underlying cause, chronicity and condition of patient.
- Lesions can progress from petechial hemorrhage to overwhelming infection and septicemia within 2–3 days.
- Acute and uncomplicated lesions usually respond to appropriate therapy.
- Untreated infections frequently progress to osteomyelitis, septicemia, and death.
- Prognosis is guarded to poor with osteomyelitis, depending on chronicity and severity.
- Neoplasia has a poor prognosis unless completely resected and with no metastasis.

MISCELLANEOUS

COMMENTS

Associated Conditions

- Osteomyelitis, sinusitis, septicemia, pneumonia and/or gastroenteritis
- Ocular or periocular disease
- Permanent tongue damage resulting in dysphagia or anorexia.
- Pharyngeal cellulitis

ZOONOTIC POTENTIAL

- Many bacteria and fungi that infect reptiles can also cause disease in humans.
- Any bites from reptiles should be treated as contaminated; immediately wash wounds with soap and water and seek medical attention; humans with open wounds on the hands should not handle reptiles or their secretions or excretions without gloves.

SYNONYMS

- Infectious stomatitis
- Mouth rot
- Ulcerative stomatitis

ABBREVIATIONS

- CBC = complete blood count
- CNS = central nervous system
- CT = computed tomography
- ICe = intracoelomic
- IM = intramuscular
- IO = intraosseous
- MRI = magnetic resonance imaging
- PO = per os
- POTZ = preferred optimal temperature zone

INTERNET RESOURCES

- Suedemeyer K, Pollock C. Presenting problem: stomatitis in reptiles. LafeberVet, November 11, 2013. https://lafeber.com/vet/presenting-problem-stomatitis-in-reptiles
- Divers SJ. Bacterial diseases of reptiles. MSD Manual Veterinary Manual, June 2020. https://www.merckvetmanual.com/exotic-and-laboratory-animals/reptiles/bacterial-diseases-of-reptiles

Suggested Reading

Jacobson ER, ed. *Infectious Diseases and Pathology of Reptiles: Color Atlas and Text.* Boca Raton, FL: CRC Press; 2007.

Mader DR, Divers SJ, eds. *Current Therapy in Reptile Medicine and Surgery*. St. Louis MO: Elsevier Saunders; 2014.

Author Sam Rivera, DVM, MS, DABVP (Avian), DACZM, DECZM (Zoo Health Management)

THERMAL BURNS

BASICS

DEFINITION/OVERVIEW

Reptiles are classified as ectothermic: they actively seek appropriate environmental temperatures to satisfy metabolic requirements. Periods of increased metabolic activity such as foraging and digestion are usually preceded and followed by actively raising core body temperature. Traditionally, heat production has been categorized into three types: radiant heat such as solar energy, convective heat such as currents of warm air, and conductive heat such as direct contact with a heat source. Reptiles usually use a combination of all three types of heat acquisition. Ventilation and humidity are also important components of thermodynamics. Most thermal burns are associated with excessive exposure to radiant and/or conductive heat.

ETIOLOGY/PATHOPHYSIOLOGY

- Thermal burns have assorted causes most of which fall into the following categories: close/direct contact with an unprotected focal heat or light source, faulty electrical equipment, or human error.
- Nociception is still poorly understood in reptiles and consequently the question remains unanswered as to why reptiles do not recognize when excessive heat is burning the integument.
- Heated simulated rocks with faulty thermostats have been associated with ventral burns in snakes. Fortunately, these devices are used with decreasing frequency today.
- Snakes that are placed outdoors for exposure to UVB light can overheat, particularly if they are not provided with areas of shade.
- Snakes that tend to burrow commonly present with severe burns on the ventrum.
- Affected snakes are exposed to thermal extremes when they lie on the glass to which a heat pad is attached.
- Overhead lights should be outside of the tank entirely, with a tank lid between the lamp and the reptile, or placed high enough in the enclosure that the reptile cannot reach it.
- Thermal burns can also occur when a reptile is weak or lethargic due to systemic disease. Therefore, a complete clinical examination should be performed to determine whether there is an underlying disease.

SIGNALMENT/HISTORY

- Thermal burns may affect reptiles of all ages and may be more prevalent during the cooler seasons when additional heating devices are used.
- History usually involves prolonged exposure to heating elements or bulbs.

CLINICAL PRESENTATION

- Clinical signs depend primarily upon severity of lesions.
- Traditionally, thermal burns have been classified according to the depth of damaged tissue.
- First-degree burns cause damage confined to the epidermis and present as erythema and sloughing of damaged scales.
- Second-degree burns involve the epidermis and dermis. This burn presents as erythema plus vesicles. The vesicles may rupture causing loss of tissue fluid and protein with a higher risk for secondary bacterial infections.
- Third-degree burns involve destruction of epidermis, dermis and underlying tissues. Secondary bacterial and/or fungal infection commonly occur.
- A more recent classification makes use of the terms "partial thickness" and "full thickness" when defining severity of burns.

RISK FACTORS

Husbandry

Exposure to inappropriate or malfunctioning heating sources is the most common cause of thermal burns.

Others

Debilitation secondary to internal disease can predispose a reptile to being too weak to move away from a heat source.

DIAGNOSIS

DIFFERENTIAL DIAGNOSIS

- Chronic dysecdysis
- Bacterial/fungal infections
- Ectoparasitism
- Trauma
- Neoplasia

DIAGNOSTICS

Diagnosis is based on history, clinical signs, and physical examination.

PATHOLOGICAL FINDINGS

- For a description of gross lesions see Clinical Presentation.
- Histopathologic findings of first-degree burns consist of dilatation of arterioles and venules, increased capillary permeability with filtration of plasma into tissue spaces and migration of erythrocytes and leukocytes.
- Second-degree burns consist of vesicles filled with an acellular transudate in addition to changes associated with first-degree burns.
- Third-degree burns are characterized by destruction of the entire integument followed by sloughing of necrotic tissue. Surrounding this zone are areas of lesser-degree burns.

TREATMENT

APPROPRIATE HEALTH CARE

N/A

NUTRITIONAL SUPPORT

- Nutritional support and proper temperatures are important factors that influence tissue regeneration.
- A 2.7–5.5 degrees C (5–10 degrees F) increase in the basking area may help improve healing; care must be taken that this does not cause additional evaporative losses.
- If the affected reptile was in a positive energy balance prior to the thermal injury and the wounds are not severe, most reptiles resume feeding as healing commences aided with the judicious use of analgesics.
- A weight loss of 10% acutely or 20% chronically should prompt nutritional intervention.
- Tube feeding with the use of an appropriate enteral, such as Oxbow Critical Care Herbivore® (Oxbow Animal Health, Omaha, NE) or EmerAid Sustain Carnivore® (EmerAid, LLC, Cornell, IL) aid in promoting anabolism and healing.
- Most snakes typically feed every 1–2 weeks and so nutritional support is typically not required.

CLIENT EDUCATION/HUSBANDRY RECOMMENDATIONS

- The owner should check the affected reptile's condition daily, implement suggested husbandry modifications, and administer medications as directed.
- Follow-up veterinary visits at prescribed intervals should be adhered to.

MEDICATIONS

DRUG(S) OF CHOICE

- If the affected reptile presents acutely after a burn (less than 30 minutes), cooling of skin is recommended with application of cold compresses for 15–20 minutes to further reduce inflammation and limit tissue swelling.
- Where blisters form, an effort should be made to minimize trauma and resultant rupture to limit tissue fluid loss and prevent secondary infection.
- For extensive wounds, a semipermeable hydrophilic wound dressing (e.g., Granuflex®, ConvaTec Inc., Oklahoma City, OK), may be used to cover defects.

THERMAL BURNS (CONTINUED)

- The use of wet-to-dry sterile bandages infused with sterile saline, or even honey, also works well and initially should be changed q24h.
- For snakes, where dressings are difficult to apply, the bandage may be sutured directly to healthy skin surrounding the wound.
- Such dressings prevent maceration of the wound by drawing fluids away from the wound surface.
- Other products that have been used widely include the porcine xenograft dressing VetBiosist® (Smiths Medical North America, Waukesha, WI), a sterile non-allergenic dressing that may be sutured over extensive wounds to provide a semipermeable membrane, protecting the granulation bed and encouraging rapid epithelialization.
- A complete blood count and biochemical analysis should also be done, especially in reptiles with third-degree burns.
- Treatment can last weeks to months, depending on the severity and extent of the burns.
- Permanent scarring with abnormal pigmentation usually occurs in the burn area.
- Chronic dysecdysis at the burn sites are a possibility.
- Topical therapy, such as dilute chlorhexidine (0.05%) and silver sulfadiazine cream, along with the use of non-adherent sterile dressings, is advised to limit secondary infection.
- Silver sulfadiazine is particularly useful due to its broad-spectrum activity and its efficacy against *Pseudomonas*, a common contaminants of burns, as well as its ability to reduce further fluid loss from evaporation.
- Ophthalmic ointments can also be used topically.
- Although analgesia of snakes is still not well elucidated, narcotic analgesics (hydromorphone 0.5-1 mg/kg IM q12–24h, tramadol 5–10 mg/kg PO, SC q24h) should be considered, NSAIDs (meloxicam 0.2–0.5 mg/kg IM, SC q24–48h), parenteral fluids (lactated Ringer's at 10–25 ml/kg IV, ICE, SC q24h), and antibiotics based upon microbiological culture and sensitivities are recommended.
- Depending on the severity of lesions, the author prefers the use of antibacterials such as piperacillin 100 mg/kg IM q24h, ceftazidime at 20 mg/kg IM q72h, or amikacin 5 mg/kg loading dose followed by 2.5 mg/kg q72h combined with metronidazole 20 mg/kg q24h.
- Patients should also be kept on non-adherent substrates to minimize further wound trauma and infection; an empty glass enclosure is the simplest to keep clean.
- SC, IV, or ICe crystalloid fluid therapy is recommended for second- and third-degree burns.

PRECAUTIONS/INTERACTIONS

- Adequate hydration should be addressed, particularly for those reptiles being treated with aminoglycosides.
- Soaking in sterile saline or water for 2–4 hours on the days when antibiotics are administered can help to provide additional hydration.
- Care must be taken when soaking reptiles in antiseptic solutions (dilute betadine, dilute chlorhexidine) due to the risk of ingestion; rather, direct application of these solutions to the wounds is recommended.

FOLLOW-UP

PATIENT MONITORING

- Affected animals should be re-evaluated every 1–2 weeks by a veterinarian.
- If this is not feasible, the owner can send pictures for appraisal until healing is progressing in a positive manner.

EXPECTED COURSE AND PROGNOSIS

- First-degree burns: damaged tissue heals in approximately 2–4 weeks.
- Second-degree burns: healing usually takes 6–8 weeks and eschar formation may develop.
- Third-degree burns: healing can take from months to years accompanied with extensive scarring. The prognosis is guarded for third-degree burns because of the possibility of sepsis.

MISCELLANEOUS

COMMENTS

Exposure to high-intensity and/or inappropriate wavelengths of UV radiation can cause signs of phototoxicity, such as photokeratoconjunctivitis and photodermatitis. Affected reptiles can present acutely with corneal and dermal opacities, excessive ecdysis, hyperkeratosis and epidermal erosions. Chronic cases may present with cataracts and cutaneous neoplasia. These cases must be differentiated from thermal burns.

ZOONOTIC POTENTIAL

N/A

SYNONYMS

N/A

ABBREVIATIONS

- ICE = intracoelomically
- IM = intramuscularly
- IV = intravenous
- NSAIDs = nonsteroidal anti-inflammatory drugs
- PO = by mouth
- SC = subcutaneously
- UVB = ultraviolet B

INTERNET RESOURCES

Divers SJ. Management and husbandry of reptiles. MSD Manual Veterinary Manual, June 2020.

Suggested Reading

Gardiner DW, Baines FM, Pandher K. Photodermatitis and photokeratoconjunctivitis in a ball python (*Python regius*) and a blue-tongue skink (*Tiliqua* spp.). *J Zoo Wildl Med* 2009;40(4):757–766.

Girling SJ, Raiti P, eds. *BSAVA Manual of Reptiles*. 2nd ed. Gloucester, UK: BSAVA; 2004.

Mader DR, ed. *Reptile Medicine and Surgery*. 2nd ed. St. Louis, MO: Elsevier Saunders; 2006.

Author Paul Raiti DVM, DABVP (Reptile and Amphibian Practice)

TICKS

BASICS

DEFINITION/OVERVIEW

Ticks are ectoparasites that feed on blood and can potentially transmit disease through their bite, along with causing local irritation, secondary infection, or rarely anemia. They are mainly seen in wild-caught animals, so any known wild-caught animals should be closely examined for their presence. Ticks may also be found on animals that are otherwise weak or debilitated. Rarely, they may be seen in captive specimens that spend time outdoors.

ETIOLOGY/PATHOPHYSIOLOGY

- Seven genera of ticks can parasitize reptiles. These include the hard ticks of the genera *Ixodes*, *Hyalomma*, *Haemaphysalis*, *Amblyomma*, and *Aponomma*, and the soft ticks *Argasidae* and *Ornithodoros*.
- Soft ticks live in nests and burrows while hard ticks live in fields or scrub areas and attach to a host as it passes by. Some are host specific.
- Ticks use their mouthparts to attach and feed on blood.
- Soft ticks become engorged and drop off within hours and may feed repeatedly while hard ticks remain attached for several days.
- Females lay eggs after a blood meal.
- Eggs hatch as a larval stage, which feed on blood from the host as well. They progress through two or more nymph stages before becoming adults, feeding on blood between each stage.
- Larvae, nymphs, and adults can live for months without a blood meal.

SIGNALMENT/HISTORY

- No predisposition for age or sex.
- Typically only seen in wild-caught animals, or those that spend significant time outdoors or are kept in unsanitary conditions with poor husbandry.

CLINICAL PRESENTATION

- Identification of tick attached to skin.
- Ticks often attach to skin folds, under scales, or around the lips, cloaca, or labial pits in snakes.
- There may be swelling, erythema, or discharge at the site of attachment from local irritation or secondary bacterial infection.
- In some cases, animals may be otherwise debilitated, weak, or have other underlying diseases.
- Animals may also soak frequently in an attempt to dislodge the parasites, and if the infestation is severe there may be signs of dysecdysis, anemia, or disease possibly transmitted by the tick.
- Ticks can serve as vectors of hemogregarines.
- Transmission by ticks of the filarid worm *Macdonaldius oschei* has been reported in snakes.

RISK FACTORS

Husbandry

- There is no specific way to avoid ticks other than regular tick control measures such as mowing the lawn regularly, removing debris piles or refuse, avoiding overwatering or standing water, limiting access by wildlife, and using tick control pesticides in the enclosure.
- Infestations can also occur in severe cases of poor husbandry and sanitation, stress and other underlying medical conditions.

Others

N/A

DIAGNOSIS

DIFFERENTIAL DIAGNOSIS

- Diagnosis is pathognomonic
- Other ectoparasites such as mites, chiggers, are significantly smaller and not confused with ticks.

DIAGNOSTICS

- Diagnosis of ticks is based on physical exam alone.
- Additional tests to evaluate the animal's overall condition may be necessary if the animal is otherwise weak or debilitated.
- This may include a fecal exam, complete blood count and chemistry panel, and/or radiography.

PATHOLOGICAL FINDINGS

- Ticks are obvious on physical exam.
- There may be evidence of inflammation or secondary bacterial colonization at the attachment site.
- Anemia is possible though because ticks are large, they are often removed before significant anemia can occur.
- Other pathologic findings could include those from a pathogen transmitted by the tick.

TREATMENT

APPROPRIATE HEALTH CARE

N/A

NUTRITIONAL SUPPORT

- Nutritional support is not needed for this condition unless the animal is otherwise debilitated.
- Snakes can be tube-fed a liquid carnivore diet at 2–3% body weight every 7–30 days depending on the species.

CLIENT EDUCATION/HUSBANDRY RECOMMENDATIONS

- Ticks must be removed from the patient and the environment for successful management.
- If ticks were obtained in an outdoor environment, then that area should be cleaned of debris and measures taken to reduce the possibility that ticks will colonize the area.
- Routine monitoring of animals and enclosures is needed.
- If the animal is wild caught and otherwise weak and debilitated, husbandry needs to be ideal to reduce stress on the animal and aid in recovery.
- Strict quarantine is necessary to avoid introducing ticks to other animals in a collection.

MEDICATIONS

DRUG(S) OF CHOICE

- Physical removal is recommended
- The tick must be grasped under the head on the mouthparts for full extraction.
- Additional treatments may be needed based on the animal's overall condition.
- If the animal is anemic due to blood loss, consider additional therapies such as B vitamins, iron dextran, or even a blood transfusion.
- Secondary infection of the attachment site can be treated with topical antibacterial ointment such as silver sulfadiazine cream, and systemic antibiotics if needed.
- FRONTLINE® Plus (Boehringer Ingelheim International GmbH, Ingelheim am Rhein, Germany) spray is effective for prevention and may aid in removal. It should never be sprayed directly on the animal; spray onto a towel and wipe the animal head to tail.
- Ivermectin 0.2 mg/kg SC may aid in tick removal, mainly for sites that are not easily accessible such as the labial pits, nostrils.
- Provent-A-Mite™ (Pro Products, Mahopac, NY) is an OTC permethrin product that appears to be both safe and effective. It can be applied to the animal or sprayed in the environment.

PRECAUTIONS/INTERACTIONS

- Use caution with any OTC remedies, particularly organophosphates or permethrins, as toxicity is possible.
- Cyfluthrin, a component of products for treating the environment, is toxic to snakes even in small amounts and should not be used.

FOLLOW-UP

PATIENT MONITORING

- None needed if ticks are physically removed.
- If secondary bacterial infection is present, resolution of clinical signs will indicate response to therapy.

TICKS (CONTINUED)

EXPECTED COURSE AND PROGNOSIS

- The prognosis for ticks themselves is excellent.
- Once the ticks are removed there should be no further complications.
- The prognosis for secondary infection of the skin is good as well.
- The main concern is if the animal is weak or debilitated overall, or if there is potential for disease transmission from the tick.
- Depending on the animal's overall condition, the prognosis may be fair to guarded.

MISCELLANEOUS

COMMENTS

- One concern with ticks on wild caught animals is potential foreign animal disease transmission.
- Any tick on a wild-caught animal from another country, and the animal itself, should be treated with suspicion.

ZOONOTIC POTENTIAL

- Ticks affecting reptiles can potentially attach to humans and cause irritation and pruritis at the site of a bite.
- Many of these can also carry and transmit disease to humans such as tularemia, Lyme disease, and other encephalitis-causing viruses.
- Use caution during removal and kill the tick immediately.

SYNONYMS

N/A

ABBREVIATIONS

- OTC = over the counter
- SC = subcutaneous

INTERNET RESOURCES

- Burridge, MJ. Controlling and Eradicating Tick Infestations on Reptiles. Veterinary Compendium, 2005. https://vetfoliovetstreet.s3.amazonaws.com/mmah/5d/12368b9df24fabb6fd86b1b65e51df/filePV_27_05_371.pdf
- PetCoach Editorial. Reptile Tick and Mite Infestation: Causes, Signs, Diagnosis, and Treatment. Petco Animal Supplies Stores, Inc. http://www.peteducation.com/article.cfm?c=17+1796&aid=2433
- Greek T. How to Recognize and Treat Reptile Ectoparasites. Reptiles, July 1, 2014. http://www.reptilesmagazine.com/Snake-Care/How-to-Recognize-and-Treat-Reptile-Ectoparasites

Suggested Reading

Burridge MJ, Simmons L. Control and eradication of exotic tick infestations on reptiles. *Proc ARAV* 2001:21–23.

Fitzgerald KT, Vera R. Acariasis. In: Mader DR, ed. *Reptile Medicine and Surgery*. 2nd ed. St. Louis, MO: Elsevier Saunders; 2006:720–738.

Jacobson ER. Parasites and parasitic disease of reptiles. In: Jacobson ER, ed. *Infectious Diseases and Pathology of Reptiles*. Boca Raton, FL: CRC Press; 2007:571–665.

Author Stacey Leonatti Wilkinson, DVM, DABVP (Reptile and Amphibian)

UPPER RESPIRATORY TRACT DISEASE

BASICS

DEFINITION/OVERVIEW

Diseases of the respiratory tract are common and often responsible for considerable morbidity and mortality in snakes. Signs of URTD in snakes can include nasal or oral discharge, respiratory sounds, and dyspnea. In snakes, primary infections of the oral cavity or esophagus can also lead to URTD. There is a wide range of pathogens and etiologies for URTD. URTD often occurs concurrently with LRTD; patients with signs of URTD must also be evaluated for LRTD. Respiratory diseases in snakes often take a long time to develop before clinical signs are evident. Snakes breathe with their mouths closed, with air entering the URT through the external nares. The air is passed from the external nares through the vestibulum nasi, the cavum nasi proprium, the conchae, the ductus nasopharyngeus, and the internal nares (choana) before reaching the trachea. The vomeronasal organ, which is usually well developed in snakes, is associated with the nose. Snakes lack a secondary palate.

ETIOLOGY/PATHOPHYSIOLOGY

- There is a wide range of etiologies associated with URTD but infectious causes are some of the most common.
- URTD may also be secondary to other diseases such as stomatitis.

Infectious

- Bacteria (*Mycobacterium chelonei*; Gram-negative such as *Pseudomonas* spp., *Aeromonas* spp., *Klebsiella* spp., *Salmonella* spp., *Proteus* spp., and anaerobic bacteria such as *Bacteroides* spp.).
- *Mycoplasma* sp. *novum* in a carpet python.
- Fungi (*Candida* spp.; *Cladosporium* sp., (synonym *Hormodendrum* sp.), in a green anaconda with mycotic stomatitis; chromomycosis combined with a fibrosarcoma in the intermandibular area of a mangrove snake).
- Viruses (ferlaviruses, arenaviruses, adenoviruses, nidoviruses, ranaviruses).
- Parasites may cause physical damage to epithelium and serve as vectors for other infections, sometimes a combination of parasitic and bacterial or viral.
- The mite *Ophionyssus natricis* has been linked to transmission of *Aeromonas hydrophila*, one of the agents associated with stomatitis in snakes and possible cause of respiratory tract infections.
- *Kalicephalus* in the nasal cavity.
- *Rhabdias*, *Kalicephalus*, renifers infecting the oral cavity or esophagus.
- Pentastomids (in oral cavity, pharynx, trachea, bronchi, lung), sometimes exiting via the glottis and then through the mouth and nares.
- Adult flukes (in oral cavity, pharynx, trachea, bronchi, lungs).

Non-Infectious

- Foreign bodies within the choana, nasal or oral cavity.
- Physical trauma/injuries affecting the nasal or oral cavity or the choana.
- Neoplasia (e.g., palatal adenoameloblastoma in an Indian python; pharyngeal squamous cell carcinoma in a Madagascar ground boa; fibrosarcoma combined with chromomycosis in the intermandibular area of a mangrove snake).
- Inhalation of dust, smoke, aerosols, or disinfectants leading to rhinotracheitis.
- Improper husbandry

SIGNALMENT/HISTORY

No age, sex, or species predisposition.

CLINICAL PRESENTATION

- Dependent on the underlying cause and snake species.
- Nasal discharge/exudate (clear to mucopurulent)
- Stridor, wheezing or clicking respiratory sounds.
- Dyspnea, open mouth-breathing
- Excess salivation or mucous secretion in the oral cavity.
- Stomatitis
- Ulceration of the nasal and buccal mucosa.
- Swelling of the face due to obstruction of the nasolacrimal duct (secondary to inflammation).
- Purulent material in the subspectacular space (provoked by bacterial infections of the spectaculocorneal space) or bullous spectaculopathy.
- Obstruction of the nostrils by retained skin, mites, dried exudate, etc.
- Elevated head and straightened cranial part of the body due to forced breathing.
- Excessive air-filled digestive tract (aerophagia) due to increased and forced inspiration.
- Nonspecific signs such as anorexia, lethargy, inactivity.

RISK FACTORS

- Inadequate husbandry
- Stressors
- Poor hygiene

Husbandry

Improper husbandry, including inappropriate temperatures and humidity, stagnant water, substrate with irritating compounds (e.g., cedar shavings), poor ventilation.

Others

- Immunosuppression, which may be caused by stress, overcrowding, relocation, concurrent disease or inappropriate husbandry.
- Sudden changes in temperature or humidity.
- Improper diet (including starvation) and endoparasitism may also be predisposing factors.

DIAGNOSIS

DIFFERENTIAL DIAGNOSIS

- Infectious diseases (bacterial, viral, fungal, parasitic)
- Trauma
- Neoplasia
- Abscess
- Foreign bodies
- Inhalation of irritating substances

DIAGNOSTICS

- Physical examination including thorough exam of the oral cavity and choana. The use of magnification may aid in identifying subtle lesions.
- Bacterial culture and sensitivity (aerobic and anaerobic) and/or fungal culture of nasal discharge, nasal flush, or inflamed tissue in the upper alimentary or respiratory tract.
- Cytology of the nasal discharge or any gross lesions of the respiratory tract or oral cavity.
- Biopsy and histopathology of nasal or oral mucosa.
- For suspected mycoplasmosis, culture and PCR of oral mucosa.
- For suspected viral infections, culture and PCR of nasal flush or nasal, oral, or pharyngeal swab.
- Diagnostic imaging (radiography, CT, MRI) for detection of foreign bodies, osteolysis, osteomyelitis, or concurrent LRTD.
- Endoscopy of the URTD (and LRTD); possibly including nasal lavage and biopsy for further diagnostics such as cytology, histopathology, virology, and electron microscopy.
- Fecal exam

PATHOLOGICAL FINDINGS

- Depending on the underlying cause, signs of mild to severe inflammation, lesions and ulcerations of the nasal and oral mucosa and submucosa may be found.
- Severe chronic ulceration of the nasal mucosa including severe chronic ulcerative rhinitis with necrotizing inflammation extending into the submucosa can be seen.
- Inflammation of the mucosa and submucosa is mostly characterized by heterophils and histiocytes; macrophages and lymphoid hyperplasia may be present.
- Granulomas can contain eosinophilic necrotic debris, mixed with heterophils and macrophages, fibrin and degenerating inflammatory cells.

UPPER RESPIRATORY TRACT DISEASE (CONTINUED)

• The palatine mucosa may be thickened and necrotic, and an accumulation of caseous material can be found in the choana in some cases.
• Purulent to caseous material in the subspectacular space(s) and bullous spectaculopathy may occur secondary to obstruction of the nasolacrimal duct.
• Osteomyelitis (with sometimes severe granulomatous inflammation of the bone marrow) and osteolysis (osteonecrosis) leading to necrotic bone tissue and bone remodeling in the adjacent structures of the skull may occur.

TREATMENT

APPROPRIATE HEALTH CARE

N/A

NUTRITIONAL SUPPORT

• Nutritional supplementation for anorexic animals is essential for recovery.
• Carnivore critical care diets can be fed once weekly until the snake starts eating on its own.

CLIENT EDUCATION/HUSBANDRY RECOMMENDATIONS

• Correct any husbandry deficiencies, with special attention to temperature, humidity, and ventilation.
• Isolate animal from others in collection, especially when viral etiology is suspected.
• It is important to ensure a full course of treatment to avoid recurrence of disease.

MEDICATIONS

DRUG(S) OF CHOICE

• Dependent on the underlying cause and the affected snake species.
• Bacteria: amikacin, ceftazidime, enrofloxacin, tylosin, preferably according to sensitivity panel for at least 4–6 weeks.
• Bacteria: systemic or nebulized antibiotics. Local instillation of antibiotics (injectable or ophthalmic solutions) in the nasal passage may also be effective.
• Fungi: systemic, local, nebulized antifungals.
• Viral: separation, strict quarantine, and intensive supportive therapy. Antiviral therapy has had low success and euthanasia is often required depending on the state of the animal and the disease.
• Parasites: antiparasitic treatment according the species.
• Foreign body within the choana, nasal/oral cavity: extraction.
• Neoplasia: surgical removal if feasible.
• Fungi: terbinafine, voriconazole, amphotericin B.
• Systemic use of itraconazole may cause severe adverse effects in some snakes.
• Fluid therapy at a fluid rate of 10–30 ml/kg/day as supportive care.

PRECAUTIONS/INTERACTIONS

Many systemic antibiotics (e.g., aminoglycosides) are excreted through the kidney or show renal toxicity, thus adequate hydration and regular monitoring of renal values is recommended.

FOLLOW-UP

PATIENT MONITORING

• Improvement of clinical signs should be expected within 1–2 weeks for bacterial and fungal infections when definitive diagnosis and treatment are employed.
• It is critical to continue treatment until clinical signs are fully resolved and repeating cultures to confirm resolution of infection if unsure.
• In cases that do not show any improvement or worsen during the first 1–2 weeks of treatment, it should be considered that the etiology and/or treatment are not accurate.
• Viral infections should also be considered in cases that do not respond to therapy or have chronic, intermittent recurrence of disease.
• Repeat diagnostics may be needed to assess resolution or progression of disease.

EXPECTED COURSE AND PROGNOSIS

• Bacterial: good prognosis depending on response to antibiotics.
• Fungal: guarded to poor prognosis.
• Viral: poor to grave prognosis especially when showing clinical signs.
• Parasitic: good prognosis
• Neoplastic: poor to grave prognosis.
• Others: depend on severity and involvement of other tissues.

MISCELLANEOUS

COMMENTS

N/A

ZOONOTIC POTENTIAL

• Dependent on the causative agent
• Mycobacteria, salmonella and pentastomids have zoonotic potential.

SYNONYMS

Upper respiratory disease syndrome

ABBREVIATIONS

• CT = computed tomography
• LRTD = lower respiratory tract disease
• MRI = magnetic resonance imaging
• PCR = polymerase chain reaction
• URT = upper respiratory tract
• URTD = upper respiratory tract disease

Suggested Reading

Jacobson E. Diseases of the respiratory system in reptiles. *Vet Med Small Anim Clin* 1978;73(9):1169–1175.

Jacobson ER. Infectious diseases of reptiles. In: Kirk RW, ed. *Current Veterinary Therapy VII. Small Animal Practice.* 7th ed. Philadelphia, PA: WB Saunders; 1980:625–633.

Jacobson ER. Overview of reptile biology, anatomy, and histology. In: Jacobson ER, ed. *Infectious diseases and pathology of reptiles.* Boca Raton, FL: CRC Press; 2007:1–130.

Junge RE, Miller RE. Reptile respiratory diseases. In: Kirk RW, Bonagura JD, eds. *Kirk's Current Veterinary Therapy XI. Small Animal Practice.* 11th ed. Philadelphia, PA: WB Saunders; 1992:1204–1210.

Wyneken J, Witherington D. Respiratory anatomy: Form and function in reptiles. *Exotic DVM* 2001;3:17–22.

Author Karina A. Mathes, DVM, Dr. med. vet., DECZM (Herpetology), European Veterinary Specialist in Zoological Medicine (Herpetology), Certified Specialist in Reptiles (Fachtieraerztin fuer Reptilien), Certified Specialist in Reptiles and Amphibians (ZB Reptilien und Amphibien)

UROLITHIASIS

BASICS

DEFINITION/OVERVIEW

Snakes do not possess urinary bladders; hence, the absence of cystic calculi. Ureteroliths and cloacoliths have occasionally been encountered in snakes.

ETIOLOGY/PATHOPHYSIOLOGY

N/A

SIGNALMENT/HISTORY

- In snakes, ureterolithiasis is associated with chronic dehydration and renal disease, which can affect animals of all ages.
- Deficiencies in husbandry such as lack of water, suboptimal ambient temperatures, and inappropriately high protein diets are commonly identified during anamnesis.

CLINICAL PRESENTATION

- Snakes with renal disease often present with anorexia, dehydration, and weight loss.
- Oral mucous membranes may contain uric acid deposits.

RISK FACTORS

Husbandry

- Hyperuricemia is commonly associated with chronic dehydration.
- Exogenous uric acid production is dependent on diet and is particularly high when the diet is rich in animal protein and fat; hence, the inappropriateness of hyperalimentation with laboratory rodents.
- Fresh water should always be present in the enclosure and supplemented with daily misting.
- Weekly soakings for most reptiles are also recommended.
- Suboptimal ambient temperatures may reduce renal blood supply and depress the immune system.

Others

N/A

DIAGNOSIS

DIFFERENTIAL DIAGNOSIS

- Space-occupying lesions of the intestinal tract including cloaca.
- Gastrointestinal foreign bodies
- Ileus
- Dystocia
- Constipation

DIAGNOSTICS

- Cloacal uroliths may be palpable.
- Hematology and plasma biochemistries should be done to evaluate renal insult (calcium, phosphorus, hematocrit, total solids and uric acid values).
- Radiography and ultrasound may be beneficial in identifying calculi in the kidneys, ureters, and cloaca.

PATHOLOGICAL FINDINGS

Necropsies have revealed concurrent renal gout, membranous glomerulopathy, renal interstitial fibrosis, glomerulonephritis and interstitial fibrosis, and renal interstitial fibrosis with mineralization.

TREATMENT

APPROPRIATE HEALTH CARE

N/A

NUTRITIONAL SUPPORT

- Reptiles that are anorexic due to renal disease may benefit from parenteral fluid therapy and tube feeding.
- More therapeutic details are discussed under RSHP management.

CLIENT EDUCATION/HUSBANDRY RECOMMENDATIONS

Husbandry parameters should be adhered to meticulously, with special emphasis on ambient temperature ranges, diet, hydration, and hygiene during the immediate and long-term convalescent period.

MEDICATIONS

DRUG(S) OF CHOICE

- Currently, there are no drugs that have been used to successfully dissolve uroliths in reptiles; however, allopurinol, a xanthine oxidase inhibitor, 10–20 mg/kg PO q24h is used to reduce uric acid levels in reptiles.
- Small cloacal uroliths can usually be passed successfully by soaking the affected snake in warm water.

PRECAUTIONS/INTERACTIONS

N/A

FOLLOW-UP

PATIENT MONITORING

Repeat physical examinations coupled with biochemical analysis will aid in evaluation of renal function.

EXPECTED COURSE AND PROGNOSIS

The prognosis in snakes with visceral gout is guarded to poor.

MISCELLANEOUS

COMMENTS

N/A

ZOONOTIC POTENTIAL

N/A

SYNONYMS

- Urinary concretions
- Uroliths

ABBREVIATIONS

PO = per os

Suggested Reading

Reavill DR, Schmidt RE. Urogenital tract diseases of reptiles. *Proc ARAV* 2013: 84–97.

Author Paul Raiti, DVM, ABVP (Reptile and Amphibian Practice)

VOMITING

BASICS

DEFINITION/OVERVIEW

Vomiting is the forcible ejection of partially or wholly digested contents from the stomach and small intestine through the mouth.

ETIOLOGY/PATHOPHYSIOLOGY

- Vomiting in reptiles is under active neural control from the autonomic and somatic nervous systems. Details of this mechanism are not completely understood, but they are likely similar to those of mammals.
- The difference between vomiting and regurgitation may be difficult to discern.

SIGNALMENT/HISTORY

- All species, ages, sexes, may be affected.
- Owner may report observing vomiting or only that vomited material was found.
- Lethargy, anorexia, weight loss, respiratory distress, or increased basking frequency.
- Ingestion of foreign material
- Neurologic signs (e.g., tremors, disorientation)

CLINICAL PRESENTATION

- No clinical signs are specific to regurgitation, and physical exam may be normal.
- Presentation varies depending on the underlying cause and chronicity.
- Dehydration and/or emaciation/cachexia.
- Hard mass on palpation of the coelomic cavity due to an obstructive lesion or organomegaly.
- Skeletal abnormalities that may include pathological fractures or abnormal growth patterns.
- Lethargy and/or obtunded mentation.
- Ulceration and accumulation of caseous material in the oral cavity.
- Secondary respiratory disease (e.g., oral/nasal discharge, abnormal respiratory sounds) or enteritis (e.g., diarrhea).
- In boids, loss of righting reflex, tremors, and disorientation may occur with suspected IBD.

RISK FACTORS

Husbandry

- Too much disturbance or lack of hiding places (increases stress/anxiety).
- Poor sanitation, overcrowding, hyper- or hypothermia, lack of quarantine for new individuals (increases stress, possibility of secondary infections, and disease transmission).
- Toxin exposure (cleaning chemicals, pesticides, heavy metals).
- Excessive/inappropriate handling (especially soon after feeding).
- Inadequate diet (incorrect calcium/phosphorus ratio, improper prey items, excessive feeding).
- Inappropriate substrate (may be accidentally ingested)

Others

- Concomitant infectious or parasitic disease.
- Snake mites (*Ophionyssus natricis*) are a potential vector for IBD.

DIAGNOSIS

DIFFERENTIAL DIAGNOSIS

- Stomatitis
- Esophagitis
- Esophageal stricture
- Gastritis
- Handling/stress (e.g., excessive pressure to coelom)
- Obstructive lesions (e.g., GI foreign body, intussusception, neoplasia, abscess, granuloma)
- Metabolic disease (e.g., nutritional secondary hyperparathyroidism, renal or hepatic dysfunction)
- Toxicoses (e.g., zinc)
- Iatrogenic (e.g., miticides, xylazine, levamisole)
- Trauma to esophagus or stomach.
- Parasites (e.g., *Cryptosporidium*, amoebiasis, ascaridiasis, cestodiasis)
- Viruses (e.g., IBD in boids)
- Bacteria/septicemia (e.g., *Chlamydophila*)
- Congenital GI defects

DIAGNOSTICS

- Husbandry review
- Physical examination
- Complete blood count and plasma biochemistries.
- Radiography with or without contrast.
- Ultrasound
- Fecal parasite exam
- Bacterial cultures from oral lesions.
- GI endoscopy or coeliotomy (direct tissue evaluation and biopsy)
- Testing for cryptosporidiosis and IBD.

PATHOLOGICAL FINDINGS

- Dependent on underlying cause
- In cryptosporidiosis, no gross pathology may be present, especially in chronic, subclinical cases.
- In clinical cases, there usually is gastromegaly due to mucosal edema and thickening, excessive mucus production, and reduction of the luminal diameter.
- Enlargement of gastric rugae, mucosal petechiae, and focal necrosis may also be present.
- For IBD, the lack of inclusion bodies does not rule out infection.

TREATMENT

APPROPRIATE HEALTH CARE

The primary goal is to identify and address the underlying cause.

NUTRITIONAL SUPPORT

- Correct fluid deficits and maintain hydration.
- Intracoelomic, subcutaneous, or intravenous routes for administration of a reptile Ringer's solution are most effective. Maintenance rate is 10–30 ml/kg/day
- Tube or assist-feeding liquid or gel diets, such as Hill's® Prescription Diet® a/d® (Hills Pet Nutrition, Inc., Topeka, KS); Mazuri® Amphibian & Carnivorous Reptile Gel (Mazuri Exotic Animal Nutrition, St. Louis, MO); Oxbow Critical Care Carnivore® (Oxbow Animal Health, Omaha, NE) may be beneficial during initial treatment/recovery.
- Gradually add normal prey items to diet as animal improves.

CLIENT EDUCATION/HUSBANDRY RECOMMENDATIONS

- Review husbandry and correct any problems.
- Avoid overfeeding and disturbing snakes 1–2 days after feeding.
- Institute quarantine procedures for new animals, including 30–60-day time period, veterinary evaluation, and 1–3-weekly fecal exams for parasites.
- Animals affected by IBD or cryptosporidiosis should be isolated from all other reptiles.

MEDICATIONS

DRUG(S) OF CHOICE

- Cimetidine 4 mg/kg IM, PO q8–12h, or famotidine 0.25–0.5 mg/kg SC, PO q24–72h
- Metoclopramide 0.06 mg/kg PO q24h for 7 days, or cisapride 0.5–2 mg/kg PO q24h
- Sucralfate 500–1000 mg/kg PO q6–8h.

PRECAUTIONS/INTERACTIONS

N/A

FOLLOW-UP

PATIENT MONITORING

Monitor for continued signs of regurgitation and possible complications.

EXPECTED COURSE AND PROGNOSIS

- Dependent on underlying cause
- Prognosis for IBD is poor, as there is no treatment.

• Prognosis for subclinical cryptosporidiosis is fair to good.
• Prognosis for clinical disease is poor to grave, and euthanasia is often indicated.

MISCELLANEOUS

COMMENTS
N/A

ZOONOTIC POTENTIAL
N/A

SYNONYMS
Emesis

ABBREVIATIONS
• GI = gastrointestinal
• IBD = inclusion body disease
• IM = intramuscular
• PO = per os
• SC = subcutaneous

Suggested Reading

Cranfield MR, Graczyk TK. Cryptosporidiosis. In: Mader DR, ed. *Reptile Medicine and Surgery*. 2nd ed. St. Louis, MO: Elsevier Saunders; 2006:756–762.

Mitchell MA, Diaz-Figueroa O. Clinical reptile gastroenterology. *Vet Clin N Am Exot Anim Pract* 2005;8:277–298.

Schumacher J. Inclusion body disease virus. In: Mader DR, ed. *Reptile Medicine and Surgery*. 2nd ed. St. Louis, MO: Elsevier Saunders; 2006:836–840.

Author Tamara Kruse, DVM, MS, and Trevor T. Zachariah, DVM, MS, DACZM

WEIGHT LOSS

BASICS

DEFINITION/OVERVIEW

For reptiles, weight loss can take the form of loss of body mass (i.e., cachexia) or fluid. In mammals, it is generally accepted that weight loss becomes clinically significant when the loss exceeds 10% of normal body weight (and when it is not completely due to fluid loss). From a clinical perspective, weight loss of more than 10–20% of a healthy, species-specific body weight is significant and must be systematically evaluated, with rapid weight loss being considered most urgent. Weight loss in reptiles may be a normal physiologic process (e.g., brumation/estivation, reproductive activity and behavior), and is not considered a primary disease, but rather, a clinical manifestation of other disease processes.

ETIOLOGY/PATHOPHYSIOLOGY

- In reptiles, normal weight loss (fluid and body mass loss) will occur during times of torpor or brumation/estivation.
- Once post-torpor normal behavior returns, the reptile will replenish lost fluids and body mass under normal circumstances or given normal access to clean water and appropriate food and environmental conditions.
- Normal weight loss may be associated with reproductive behavior or gravidity.
- Pathologic weight loss may be associated with a variety of non-infectious and infectious disease processes.
- In pet reptiles, inappropriate husbandry is the most common underlying cause of pathologic weight loss.
- Poor husbandry may frequently lead to metabolic diseases of secondary infectious diseases due to immune system compromise of the animal.
- Infectious diseases, and debilitating non-infectious diseases, will commonly result in weight loss due to both body mass and fluid loss.
- In some cases, reptiles succumb to a non-specific disease process referred to as "maladaptation or failure to thrive syndrome," which is characterized by the failure of a captive reptile to adapt to its current conditions, or a wild-caught reptile unable to adapt to the captive environment.
- Many of these animals will lose weight and die, and a specific disease process is not diagnosed.

SIGNALMENT/HISTORY

- Weight loss in reptiles has no specific signalment, and can affect males or females of any species and any age.
- A typical history suggests rapid weight loss of ≥ 10% acutely or ≥ 20% chronically.
- Weight loss in reptiles typically includes some degree of dehydration, in addition to loss of body mass and/or fat stores.
- If the individual or species normally brumates/estivates, weight loss can be expected as a normal physiologic process.
- With pathologic weight loss, the husbandry and environment must be evaluated thoroughly, and infectious and noninfectious diseases must be considered as underlying causes to the weight loss.

CLINICAL PRESENTATION

- Reptiles presenting with weight loss typically show observable loss of muscle mass.
- The vertebral column and become more readily apparent, with the body of the snake taking on a more triangular appearance.
- In severe cases, the coelomic cavity may appear sunken.
- With dehydration, the eyes may sink into the bony orbits, and the severe tenting or wrinkling of the skin may become distinct, depending on the species.

RISK FACTORS

Husbandry

- Poor husbandry is the most common contributing factor to pathologic process in reptiles, including weight loss.
- Inappropriate housing type or improper placement within a client's household or other facility.
- Inappropriate ambient temperature and humidity
- Lack of access to clean water.
- Inappropriate type, quality and quantity of food offered for the species.
- Type of substrate, cage furniture, and frequency of cleaning/replacing substrate.
- Toxicity associated with environmental cleaning solutions.
- Foreign body ingestion and GI impaction.
- Thermal burns
- Dental disease
- Chronic renal disease
- Exposure to toxic chemicals
- In some cases, maladaptation syndrome or failure to thrive syndrome should also be considered as an underlying cause of weight loss.

Others

N/A

DIAGNOSIS

DIFFERENTIAL DIAGNOSIS

Normal Behavior

- Periods of torpor, brumation and estivation are normal for some species and may be associated with weight loss (loss of body mass and fluids).
- In some species, fluid loss during brumation/estivation can contribute to more than 10% of total weight loss.
- Reproductive activity, behavior and gravidity may contribute to normal seasonal weight loss.

Non-Infectious Diseases

- Exposure to toxic substances
- Developing disease processes secondary to poor husbandry or nutrition.

Neoplasia

- A number of neoplastic diseases have been identified in reptile species, with many different organ systems affected.
- Most of these neoplastic diseases have an expected clinical sequela of hyporexia, dehydration, and weight loss.

Infectious Diseases

- Reptiles are susceptible to many infectious diseases, all of which can contribute to hyporexia, dehydration, and weight loss.
- Common reptile diseases observed in clinical practice, include endoparasites (GI protozoa, nematodes, amoebae, and hemoparasites); ectoparasites (mites, ticks); Gram-negative bacterial infections and septicemia; *Chrysosporium* species and other fungal infections; viruses.

DIAGNOSTICS

- Since weight loss is not a specific disease, a significant clinical diagnostic workup will be necessary.
- A thorough history, including the following will be useful: housing; feeding practices; maintenance temperature and humidity; presence of other animals; ad libitum access to water and water quality.
- Comparison to conspecifics housed in the same environment may confirm individual or group disease.
- A complete physical examination is critical to identify obvious lesions on the skin, within the oral cavity, or associated with the eyes.
- A fecal sample should be evaluated by direct smear and fecal float, if possible.
- A complete blood count and biochemical profile, along with imaging modalities (radiography, ultrasound, and/or CT), should be considered.
- Aerobic and anaerobic bacterial cultures of blood samples may be useful in debilitated reptiles due to the possibility of sepsis.
- Intracoelomic or GI endoscopy, with or without biopsy and histopathology, may help with the diagnosis.
- In cases of obvious skin disease, a biopsy with histopathologic examination is important.

PATHOLOGICAL FINDINGS

- Pathologic findings are non-specific for weight loss, but the underlying cause may be associated with obvious gross pathologic or histopathologic lesions.
- Gross pathology of non-specific weight loss might include loss of intracoelomic fat bodies, lack of intracoelomic organ-associated fat, and generalized muscle wasting.

TREATMENT

APPROPRIATE HEALTH CARE

N/A

NUTRITIONAL SUPPORT

- Nonspecific nutritional support may include regular force-feeding of an appropriate commercial diet.
- The directions on the label of the commercial diet can be followed for appropriate volume per feeding and frequency.
- Alternatively, force-feeding whole prey items (e.g., pinkie mice or small fish) may be useful.

CLIENT EDUCATION/HUSBANDRY RECOMMENDATIONS

N/A

MEDICATIONS

DRUG(S) OF CHOICE

- Based on the diagnosis of the underlying cause of weight loss, treatment should be focused on the primary disease process.
- Correct hydration status by soaking or administering appropriate fluid therapy due to fluid loss (typically an isotonic solution), as any debilitated reptile will likely be moderately to severely dehydrated.
- Based on the primary disease process underlying the weight loss, antimicrobial and anti-inflammatory drugs may be warranted.
- Vitamin and mineral supplements (e.g., calcium in the form of parenteral calcium gluconate or oral calcium glubionate) may be beneficial if nutritional deficiencies underlie the weight loss; or oversupplementation of vitamins and minerals may need to be discontinued if this appears to be causing primary disease.

PRECAUTIONS/INTERACTIONS

N/A

FOLLOW-UP

PATIENT MONITORING

- Correction of inappropriate husbandry and/or feeding practices will significantly benefit the patient.
- If medical treatment is necessary, the body weight can be measured and the body condition assessed daily.
- If appropriate, medical therapy can be initiated and the patient monitored for improving condition.

EXPECTED COURSE AND PROGNOSIS

- Replenishing lost fluids from normal physiologic processes, such as brumation/estivation, may be warranted and should improve the reptiles' condition and provide a good prognosis.
- Depending on the primary underlying disease process and duration, the prognosis will range from poor to good for re-establishing normal body weight and condition.
- If husbandry problems can be corrected in a relatively short amount of time, the prognosis may be good.
- If the underlying disease process is progressive and debilitating, the prognosis will be poor.
- In cases of some infectious diseases, antimicrobials can be administered for bacterial or fungal diseases using topical, parenteral, or oral solutions.

MISCELLANEOUS

COMMENTS

N/A

ZOONOTIC POTENTIAL

N/A

SYNONYMS

- Cachexia
- Wasting

ABBREVIATIONS

- CT = computed tomography
- GI = gastrointestinal

Suggested Reading

Mader DR, ed. *Reptile Medicine and Surgery*. 2nd ed. St. Louis, MO: Elsevier Saunders; 2006.

Author Kurt K. Sladky, MS, DVM, DACZM, DECZM (Zoo Health Management & Herpetology)

YEAST INFECTIONS

BASICS

DEFINITION/OVERVIEW

Infection with *Candida* spp., *Cryptococcus* spp., or exceptionally other yeasts is rare in reptiles, in comparison with mammals and birds.

ETIOLOGY/PATHOPHYSIOLOGY

- Many yeasts, especially *Candida* species, are normal constituents of reptile GI and even respiratory tracts.
- Typically secondary to concurrent condition or infection.

SIGNALMENT/HISTORY

Any reptile species, any sex, any age.

CLINICAL PRESENTATION

- Anorexia, diarrhea, weight loss, debilitation.
- Signs may be non-specific or depend on affected organ system.
- Cryptococcosis has manifested as a granulomatous pneumonia and meningoencephalitis in an anaconda, but as a cutaneous swelling in a skink.

RISK FACTORS

Husbandry

Poor husbandry is likely a factor with these often opportunistic pathogens.

Others

- Breaches in mucosal epithelia from concurrent issues/infections may allow deep tissue access to yeast.
- Prolonged antibiotic treatment may also favor yeast proliferation.

DIAGNOSIS

DIFFERENTIAL DIAGNOSIS

- Viral and/or bacterial stomatitides and enteritides, or even protozoal GI infections.
- Viral, bacterial, parasitic, or other respiratory infections.

DIAGNOSTICS

- Cytology of swabs or washes that demonstrate budding yeast, and ideally inflammatory cells.
- Culture of swabs, exudates, and biopsies are needed but the isolation of *Candida* is insufficient to confirm causality.
- Concurrent histopathological evidence of yeast infection in biopsy/tissue sections essential to establish causality.

PATHOLOGICAL FINDINGS

Necrosis, inflammation, and budding yeast with pseudohyphae.

TREATMENT

APPROPRIATE HEALTH CARE

- Systemic antifungals, fluid therapy, thermal and nutritional support.
- Isolation of sick animals
- Review of captive husbandry

NUTRITIONAL SUPPORT

Assist-feeding if needed

CLIENT EDUCATION/HUSBANDRY RECOMMENDATIONS

- Isolation of sick animals and thorough hygiene.
- Critical review of husbandry

MEDICATIONS

DRUG(S) OF CHOICE

- Fluconazole may be efficient in treating yeast infections, but some *Candida* species are inherently fluconazole resistant.
- Superficial gastric or intestinal mucosal infections may respond to nystatin.
- Probably better to use broader-spectrum, systemically absorbed triazoles such as itraconazole.

PRECAUTIONS/INTERACTIONS

N/A

FOLLOW-UP

PATIENT MONITORING

- Might require intensive care
- Monitor response to antifungal therapy and supportive measures.

EXPECTED COURSE AND PROGNOSIS

- Variable, depending on duration and severity of disease, affected organ systems, and extent of lesions.
- As these infections are often diagnosed late in the disease process, prognosis should be guarded.

MISCELLANEOUS

COMMENTS

- A presumptive diagnosis of candidiasis or other yeast infection may be possible cytologically from clinical samples, but every effort should be made to pursue identification of these yeast to species.
- Yeast identification may carry treatment implications, as sensitivity panels can be determined.
- Only with proper identification can we understand which yeast carry pathogenic potential.

ZOONOTIC POTENTIAL

- Cryptococcosis, a zoonotic disease, has been documented in reptiles.
- Candidiasis is rare in reptiles, but also is a potential zoonosis.

SYNONYMS

N/A

ABBREVIATIONS

GI = gastrointestinal

Suggested Reading

Paré JA, Jacobson ER. Mycotic diseases of reptiles. In: Jacobson ER, ed. *Infectious Disease and Pathology of Reptiles, Color Atlas and Text.* Boca Raton, FL: CRC Press; 2007:527–570.

Author Jean A. Paré, DMV, DVSc, DACZM, DECZM (Zoo Health Management)

Section V

Crocodilians

AFLATOXICOSIS

BASICS

DEFINITION/OVERVIEW

Aflatoxicosis is caused by infection with certain strains of toxin-producing fungi. Exposure occurs through ingestion of contaminated cereals, grains, and other plant products that have been exposed to high temperature and moisture.

ETIOLOGY/PATHOPHYSIOLOGY

- *Aspergullis flavus*, *A. parasiticus*, and *Penicillium puberulum* are some of the most commonly reported toxicogenic species.
- The mere presence of these fungi does not indicate that aflatoxicosis will occur but rather the potential for mycotoxin production under the right environmental conditions.
- These toxins are then ingested by the animals leading to aflatoxicosis, which has is primary pathologic effects in then liver.

SIGNALMENT/HISTORY

- Affected animals can be of any age or sex, but younger animals may be more severely affected.
- There is usually a history of food stored in a silo, thawed whole chickens, or a slow turnover of bagged feed.
- Improper food storage or handling of thawed whole prey is a key element.

CLINICAL PRESENTATION

- Aflatoxicosis can have an either subacute, acute, or chronic presentation, although these may be more difficult to differentiate when working with animals in commercial farms.
- Subacute and acute toxicosis may lead to inappetence, lethargy, weakness, hemorrhage, icterus, and increased mortality in a noticeable subset of animals.
- The chronic toxicosis may present with the same signs but may be more sporadic and with less noticeable mortality.
- It should be noted that icterus does occur in crocodilians as they are capable of producing bilirubin.

RISK FACTORS

Husbandry

- Improperly stored feed at high temperatures and humidity is an important source of aflatoxins.
- Feeding whole chickens with feed ingesta within the intestinal tract was a source of aflatoxicosis in *A. mississippiensis*.
- Poor hygiene and failure to clean up any food remnants from the dry areas of the housing pens is also a potential source.

Others

N/A

DIAGNOSIS

DIFFERENTIAL DIAGNOSIS

- West Nile virus
- Adenovirus

DIAGNOSTICS

- Definitive diagnosis is obtained by necropsy and aflatoxin testing of liver tissue.
- Clinical signs of icterus, gross hepatic changes including necrosis and fibrosis, and a history of feeding whole chickens or improper food storage are all supportive of a diagnosis.
- There are often elevations of bilirubin and AST if enough functional liver tissue still remains.

PATHOLOGICAL FINDINGS

- Gross changes include icterus of the skin, tongue, mucous membranes, sclera, and great vessels.
- Hepatic nodules, fibrosis, and necrosis is also observed.

TREATMENT

APPROPRIATE HEALTH CARE

- There is no known treatment.
- The best course of action is removal of contaminated feed.

NUTRITIONAL SUPPORT

Replace contaminated feed with a new source.

CLIENT EDUCATION/HUSBANDRY RECOMMENDATIONS

- Feeding of whole chickens should be discouraged.
- Food storage, handling, and use should be reviewed.
- Bagged feed should be stored in a dry, cool area, preferably a climate-controlled space in warmer climates.
- Any silos should be inspected and regularly maintained to ensure that water cannot enter the storage tank and is not holding excess humidity.

MEDICATIONS

DRUG(S) OF CHOICE

N/A

PRECAUTIONS/INTERACTIONS

N/A

FOLLOW-UP

PATIENT MONITORING

Clinically affected animals are unlikely to recover; euthanasia/slaughter should be considered.

EXPECTED COURSE AND PROGNOSIS

- Infected animals have a grave prognosis and will often die.
- Once the contaminated feed is removed and husbandry practices improved, the prognosis for non-clinical animals is excellent.

MISCELLANEOUS

COMMENTS

N/A

ZOONOTIC POTENTIAL

N/A

SYNONYMS

- Aspergillus toxicosis
- Moldy corn toxicity

ABBREVIATIONS

AST = aspartate aminotransferase

Author Javier G. Nevarez, DVM, PhD, DACZM, DECZM (Herpetology)

ANOREXIA

BASICS

DEFINITION/OVERVIEW

Anorexia is the lack of appetite or intake of food, and does not define an underlying cause. Many pathological and even physiological conditions can result in decreased food intake. Anorexia is distinct from decreased appetite, which is also known as hypophagia.

ETIOLOGY/PATHOPHYSIOLOGY

- Anorexia may be a normal physiologic/behavioral occurrence during certain times of the year (e.g., brumation, estivation, reproductive season).
- Pathologic causes of anorexia may stem from either GI or extra-GI disease (e.g., any painful condition or systemic illness).
- Improper husbandry and offering the wrong type and size of food may also lead to anorexia.
- Anorexia may often result in dehydration, as many reptile's primary fluid intake is through food items.
- Prolonged anorexia may lead to hepatic lipidosis, which may result in nausea, leading to continued lack of food intake.
- Nutritional imbalances and metabolic derangements can occur with chronic anorexia and cachexia may ensue.
- Primarily, the GI and musculoskeletal systems are affected with anorexia.
- Animals that are not consuming food for prolonged periods of time may not defecate significant amounts.
- As the body begins to break down adipose tissue stores and muscle, bony prominences become more obvious as body condition decreases.

SIGNALMENT/HISTORY

- Anorexia has no age or sex predilection.
- It is important to differentiate physiologic/behavioral anorexia from that caused by an underlying pathology or disease process.

CLINICAL PRESENTATION

- An isolated incident or occasional episodes of anorexia in otherwise healthy animals may be inconsequential, especially in animal presenting in good body condition.
- Decreased food intake over an extended period.
- Clients may report repeated attempts at feeding.
- Clinical signs of chronic anorexia include a decreased body condition score with prominent bony protuberances, dehydration, and muscle wasting.

RISK FACTORS

- Any disease process could result in anorexia.
- Different types of stress may also result in decreased food intake.

Husbandry

- Adjusting to captivity: often seen in newly acquired animals. A period for acclimation may be necessary prior to an animal feeling secure enough to start eating on its own.
- Improper husbandry: inappropriate environmental temperature or humidity, inappropriate food items (type and/or size), malnutrition, inadequate exposure to UVB lighting, poor water quality, overcrowding, rapid change of diet, lack of provision of hiding areas.
- Stress: social or environmental

Others

- Physiologic
- Cardiovascular disease: cardiomyopathy, congestive heart failure.
- Reproductive activity: gravid females, breeding males.
- Reproductive disease: pre- or postovulatory dystocia.
- Respiratory infections: bacterial pneumonia, mycoplasmosis.
- Any infectious disease
- Systemic illness: septicemia
- GI disease: stomatitis, foreign bodies, neoplasia, intussusception, gastroenteritis, prolapses.
- Parasitic disease
- Neurologic disease
- Toxic diseases: lead intoxication
- Metabolic: nutritional secondary hyperparathyroidism.
- Any potentially painful condition

DIAGNOSIS

DIFFERENTIAL DIAGNOSIS

- Conditions that result in failed food prehension (disorders of the tongue or oral cavity) or processing may result in animals that attempt to eat (have an appetite) but are unable to do so successfully.
- Hypophagia may be mistaken for anorexia in certain circumstances.

DIAGNOSTICS

Diagnostic procedures should be tailored towards identifying the underlying cause of the anorexia and identifying potential negative sequelae (e.g., hepatic lipidosis).

Baseline Blood Work

- CBC, PCV, transferrin saturation, biochemistry.
- Findings on CBC and biochemistry panels are usually non-specific but may be suggestive of underlying disease process(es) resulting in the observed anorexia.
- Bile acids and liver leakage enzymes (AST) may be increased if hepatic lipidosis is present secondary to prolonged anorexia.

Imaging

- Radiography can help identify abnormalities of the GI tract such as foreign bodies and masses.
- Ultrasound and CT can provide more detailed information about possible hepatic lipidosis, ileus, and coelomic masses.

Other Tests

Additional diagnostics, including infectious or parasitic disease testing, may be warranted based on patient history and physical examination findings. The presumed underlying causes should be thoroughly investigated.

PATHOLOGICAL FINDINGS

- Findings depend on underlying cause of the anorexia.
- Hepatic lipidosis may be suspected based on the findings of advanced imaging or biochemistry evaluation.

TREATMENT

APPROPRIATE HEALTH CARE

N/A

NUTRITIONAL SUPPORT

- Nutritional support should be started in anorectic animals that have lost 10% of their body weight acutely (7 days or less) or 20% chronically (longer than 7 days).
- This weight loss must also be monitored together with an assessment of BCS.
- Anorectic animals with a BCS of 2/5 or lower may be immediate candidates for nutritional support.
- Animals should be housed in appropriate environments and maintained at their preferred optimum temperature zones to facilitate proper takeup of the provided nourishment.
- Placement of an esophagostomy tube should be considered for long-term support and to minimize stress of force-feeding.
- Although poorly understood in veterinary medicine, the potential exists for refeeding syndrome in chronically anorectic patients, necessitating careful planning of nutritional support in these animals.
- Recommendations include feeding chronically anorectic animals half of their calculated energy requirements initially, then slowly increasing up to the full energy requirement over 7–10 days.

ANOREXIA (CONTINUED)

CLIENT EDUCATION/HUSBANDRY RECOMMENDATIONS

- The clinician should perform a thorough review the patient's current husbandry, including feeding regimen.
- It is important to ensure that a proper diet of appropriate size is being offered.
- The diet must be presented to the animal appropriately (e.g., feeding diurnal animals during daylight hours, offering prey on land vs. in the water or vice versa). Any husbandry or dietary deficiencies should be corrected.
- Clients should be notified that offering live food items to anorectic animals could result in rapid, serious injury secondary to prey attacks.
- For most cases, live mammalian prey should not be offered to crocodilians without direct supervision.

MEDICATIONS

DRUG(S) OF CHOICE

- Commercial, high-calorie formulations designed for nutritional support in reptiles are recommended when feeding anorectic crocodilians.
- A slurry can be made with a commercial pelleted diet.

PRECAUTIONS/INTERACTIONS

- Exercise caution when force-feeding in order to prevent dental and mandibular trauma.
- Be careful not to administer too large a volume of nutritional formula in small patients.
- Feed 1–3% of body weight initially to ensure that the animal will tolerate the feedings.

FOLLOW-UP

PATIENT MONITORING

- Individuals should be monitored for resolution of anorexia following correction of any husbandry and dietary deficiencies.
- Serial imaging and blood chemistry evaluation may be considered to monitor for development or resolution of secondary liver insult.
- In patients with esophagostomy tubes, the tube should be monitored for clogging and the stoma regularly evaluated for signs of infection.

EXPECTED COURSE AND PROGNOSIS

- Anorexia may continue until the underlying reason is identified and treated.
- Prognosis for resolution of anorexia depends on the severity of the underlying cause.

MISCELLANEOUS

COMMENTS

- Simply providing appropriate husbandry will help prevent many causes of anorexia in crocodilians.
- Prompt diagnosis of true anorexia enables initiation of proper nutritional support and may prevent formation of hepatic lipidosis, which can perpetuate the lack of appetite.
- Supportive care should be continued while an underlying cause for the anorexia is identified and corrected.
- Gravid individuals may decrease their amount of food consumption from lack of coelomic space for GI distension.
- Animals that are anorectic from an underlying pathologic condition may cease or abort reproductive activity due to preferential allotment of energy for other physiologic functions.

ZOONOTIC POTENTIAL

N/A

SYNONYMS

- Anophagia
- Aphagia
- Inappetence

ABBREVIATIONS

- AST = aspartate aminotransferase
- BCS = body condition score
- CBC = complete blood count
- CT = computed tomography
- GI = gastrointestinal
- PCV = packed cell volume
- UVB = ultraviolet B

Suggested Reading

De Voe RS. Nutritional support of reptile patients. *Vet Clin North Am Exot Anim Pract* 2014;17:249–261.

Divers SJ, Stahl S, eds. *Mader's Reptile and Amphibian Medicine and Surgery*. 3rd ed. St. Louis, MO: Elsevier; 2019.

Author Grayson Doss, DVM, DACZM

CHLAMYDIOSIS

BASICS

DEFINITION/OVERVIEW

Chlamydiosis has been a chronic problem of farmed Nile crocodiles (*Crocodylus niloticus*) in South Africa and Zimbabwe and in American alligator (*Alligator mississippiensis*) farms in the United States. Outbreaks are also reported from Indo-Pacific crocodiles (*C. porosus*) in Australia and Papua New Guinea and Siamese crocodiles (*C. siamensis*) in Thailand. Reports in crocodiles are of acute hepatitis and chronic conjunctivitis affecting hatchling and juveniles. In alligators, clinical cases of conjunctivitis have been limited to hatchlings; chronic hepatitis is more common in juveniles.

ETIOLOGY/PATHOPHYSIOLOGY

- The specific chlamydial organism causing disease in crocodilians has yet to be definitively identified.
- *Chlamydophila psittaci* has been proposed as the closest species to the one pathogenic in crocodilians but it is suspected that the chlamydial species infecting crocodiles and alligators is likely a novel one.
- Besides knowing that it causes hepatitis and conjunctivitis, the pathophysiology in crocodilians is not fully understood.
- The source/origin of the chlamydial organisms affecting crocodilians is also unknown at this time.
- In alligators, typical outbreaks are characterized by animals eating less and increased mortality, which typically subsides within a week.
- These outbreaks are usually in alligators approaching 1 year of age and overall cause high morbidity but low mortality.
- Surviving animals may become subclinical carriers. In crocodiles, high mortality of hatchlings is more commonly reported.

SIGNALMENT/HISTORY

- Reports are restricted to captive reared/housed, juvenile (< 3 years) crocodilians.
- Repeat outbreaks are a common occurrence at affected farms.

CLINICAL PRESENTATION

- In crocodiles, sudden mortalities of hatchlings with no clinical signs are reported.
- Severe conjunctivitis is seen as a chronic process.
- In American alligators, conjunctivitis has been observed in hatchlings only, with the juveniles being affected by hepatitis as an apparently chronic process.
- Animals with conjunctivitis become anorexic due to inability to see food and this is followed by increased mortality.

RISK FACTORS

- Thus far, clinical disease has been limited to crocodilians in captivity.
- No specific risk factors have been identified.
- Biosecurity is critical to prevent the spread of the disease.

Husbandry

- A lack of quarantine and biosecurity can lead to spread of the disease within a facility.

Others

N/A

DIAGNOSIS

DIFFERENTIAL DIAGNOSIS

- West Nile virus
- Pneumonia
- Mycoplasmosis

DIAGNOSTICS

- PCR: A generic *Chlamydia* PCR can be used to identify infected animals, but species identification is not currently possible. Liver and spleen are the ideal tissues to be tested.
- Histopathology helps to characterize the hepatitis as consistent with chlamydial infection.
- Culture: these are difficult organisms to grow in culture. Nonetheless, culture should be attempted as it could help in the identification of the suspected novel species.
- Electron microscopy can help confirm the presence of a chlamydial organism within tissues.

PATHOLOGICAL FINDINGS

- Grossly, the liver can appear enlarged, pale and mottled.
- Splenomegaly and ascites can also be found.
- On histology, there is severe lymphoplasmacytic hepatitis and necrosis.
- When present, severe blepharoconjunctivitis with a fibrinous membrane covering the cornea and nictitans.

TREATMENT

APPROPRIATE HEALTH CARE

- Treatment of an unknown chlamydial species that is possibly zoonotic is debatable.
- The potential impact of antimicrobial resistance development and how this could affect treatment of humans must be considered.

NUTRITIONAL SUPPORT

Due to the nature of crocodilians and the large number of animals affected at once, force-feeding is not a practical approach.

CLIENT EDUCATION/HUSBANDRY RECOMMENDATIONS

It is critical to implement quarantine and biosecurity protocols to prevent spread of the disease during an outbreak.

MEDICATIONS

DRUG(S) OF CHOICE

- Oxytetracycline 75–100 mg/kg IM, PO; typically must be mixed with feed when treating thousands of animals.
- There is an anecdotal report of effectiveness in crocodiles but pharmacokinetic data do not support oral administration of oxytetracycline in alligators.

PRECAUTIONS/INTERACTIONS

Pharmacokinetics of oral tetracycline in American alligators did not reach MIC, so treatment with oral tetracycline is not recommended for alligators.

FOLLOW-UP

PATIENT MONITORING

PCR of liver tissue can be performed from animals at time of slaughter to determine whether they are indeed carriers and the disease is present within a farm.

EXPECTED COURSE AND PROGNOSIS

- Prognosis for clinically ill animals is grave, as mortalities can be high and sudden.
- Those that survive an outbreak appear to do well but are suspected to be carriers.

MISCELLANEOUS

COMMENTS

N/A

ZOONOTIC POTENTIAL

- A number of chlamydial species are zoonotic.
- The zoonotic potential of the species causing disease in crocodilians is unknown, but it should be assumed that it could be.
- Proper precautions should be taken when working with infected animals, especially during necropsy.

SYNONYMS

N/A

ABBREVIATIONS

- IM = intramuscular
- MIC = minimum inhibitory concentration
- PCR = polymerase chain reaction
- PO = per os

CHLAMYDIOSIS (CONTINUED)

Suggested Reading

Huchzermeyer FW, Gerdes GH, Foggin CM, et. al. Hepatitis in farmed hatchling Nile crocodiles (*Crocodylus niloticus*) due to chlamydial infection. *S Afr Vet Ver* 1994;65(1):20–22.

Huchzermeyer FW. Transmissible diseases. In: Huchzermeyer FW (ed.). *Crocodiles: Biology, Husbandry, and Diseases.* Cambridge, MA: CABI Publishing; 2003:167–170.

Sariya L, Kladmanee K, Bhusri B, et. al. Molecular evidence for genetic distinctions between Chlamydiaceae detected in Siamese crocodiles (*Crocodylus siamensis*) and known Chlamydiaceae species. Japan J *Vet Res* 2015;63(1):5–14.

Author Javier G. Nevarez, DVM, PhD, DACZM, DECZM (Herpetology)

CLOACAL PROLAPSE

BASICS

DEFINITION/OVERVIEW

A prolapse is the moving or slipping of a body part from its usual position or anatomic relation. In the reptile, a prolapse from the vent may be of cloacal, rectal, phallus, oviductal, or bladder in origin.

ETIOLOGY/PATHOPHYSIOLOGY

- The underlying causes for prolapse is often unknown.
- See Differential Diagnosis for a list of possible etiologies.

SIGNALMENT/HISTORY

- There appear to be no specific signalment or predilections noted for the various reptilian prolapses.
- Female reptilians may be overrepresented due to occurrences of dystocia.

CLINICAL PRESENTATION

- A prolapse is easy to visualize as abnormal tissue protruding from the cloacal/vent region.
- In reptiles housed outdoors and in case of small prolapses, the owners may not notice a problem until days after it has occurred.
- A prolapse should be considered an emergency and evaluated promptly.
- The tissue should be kept moist either through gentle washing the area with water and loosely wrapped in a damp cloth or paper towel until the animal can be evaluated a veterinarian.
- The extruded tissue should be identified to the tissue(s) involved, such as cloacal with/without bladder, oviduct, proctodeum, colon, phallus.
- Once the issues are identified, the clinician may be able to narrow the diagnosis to determine the course of diagnostics and therapeutics.

RISK FACTORS

- In cases of nutritional secondary hyperparathyroidism, the muscle tone around the cloacal opening is decreased, leading to potential tissue exposure.
- Any generalized physical straining of the patient can lead to tissue exposure through the cloaca, such as dyspnea, obstipation, parasites, infection.
- Space-occupying lesions located in the coelomic cavity, such as, neoplasia, hepato/renomegaly, eggs, may also cause increase straining and cloacal prolapse.

Husbandry

- Several factors of husbandry may lead to one of the clinical conditions listed in the Differential Diagnosis section.
- Corrections of the deficient aspects of the husbandry can lead to reversal of some of those listed conditions.

Others

- Some cloacal tissue may prolapse during normal oviposition.
- Iatrogenic prolapses may occur when owners attempt to manually manipulate ova in suspected cases of dystocia or feces in constipated animals.

DIAGNOSIS

DIFFERENTIAL DIAGNOSIS

- Parasites
- Hypocalcemia
- Dehydration
- Metabolic disease
- Neoplasia
- Impaction
- Obstruction
- Trauma
- Coelomic space-occupying lesion
- Obesity
- Bacterial infection
- Intoxication

DIAGNOSTICS

- Radiography and ultrasound may be useful in determining internal abnormalities (e.g., impactions, masses, obstructions).
- The small size of some reptiles may lead to reduced imaging detail, which makes interpretation challenging. Dental radiography may be a better alternative in smaller species (< 100 g).
- A fecal examination should be performed in all cases. This can be directly from the feces, a saline cloacal wash, or direct impression smear of the prolapsed tissue may reveal the presence of parasites such as nematode larvae or eggs.
- A complete blood count and chemistry panel may assist in the determination of underlying physiologic abnormalities.

PATHOLOGICAL FINDINGS

- Protozoal infections affecting the gastrointestinal tract may be diagnosed on histopathology.
- Other findings will be consistent with the underlying cause, but often no specific cause or pathology can be identified.

TREATMENT

APPROPRIATE HEALTH CARE

- Treatment often involves direct replacement of the tissue back into normal anatomic position either by manual or surgical means in combination with correction of the underlying etiology.
- The patient should be fully evaluated for general health status and treated accordingly.
- The prolapsed tissue should be evaluated for presence of devitalization, which must be surgically or medically addressed prior to prolapse reduction.
- In cases of reproductive system prolapse (i.e., oviduct), the tissue may be replaced but damage to the suspensory ligaments and internal vasculature may be present.
- In severe oviductal prolapses, discussion with the owner about desired reproductive status should take place with a potential for coeliotomy and ovariosalpingectomy.
- In some cases, the internal reproductive structures may be medically or surgically repaired; however, further reproductive events could result in dystocia.
- The prolapse may be reduced in size by coating with a hyperosmotic solution such as 2–5% ophthalmic saline or concentrated sugar solution.
- Direct application of dry salt or sugar may be attempted, but the extreme osmolar difference could lead to direct tissue damage and should be closely monitored.
- After several minutes of application, the prolapsed tissue should become less edematous and capable of reduction back into the body cavity.
- A moistened and lubricated (water soluble) cotton tip applicator or metal probe is used to gently push the tissue back inside the body cavity aligning the lumen.
- A purse-string suture around the cloaca or lateral sutures across the cloacal margin may be placed for 10–14 days to allow for the tissue swelling to resolve in place.
- Surgical options such as resection of the diseased tissue and double-layer closure can be performed prior to tissue replacement.
- In more extensive cases, a coeliotomy may be performed with the tissue resection performed within the coelomic cavity where the tissue is in approximate "normal" anatomic position.
- Colonic prolapses may require a colopexy where sutures are placed to facilitate the "tacking" of the colon to the dorsolateral body wall.

NUTRITIONAL SUPPORT

The reptilian patient may need weight and body condition monitoring to determine if additional caloric supplementation is needed.

CLIENT EDUCATION/HUSBANDRY RECOMMENDATIONS

- If surgical correction of the prolapse is undertaken, the client should be directed on postoperative care of any surgical sites, suture, etc.

CLOACAL PROLAPSE (CONTINUED)

- A detailed log of activity, as well as food intake/defecations, should be maintained and related back to the veterinarian.
- If any changes to the husbandry are determined, the owner should correct the husbandry prior to the patient returning home, such as changes to temperature and/or humidity, exposure ultraviolet lighting.

MEDICATIONS

DRUG(S) OF CHOICE

- NSAIDs or opioids may be used in management of the inflammation and pain associated with the physical discomfort of the prolapse or surgery.
- Depending on the determined etiology, antibiotics or antiparasiticides may be indicated.

PRECAUTIONS/INTERACTIONS

- When replacing the prolapse, extreme care must be taken not to tear or perforate the delicate, inflamed tissue.
- After the sutures are removed, the tissue may re-prolapse if swelling/inflammation are still present or the underlying etiology has not been corrected. Placement of additional sutures may be required.
- Hydration status of the patent must be considered before use of NSAIDs.

FOLLOW-UP

PATIENT MONITORING

- The patient should be followed up daily after clinical repair of the prolapse for reoccurrence.
- The owner should monitor and record all food intake and defecations during this time.
- Any abnormal changes should be related back to the veterinarian to determine any further changes to the therapy.

EXPECTED COURSE AND PROGNOSIS

- Prolapses of the oviduct and bladder tend to have a guarded to grave prognosis due to the degree of underlying physical damage to the affected tissues and cloaca.
- Rectal and cloacal prolapses tend to have a fair prognosis if treated promptly.
- Phallus/hemipenal prolapses have excellent to good prognosis, as these are purely copulatory organs.
- The length of time the prolapse presents has an inverse effect on the prognosis.
- When treated early in the disease process and the tissue appears viable, cloacal prolapse replacement may lead to clinical resolution if the underlying etiology is addressed.
- Once the tissue begins to desiccate and become devitalized, there is a guarded to grave prognosis.

MISCELLANEOUS

COMMENTS

N/A

ZOONOTIC POTENTIAL

N/A

SYNONYMS

N/A

ABBREVIATIONS

NSAIDs = nonsteroidal anti-inflammatory drugs

Suggested Reading

Barten, SL. Penile prolapse. In: Mader DR, ed. *Reptile Medicine and Surgery*. 2nd ed. St. Louis, MO: Elsevier Saunders; 2006:862–864.

Bennett, RA. Cloacal prolapse. In: Mader DR, ed. *Reptile Medicine and Surgery*. 2nd ed. St. Louis, MO: Elsevier Saunders; 2006:751–755.

Author Rob L. Coke, DVM, DACZM, DABVP (Reptile & Amphibian), CVA

CONJUNCTIVITIS

BASICS

DEFINITION/OVERVIEW

Conjunctivitis is inflammation of the conjunctiva. In reptiles, conjunctivitis often presents concurrently with blepharedema, which is edema and swelling of the eyelids. In many cases, the blepharedema is severe enough to impede proper evaluation of the eye and hence identification of conjunctivitis. Blepharoconjunctivitis is a common presentation.

ETIOLOGY/PATHOPHYSIOLOGY

- In crocodilians, conjunctivitis is more often associated with chlamydiosis or mycoplasmosis.
- Other bacterial, viral, fungal or parasitic etiologies are also possible.
- Poor air quality, environmental irritants or toxins should also be considered, especially when housed indoors.
- Trauma should be considered, especially in cases of unilateral conjunctivitis.

SIGNALMENT/HISTORY

- There is no specific signalment for the occurrence of conjunctivitis.
- The focus should be on obtaining a thorough history of the husbandry.

CLINICAL PRESENTATION

- In addition to the conjunctivitis itself, crocodilians may present with blepharedema, blepharospasm, and/or periocular swelling usually affecting both eyes and causing blepharoconjunctivitis.
- Animals may also present with anorexia, depression and lethargy due to either the systemic effects of the underlying etiology or simply from their inability to see properly.

RISK FACTORS

Husbandry

Poor cleanliness and hygiene of the enclosure can also lead to increased environmental bacterial load that can contribute to conjunctivitis.

Others

N/A

DIAGNOSIS

DIFFERENTIAL DIAGNOSIS

- Mycoplasmosis
- Chlamydiosis
- Trauma

DIAGNOSTICS

- A complete ophthalmic examination with the use of magnification by direct or indirect ophthalmoscopy including fluorescein test to detect corneal ulcers.
- Sampling of the conjunctiva for bacterial culture and sensitivity.
- A generic *Chlamydia* PCR can be used to identify infected animals, but species identification is not currently possible. Liver and spleen are the ideal tissues to be tested but conjunctiva may be used also. For suspected *Mycoplasma alligatoris* or *M. crocodyli*, PCR of lung, trachea, and other affected tissues is the most sensitive method of diagnosis.

PATHOLOGICAL FINDINGS

- Blepharoconjunctivitis is a common presentation.
- Plaques or caseous material may be observed within the fornix or even covering the corneal surface.
- Mucopurulent discharge

TREATMENT

APPROPRIATE HEALTH CARE

- Treatment will be based on the underlying etiology; anti-inflammatories and analgesics should be considered in most cases.
- Treatment of an unknown chlamydial species that is possibly zoonotic is debatable.
- The potential impact of antimicrobial resistance development and how this could affect treatment of humans must be considered.
- Concurrent systemic and ophthalmic therapy is recommended for best response in cases of infectious etiologies.
- Treatment of viral infections is often unrewarding.
- Flushing and cleaning of the eyes is also necessary to remove any adhered material or plaques that may be harboring organisms.
- A solution of 1 part povidone iodine to 50 parts saline can be used.
- When blepharoedema is present, a pipette tip, tomcat catheter, or intravenous catheter can be inserted between the eyelids to flush the eyes.
- Treatment of large number of animals, as in commercial operations, is less likely to result in resolution.

NUTRITIONAL SUPPORT

- In cases of anorectic animals, force-feeding with easily digestible proteins should be initiated.
- Direct feeding by stomach tube or gavage needle can be performed in some species.
- Placement of an esophagostomy tube should be considered for chronic management.
- Supportive fluid therapy should be provided.

CLIENT EDUCATION/HUSBANDRY RECOMMENDATIONS

- Remove and isolate sick individuals and reduce stress by providing optimal living conditions, and hygiene.
- Thorough cleaning of cage to reduce environmental load of infectious organisms.
- Ensure quarantine protocols have been implemented for all new arrivals.
- Treatment compliance is key for response to therapy.

MEDICATIONS

DRUG(S) OF CHOICE

Systemic Therapy

- Meloxicam 0.5 mg/kg IM, PO q24h
- Dexamethasone sodium phosphate 0.1–0.3 mg/kg IM, SC, IV q24h for 3 days
- Tetracyclines: long-acting tetracycline administered IV and IM 10 mg/kg q5d maintained MIC in *A. mississippiensis*. However, oral administration at 50 mg/kg did not result in appropriate levels. Anecdotal use of tetracyclines in crocodile species suggests a response to therapy, so species variability may exist for its oral bioavailability.
- Oxytetracycline 75–100 mg/kg IM, PO; typically has to be mixed with feed when treating thousands of animals. An anecdotal report of effectiveness in crocodiles but pharmacokinetic data do not support oral administration in alligators.
- Enrofloxacin 5 mg/kg IV q36h in *A. mississippiensis* (PO dosing ineffective).

Ophthalmic Therapy

- Ophthalmic antibiotics applied 3–4 times daily.
- Ophthalmic ant inflammatory applied 3–4 times daily.
- Ophthalmic itraconazole applied 3–4 times daily.

PRECAUTIONS/INTERACTIONS

Vitamin A must be administered parenterally only in cases with clear indication of hypovitaminosis A, otherwise there is a risk of causing hypervitaminosis A.

FOLLOW-UP

PATIENT MONITORING

Weekly to two-weekly re-evaluation is recommended to determine response to therapy.

EXPECTED COURSE AND PROGNOSIS

- Course and prognosis will vary according to the etiology.
- Prognosis for viral infections is grave, as these animals typically become progressively worse over time.
- For other etiologies prognosis is good to excellent.

CONJUNCTIVITIS (CONTINUED)

MISCELLANEOUS

COMMENTS

N/A

ZOONOTIC POTENTIAL

Unknown for chlamydiosis; use caution.

SYNONYMS

N/A

ABBREVIATIONS

- IM = intramuscular
- IV = intravenous
- MIC = minimum inhibitory concentration
- PCR = polymerase chain reaction
- PO = per os
- SC = subcutaneous

Suggested Reading

Brown DR, Farley JM, Zacher LA, et al. *Mycoplasma alligatoris* sp. *nov.*, from American alligators. *Int J Syst Evol Microbiol* 2001;51:419–424.

Huchzermeyer FW. Transmissible diseases. In: Huchzermeyer FW (ed.). *Crocodiles: Biology, Husbandry, and Diseases.* Cambridge, MA: CABI Publishing; 2003:167–170.

Lawton, MPC. Reptilian ophthalmology. In: Mader DR, ed. *Reptile Medicine and Surgery*. 2nd ed. St. Louis, MO: Elsevier Saunders; 2006:334–336.

Rivera S, Nevarez JG, Maxwell LK, Barker SA. Pharmacokinetics of tetracycline after single-dose oral administration in the American alligator (*Alligator mississippiensis*). *J Zoo Wildl Med* 2012;43(4):858–863.

Author Javier G. Nevarez, DVM, PhD, DACZM, DECZM (Herpetology)

CRYPTOSPORIDIUM

BASICS

DEFINITION/OVERVIEW

Cryptosporidia are apicomplexan parasites typified by possessing an apical complex, and with four naked sporozoites within each oocyte. *Cryptosporidium* spp. can be distinguished from other coccidian parasites by the location that they occupy within the host cell membrane, their capacity for autoinfection, and their resistance to antiparasitic medication. Possessing a durable oocyst wall consisting of a double layer of a protein–lipid–carbohydrate matrix, *Cryptosporidium* is highly resistant to environmental degradation and chemical disinfection. Historically, oocyst morphology has been used for species identification, but this is considered unreliable and species assignment is now determined by molecular characteristics. *Cryptosporidium* spp. are ubiquitous in the environment and are globally distributed.

ETIOLOGY/PATHOPHYSIOLOGY

- There has only been one documented case of an unspecified *Cryptosporidium* sp. isolated from a captive Nile crocodile in Egypt.
- The infection may have originated from an infected keeper or rodents fed to the animal.
- The infected crocodile did not show any clinical signs.

SIGNALMENT/HISTORY

No apparent clinical signs

CLINICAL PRESENTATION

Subclinical infection

RISK FACTORS

The greatest risk factor for developing infection is poor quarantine of new animals entering a collection or from infected prey items.

Husbandry

N/A

Others

N/A

DIAGNOSIS

DIFFERENTIAL DIAGNOSIS

Enteritis: bacterial or other protozoal disease.

DIAGNOSTICS

Examination of Feces

- Unstained smears are useful
- Sensitivity of detection increases with an acid-fast stain and is greatest with an IFA stain.
- Sensitivity may be increased if performed postprandially.
- An important limitation of these tests is their lack of specificity to differentiate *Cryptosporidium* spp.
- False positive results can occur in animals that have ingested prey items (i.e., mice) infected with other *Cryptosporidium* spp. that are not pathogenic to reptiles.

Polymerase Chain Reaction

- A highly sensitive test that can be used for either fecal or lavage samples.
- Can also differentiate between *Cryptosporidium* spp.

PATHOLOGICAL FINDINGS

N/A

TREATMENT

APPROPRIATE HEALTH CARE

None attempted

NUTRITIONAL SUPPORT

Stomach tubing with easily digestible proteins and supportive fluid therapy may be important for instances of clinical disease.

CLIENT EDUCATION/HUSBANDRY RECOMMENDATIONS

Clients should be made aware of the insidious nature of infection, the unlikelihood of successful treatment, the risks that affected animals pose to the remaining collection, and the known zoonotic potential of some *Cryptosporidium* spp.

MEDICATIONS

DRUG(S) OF CHOICE

N/A

PRECAUTIONS/INTERACTIONS

- Euthanasia should be strongly considered for clinically affected animals to limit spread.
- If this is not an option, diseased reptiles should be separated from the remaining collection and strict barrier nursing protocols enacted to prevent spread.

FOLLOW-UP

PATIENT MONITORING

- Regular fecal examination and ELISA assays for suspected at-risk animals.
- Monitor for signs of disease (i.e., wasting, diarrhea, persistent regurgitation).

EXPECTED COURSE AND PROGNOSIS

No disease seen

MISCELLANEOUS

COMMENTS

N/A

ZOONOTIC POTENTIAL

Unknown, but it should be remembered that prey items fed to reptiles may harbor *Cryptosporidium*, which can pose a risk to immunocompromised individuals.

SYNONYMS

N/A

ABBREVIATIONS

- ELISA = enzyme-linked immunosorbent assay
- IFA = immunofluorescent antibody
- PCR = polymerase chain reaction

Suggested Reading

Cranfield MR, Graczyk TK. Cryptosporidiosis. In: Mader DR, ed. *Reptile Medicine and Surgery*. 2nd ed. St. Louis, MO: Elsevier Saunders; 2006: 756–762.

Graczyk TK, Owens R, Cranfield MR. Diagnosis of subclinical cryptosporidiosis in captive snakes based on stomach lavage and cloacal sampling. *Vet Parasitol* 1996;67:143–151.

Huchzermeyer FW. Crocodiles: *Biology, Husbandry and Diseases*. Cambridge, MA: CABI Publishing; 2003.

Plutzer J, Karanis P. Genetic polymorphism in *Cryptosporidium* species: an update. *Vet Parasitol* 2009;165(3–4):187–199.

Author T. Franciscus Scheelings, BVSc, MVSc, PhD, MANCVSc (Wildlife Health), DECZM (Herpetology)

DERMATITIS

BASICS

DEFINITION/OVERVIEW

Dermatitis is a general term referring to inflammation of the skin. Information presented here focuses on dermatitis observed in captive crocodilians in commercial operations.

ETIOLOGY/PATHOPHYSIOLOGY

- Mixed bacterial and fungal dermatitis are the most common type observed in farms.
- Dermatitis is often caused by a high bacterial and/or fungal growth in the biofilm on the water and other surfaces of the enclosure.

SIGNALMENT/HISTORY

- Can affect all crocodilians of any age and sex.
- Usually associated with history of feeding fatty foods, low frequency of water exchange, poor hygiene, or overfeeding.

CLINICAL PRESENTATION

- The most prevalent dermatitis of concern presents as a white film on the dorsal body surfaces, primarily the head, back, and base of the tail.
- This white film can be manually removed; the underlying skin may appear normal to ulcerated depending on chronicity and severity.
- The skin over the inguinal and axillary regions may also be erythematous.
- As the disease progresses some animals may develop secondary conjunctivitis, subsequent anorexia, and ultimately may die.
- Others may die from development of systemic infection.

RISK FACTORS

Husbandry

Poor hygiene, overfeeding, and feeding of fatty foods are all predisposing factors that contribute to bacterial/fungal overgrowth.

Others

- Immunosuppression due to stressors may also make animals more susceptible to infection.
- While not proven through any controlled studies, the author has observed certain materials used to manufacture pens or to line the pens to develop a biofilm in a short period of time.
- The pen/liner material may also be an important contributing factor.

DIAGNOSIS

DIFFERENTIAL DIAGNOSIS

- Bacterial dermatitis
- Fungal dermatitis
- Mixed bacterial and fungal dermatitis.

DIAGNOSTICS

- Histology: Definitive diagnosis is accomplished by histologic evaluation of the skin to confirm the presence of bacteria and/or fungi and the inflammatory response associated with their presence in the skin.
- Cytology: Cytologic examination of skin impressions may reveal an abundance of bacteria and/or fungi. However, this does not confirm causation as it is usual for aquatic animals to have an abundant number of organisms on the skin.
- Culture: Bacterial and/or fungal culture are likely to yield a mixture of organisms, making it difficult to interpret results and determine pathogenicity. For this reason, it is often unrewarding and of less clinical value.

PATHOLOGICAL FINDINGS

- Grossly, the skin may have a white film or discoloration.
- Once the skin is dry, it can be difficult to observe the film, so animals are best kept moist until the time of necropsy.
- Skin erythema and ulceration may be present.

TREATMENT

APPROPRIATE HEALTH CARE

- Treatment largely relies on improvement of husbandry and hygiene. This includes eliminating high-fat diets such as chicken or other fatty meat products.
- When possible, a commercial pelleted diet should be used instead. However, even commercial diets can be high in fat.
- Proper cleaning of the enclosures is key for prevention and treatment. This includes flushing and cleaning the pens more frequently and using a brush to help remove the biofilm from all solid the surfaces in the pen.
- Certain water treatments may also help prevent or manage the disease, but their effectiveness is not consistent. It must also be considered that water treatments are ineffective in the presence of a large amount of organic matter.
- Antibiotics should never be used to treat the water as they are ineffective in this manner and such use will contribute to antimicrobial resistance.

NUTRITIONAL SUPPORT

N/A

CLIENT EDUCATION/HUSBANDRY RECOMMENDATIONS

- Implementation of proper feeding and hygiene is critical for prevention of dermatitis.
- The speed at which animals consume all food should be evaluated to avoid overfeeding, which leads to food remnants that deteriorate water quality.
- All solid surfaces should be assessed for the presence of a slime film, which likely harbors the organisms responsible for dermatitis. This film should be removed with a brush.
- Porous materials such as wood should be avoided as they cannot be disinfected and are ideal for harboring bacteria and fungi.
- A monitoring plan should be developed to determine what cleaning frequency is best suited to prevent buildup of bacteria and fungi while also causing minimal stress to the animals.

MEDICATIONS

DRUG(S) OF CHOICE

- The use of automated chlorinators is used by some facilities to help maintain water hygiene. Safe chlorine rates and levels have not been established. Anecdotal evidence suggests 2–4 ppm (2–4 mg/l) is safe for crocodiles.
- NaCl: *Alligator mississippiensis* tolerated exposure of 5 ppt (5 g/L of water) up to 4 weeks without detrimental effects. At concentrations beyond 10 ppt, weight loss and decrease in growth were observed. Mortality was observed at 15 ppt and beyond. Crocodile species that normally inhabit estuarine areas (*Crocodylus acutus*, *C. porosus*, *C. niloticus*, and *C. johnstoni*) may have a higher tolerance for NaCl but still experience physiologic effects with a high dose and/or long-term exposure.
- Potassium permanganate 5–10 ppm (5–10 mg/) in clean water for 3–4 hours.
- Iodine: a 1-part iodine to 50-parts water of a 1% iodine solution can be used to soak animals for 4–5 hours. The solution can also be sprayed on affected animals when out of the water.
- Soap: Dish soap may be used as a surfactant to help break the fat layer and biofilm at the water surface. This is not an effective standalone therapy, but is rather an adjunct approach to a comprehensive management plan.
- Copper sulfate: immersion in water with 1 ppm copper sulfate for 15 minutes q12h for 6 weeks or until lesions resolve. Topical application of 0.5% copper sulfate.
- Topical application of F10® (Health and Hygiene (Pty) Ltd., Stormill, South Africa) or 0.5% zinc sulfate.

PRECAUTIONS/INTERACTIONS

- Potential for copper or zinc toxicity is not known when performing topical or immersion treatments.
- Animals must be monitored during treatment for any evidence of distress and rinsed thoroughly afterwards.
- These treatments must be done carefully, especially in endangered species.

FOLLOW-UP

PATIENT MONITORING

Once feeding and hygiene practice changes have been implemented, it may take 4–6 weeks to see improvement in mildly affected animals.

EXPECTED COURSE AND PROGNOSIS

- The overall prognosis is fair to grave due to the damage to the skin, especially once it has become ulcerated, and variable response to therapy when applied in a large scale.
- Prognosis may be better when treating a small number of animals.
- Even with treatment, reoccurrence of skin lesions may occur.
- It is possible for mildly affected animals to recover once hygiene and management practices are improved.

MISCELLANEOUS

COMMENTS

Dermatitis devalues the crocodilian skin and can have significant economic consequences.

ZOONOTIC POTENTIAL

- Depending on the specific etiology, zoonosis is possible.
- Appropriate precaution must be taken accordingly.

SYNONYMS

- Greasy alligator disease
- White film disease
- White head
- White slime diseases

ABBREVIATIONS

- ppm = parts per million
- ppt = parts per thousand

Suggested Reading

Lauren DJ. The effect of chronic saline exposure on the electrolyte balance, nitrogen metabolism, and corticosterone titer in the American alligator, *Alligator mississippiensis. Comp Biochem Physiol* 1985; 81A(2):217–223.

Author Javier G. Nevarez, DVM, PhD, DACZM, DECZM (Herpetology)

DERMATOPHILOSIS

BASICS

DEFINITION/OVERVIEW

Dermatophilosis is an infection affecting the skin of various animal species, including crocodilians. It causes an exudative dermatitis with scabs starting between the scales, more often identified on the ventral skin. It is commonly called "brown spot" disease in crocodilians due to the gross appearance of the lesions.

ETIOLOGY/PATHOPHYSIOLOGY

- *Dermatophilus congolensis* was thought to be the only species, but *D. chelonae* has been described from chelonians and snakes, and a new species, *D. crocodyli*, has also been proposed in crocodiles.
- *Dermatophilus* spp. are Gram-positive, facultative anaerobic, non-acid-fast actinomycetes.
- *Dermatophilus* can occur as filamentous hyphae or a motile zoospore.

SIGNALMENT/HISTORY

- More commonly reported in captive, farmed crocodilian species.
- No age or sex predilection.

CLINICAL PRESENTATION

Infected animals have tan to brown crusts and scabs that originate on the junction of the ventral scales and spread outwards.

RISK FACTORS

- Poor hygiene appears to be the predominant predisposing factor.
- Other factors causing immunosuppression such as overcrowding may also play a role.

Husbandry

Improving the overall hygiene by cleaning more frequently, recirculating water, and keeping the facilities clean are the most important husbandry aspects.

Others

N/A

DIAGNOSIS

- Definitive diagnosis is best achieved by histological examination of affected skin.
- Other diagnostics include cytologic examination of impression smears from lesions or minced lesions stained with *Giemsa* stains.
- The bacteria appear filamentous with a segmented, railroad track like appearance.
- Bacterial culture may also be attempted but the organism is challenging to grow consistently.

DIFFERENTIAL DIAGNOSIS

- Pox virus
- Herpesvirus

DIAGNOSTICS

- Histology from affected skin
- Cytology of scabs
- Bacterial culture

PATHOLOGICAL FINDINGS

- Grossly, lesions are characterized as tan to brown coalescing crusts and scabs on the epidermis and dermis.
- Disease is limited to the skin and some cases may be self-limiting, but this is less likely in humid environments.
- Histologically, the characteristic branching hyphae with septation, zoospores and coccoidal cells can be observed in active lesions.
- Organisms may be absent in chronic lesions.

TREATMENT

APPROPRIATE HEALTH CARE

Strict hygiene is the most effective preventative measure.

NUTRITIONAL SUPPORT

Due to the nature of crocodilians and the large number of animals affected at once, force-feeding is not a practical approach.

CLIENT EDUCATION/HUSBANDRY RECOMMENDATIONS

- Maintaining strict hygiene measures is the key to preventing the occurrence of dermatophilosis.
- Water must be changed frequently and the pens scrubbed to eliminate organic matter.

MEDICATIONS

DRUG(S) OF CHOICE

- Topical application of F10® (Health and Hygiene (Pty) Ltd., Stormill, South Africa), 0.5% copper sulfate or 0.5% zinc sulfate.
- Immersion in water with 1 ppm copper sulfate for 15 minutes q12h for 6 weeks or until lesions resolve.

PRECAUTIONS/INTERACTIONS

- Animals must be monitored during treatment for any evidence of distress and rinsed thoroughly afterwards.
- Potential for copper or zinc toxicity is not known when performing topical or immersion treatments.
- These treatments must be done carefully, especially in endangered species.

FOLLOW-UP

PATIENT MONITORING

- Monitor daily during treatment period to determine response to therapy based on resolution of skin lesions.
- Those with resolved lesions should be removed from the treatment group and kept separate.

EXPECTED COURSE AND PROGNOSIS

- When affecting a large number of crocodilians, the overall prognosis is fair to grave, due to the damage to the skin and variable response to therapy when applied in a large scale.
- Prognosis may be better when treating a small number of animals. Even with treatment, reoccurrence of skin lesions may occur.

MISCELLANEOUS

COMMENTS

- Dermatophilosis devalues the crocodilian skin and can have significant economic consequences.
- Figure 1a & b – see web image supplementary content for Section V (Crocodilians).

ZOONOTIC POTENTIAL

Dermatophilosis is zoonotic and humans may contract it after handling infected tissues.

SYNONYMS

Brown spot disease

ABBREVIATIONS

ppm = parts per million

INTERNET RESOURCES

Buenviaje, G. Studies on skin diseases of crocodiles. PhD Thesis, James Cook University; 2000. https://researchonline.jcu.edu.au/27713

Suggested Reading

Buenviaje GN, Hirst RG, Ladds PW, et al. Isolation of *Dermatophilus* sp from skin lesions in farmed saltwater crocodiles (*Crocodylus porosus*). *Aust Vet J* 1997;75(5):365–367.

Buenviaje GN, Ladds PW, Martin Y. Pathology of skin diseases in crocodiles. *Aust Vet J* 1998;76(5):357–363.

Author Javier G. Nevarez, DVM, PhD, DACZM, DECZM (Herpetology)

DYSTOCIA

BASICS

DEFINITION/OVERVIEW

Dystocia is difficulty laying eggs.

ETIOLOGY/PATHOPHYSIOLOGY

- The reproductive cycle of crocodilians is well studied compared with other reptile species.
- Crocodilians are very strong seasonal breeders and the hormone cycle has been described in various species.
- A multitude of environmental and behavioral factors are known to contribute to female reproductive behaviors such as nest building.
- It is reported that young females build nests yet lay no eggs for a few seasons until they reach full sexual maturity.
- A lack of breeding and exposure to males has a negative impact on crocodilians ability to produce follicles and ovulate.
- In addition to basic husbandry aspects such as temperature, humidity, and a proper diet, female reptiles also have a need for appropriate substrate and environment that is conductive for egg laying and crocodilians are thought to be exquisitely sensitive to environmental cues.
- All these reasons explain why dystocia is rare in crocodilians, since they will often not even produce follicles unless the right combination of environmental cues are present.

SIGNALMENT/HISTORY

- Dystocia occurs in female crocodilians of reproductive age or size.
- Most animals have a history of inadequate nutrition and husbandry lacking an appropriate area for laying eggs.

CLINICAL PRESENTATION

- Signs of dystocia may include coelomic distention, straining with or without vocalization, decreased fecal production, cloacal prolapse, hind limb weakness/paresis, lethargy, and anorexia.
- Some animals may also appear restless and be observed attempting to dig.
- In some instances, the eggs may be palpable through the lateral coelomic cavity. This should be done carefully to avoid rupturing the eggs.
- Other abnormalities identified in physical exam may include dehydration, poor body condition score, and pliable bones.

RISK FACTORS

Husbandry

- Inappropriate husbandry is likely a significant contributing factor to the occurrence of dystocia.
- Beyond temperature and humidity, inadequate diet and calcium supplementation is key in the development of NSHP, which in turn can have a significant impact in calcium availability, egg calcification, and contractions of the reproductive tract.
- Crocodilians presenting for dystocia may also have concurrent NSHP.
- An often-forgotten aspect of the husbandry of reproductive female crocodilians is the provision of adequate substrate material for building a nest.
- Crocodilians are known for their nest building and lack of ability to do so is likely to result in dystocia.
- Reptiles that may not perceive the environmental conditions as adequate for successful oviposition may not have the proper stimuli to lay their eggs.

Others

- A less discussed topic is the effect that lack of exposure to males may have on the reproductive cycle of reptiles.
- Crocodilians have well-known courtship and breeding behaviors that likely influence the proper hormonal stimulation of prospective females.
- Female crocodilians kept alone without the benefit of behavioral cues from a male counterpart are likely to have an abnormal reproductive cycle.
- The possibility of a behavioral effect must be considered, especially when animals are maintained in proper husbandry and are otherwise healthy.

DIAGNOSIS

DIFFERENTIAL DIAGNOSIS

- Follicular stasis
- Neoplasia
- Egg yolk coelomitis
- Ovarian cysts
- GI obstruction

DIAGNOSTICS

Imaging

- Radiography: the eggs appear calcified and ovoid.
- Ultrasound appearance of calcified eggs is a well-delineated hyperechogenic eggshell membrane to significant acoustic shadowing.
- Ultrasound may be more sensitive than radiography at diagnosing broken eggs, which may be associated with egg yolk coelomitis.
- CT scan and MRI are extremely sensitive at identifying eggs and can better assess their structure, integrity, and location.

Coelioscopy

- Coelioscopic examination allows for confirmation of the presence of eggs and ruling out egg yolk coelomitis.
- The presence of eggs makes coelioscopy more difficult due to their space-occupying nature.
- Coelioscopy can also be used to assess the viability of the oviduct, based on appearance and coloration.

Hematology and Biochemistry

- A chemistry panel is essential to help in identifying other possible underlying disease processes, such as dehydration and NSHP.
- In addition to Ca and P, Mg levels should be documented as Mg also plays an important role in Ca homeostasis.
- Levels of Mg below 1 mg/dl and/or ionized Ca below 1 mmol/l should be considered deficient.
- Hypercalcemia and hyperphosphatemia are common findings in reproductively active female crocodilians.
- CBC: a leukocytosis indicates a significant inflammatory response that may suggest an additional underlying disease like egg yolk coelomitis.

PATHOLOGICAL FINDINGS

- Grossly, dystocia can be identified by the presence of eggs within the oviduct.
- Pathologic findings may include variation in eggs size, calcification, malformations, broken eggshells, and oviduct torsions.
- Healthy eggs should be smooth, uniform in shape and white in color.
- A deviation from this appearance (i.e., dark, shriveled) is indicative of pathology.

TREATMENT

- It is critical to provide an appropriate nesting area with materials that are found in their natural environment.
- If the crocodilian appears to be stable, medical therapy alone can be attempted and the animal monitored for evidence of egg laying.
- There are no specific timelines as to how quickly egg laying should occur once medical therapy is initiated.

APPROPRIATE HEALTH CARE

- The treatment approach to dystocia is based on the clinical condition at presentation, amount and appearance of the eggs based on imaging or coelioscopy, and the ability to provide a suitable environment for egg laying.
- All crocodilians will benefit from medical treatment, even if surgery is ultimately required.
- Medical therapy consists of correcting the husbandry, providing an appropriate nesting area, and supportive therapy with emphasis on correcting calcium deficiencies.
- Oxytocin or arginine vasotocin can be administered, as long as an obstructive process is not suspected.
- Some recommend the use of beta-adrenergic blockers such as propranolol or atenolol before administration of oxytocin, as these drugs have been shown to potentiate the effects of oxytocin in humans due to their ability to increase uterine activity.

DYSTOCIA (CONTINUED)

- The majority of cases in which there are broken or malformed eggs require surgical intervention.
- Surgery is best performed before dystocia progresses, while the animal is metabolically stable.
- Surgery should be an immediate consideration for animals with documented chronic dystocia, metabolic derangements, and when egg yolk coelomitis is suspected.
- The goal of surgery is to remove the eggs and perform an ovariosalpingectomy to avoid reoccurrence.
- Extreme care must be taken to not rupture the eggs in the coelomic cavity, as the yolk is extremely antigenic and will cause a severe inflammatory response.
- If leakage occurs, the coelomic cavity should be thoroughly lavaged before closure.

NUTRITIONAL SUPPORT

Dietary deficiencies must be corrected with special emphasis on UVB light and oral Ca supplementation.

CLIENT EDUCATION/HUSBANDRY RECOMMENDATIONS

- It is important to establish individual animal baseline values and to confirm the sex of the animal.
- Dystocia likely has a multifactorial cause; all husbandry deficiencies must be corrected, with emphasis on UVB light, calcium supplementation, nutrition, temperature, humidity, and provision of adequate nesting substrate.
- When possible, the animal should be weighed at least weekly to document any sudden weight increases that may be indicative of egg development.
- The possible stressor of these weigh-ins on the animal must be assessed.

MEDICATIONS

DRUG(S) OF CHOICE

- Propranolol 1 mg/kg PO once, at least 3 hours prior to administration of oxytocin or arginine vasotocin.
- Atenolol 7 mg/kg PO once, at least 3 hours prior to administration of oxytocin or arginine vasotocin.
- Arginine vasotocin 0.5–1 µg/kg IV, IO, IM, ICe q12–24h should be administered 30–60 minutes after IM or SC injection of calcium gluconate.
- Oxytocin 5–10 iu/kg IM, IV, IO q4–8h (IV administration may be more efficacious but must be done slowly).
- Calcium: start with calcium gluconate 100 mg/kg IM, SC q12–24h, followed by calcium glubionate 10–100 mg/kg PO q4–24h long term.
- Magnesium sulfate 20 mg/kg IM, SC q24–72h or magnesium lactate (Rescue Cal+, Repashy Ventures, Saskatoon, SK) 20 mg/kg PO q24h.
- Crystalloid fluids 20–30 ml/kg SC, IV, IO q24h
- Meloxicam 0.5 mg/kg PO, IM, SC q 24–48h

PRECAUTIONS/INTERACTIONS

- There is scant information about the safety and efficacy of oxytocin and arginine vasotocin when used for prolonged periods over 2–3 days.
- IV administration of both these drugs should be done slowly as they can cause life-threatening hypotension.
- Beta-adrenergic blockers also may cause bradycardia and hypotension.

FOLLOW-UP

PATIENT MONITORING

- If performing medical therapy alone, especially with oxytocin or arginine vasotocin, the animals should be monitored closely to identify any signs of distress, although this is a rare occurrence.
- If an underlying disease process was diagnosed, appropriate follow-up diagnostics should be performed to determine improvement of that condition or the need to alter therapy.
- For those undergoing surgery, a re-evaluation within 1–2 weeks is recommended to evaluate the surgical site and overall recovery.

EXPECTED COURSE AND PROGNOSIS

- Ultimately, the prognosis will depend on the underlying cause of dystocia and the response to therapy.
- Cases with underlying infectious or metabolic disease that respond to medical therapy have a good prognosis.
- Many cases requiring surgical therapy have a good to guarded prognosis.

MISCELLANEOUS

COMMENTS

- The ultimate diagnosis of dystocia is based on interpretation of clinical signs, history, and results of physical exam and diagnostics.
- In all cases, it is essential to have at least one confirmatory test that there are indeed eggs present in the coelomic cavity.
- It must be mentioned that the sex of the animals must be confirmed as female before surgery is performed since males may present with coelomic neoplasias or GI obstructions that clinically appear very similar to follicular stasis.
- While this may seem obvious, in crocodilians sex determination can be erroneous if done hastily as females possess a large clitoris that may be confused for a phallus.
- To be sure of the sex, the phallus is easily extracted from the cloaca in males while the clitoris remains immobile.

ZOONOTIC POTENTIAL

N/A

SYNONYMS

- Egg bound
- Postovulatory follicular stasis

ABBREVIATIONS

- Ca = calcium
- CBC = complete blood count
- CT scan = computed tomography
- GI = gastrointestinal
- ICe = intracoelemic
- IM = intramuscular
- IO = intraosseous
- IV = intravenous
- Mg = magnesium
- MRI = magnetic resonance imaging
- NSHP = nutritional secondary hyperparathyroidism
- P = phosphorus
- PO = per os
- SC = subcutaneous
- UVB = ultraviolet B

Suggested Reading

Grigg G. Reproduction. In: Grigg G and Kirshner D, eds. *Biology and Evolution of Crocodylians*. Ithaca, NY: Cornell University Press; 2015:431–476.

Hochleithner C, Holland M. Ultrasonography. In: Mader D, Divers SJ, eds. *Current Therapy in Reptile Medicine and Surgery*. St. Louis, MO: Elsevier Saunders, 2014:107–127.

Jacobson ER. Overview of reptile biology, anatomy, and histology. In: Jacobson ER, ed. *Infectious Diseases and Pathology of Reptiles: Color Atlas and Text*. Boca Raton, FL: CRC Press; 2007:14–17.

Author Javier G. Nevarez, DVM, PhD, DACZM, DECZM (Herpetology)

EGG YOLK COELOMITIS

BASICS

DEFINITION/OVERVIEW

Egg yolk coelomitis occurs when yolk material is released into the coelomic cavity as a result of a ruptured follicle or egg due to oophoritis, follicular stasis, dystocia, salpingitis, or aggressive palpation. Egg yolk coelomitis is rare in crocodilians but has been diagnosed in captive and free-ranging animals.

ETIOLOGY/PATHOPHYSIOLOGY

- In all cases, yolk coelomitis is a result of yolk material free within the coelomic cavity overwhelming the body's activity to resorb the material.
- This leads to an intense inflammatory response that is often sterile but can also be associated with secondary bacterial infection.
- It can progress to adhesions throughout the coelomic cavity, septicemia, and death.

SIGNALMENT/HISTORY

- Egg yolk coelomitis occurs in female crocodilians of reproductive age or size.
- Most animals have a history of inadequate husbandry, being housed alone without access to a male, and lacking an appropriate area for laying eggs or giving birth.

CLINICAL PRESENTATION

- Crocodilians with yolk coelomitis often present with non-specific clinical signs like anorexia and lethargy.
- Some animals may present with coelomic distention.
- Other abnormalities identified in physical exam may include hind limb weakness/paresis, dehydration, poor body condition score, and pliable bones.
- Some animals may present obtunded due to rapid progression of the disease.

RISK FACTORS

Husbandry

- Any factors that may results in follicular stasis or dystocia are also contributing factors to yolk coelomitis.
- These include inadequate husbandry, nutrition, brumation, and nesting environment.

Others

- A less discussed topic is the effect that lack of exposure to males may have on the reproductive cycle of reptiles.
- Crocodilians have well known courtship and breeding behaviors that likely influence the proper hormonal stimulation of prospective females.
- Female crocodilians in kept alone without the benefit of behavioral cues from a male counterpart are likely to have an abnormal reproductive cycle.
- This possibility of a behavioral effect must be considered, especially when animals are maintained in proper husbandry and are otherwise healthy.

DIAGNOSIS

DIFFERENTIAL DIAGNOSIS

- Follicular stasis
- Dystocia
- Neoplasia
- Ovarian cysts
- GI obstruction
- Septicemia

DIAGNOSTICS

Imaging

- Radiographs: Radiographic findings may include free fluid, follicles, or ruptured eggs.
- Ultrasound: aspiration of any free fluid can be used to diagnose egg yolk coelomitis.
- CT scan and MRI: Both these modalities are extremely sensitive for evaluation of the reproductive tract. They can also help assess damage to other organs.

Cytology

- Evaluation of free fluid in the coelomic cavity will be a confirmatory test of yolk coelomitis.
- In acute cases, the fluid is yellow to white with high amount of proteinaceous material and inflammatory cells.
- In chronic cases, the fluid may appear cloudier.
- Blood and bacteria may also be observed with either presentation.

Coelioscopy

- Coelioscopic examination allows for confirmation of yolk coelomitis but may be confounded by changes in anatomy due to adhesions.

Hematology and Biochemistry

- A chemistry panel is essential to help identify other possible underlying disease processes such as dehydration and NSHP.
- In addition to Ca and P, Mg levels should be documented as Mg also plays an important role in Ca homeostasis.
- Levels of Mg below 1 mg/dl and/or ionized Ca below 1 mmol/l should be considered deficient.
- Hypercalcemia and hyperphosphatemia are common findings in reproductively active female lizards. Hyperproteinemia, anemia, and hypoglycemia may also be identified.
- CBC: a leukocytosis may be observed but does not always occur, especially in chronic cases.
- Leukopenia may be present if sepsis has ensued.

PATHOLOGICAL FINDINGS

- During the acute stages, egg yolk coelomitis presents as yellow to white, viscous, free fluid within the cavity.
- Fragments of more solid yolk may also be free-floating within the cavity.
- Chronically more adhesions develop and form a white fibrinous to fibrotic membrane on the serosal surfaces of the organs.
- The lesions are often severe enough that surgical repair is not possible.
- Many cases are diagnosed postmortem.

TREATMENT

APPROPRIATE HEALTH CARE

- Any underlying abnormalities (e.g., NSHP, dehydration, anemia) must be treated accordingly.
- These animals must also receive anti-inflammatories and analgesics as the reaction to the yolk and subsequent adhesions are extremely painful.
- Animals with yolk coelomitis must undergo surgery in an attempt to correct the condition but it is often fatal.
- The goal of exploratory coeliotomy is to determine the severity of the diseases and whether successful lavage and cleaning of the cavity can be performed.
- Any free-floating material must be removed and the cavity lavaged copiously to remove the protein. If this can be accomplished, an ovariosalpingectomy is performed.

NUTRITIONAL SUPPORT

Dietary deficiencies must be corrected with special emphasis on UVB light and oral Ca supplementation.

CLIENT EDUCATION/HUSBANDRY RECOMMENDATIONS

- It is important to establish individual baseline values and confirm the sex of the animal.
- Egg yolk coelomitis occurs as a sequel to multifactorial causes, therefore all husbandry deficiencies must be corrected with emphasis on UVB light, calcium supplementation, nutrition, temperature, humidity, and provision of adequate nesting substrate for oviparous species.
- When possible, the animal should be weighed at least weekly to document any sudden weight increases that may be indicative of egg development.
- The possible stressor of these weigh-ins on the animal must be assessed.

EGG YOLK COELOMITIS (CONTINUED)

MEDICATIONS

DRUG(S) OF CHOICE

- Meloxicam 0.5 mg/kg PO, IM, SC q24–48h
- Morphine 1–10 mg/kg IM, SC q24h
- Hydromorphone 0.2–0.5 mg/kg IM, SC q12–24h

PRECAUTIONS/INTERACTIONS

- Morphine and hydromorphone can cause sedation and respiratory depression.
- Dose and frequency of administration should be refined based on the patient's response.

FOLLOW-UP

PATIENT MONITORING

- If an underlying disease process was diagnosed, appropriate follow-up diagnostics should be performed to determine improvement of that condition or the need to alter therapy.
- A re-evaluation within 1–2 weeks of surgery is recommended to evaluate the surgical site and overall recovery.

EXPECTED COURSE AND PROGNOSIS

- The overall prognosis will depend on the speed with which the diseases is recognized by the caretakers and diagnosed and treated by the veterinarian.
- Per-acute to acute cases have a fair prognosis.
- Chronic cases have a grave prognosis.

MISCELLANEOUS

COMMENTS

N/A

ZOONOTIC POTENTIAL

N/A

SYNONYMS

- Egg coelomitis/peritonitis
- Yolk coelomitis/peritonitis

ABBREVIATIONS

- Ca = calcium
- CT scan = computed tomography
- GI = gastrointestinal
- IM = intramuscular
- Mg = magnesium
- MRI = magnetic resonance imaging
- NSHP = nutritional secondary hyperparathyroidism
- P = phosphorus
- SC = subcutaneous
- UVB = ultraviolet B

INTERNET RESOURCES

Pollock C. Reproductive disease in reptiles: twelve key facts. https://lafeber.com/vet/reproductive-disease-in-reptiles-twelve-key-facts

Suggested Reading

Grigg G. Reproduction. In: Grigg G and Kirshner D, eds. *Biology and Evolution of Crocodylians*. Ithaca, NY: Cornell University Press; 2015:431–476.

Taylor HW, McDonald MM. Egg yolk serositis in an American alligator (*Alligator mississippiensis*). *J Wild Dis* 1988;24(4):700–702.

Author Javier G. Nevarez, DVM, PhD, DACZM, DECZM (Herpetology)

EIMERIA

BASICS

DEFINITION/OVERVIEW

Eimeria is a genus of apicomplexan parasites characterized by oocytes having four sporocysts that each contain two sporozoites. *Eimeria* spp. are typically intracytoplasmic parasites, but some have been described as having intranuclear development. They rarely cause disease and commonly form a normal component of the gastrointestinal flora of reptiles.

ETIOLOGY/PATHOPHYSIOLOGY

- Over 200 species of *Eimeria* have been described in reptiles.
- With the advent of molecular techniques, the rate of species discovery is increasing exponentially.
- *Eimeria* spp. have a direct life cycle with infective stages passed in the feces of the host.
- *Eimeria* can be found in the gallbladder, bile ducts, and intestinal epithelium of snakes, lizards, and crocodilians.
- Most reports of illness associated with *Eimeria* infection are from captive animals that have been housed under suboptimal conditions.
- Virulence may be exacerbated by a range of intrinsic and extrinsic factors such as concurrent disease and infective dose.
- Although a range of *Eimeria* spp. have been identified from crocodilians, none has been associated with disease.

SIGNALMENT/HISTORY

- Animals kept at high stocking density.
- Unsanitary conditions
- Maladaptation of wild animals entering captive situations.

CLINICAL PRESENTATION

No disease known

RISK FACTORS

Husbandry

New (captive or wild) animals entering a collection with poor hygiene and high stocking densities.

Others

N/A

DIAGNOSIS

DIFFERENTIAL DIAGNOSIS

Other gastrointestinal disease such as bacterial or protozoal infections (i.e., *Isospora*).

DIAGNOSTICS

- Examination of feces for presence of oocysts using light microscopy is the most reliable test.
- Molecular techniques such as PCR may aid in species delineation but are unlikely to improve treatment efficacy or prognosis.
- Protozoa may also be seen in biopsy or necropsy samples.
- For preservation of coccidia for future diagnostics, fecal samples should be stored in 2–3% aqueous (w/v) potassium dichromate ($K_2Cr_2O_7$).

PATHOLOGICAL FINDINGS

None reported

TREATMENT

APPROPRIATE HEALTH CARE

- Because *Eimeria* spp. are not reported pathogens in crocodilians, prophylactic therapy or treatment based on the identification of *Eimeria* spp. alone should not be performed, to avoid development of resistance.
- If clinical disease is confirmed, treatment can be performed with protocols used in other reptile species.

NUTRITIONAL SUPPORT

N/A

CLIENT EDUCATION/HUSBANDRY RECOMMENDATIONS

- Monitor infected individuals for development of any clinical signs.
- Reduce stress by providing optimal living conditions, and hygiene.
- Thorough cleaning of cage to reduce environmental contamination of oocysts.
- Ensure that quarantine protocols have been adopted for all new arrivals and during quarantine all animals should be subjected to repeated clinical and fecal examinations.

MEDICATIONS

DRUG(S) OF CHOICE

N/A

PRECAUTIONS/INTERACTIONS

N/A

FOLLOW-UP

PATIENT MONITORING

Repeat fecal examination at monthly intervals.

EXPECTED COURSE AND PROGNOSIS

Since no clinical disease has been reported in crocodilians, prognosis is excellent.

MISCELLANEOUS

COMMENTS

N/A

ZOONOTIC POTENTIAL

Due to their high host-specificity there is no known zoonotic risk with any *Eimeria* species.

SYNONYMS

N/A

ABBREVIATIONS

PCR = polymerase chain reaction

Suggested Reading

Jacobson ER. Parasites and parasitic diseases of reptiles. In: Jacobson ER, ed. *Infectious Diseases and Pathology of Reptiles: Color Atlas and Text.* Boca Raton, FL: CRC Press; 2008:571–665.

Author T. Franciscus Scheelings, BVSc, MVSc, PhD, MANCVSc (Wildlife Health), DECZM (Herpetology)

FOLLICULAR STASIS

BASICS

DEFINITION/OVERVIEW

Follicular stasis is the retention of ovarian follicles. Normally, follicles ovulate into the oviduct or undergo atresia. If neither happens, the reptile is considered to be in follicular stasis. Identifying whether the presence of follicles is pathologic or physiologic is difficult, given that, most of the time, the stage of the reproductive cycle in an individual animal is unknown. A diagnosis of follicular stasis is often made once the animal starts showing clinical signs of illness or follicles are present for a longer period than expected for the species. Follicular stasis is an uncommon presentation in crocodilians.

ETIOLOGY/PATHOPHYSIOLOGY

- Follicles can fail to ovulate and undergo atresia for a number of reasons, but in most cases an abnormal hormonal status can be assumed.
- The reproductive cycle of crocodilians is well studied compared with other reptile species.
- Crocodilians are very strong seasonal breeders and the hormone cycle has been described in various species.
- A multitude of environmental and behavioral factors are known to contribute to female reproductive behaviors such as nest building.
- It is reported that young females build nests yet lay no eggs for a few seasons until they reach full sexual maturity.
- A lack of breeding and exposure to males has a negative impact on crocodilians ability to produce follicles and ovulate.
- In addition to basic husbandry aspects such as temperature, humidity and a proper diet, female reptiles also have a need for appropriate substrate and environment that is conductive for egg laying and crocodilians are thought to be exquisitely sensitive to environmental cues.
- All these reasons explain why follicular stasis is rare in crocodilians, since they will not even produce follicles unless the right combination of environmental cues is present.

SIGNALMENT/HISTORY

- Follicular stasis occurs in female crocodilians of reproductive age or size.
- It is likely more common in older females but there are not enough data to confirm an age predisposition.
- A history of inadequate husbandry, being housed alone without access to a male, and lacking an appropriate area/substrate for building a nest may be part of the presenting history.
- There may also be crocodilians with appropriate husbandry that still suffer from follicular stasis for unknown reasons.

CLINICAL PRESENTATION

- Crocodilians with follicular stasis often present for non-specific clinical signs like anorexia and lethargy.
- These could be due to the pathologic effects of the retained follicles, an underlying disease, or both.
- Some animals may present with coelomic distention but follicles are not easily palpable.
- Palpation of the coelomic cavity must be done gently to avoid rupturing the follicles.
- In the majority of cases, the caretakers are not aware of the fact that the crocodilian is in follicular stasis.
- Other abnormalities identified in physical exam may include dehydration, poor body condition score, and significant weight gain that does not match with the growth of the animal.
- Because of their strong seasonality, it is easier to determine when a crocodilian may be in follicular stasis by simply looking at the time of the year and the expected cycle for the animal at that period.

RISK FACTORS

Husbandry

- Inappropriate husbandry is likely a significant contributing factor to the occurrence of follicular stasis.
- Beyond temperature and humidity, inadequate nutrition such as UVB light exposure, vitamin D3 intake, and calcium supplementation are key in the development of NSHP, which in turn can have a significant impact in calcium availability and follicular development.
- Crocodilians presenting with follicular stasis should be evaluated for concurrent NSHP.
- An often-forgotten aspect of the husbandry of reproductive female reptiles is the provision of an adequate substrate for nesting/oviposition. This is a critical aspect for crocodilian species.
- It is often accepted that reptiles that may not perceive the environmental conditions are adequate for successful reproduction will resorb the follicles through atresia.
- Crocodilians may not even produce follicles if the conditions are not adequate.
- In captivity, there may be a combination of factors that do not allow for normal follicular atresia.

Others

- A less discussed topic is the effect that lack of exposure to males may have on the reproductive cycle of reptiles.
- Crocodilians have well known courtship and breeding behaviors that likely influence the proper hormonal stimulation of prospective females.
- Female crocodilians in kept alone without the benefit of behavioral cues from a male counterpart are likely to have an abnormal reproductive cycle.
- This possibility of a behavioral effect must be considered, especially when animals are maintained in proper husbandry and are otherwise healthy.

DIAGNOSIS

DIFFERENTIAL DIAGNOSIS

- Dystocia
- Neoplasia
- Egg yolk coelomitis
- Ovarian cysts
- GI obstruction

DIAGNOSTICS

Imaging

- Radiography: follicles appear as non-calcified, round to ovoid, variably sized soft tissue opacities in the caudal coelom. At times, the follicles may either be large enough or of large enough numbers to encompass over 50% of the coelomic cavity.
- Ultrasound: early follicles appear as anechoic and progress to have more echogenicity as they mature or fail to ovulate. Follicles with a more heterogeneous distribution within the lumen should be highly suspicious of being retained follicles as the material within becomes firmer and inspissated.
- Ultrasound examination and aspiration of any free fluid can also be used to rule out egg yolk coelomitis.
- CT and MRI are extremely sensitive at identifying follicles and can better assess the differences in size, shape and content of the follicles.

Coelioscopy

Coelioscopic examination allows for confirmation of the presence of follicles and evaluation of their color and size to help determine whether the presentation may be pathologic.

Hematology and Biochemistry

- A chemistry panel is essential to help identify other possible underlying disease processes such as dehydration and NSHP. In addition to Ca and P, Mg levels should be documented as Mg also plays an important role in Ca homeostasis.
- Levels of Mg below 1 mg/dl should be considered deficient.
- Hypercalcemia and hyperphosphatemia are common findings in reproductively active female crocodilians.

- CBC: a leukocytosis indicates a significant inflammatory response that may suggest an additional underlying disease like egg yolk coelomitis.

PATHOLOGICAL FINDINGS

- Grossly, follicular stasis can be differentiated from dystocia by the presence of follicles outside of the oviduct.
- At times, the follicles may be large enough to appear to be in chains but are surrounded by the ovarian membrane rather than the oviduct.
- Healthy follicles should be smooth and white to yellow in color.
- A deviation from this appearance (i.e., dark, shriveled or cystic follicles) is indicative of pathology.

TREATMENT

- Surgery is best performed before stasis progresses while the animal is metabolically stable.
- Surgery should be an immediate consideration for crocodilians with documented chronic stasis, metabolic derangements, and when egg yolk coelomitis is suspected.
- The goal of surgery is to remove the follicles and perform an ovariectomy in order to avoid reoccurrence.
- Follicular stasis is commonly associated with follicles on both ovaries but even if only one is affected, bilateral ovariectomy is recommended.
- Extreme care must be taken to not rupture the follicles in the coelomic cavity, as the yolk is extremely antigenic and will cause a severe inflammatory response.
- If leakage occurs, the coelomic cavity should be thoroughly lavaged before closure.

APPROPRIATE HEALTH CARE

- The treatment approach to follicular stasis is based on diagnosis and treatment of contributing factors leading to the stasis and treatment of the stasis itself.
- The clinical condition at presentation, time of the year, amount and appearance of the follicles based on imaging or coelioscopy, and ability to provide a suitable environment all contribute to the decision-making process.
- When housed in unnatural climates for the species, the normal cycle may be altered.
- All crocodilians will benefit from medical treatment even if surgery is ultimately required.
- Medical therapy consists of correcting the husbandry, providing an appropriate nesting area and substrate, and supportive therapy with emphasis on calcium supplementation.
- If the crocodilian appears to be stable, medical therapy alone can be attempted and the animal monitored for evidence of follicular atresia.
- By the end of the reproductive season, it would be expected that follicular atresia would occur.

NUTRITIONAL SUPPORT

Dietary deficiencies must be corrected with special emphasis on UVB light exposure/vitamin D3 intake and oral Ca supplementation.

CLIENT EDUCATION/HUSBANDRY RECOMMENDATIONS

- Caretakers should be encouraged to seek veterinary care of crocodilians early on to establish individual baseline values and confirm the sex of the animal.
- Follicular stasis likely has a multifactorial cause, so all husbandry deficiencies must be corrected, such as nutrition, temperature, humidity, and provision of adequate nesting substrate and environment.
- Sudden, unexplained, weight increases and/or coelomic distention may be indicative of follicular development.

SURGICAL CONSIDERATIONS

Surgical intervention is required if atresia has not occurred within a few weeks of the end of the reproductive cycle.

MEDICATIONS

DRUG(S) OF CHOICE

- Calcium: start with calcium gluconate 100 mg/kg IM, SC q 12–24h, followed by calcium glubionate 10–100 mg/kg PO q4–24h long term.
- Magnesium sulfate 20 mg/kg IM, SC q24–72h, or magnesium lactate (Rescue Cal+, Repashy Ventures, Saskatoon, SK) 20 mg/kg PO q24h.
- Crystalloid fluids 20–30 ml/kg SC, IV q24h
- Meloxicam 0.5 mg/kg PO, IM, SC q24–48h
- Morphine 1–10 mg/kg IM, SC q24 h
- Hydromorphone 0.2–0.5 mg/kg IM, SC q12–24h

PRECAUTIONS/INTERACTIONS

- Morphine and hydromorphone can cause sedation and respiratory depression.
- Dose and frequency of administration should be refined based on the patient's response.

FOLLOW-UP

PATIENT MONITORING

- If performing medical therapy alone, the weight of the crocodilian should be recorded weekly, if possible, to provide an early indication that follicle atresia may be occurring.
- Any acute weight losses beyond 10% of the body weight should prompt re-evaluation by a veterinarian.
- If an underlying disease process was diagnosed, appropriate follow up diagnostics should be performed to determine improvement of that condition or the need to alter therapy.
- For those undergoing surgery, a re-evaluation with 1–2 weeks is recommended to evaluate the surgical site and overall recovery.

EXPECTED COURSE AND PROGNOSIS

- Ultimately, the prognosis will depend on the underlying cause of follicular stasis and the required therapy.
- Cases with underlying infectious or metabolic disease that respond to medical therapy have a good prognosis.
- Many cases requiring surgical therapy have a good to guarded prognosis.

MISCELLANEOUS

COMMENTS

- The ultimate diagnosis of follicular stasis is based on interpretation of clinical signs, history, and results of physical exam and diagnostics.
- Before ovariectomy is performed, it is essential to have at least one confirmatory test that there are indeed follicles present in the coelomic cavity.
- It must be mentioned that the sex of the animals must be confirmed as female before surgery is performed since males may present with coelomic neoplasias or GI obstructions that clinically appear very similar to follicular stasis.
- While this may seem obvious, in crocodilians sex determination can be erroneous if done hastily, as females possess a large clitoris which may be confused with a phallus.
- To be sure of the sex, the phallus is easily extracted from the cloaca in males, while the clitoris remains immobile.

ZOONOTIC POTENTIAL

N/A

SYNONYMS

Preovulatory follicular stasis

ABBREVIATIONS

- Ca = calcium
- CT scan = computed tomography
- GI = gastrointestinal
- IM = intramuscular
- Mg = magnesium
- MRI = magnetic resonance imaging

FOLLICULAR STASIS (CONTINUED)

- NSHP = nutritional secondary hyperparathyroidism
- P = phosphorus
- PO = per os
- SC = subcutaneous
- UVB = ultraviolet B

Suggested Reading

Grigg G. Reproduction. In: Grigg G and Kirshner D, eds. *Biology and Evolution of Crocodylians*. Ithaca, NY: Cornell University Press; 2015:431–476.

Jacobson ER. Overview of reptile biology, anatomy, and histology. In: Jacobson ER, ed. *Infectious Diseases and Pathology of Reptiles: Color Atlas and Text*. Boca Raton, FL: CRC Press; 2007:14–17.

Author Javier G. Nevarez, DVM, PhD, DACZM, DECZM (Herpetology)

HYPERGLYCEMIA

BASICS

DEFINITION/OVERVIEW
Hyperglycemia is abnormally high blood glucose concentration. In most species, glucose concentrations fluctuate. Normal glucose concentration ranges from 60 mg/dl to 200 mg/dl (3.3–11 mmol/l).

ETIOLOGY/PATHOPHYSIOLOGY
- The etiology is largely unknown.
- Transient hyperglycemia may be postprandial or stress induced.
- Elevated glucose may be seen during ovulation and with certain neoplastic processes.
- Iatrogenic from prior glucose or glucocorticosteroid administration.
- It is speculated that endocrine pancreas disease may lead to insulin deficiency resulting in a diabetes mellitus-like syndrome, but this has not been documented.

SIGNALMENT/HISTORY
N/A

CLINICAL PRESENTATION
- Unspecific
- Possibly increased water consumption, increased urine (urate) production, and weight loss.

RISK FACTORS
- Largely unknown
- Stress from handling or improper housing may predispose.

Husbandry
N/A

Others
N/A

DIAGNOSIS
- Blood glucose analysis
- Levels above 200 mg/dl (11 mmol/l) indicate hyperglycemia.

DIFFERENTIAL DIAGNOSIS
N/A

DIAGNOSTICS
- Blood glucose measurements should be repeated, as a single elevated value likely is insignificant.
- Persistent hyperglycemia is a more relevant finding.
- Glucosuria should be evaluated to identify chronic hyperglycemia.
- Underlying causes should be investigated: ovarian activity, neoplasia, metabolic disease.

PATHOLOGICAL FINDINGS
The etiology for persistent hyperglycemia is unknown, but the endocrine pancreas should be thoroughly evaluated.

TREATMENT

APPROPRIATE HEALTH CARE
N/A

NUTRITIONAL SUPPORT
N/A

CLIENT EDUCATION/HUSBANDRY RECOMMENDATIONS
N/A

MEDICATIONS

DRUG(S) OF CHOICE
- In cases with persistent hyperglycemia, where systemic disease has been ruled out, experimental insulin treatment may be attempted.

Suggested starting dose: 5–10 iu q24–48h

PRECAUTIONS/INTERACTIONS
N/A

FOLLOW-UP

PATIENT MONITORING
- Follow up with repeated glucose measurements.
- Monitor general health of patient.

EXPECTED COURSE AND PROGNOSIS
- Transient hyperglycemia is likely insignificant.
- Chronically elevated levels carry a poor prognosis.

MISCELLANEOUS

COMMENTS
N/A

ZOONOTIC POTENTIAL
N/A

SYNONYMS
N/A

INTERNET RESOURCES
Kaplan M. Hypoglycemia and Hyperglycemia in Reptiles. Melissa Kaplan's Herp Care Collection, January 1, 2014. http://www.anapsid.org/diabetes.html

Suggested Reading
Campbell TW. Clinical pathology. In: Mader DR, Divers SJ, eds. *Current Therapy in Reptile Medicine and Surgery*. St. Louis, MO: Elsevier; 2014:70–92.

Stahl SJ. Hyperglycemia in reptiles. In: Mader DR, ed. *Reptile Medicine and Surgery*. 2nd ed. St. Louis, MO: Elsevier Saunders; 2006:822–830.

Author Mads F. Bertelsen, DVM, DVSc, DACZM, DECZM (Zoo Health Management)

HYPOGLYCEMIA

BASICS

DEFINITION/OVERVIEW
Hypoglycemia is abnormally low blood glucose concentration. In most species, glucose concentrations fluctuate, and normal concentrations range from 60 mg/dl to 200 mg/dl (3.3–11 mmol/l), although lower values may be normal.

ETIOLOGY/PATHOPHYSIOLOGY
- Exhaustion, starvation, malnutrition
- Septicemia
- Hepatobiliary disease
- Pancreatic disease
- Possibly stress-induced syndrome

SIGNALMENT/HISTORY
- Animals with severe systemic disease may be predisposed.
- Long-lasting anorexia

CLINICAL PRESENTATION
- Weakness
- Tremors
- Loss of righting reflex
- Torpor
- Unresponsiveness

RISK FACTORS
- Systemic disease
- Poor nutritional status

Husbandry
N/A

Others
N/A

DIAGNOSIS

DIFFERENTIAL DIAGNOSIS
N/A

DIAGNOSTICS
- Blood glucose levels below 20 mg/dl (1.1 mmol/l) indicate hypoglycemia.
- Detection of hypoglycemia in a clinically healthy animal should not cause concern.
- In animals with clinical signs and hypoglycemia, attempts should be made to rule out septicemia, hepatobiliary disease, and pancreatic neoplasia.
- Glucose may be artificially low in blood samples stored for a prolonged period prior to separation of plasma/serum.

PATHOLOGICAL FINDINGS
- Depends on underlying etiology
- The pancreas should be thoroughly evaluated.

TREATMENT

APPROPRIATE HEALTH CARE
Treat underlying disease

NUTRITIONAL SUPPORT
Consider energy-rich nutritional support by stomach tube in cases of anorexia.

CLIENT EDUCATION/HUSBANDRY RECOMMENDATIONS
If related to poor nutrition and management, educate client on appropriate feeding practices.

MEDICATIONS

DRUG(S) OF CHOICE
Supportive administration of glucose or dextrose parenterally (e.g., 2.5% in 0.45% saline, 20–40 ml/kg SC) or orally (3 g/kg PO) may be indicated.

PRECAUTIONS/INTERACTIONS
N/A

FOLLOW-UP

PATIENT MONITORING
Monitor glucose levels and clinical signs.

EXPECTED COURSE AND PROGNOSIS
- If related to nutritional status prognosis is good.
- If secondary to severe systemic disease prognosis is poor.

MISCELLANEOUS

COMMENTS
N/A

ZOONOTIC POTENTIAL
N/A

SYNONYMS
N/A

ABBREVIATIONS
- PO = per os
- SC = subcutaneous

INTERNET RESOURCES
Kaplan M. Hypoglycemia and Hyperglycemia in Reptiles. Melissa Kaplan's Herp Care Collection, January 1, 2014. http://www.anapsid.org/diabetes.html

Suggested Reading

Campbell T. Clinical Pathology. In: Mader DR, Divers SJ, eds. *Current Therapy in Reptile Medicine and Surgery*. St. Louis, MO: Elsevier; 2014:70–92.

Stahl SJ. Hyperglycemia in reptiles. In: Mader DR, ed. *Reptile Medicine and Surgery*. 2nd ed. St. Louis, MO: Elsevier Saunders; 2006: 822–830.

Author Mads F. Bertelsen, DVM, DVSc, DACZM, DECZM (Zoo Health Management)

HYPOXIA

BASICS

DEFINITION/OVERVIEW

Suspected cases of hypoxia are known to occur in captive crocodilian operations due to low levels of oxygen in the air. In some cases, increased ammonia levels are suspected to be a concurrent or contributing factor.

ETIOLOGY/PATHOPHYSIOLOGY

- The full pathophysiology has not been studied at this point.
- Clinical impressions are that increased temperatures within the buildings, in conjunction with high levels of ammonia and fermentable food, lead to oxygen depletion in the air.

SIGNALMENT/HISTORY

- Can affect any age and sex.
- Occurs most commonly during warmer months of the year.
- Part of the historical information may involve having skipped a cleaning day, overfeeding, or observation of remnant food in the buildings.

CLINICAL PRESENTATION

- Animals present with neurologic signs including difficulty swimming and walking, head tilt, and being obtunded.
- Animals may also appear to have difficulty breathing.
- Per acute to acute death may also be observed.

RISK FACTORS

High environmental temperatures, infrequent cleaning of the pens, and increased amount of left-over, uneaten food are all factors that appear to be associate with occurrence of this problem.

Husbandry

N/A

Others

N/A

DIAGNOSIS

Diagnosis is based on clinical presentation, history, response to management changes, and ruling out other diseases.

DIFFERENTIAL DIAGNOSIS

- West Nile virus
- Aflatoxicosis
- Pneumonia

DIAGNOSTICS

- Histopathology: Necropsy and histopathological evaluation should be performed to rule out any other disease factor.
- WNV RT-PCR: Animals should be tested to rule out West Nile virus, as it can have a very similar presentation.
  - Liver and brain tissue (pooled samples) can be used for fast diagnosis using RT-PCR.

PATHOLOGICAL FINDINGS

There is usually an absence of specific histopathologic lesions, other than inflammation of the respiratory tract.

TREATMENT

APPROPRIATE HEALTH CARE

- Allow fresh air into the building.
- Improve hygiene by changing the water and cleaning any food remnants.

NUTRITIONAL SUPPORT

N/A

CLIENT EDUCATION/HUSBANDRY RECOMMENDATIONS

- It is critical to ensure that water changes are performed frequently.
- Any food remnants must be removed, especially during warm weather.
- Fresh air should be allowed to circulate through the buildings.
- Installing ventilation fans can help to eliminate the occurrence of this condition.

MEDICATIONS

DRUG(S) OF CHOICE

N/A

PRECAUTIONS/INTERACTIONS

N/A

FOLLOW-UP

PATIENT MONITORING

Within 24–48 hours of addressing the problem, animals should return back to normal and clinical signs dissipate completely.

EXPECTED COURSE AND PROGNOSIS

- The majority of animals recover once treatment is applied, with the allowance of fresh air into the building having a significant impact within hours.
- In most cases, there is a high morbidity with low mortality.

MISCELLANEOUS

COMMENTS

N/A

ZOONOTIC POTENTIAL

- While there is no disease per se, workers do often report a strong odor upon entering the building and sometimes feeling short of breath.
- It is recommended that the building doors be opened to allow air exchange before working in the building when this situation is encountered.

SYNONYMS

- Bad air
- Toxic air

ABBREVIATIONS

- RT-PCR = reverse transcriptase polymerase chain reaction
- WNV = West Nile virus

Author Javier G. Nevarez, DVM, PhD, DACZM, DECZM (Herpetology)

ISOSPORA

BASICS

DEFINITION/OVERVIEW

Isospora is an apicomplexan parasite with two sporocysts containing four sporozoites. *Isospora* spp. are typically intracytoplasmic parasites, but some may have intranuclear development.

ETIOLOGY/PATHOPHYSIOLOGY

- *Isospora* has a direct life cycle with infective stages passed in the feces of the host.
- Infections are confined to the intestines.
- Most reports of illness associated with *Isospora* infection are from captive animals that have been housed under suboptimal conditions, with infection often further complicated by concurrent disease such as dependoviruses and adenoviruses.
- *Isospora* spp. have been isolated from crocodilians but have not been associated with clinical disease.

SIGNALMENT/HISTORY

- High stocking density
- Unsanitary conditions
- Maladaptation of wild animals entering captivity.

CLINICAL PRESENTATION

None reported, but may relate to GI upset.

RISK FACTORS

Husbandry

- Breeding colonies at high stocking density are at greatest risk.
- Poor hygiene and stress are likely to predispose to infection and disease.

Others

Concurrent disease or excessive stress may cause immunosuppression, increasing risks of disease expression.

DIAGNOSIS

DIFFERENTIAL DIAGNOSIS

Other GI disease such as bacterial or protozoal infections (i.e., *Eimeria*).

DIAGNOSTIS

- Examination of feces for presence of oocysts using light microscopy.
- Molecular techniques such as PCR may aid in species delineation but are unlikely to improve treatment efficacy or prognosis.
- Protozoa may also be seen in biopsy or necropsy samples.
- Fecal samples should be stored in 2–3% of aqueous (w/v) potassium dichromate ($K_2Cr_2O_7$).

PATHOLOGICAL FINDINGS

- Gross lesions may be mild and unapparent in many cases.
- Histologically, there may be small intestinal villous atrophy with intracytoplasmic coccidia within enterocytes.

TREATMENT

APPROPRIATE HEALTH CARE

- Because *Isospora* spp. are not reported pathogens in crocodilians, prophylactic therapy or treatment should not be based on the identification of *Isospora* spp. alone, to avoid development of resistance.
- If clinical disease is confirmed, treatment with protocols used in other reptile species can be adopted.

NUTRITIONAL SUPPORT

N/A

CLIENT EDUCATION/HUSBANDRY RECOMMENDATIONS

- Monitor infected individuals for development of any clinical signs.
- Reduce stress by providing optimal living conditions, and hygiene.
- Thoroughly clean the cage to reduce environmental contamination of oocysts.
- Ensure that quarantine protocols have been adopted for all new arrivals.
- During quarantine all animals should be subjected to repeated clinical and fecal examinations.
- Keep stocking densities as low as possible, especially in stressful conditions such as breeding colonies.

MEDICATIONS

DRUG(S) OF CHOICE

N/A

PRECAUTIONS/INTERACTIONS

N/A

FOLLOW-UP

PATIENT MONITORING

Repeat fecal examination at monthly intervals.

EXPECTED COURSE AND PROGNOSIS

Since no clinical disease has been reported in crocodilians, prognosis is excellent.

MISCELLANEOUS

COMMENTS

N/A

ZOONOTIC POTENTIAL

N/A

SYNONYMS

N/A

ABBREVIATIONS

- GI = gastrointestinal
- PCR = polymerase chain reaction

Suggested Reading

Jacobson ER. Parasites and parasitic diseases of reptiles. In: Jacobson ER, ed. *Infectious Diseases and Pathology of Reptiles: Color Atlas and Text*. Boca Raton, FL: CRC Press; 2008: 571–665.

Kim DY, Mitchell MA, Bauer RW, et al. An outbreak of adenoviral infection in inland bearded dragons (*Pogona vitticeps*) coinfected with *Dependovirus* and coccidial protozoa (*Isospora* sp.). *J Vet Diagn Invest* 2002;14:332–334.

Wolf D, Vrhovec MG, Failing K, et al. Diagnosis of gastrointestinal parasites in reptiles: comparison of two coprological methods. *Acta Vet Scand* 2014;56:1–13.

Author T. Franciscus Scheelings, BVSc, MVSc, PhD, MANCVSc (Wildlife Health), DECZM (Herpetology)

MYCOPLASMOSIS

BASICS

DEFINITION/OVERVIEW
Mycoplasmosis has been reported in naturally and experimentally infected American alligators (*Alligator mississippiensis*) and experimentally infected broad-nosed caimans (*Caiman latirostris*). Siamese crocodiles (*Crocodylus siamensis*) did not develop disease upon experimental infection, but antibodies could be detected in all three species. Naturally occurring mycoplasmosis has also been reported in Nile crocodiles (*C. niloticus*).

ETIOLOGY/PATHOPHYSIOLOGY
- *Mycoplasma alligatoris* causes natural infection in *A. mississippiensis*.
- *M. crocodyli* causes infection in *C. niloticus*.

SIGNALMENT/HISTORY
- No sex or age predilection
- Natural infection only reported in *A. mississippiensis* and *C. niloticus*, but other species are suspected to be susceptible.

CLINICAL PRESENTATION
- Signs are usually non-specific, including weakness, lethargy, and anorexia.
- Ocular discharge, paresis, and edema of the face, cervical region and limbs may also be observed.

RISK FACTORS
- There are no specific risk factors known at this time.
- Reports of *M. alligatoris* are limited to animals originating from Florida and *M. crocodyli* to Zimbabwe, so the origin source of the animals could be a risk factor.

Husbandry
Owing to the contagious nature of the disease, harboring animals in close quarters is likely to contribute to spread of the diseases.

Others
N/A

DIAGNOSIS
Due to the severity of the disease and potential for spread through a facility, suspect animals should be euthanized for a full diagnostic workup.

DIFFERENTIAL DIAGNOSIS
- Septic arthritis
- Gout
- West Nile virus

DIAGNOSTICS
- Serology: antibodies to *M. alligatoris* and *M. crocodyli* in clinically ill animals are suggestive of infection.
- PCR: PCR of lung, trachea, and other affected tissues is the most sensitive method of diagnosis.
- Culture: A positive culture in conjunction with clinical signs would confirm infection.
- Immunohistochemistry: Can identify the presence of the organism within tissues as an adjunct to other diagnostics.

PATHOLOGICAL FINDINGS
Pneumonia, pericarditis, and polyarthritis are the most common findings in infected animals.

TREATMENT

APPROPRIATE HEALTH CARE
Oral antibiotic therapy

NUTRITIONAL SUPPORT
The nature of crocodilians and the large number of animals affected at once means that force-feeding is not a practical approach.

CLIENT EDUCATION/HUSBANDRY RECOMMENDATIONS
- Isolation of affected animals is critical to prevent further spread.
- All enclosure smuts be cleaned and disinfected before new animals are introduced.
- New animals must be quarantined for at least 60 days before mixing with current stocks.

MEDICATIONS

DRUG(S) OF CHOICE
- Long-acting tetracycline administered IV and IM 10 mg/kg q5d maintained MIC in *A. mississippiensis*. Oral administration at 50 mg/kg did not result in appropriate levels.
- Anecdotal use of tetracyclines in crocodile species suggests a response to therapy, so species variability may exist for their oral bioavailability.
- Enrofloxacin 5 mg/kg IV q36h in *A. mississippiensis* but PO dosing was ineffective.

PRECAUTIONS/INTERACTIONS
N/A

FOLLOW-UP

PATIENT MONITORING
N/A

EXPECTED COURSE AND PROGNOSIS
- When treating a large number of animals with oral therapy, once they are clinically ill, prognosis is grave due the variable response when applied in a large scale.
- Prognosis may be better when treating a small number of animals via the IM route.
- It is possible that some animals may be subclinical carriers even after recovery.

MISCELLANEOUS

COMMENTS
N/A

ZOONOTIC POTENTIAL
Unknown at this point but should be treated as potentially zoonotic.

SYNONYMS
N/A

ABBREVIATIONS
- IM = intramuscular
- IV = intravenous
- MIC = minimum inhibitory concentration
- PCR = polymerase chain reaction
- PO = per os

Suggested Reading

Brown DR, Farley JM, Zacher LA, et al. *Mycoplasma alligatoris* sp. *nov.*, from American alligators. *Int J Syst Evol Microbiol* 2001;51:419–424.

Brown DR, Zacher LA, Carbonneau DA. Seroprevalence of *Mycoplasma alligatoris* among free-ranging alligators (*Alligator mississippiensis*) in Florida, *2003. J Zoo Wildl Med* 2005;36(2):340–341.

Mohan K, Foggin CM, Muvavarirwa P, et al. *Mycoplasma*-associated polyarthritis in farmed crocodiles (*Crocodylus niloticus*) in Zimbabwe. *Onderstepoort J Vet Res* 1995;62(1):45–49.

Pye GW, Brown DR, Nogueira MF, et al. Experimental inoculation of broad-nosed caimans (*Caiman latirostris*) and Siamese crocodiles (*Crocodylus siamensis*) with *Mycoplasma alligatoris. J Zoo Wildl Med* 2001;32(2):196–201.

Rivera S, Nevarez JG, Maxwell LK, Barker SA. Pharmacokinetics of tetracycline after single-dose oral administration in the American alligator (*Alligator mississippiensis*). *J Zoo Wildl Med* 2012;43(4):858–863.

Author Javier G. Nevarez, DVM, PhD, DACZM, DECZM (Herpetology)

NANNIZZIOPSIS MYCOSES

BASICS

DEFINITION/OVERVIEW

Nannizziopsis mycoses causes dermatomycosis in farmed saltwater crocodiles in Australia. Sometimes disseminates to internal organs.

ETIOLOGY/PATHOPHYSIOLOGY

- *N. crocodili* infects young farmed saltwater crocodiles in Australia.
- Spores/conidia from infected animals on intact skin or cutaneous breaches lead to hyphal proliferation in the epidermal stratum corneum, and necrosis and hyphae in the dermis and deeper structures.
- Rarely disseminates to internal organs.

SIGNALMENT/HISTORY

- YFD is a contagious cutaneous infection that is common in North America and Europe, and maybe elsewhere.
- Focal to multifocal, progressive necrosis and crusting, and even sloughing of the epidermis over the head, body, or limbs.
- Deeper infection may cause granulomatous inflammation in muscles and bones.

CLINICAL PRESENTATION

- Focal/multifocal often extensive necrotic skin lesions.
- Discolored and/or thickened scales, coalescing necrotic and/or crusty scales, ulcers.
- Most often over the head/face/rostrum, but also over the body.
- Facial features may be distorted from deeper infection.
- Often ultimately fatal

RISK FACTORS

Husbandry

- *N. dermatitidis* is a primary pathogen, as probably are other lizard *Nannizziopsis* species.
- Can occur even when captive husbandry seems adequate.
- Proper quarantine of incoming animals is warranted.

Others

Most often seen in bearded dragons purchased from large pet store chains.

DIAGNOSIS

DIFFERENTIAL DIAGNOSIS

- Trauma
- Thermal injuries/burns
- Papillomas
- Dermatophilosis
- Devriesea agamarum infection
- Other bacterial dermatitides
- Abscesses, parasites, and tumors when presenting with dermal and/or deep granulomas.

DIAGNOSTICS

- Presentation is often suggestive
- When present, arthroconidia on stained impression smears of skin lesions are very suggestive.
- A combination of histopathology and culture of skin biopsies are essential for definitive diagnosis.
- PCR on fungal isolate or on biopsy/tissue sections required.

PATHOLOGICAL FINDINGS

- Epidermal/dermal hyalohyphomycosis with extensive epidermal necrosis, often hyperkeratosis, heterophilic, and then mixed inflammatory cell infiltration, with or without dermal or deeper granulomas.
- PAS or silver stains may be needed to identify fungal elements.
- Rarely, systemic involvement

TREATMENT

APPROPRIATE HEALTH CARE

- Review and improvement of captive husbandry.
- Supportive measures (fluids, assist-feeding, thermal support).
- Surgical debridement of necrotic/crusty lesions indicated to decrease fungal load.
- Topical antiseptic or antifungal
- Systemic antifungal drugs almost always indicated.

NUTRITIONAL SUPPORT

Assist-feeding if needed

CLIENT EDUCATION/HUSBANDRY RECOMMENDATIONS

- Closely inspect the integument
- Quarantine new animals being added to the collection.
- Isolation of sick animals and use of strict hygiene.
- Thorough review of husbandry and adjustments when needed.

MEDICATIONS

DRUG(S) OF CHOICE

- *N. dermatitidis* and *N. crocodili* equally susceptible in vitro to itraconazole, terbinafine, and voriconazole but MICs for itraconazole higher for *N. guarroi.*
- Itraconazole and terbinafine may be synergistic and both accumulate and persist in the epidermis.

PRECAUTIONS/INTERACTIONS

- Interactions of triazoles and/or allylamines with other drugs possible.
- Itraconazole and terbinafine may be synergistic.

FOLLOW-UP

PATIENT MONITORING

- Monitor appetite, demeanor, and skin improvement with treatment.
- Blood work to monitor liver enzymes while on antifungals.

EXPECTED COURSE AND PROGNOSIS

- Variable
- Good if lesions are mild and/or superficial and addressed early.
- Guarded or poor if deeper lesions (e.g., myositis, osteomyelitis) present or in chronic and/or severe cases.

MISCELLANEOUS

COMMENTS

N/A

ZOONOTIC POTENTIAL

- None identified to date
- *Nannizziopsis* isolates from humans belong to species distinct from those infecting reptiles.

SYNONYMS

Practically all *Chrysosporium* anamorph of *Nannizziopsis vriesii* lizard isolates deposited over decades in fungal collections were reassigned to the above novel *Nannizziopsis* species when molecular probes were used.

ABBREVIATIONS

- MIC = minimum inhibitory concentration
- PAS = periodic acid–Schiff
- PCR = polymerase chain reaction
- YFD = yellow fungus disease

Suggested Reading

Paré JA, Sigler L. An overview of reptile fungal pathogens in the genera *Nannizziopsis, Paranannizziopsis,* and *Ophidiomyces. J Herp Med Surg* 2016;26:46-53.

Sigler L, Hambleton S, Paré JA. Molecular characterization of reptile pathogens currently known as members of the *Chrysosporium* anamorph of *Nannizziopsis vriesii* complex and relationship with some human-associated isolates. *J Clin Microbiol* 2013;51:3338–3357.

Author Jean A. Paré, DMV, DVSc, DACZM, DECZM (Zoo Health Management)

NUTRITIONAL SECONDARY HYPERPARATHYROIDISM

BASICS

DEFINITION/OVERVIEW

NSHP is one of the most common disorders in captive reptiles. The disease is characterized by hypocalcemia, which is caused by deficiency of calcium and/or vitamin D in the diet or a lack of UVB light exposure. This results in increased PTH production, leading to increased calcium resorption from the bones. Affected reptiles typically present with functional and morphological bone changes including pathological fractures and/or with tetany, seizure-like activity and muscle tremors.

ETIOLOGY/PATHOPHYSIOLOGY

- The etiology of NSHP is considered multifactorial. In carnivorous reptiles, a diet poor in calcium and vitamin D3 is a common cause of NSHP.
- Low calcium intake results in low blood calcium concentrations. A concentration below 2.3 mmol/l triggers the parathyroid glands to produce PTH to raise the level.
- PTH stimulates osteoclastic activity, resulting in different degrees of bone depletion. It also stimulates calcium reabsorption in the kidneys.
- A lack of dietary vitamin D3 or UVB light exposure from the sun or UVB bulbs is another critical factor in the development of NSHP.
- The active form of vitamin D3 is 1,25 dihydroxycholecalciferol, which is mediated in most species by exposure to UVB light in the range of 280–315 nm. The 1,25-dihydroxycholecalciferol increases intestinal calcium absorption and renal calcium reabsorption.

SIGNALMENT/HISTORY

- NSHP is the most common nutritional disorder of captive reptiles.
- Carnivores offered whole prey are rarely affected by NSHP because whole vertebrate prey contains adequate amounts of calcium and vitamin D3.
- Reptiles in life stages experiencing intensive growth are most affected from the chronic form of the disease (i.e., skeletal deformities) because of the increased demands of calcium during this period.
- Reptiles in life stages experiencing high demands of calcium for a short period (e.g., reproductive females), are usually presented with the acute form of the disease (i.e., hypocalcemia and tetany).

CLINICAL PRESENTATION

- Clinical signs vary depending on the severity of the disease.
- Softening of the mandible and/or maxilla (rubber jaw).
- Deformation of long bones
- Tetany
- Seizure-like activity
- Muscle tremors
- Decreased activity and anorexia

RISK FACTORS

Husbandry

- Insufficient calcium intake
- Excessive phosphorus intake
- Insufficient vitamin D intake
- Excessive vitamin A intake
- Insufficient exposure to UVB radiation in the range of 280–315 nm.
- Lack of hibernation in hibernating species, which results in excessive growth rates.

Others

Concurrent parasitism may exacerbate NSHP.

DIAGNOSIS

DIFFERENTIAL DIAGNOSIS

- RSHP
- Primary hyperparathyroidism

DIAGNOSTICS

- In most cases, NSHP is diagnosed based on clinical presentation and history of inappropriate diet and/or management.
- Radiography, blood work and fecal exams are indicated to confirm the clinical suspicion, determine the severity of the disease and formulate a prognosis.
- These diagnostic tests are also useful to rule out concomitant conditions like egg dystocia, endoparasitism, and constipation.

Radiography

- Decreased bony cortices and pathologic fractures may be observed.
- Depending on the duration of the disease, crocodilians may present long bone deformities.

Hematology and Biochemistry

- Chemistry panel: Hypocalcemia is usually observed in the early and late stages of the disease. It is common to have animals with NSHP be normocalcemic or even hypercalcemic due to the active resorption of calcium from the bones.
- Hyperphosphatemia may be observed concurrently, especially when hypocalcemia is present.
- A chemistry panel is particularly indicated in reptiles presenting with seizure-like activity or muscle tremors.
- They are also useful for monitoring response to therapy.
- Analysis should include measurement of ionized calcium. In general, values of ionized calcium lower than 1.0–1.2 mmol/l are abnormal.
- The calcium to phosphorus ratio is expected to be 1 : 5 to 2 : 1, and a decrease is suggestive of calcium depletion (e.g., NSHP, RSHP or renal disease).

Fecal Exams

Endoparasites may be a confounding factor in the development of this disease, as they can contribute to depletion of nutrients.

PATHOLOGICAL FINDINGS

- Gross pathological findings include deformity and softening of bone tissue, including jaws and/or long bones.
- Alterations of parathyroid glands may be present in form of generalized or focal enlargements.
- Histopathological lesions may range from increased osteoclastic resorption of otherwise well-formed and mineralized bone laminae to thinning of laminae and widening of medullary cavities, with scalloped endosteal surfaces due to massive resorptive activity.
- The cortices may be thinned and layers of osteoblasts and unmineralized osteoid on the periosteal surface may be present.

TREATMENT

APPROPRIATE HEALTH CARE

N/A

NUTRITIONAL SUPPORT

- Reptiles with chronic NSHP are often anorectic.
- The anorexia is usually transient and improves once the management is corrected.
- Reptiles with severe NSHP may not be able to ingest food due to the changes in the mandibular bones or concurrent diseases.
- In such cases, gavage-feeding or placement of an esophagostomy tube is indicated.

CLIENT EDUCATION/HUSBANDRY RECOMMENDATIONS

- NSHP is caused by improper diet and husbandry.
- Despite the efforts made to educate owners on adequate husbandry practices, NSHP is still one of the most common disorders of captive reptiles.
- Dietary issues to consider to prevent NSHP are provision of whole prey diet or balanced commercial diet that has the proper quantity of vitamins, especially vitamin A and D.
- Husbandry issues to consider to prevent NSHP are exposure to unfiltered sunlight (or as an alternative UVB through a UVB-emitting lamp), and provision of an environment adequate for brumation in brumating species.
- When provided with a complete, balanced diet, exposure to UVB has less of an effect in the development of NSHP.

NUTRITIONAL SECONDARY HYPERPARATHYROIDISM (CONTINUED)

MEDICATIONS

DRUG(S) OF CHOICE

- Fluid administration is required, as reptiles presenting with this condition are usually severely dehydrated.
- In reptiles presented with acute hypocalcemic crisis, calcium should be administered IV, or IM when an IV line is not available.
- There is no dosage that has been evaluated for effectiveness and safety in reptiles.
- In general, dosages of 50–100 mg/kg of calcium gluconate are considered effective.
- In reptiles presented with chronic NSHP, the mainstay of the therapy is an improvement in husbandry and diet.
- Feeding whole prey with organs, particularly liver, is critical for proper calcium and vitamin D3 ingestion.
- While UVB light exposure may not be an absolute requirement for carnivorous reptiles, it is still advisable when possible.
- Exposure to unfiltered sunlight for basking species is preferred over artificial UVB lights.
- When sunlight exposure is not possible or ideal (e.g., winter time), proper selection and use of UVB lights is necessary.
- A gradual change to a diet that contains the appropriate levels of calcium, vitamin D, and fibers, with low level of phosphorus is also required.
- Administration of oral calcium may assist in the recovery, but it must not be used as a stand-alone treatment.
- Calcium supplements containing vitamin D should be carefully dosed to avoid hypervitaminosis D.
- Calcium gluconate 50–100 mg/kg SC, IM, IV q6–24h
- Calcium glubionate 50–360 mg/kg PO q12–24h

PRECAUTIONS/INTERACTIONS

- It is presumed that, as in other vertebrates, parenteral calcium administration may provoke cardiac arrhythmias.
- Administration of exogenous vitamin D3 may result in excessive concentrations, resulting in intoxication and metastatic calcification of tissues.
- The only cases where exogenous vitamin D3 should be administered is when renal and/or hepatic functions are impaired, and endogenous vitamin D3 cannot be produced.
- Liver and fish oil are natural sources of vitamin D3.

FOLLOW-UP

PATIENT MONITORING

- In cases of acute hypocalcemic crisis, the reptile requires intensive care and monitoring of ionized calcium levels and ECG activity.
- In cases of chronic NSHP, if the reptile is eating on its own, a physical exam once every 7–14 days, accompanied by radiography and blood work, is usually adequate to assess response to therapy.

EXPECTED COURSE AND PROGNOSIS

- The prognosis of the disease is strictly dependent on the chronicity of the improper husbandry and on the severity of clinical signs and pathology upon presentation.
- Young animals, even if presented with hypocalcemic crisis, may have a favorable outcome if treated aggressively.
- Older animals, that present with chronic bone tissue depletion, may have a worse prognosis.
- Animals with multiple fractures and decreased cortices across the majority of the long bones tend to have a worse prognosis for recovery.

MISCELLANEOUS

Currently, there is a lack of information as to the proper amounts of calcium, vitamin D and other nutrients required for proper health of reptiles. The source of these nutrients may also influence their ability to be properly absorbed through the intestinal tract. It is possible that supplementation of these nutrients is not as effective as the natural ingestion via proper foods.

COMMENTS

N/A

ZOONOTIC POTENTIAL

N/A

SYNONYMS

- Fibrous osteodystrophy
- Metabolic bone disease
- Nutrition-related metabolic bone disease

ABBREVIATIONS

- ECG = electrocardiogram
- IM = intramuscular
- IV = intravenous
- NSHP = nutritional secondary hyperparathyroidism
- PO = per os
- PTH = parathyroid hormone
- RSHP = secondary hyperparathyroidism
- SC = subcutaneous
- UVB = ultraviolet B

INTERNET RESOURCES

- Additional information on reptile endocrinology from Carl Gans Collections: BiologyoftheReptilia.http://carlgans.org/bor-view/?borv=3&borp=7
- Information on secondary hyperparathyroidism in humans: Kim L. Hyperparathyroidism. Medscape, August 18, 2020. http://emedicine.medscape.com/article/127351-overview?pa=mcKd1JF66kULHOzxxIxn2fK%2Bx5xE5kE6dUeU7dvJSrcnjyhACchqCtq5rNZR2UhkQPQxex%2Bo7mr5pATtx84gCBXKySxof3ndUJD5aivxmIc%3D#a4

Suggested Reading

Mans C, Braun J. Update on common nutritional disorders of captive reptiles. *Vet Clin North Am Exot Anim Pract* 2014;17(3):369–395.

Author Paolo Selleri, DMV, PhD, SpecPACS, DECZM (Herpetology & Small Mammals), and Nicola Di Girolamo, DMV, MSc, PhD, DECZM (Herpetology)

OTHER HYALOHYPHOMYCOSES

BASICS

DEFINITION/OVERVIEW

Other infections are seen with non-pigmented (hyaline) filamentous fungi, such as *Aspergillus*, *Purpureocillium lilacinum* (formerly *Paecilomyces lilacinum*), *Fusarium*, *Metarhizium*, and many others fungi in genera other than *Chamaeleomyces*, *Nannizziopsis*, *Paranannizziopsis*, and *Ophidiomyces*.

ETIOLOGY/PATHOPHYSIOLOGY

- Ubiquitous environmental fungi that act as opportunistic pathogens in stressed/immunocompromised, or otherwise sick or debilitated animals.
- Some, like *Fusarium incarnatum* (formerly *F. semitectum*) in Texas tortoises or *Schizangiella serpentis* in snakes, may act as true pathogens while others, like *Purpureocillium lilacinum* or *F. solani*, seem to need little help in causing infection.
- Some are known insect pathogens, like *Metarhizium anisopliae* or *Beauveria bassiana*.

SIGNALMENT/HISTORY

- Any reptile, any age, any sex.
- History usually discloses substandard to outright deficient husbandry, poor hygiene, concurrent disease or infection, climactic extreme conditions (e.g., cold stunning in sea turtles) or life support system failure in captive animals (e.g., loss of heat from power failure) that result in immune suppression.

CLINICAL PRESENTATION

- Reflects the organ system affected
- Dermatomycoses with epidermal necrosis, respiratory signs common in crocodilians subject to hypothermia.
- Systemic, disseminated disease also often a consequence of prior hypothermia.

RISK FACTORS

Husbandry

- Poor or deficient husbandry is probably single most important predisposing factor.
- Climactic events in wild reptiles.

Others

- Chronic debilitating disease process
- Concurrent bacterial or other infections.
- Prolonged antibiotic therapy

DIAGNOSIS

DIFFERENTIAL DIAGNOSIS

- Differential diagnosis depends on presentation and targeted organ system.
- Bacterial/mycobacterial, viral, and parasitic diseases.
- Neoplasia when disseminated granulomas

DIAGNOSTICS

- Culture and cytology of material/clinical samples.
- Biopsy of lesions and histopathology to confirm causation.
- Blood work and imaging to determine extent of disease/lesions.

PATHOLOGICAL FINDINGS

Hyaline hyphae or other fungal elements within inflamed and/or necrotic tissue or within granulomas, consistent in morphology (e.g., diameter, septation, branching) with those of the hyaline fungus isolated from the lesion.

TREATMENT

APPROPRIATE HEALTH CARE

- Wide spectrum antifungal drugs
- Fluids, antibiotic coverage, thermal and nutritional support.
- Correct perceived husbandry deficiencies
- Debulking of lesions, when possible.

NUTRITIONAL SUPPORT

Assist-feeding if needed

CLIENT EDUCATION/HUSBANDRY RECOMMENDATIONS

- Quarantine of incoming animals
- Thorough and meticulous captive husbandry.

MEDICATIONS

DRUG(S) OF CHOICE

- Ideally based on fungal identification and known susceptibility of the causative fungus to the various antifungal drugs.
- In vitro assays might be available.
- Broad-spectrum antifungals that are efficacious against molds (itraconazole, voriconazole, terbinafine) probably indicated, pending culture and sensitivity results.

PRECAUTIONS/INTERACTIONS

- Triazole antifungal and terbinafine possibly synergistic.
- Interactions with other drugs possible.

FOLLOW-UP

PATIENT MONITORING

- Monitor appetite, demeanor, and skin improvement with treatment.
- Blood work to monitor liver enzymes and other parameters while on antifungals and/or to assess immune status indicated.

EXPECTED COURSE AND PROGNOSIS

- Often diagnosed late in the course of disease.
- Early infection often subclinical in reptiles, which tend to be stoic, and fungal etiology often unsuspected by clinicians.
- Prognosis is usually guarded to very poor, but may vary depending on duration, severity, and extent of lesions, and on the sensitivity pattern of the offending fungus.

MISCELLANEOUS

COMMENTS

N/A

ZOONOTIC POTENTIAL

Many fusaria and aspergilli carry some mild zoonotic impact.

SYNONYMS

Necrotizing Scute Disease refers to *Fusarium incarnatum* infection of the shell in Texas tortoises.

Suggested Reading

Paré JA, Jacobson ER. Mycotic diseases of reptiles. In: Jacobson ER, ed. *Infectious Disease and Pathology of Reptiles: Color Atlas and Text.* Boca Raton, FL: CRC Press; 2007:527–570.

Author Jean A. Paré, DMV, DVSc, DACZM, DECZM (Zoo Health Management)

PENTASTOMIDS

BASICS

DEFINITION/OVERVIEW

Pentastomids are crustacean endoparasites of the respiratory system, primarily of carnivorous reptiles. Approximately 90% of pentastomids use carnivorous reptiles as their definitive hosts, with 70% being found in snakes. Pentastomiasis occurs on all continents except Antarctica.

ETIOLOGY/PATHOPHYSIOLOGY

- Most adult crocodilian pentastomids live in the lungs, and bronchioles.
- *Leiperia* spp. inhabit the trachea and bronchi (females), bronchi, aorta, and pulmonary artery (males and immature parasites).
- *Subtriquetra* spp. inhabits the nasopharynx
- Females are larger and longer lived than males.
- Eggs are coughed up from the lungs or ingested and passed in feces.
- Intermediate hosts, primarily fish, but also possibly insects, anurans, reptiles, birds or mammals, ingest pentastomid eggs, which hatch, and go through two instars (growth periods between molts), before becoming encysted somewhere in the intermediate host's body.
- When the intermediate host is eaten by the definitive host, third-stage larvae emerge from the cyst and migrate to the host's lungs, where they feed on blood through the lung wall (hematophagous).
- Pentastomids damage the respiratory system which may lead to secondary bacterial or fungal colonization, pneumonia, septicemia, or death.
- Heavy infestations can severely scar the lungs and bronchi.
- Pentastomid genera parasitizing crocodilians are primarily Sebekidae (including *Agema*, Alofia, *Selfia*, *Sebekia*, *Leiperia*), but also Subtriquetridae (*Subtriquetra*).

SIGNALMENT/HISTORY

Farm raised or wild crocodilians, especially those eating mosquito fish, *Gambusia affinis*.

CLINICAL PRESENTATION

- Can be subclinical or have subcutaneous swellings, respiratory tract disease, pneumonia, dyspnea, weight loss, or poor growth.
- One study found 90–100% of clinically healthy American alligators, *Alligator mississippiensis*, in northern Florida, to be infected with *Sebekia mississippiensis*.

RISK FACTORS

- Feeding live or fresh fish
- Freeze or boil fish to kill parasitic larvae.
- Mosquito fish, were intermediate hosts (60–86% infected) for *Sebekia* spp. in American alligators.
- Freezing mosquito fish at –10°C (14°F) for 72 hrs was found to kill *Sebekia oxycephala* larvae.
- Many different fish species are intermediate host for pentastomids, fish are the primary vector in crocodilians.
- Male crocodilians more commonly affected than females.

Husbandry

Yet another compelling reason for quarantine and fecal examinations.

Others

N/A

DIAGNOSIS

- Detection of pentastomid eggs on fecal flotation, lung or cloacal washes, or tracheal discharge.
- Adult pentastomids are sometimes visible on radiography or via pulmonoscopy.
- They may also be observed in tissues via ultrasound examination.
- Adults may be found on exploratory surgery, necropsy, or histopathology.
- Suspected *Sebekia* spp. infections resulted in multifocal sub-pleural black foci up to 1.5 cm in diameter in New Guinea crocodiles (*Crocodylus novaeguineae*).

DIFFERENTIAL DIAGNOSIS

Respiratory signs may also be caused by:

- Other parasites
- Viruses
- Bacteria
- Fungi
- Neoplasia
- Trauma
- Foreign bodies

DIAGNOSTICS

- Fecal examination revealing thin walled, large (up to 130 µm in diameter), distinct ova, containing larvae with four claw-like hooklets.
- A complete blood count might reveal anemia or eosinophilia.

PATHOLOGICAL FINDINGS

- Pentastomids are medium to large (0.25–15 cm), superficially segmented, wormlike parasites, with two compound pairs of hooks surrounding the mouth.
- Adults may be recovered from the mouth, trachea, bronchioles, and lungs.
- Encysted instars may be found in the liver and lungs.
- In tissues, pentastomids are identified histologically by the presence of acidophilic glands adjacent to the intestine, and black sclerotized openings in the body wall.
- Inflammatory response in the lung may be mild with pentastomids because all life stages secrete surfactant very similar to host surfactant, which is thought to help them evade the host's immune system.
- Degrading molted pentastomid cuticles shed into the lung lumen may induce putrid pneumonia.
- Feed attachment sites on the lung surface can cause multiple crateriform ulcers with heterophilic or mixed inflammation.
- Pulmonary hemorrhage, edema, necrosis, fibrosis, granulomatous or interstitial pneumonia, bronchiectasis, and lung consolidation have been observed.
- In fresh dead crocodiles, the suffocating pentastomes will come crawling out of cuts made into the lungs.
- Pentastomids can be identified by morphological and molecular techniques.

TREATMENT

APPROPRIATE HEALTH CARE

Stabilize the patient first with antibiotics, if indicated.

NUTRITIONAL SUPPORT

N/A

CLIENT EDUCATION/HUSBANDRY RECOMMENDATIONS

- Do not feed fresh or live fish.
- Freeze fish for at least 3 days first to kill pentastomid larvae.

MEDICATIONS

DRUG(S) OF CHOICE

- Doramectin at 1 ml/50 kg of body mass IM has been recommended as a safe and effective treatment for pentastomids in Nile crocodiles (*C. niloticus*) (Huchzermeyer, 2003).
- Ivermectin at one half the mammalian dose caused paralysis of Nile crocodiles and was not recommended.

PRECAUTIONS/INTERACTIONS

Living pentastomids secrete surfactant that helps them to evade the host's immune system, but upon their death in tissue or lungs, a severe antigenic release or putrefaction, with serious and potential lethal complications can occur.

FOLLOW-UP

PATIENT MONITORING

Perform serial fecal examinations post treatment to gauge effectiveness.

EXPECTED COURSE AND PROGNOSIS

- Highly variable dependent on parasitic burden, chronicity, condition of patient and husbandry.
- Chronic infections severely scar the lungs of crocodilians.

MISCELLANEOUS

COMMENTS

N/A

ZOONOTIC POTENTIAL

- Species infecting humans belong to the families Linguatulidae, Armilliferidae, Porocephalidae, and Raillietiellidae, which have not been reported in crocodilians.
- All pentastomids should be considered potentially zoonotic.
- In the intermediate hosts, pentastome larvae often hatch and bore through the stomach wall and encyst in nearby mesentery, peritoneum or viscera.
- *Sebekia* spp. can cause a parasitic dermatitis in humans.

SYNONYMS

- Pentastomiasis
- Tongue worms

ABBREVIATIONS

IM = intramuscular

Suggested Reading

Boyce WM, Cardeilhac P, Lane T, et al. Sebekiosis in captive alligator hatchlings. *J Am Vet Med Assoc* 1984;185(11):419–1420.

Boyce WM. The prevalence of *Sebekia mississippiensis* (pentastomida) in American alligators (*Alligator mississippiensis*) in north Florida and experimental infection of paratenic hosts. *Proc Helminthol Soc Wash* 1985;52(2):278–282.

Huchzermeyer FW. Transmissible diseases. In: Huchzermeyer FW, ed. *Crocodiles: Biology, Husbandry and Diseases.* Cambridge, MA: CABI Publishing; 2003;89:167–170.

Jacobson ER. Parasites and parasitic diseases of reptiles. In: Jacobson ER, ed. *Infectious Disease and Pathology of Reptiles: Color Atlas and Text.* Boca Raton, FL: CRC Press; 2007:571–665.

Junker K, Boomker J. A check-list of the pentastomid parasites of crocodilians and freshwater chelonians. *Onderstepoort J Vet Res* 2006;73:27–36.

Paré JA. An overview of pentastomiasis in reptiles and other vertebrates. *J Exot Pet Med* 2008;17:285–294.

Author Thomas H. Boyer, DVM, DABVP (Reptile and Amphibian Practice)

PHAEOHYPHOMYCOSES

BASICS

DEFINITION/OVERVIEW

Phaeohyphomycosis refers to any infection with dematiaceous (pigmented) fungi such as *Exophiala*, *Cladosporium*, *Ochroconis*, *Ulocladium*, *Trichoderma*, and many others. The cell wall of these fungi contains variable amounts of melanin, and hyphae are therefore easily seen on routine H&E histological sections. These infections are relatively uncommon in reptiles.

ETIOLOGY/PATHOPHYSIOLOGY

- Phaeohyphomycoses are environmental fungi often found in soil and/or water that usually infect cutaneous wounds, or less often sick or debilitated animals.
- These opportunistic pathogens typically cause deep granulomatous infections of the feet, and rarely disseminate.
- *Exophiala* spp., in particular, have been isolated with some regularity from reptiles with phaeohyphomycosis.

SIGNALMENT/HISTORY

Any reptile, any age or sex.

CLINICAL PRESENTATION

- Swellings, nodules, wounds, often on the feet or ventrum (body parts in contact with soil).
- Slow progression; tends to not disseminate.

RISK FACTORS

Husbandry

- Substandard or otherwise deficient husbandry.
- Soil substrate
- Poor water quality

Others

Open wounds or other cutaneous breaches may facilitate invasion by these opportunistic fungi.

DIAGNOSIS

DIFFERENTIAL DIAGNOSIS

- Other fungal infections
- Mycobacteriosis
- Abscesses
- Neoplasia.

DIAGNOSTICS

- Biopsy and histopathology
- Culture of biopsy tissue or PCR.
- Pigmented fungi associated with inflammation/necrosis in histological section, and morphology of fungi in tissues consistent with morphology of putative isolate cultured from biopsy.

PATHOLOGICAL FINDINGS

Pigmented hyphae or other fungal elements within inflamed and/or necrotic tissue or within granulomas, consistent in morphology (e.g., pigmentation, diameter, septation, branching) with those of fungal isolates from the lesion.

TREATMENT

Debulking of lesions, when possible.

APPROPRIATE HEALTH CARE

- Fluids, antibiotic coverage, thermal and nutritional support.
- Correct perceived husbandry deficiencies

NUTRITIONAL SUPPORT

Assist-feeding if needed

CLIENT EDUCATION/HUSBANDRY RECOMMENDATIONS

- Quarantine incoming animals
- Thorough and meticulous captive husbandry.

MEDICATIONS

DRUG(S) OF CHOICE

- Many, if not most, pigmented fungi display resistance to triazoles and allylamines.
- Ideally based on fungal identification and known susceptibility of the causative fungus to the various antifungal drugs.
- In vitro assays might be available.

PRECAUTIONS/INTERACTIONS

N/A

FOLLOW-UP

PATIENT MONITORING

- Monitor appetite, demeanor, and skin improvement with treatment.
- Blood work to monitor liver enzymes and other parameters while on antifungals.
- Assess immune status

EXPECTED COURSE AND PROGNOSIS

- Often diagnosed late in the course of disease, when lesions are chronic and/or extensive.
- Amputation may be indicated when lesion is located on/in feet.
- Prognosis usually guarded, but may vary depending on duration, severity, and extent of lesions, and on the sensitivity pattern of the offending fungus.

MISCELLANEOUS

COMMENTS

N/A

ZOONOTIC POTENTIAL

- Minimal
- Some pigmented fungi can cause local infections and onychomycosis in humans, and rarely fungemia and disseminated disease.

SYNONYMS

N/A

ABBREVIATIONS

- H&E = hematoxylin and eosin
- PCR = polymerase chain reaction

Suggested Reading

Paré JA, Jacobson ER. Mycotic diseases of reptiles. In: Jacobson ER, ed. *Infectious Disease and Pathology of Reptiles: Color Atlas and Text*. Boca Raton, FL: CRC Press; 2007:527–570.

Author Jean A. Paré, DMV, DVSc, DACZM, DECZM (Zoo Health Management)

POXVIRUS

BASICS

DEFINITION/OVERVIEW

Poxviruses infecting crocodilians are unclassified members of the subfamily Chordopoxvirinae within the family Poxviridae. They affect crocodilian species worldwide with reports restricted to captive animals. It has been reported from spectacled caiman (*Caiman crocodilus fuscus*), Brazilian caiman (*C. crocodilus yacare*), Nile crocodile (*Crocodylus niloticus*), Saltwater crocodile (*C. porosus*), and Freshwater crocodile (*C. johnstoni*). Individual clinical cases in other species are also known to occur.

ETIOLOGY/PATHOPHYSIOLOGY

- Two different viruses are reported, crocodile poxvirus and caiman poxvirus.
- The epidemiology is not known at this time.

SIGNALMENT/HISTORY

Primarily affects captive, young crocodilians.

CLINICAL PRESENTATION

- Crocodile poxvirus is reported to cause 2–8 mm, yellow to brown lesions that can be wart-like, raised to unraised nodules, or ulcerated.
- Caiman poxvirus is reported to cause 1–3 mm, gray to white, coalescing to macular lesions.
- Lesions have been observed on the head, palpebrae, oral cavity, tongue, nostrils, and throughout the skin.
- Morbidity can be high but with low mortality.

RISK FACTORS

Specific risk factors are unknown, but a weakened immune system likely plays a role since it mostly affects young animals.

Husbandry

Poor hygiene and overcrowding can exacerbate the severity of the diseases.

Others

N/A

DIAGNOSIS

DIFFERENTIAL DIAGNOSIS

Squamous cell carcinoma

DIAGNOSTICS

- Histopathology: identification of characteristic lesions and possibly Borrel or Bollinger's bodies.
- PCR and DNA sequencing: definitive diagnosis is best achieved by PCR and DNA sequencing. Sequencing may also help in identifying new poxviruses in unreported species.
- Electron microscopy as an adjunct diagnostic to histopathology.

PATHOLOGICAL FINDINGS

- Histologic evaluation of affected tissues reveals epithelial hyperplasia, hyperkeratosis, acanthosis, and necrosis.
- Borrel and Bollinger's bodies may also be observed.

TREATMENT

APPROPRIATE HEALTH CARE

- There is no treatment for poxvirus in crocodilians.
- Animals appear to recover regardless of any changes in management, but improved hygiene is suspected to reduce viral load in the environment.
- If dealing with a small number of animals, supportive care can be provided.

NUTRITIONAL SUPPORT

Due to the nature of crocodilians and the large number of animals affected at once, force-feeding is not a practical approach.

CLIENT EDUCATION/HUSBANDRY RECOMMENDATIONS

Improvements in hygiene and reducing stressors on the animals are factors that can help to reduce the occurrence and/or severity of the clinical disease.

MEDICATIONS

DRUG(S) OF CHOICE

N/A

PRECAUTIONS/INTERACTIONS

N/A

FOLLOW-UP

PATIENT MONITORING

Animals appearing weak and debilitated should be separated as they may be less likely to survive infection and can serve as a source of virus.

EXPECTED COURSE AND PROGNOSIS

- Morbidity is high but mortality is typically low.
- Animals recover with little to no supportive care.
- In some instances, pox lesions may lead to skin defects affecting the quality and value of the hides.

MISCELLANEOUS

COMMENTS

N/A

ZOONOTIC POTENTIAL

Unknown

SYNONYMS

N/A

ABBREVIATIONS

PCR = polymerase chain reaction

Suggested Reading

Buenviaje GN, Ladds PW, Melville L: Poxvirus infection in two crocodiles, *Aust Vet J* 1992;69(1):15–16.

Horner RF: Poxvirus in farmed Nile crocodiles. *Vet Rec* 1990;122(19):459–462.

Huchzermeyer FW, Huchzermeyer KD, Putterill JF. Observations on a field outbreak of pox virus infection in young Nile crocodiles (*Crocodylus niloticus*). *J S Afr Vet Assoc.* 1991;62(1):27–29.

Jacobson ER, Popp JA, Shields RP, Gaskin JM. Poxlike skin lesions in captive caimans. *J Am Vet Med Assoc* 1979;175(9):937–940.

Pandey GS, Inoue N, Ohshima K, et. al. Poxvirus infection in Nile crocodiles (*Crocodylus niloticus*). *Res Vet Sci* 1990;49(2):171–176.

Penrith ML, Nesbit JW, Huchzermeyer FW. Pox virus infection in captive juvenile caimans (*Caiman crocodilus fuscus*) in South Africa. *J S Afr Vet Assoc* 1991;62(3):137–139.

Ramos MC, Coutinho SD, Matushima ER, Sinhorini IL. Poxvirus dermatitis outbreak in farmed Brazilian caimans (*Caiman crocodilus yacare*). *Aust Vet J* 2002;80(6):371–372.

Author Javier G. Nevarez, DVM, PhD, DACZM, DECZM (Herpetology)

SALMONELLOSIS

BASICS

DEFINITION/OVERVIEW

Salmonellosis is a cosmopolitan disease that can infect all vertebrates. While salmonellosis can occur in crocodilians, most serve as latent carriers or reservoirs of *Salmonella* spp. and pose a zoonotic concern for workers. *Salmonella* spp. should be considered a component of the indigenous microflora of crocodilians. Because these animals can naturally harbor this pathogen, those working with them should be made aware of the risks and provided information regarding best hygiene practices to minimize their exposure.

ETIOLOGY/PATHOPHYSIOLOGY

- Anaerobic, Gram-negative, straight rods, flagellated.
- Species: *Salmonella enterica* and *S. bongori*; subsp. *S. enterica* [I], *S. salamae* [II], *S. arizonae* [IIIa], *S. diarizonae* [IIIb], *S. houtenae* [IV], and *S. indica* [VI].
- Reptiles are most likely to be carriers of *S. arizonae* [IIIa] and *diarizonae* [IIIb].
- There are over 2,637 extant *Salmonella* serovars.
- All *Salmonella* serovars should be considered pathogenic.
- Serovars are characterized by their somatic (O) and flagellar (H) antigens.
- A wide range of serovars have been reported from crocodilians, some common ones include Poona, Singapore, Enteritidis, Cerro, and Pomona.
- Serovar identification is still used to identify sources of salmonellosis.
- Antimicrobial resistance patterns and pulse-field gel electrophoresis are used to confirm the sources of salmonellosis for human patients.

SIGNALMENT/HISTORY

Outbreaks of salmonellosis are usually reported in young animals that have undergone a recent stressor.

CLINICAL PRESENTATION

- Crocodilians that are carriers of *Salmonella* spp. typically appear healthy on physical examination or present for another illness; thus, it is important to recognize that these animals may serve as a potential source of infection and that the treatment used (e.g., antibiotics) could alter the pathogenicity of the *Salmonella* spp.
- Crocodilians with salmonellosis may present with nonspecific clinical signs: lethargy, anorexia, weakness, failure to thrive, weight loss, decreased body condition.
- A low level of increased mortality may be observed.

RISK FACTORS

Husbandry

Overcrowding and suboptimal husbandry conditions can lead to infection or increased shedding of *Salmonella* spp.

Others

Stressors can also precipitate salmonellosis.

DIAGNOSIS

DIFFERENTIAL DIAGNOSIS

- Enteritis (other species of Enterobacteriaceae)
- Renal disease
- Liver disease
- Primary and secondary bacterial infections.
- Fungal infections
- Neoplasia
- Osteomyelitis

DIAGNOSTICS

- Necropsy and histopathological evaluation is the best approach for diagnosis in commercial operations.
- Microbiological culture of a gastrointestinal sample or abscess can be used to confirm the presence of *Salmonella* spp.
- Positive fecal cultures in clinically normal animals are not uncommon. These animals should not be treated for *Salmonella*, as this can lead to the development of antimicrobial resistance in the *Salmonella* sp.
- Culture of *Salmonella* spp. requires special consideration, as the organism can be outcompeted by other Enterobacteriaceae under standard culture methods. Thus, it is important to specifically request a *Salmonella* spp. culture from the diagnostic laboratory if the organism is suspected. Enrichment with selenite or tetrathionate is required. Samples are then plated on to specific agars such as XLD, Salmonella–Shigella agar, or XLT-4 agar. XLD and XLT-4 agars have a hydrogen sulfide indicator system to detect lactose-fermenting *Salmonella* spp.
- Factors that influence the reliability of culture include the collection method, quantity and/or type of sample collected, temporal variation in shedding, and culture methods. Time to perform culture can delay appropriate antimicrobial therapy and control/mitigation procedures.
- PCR can be used to confirm the presence of *Salmonella* spp. in a sample. This test is considered more sensitive than culture and provides faster turnaround times. One limitation of PCR is that it cannot provide an antibiotic sensitivity profile to guide treatment.
- Parallel testing with PCR and culture is recommended to increase the sensitivity of the testing methods.
- Complete blood counts can be used to confirm an inflammatory leukogram or toxic changes that might occur with salmonellosis.

PATHOLOGICAL FINDINGS

- *Salmonella* spp. are commonly isolated from the gastrointestinal tract of crocodilians on postmortem examinations as an incidental finding.
- Animals that have clinical salmonellosis will have typical inflammatory signs associated with the pathogen causing an enteritis or systemic infection.

TREATMENT

APPROPRIATE HEALTH CARE

- Crocodilians that are clinically normal and not showing signs of disease should never be treated for *Salmonella* spp.
- Treating animals that are latent carriers could potentiate antimicrobial resistance.
- Treatment of salmonellosis in commercial crocodilian operations is not recommended as it may lead to increased bacterial resistance and the effectiveness in large scale can be unrewarding.
- If treatment is elected, it should only be performed after obtaining results of an antibiotic sensitivity profile.

NUTRITIONAL SUPPORT

Due to the nature of crocodilians and the large number of animals affected at once, force-feeding is not a practical approach.

CLIENT EDUCATION/HUSBANDRY RECOMMENDATIONS

Improvements in hygiene and reducing stressors on the animals are factors that can help reduce the occurrence and/or severity of the clinical disease.

MEDICATIONS

DRUG(S) OF CHOICE

Based on sensitivity profile

PRECAUTIONS/INTERACTIONS

N/A

FOLLOW-UP

PATIENT MONITORING

Animals appearing weak and debilitated should be separated as they may be less likely to survive infection and can serve as a source of *Salmonella* sp.

EXPECTED COURSE AND PROGNOSIS

- Crocodilians diagnosed with salmonellosis from culture or PCR may not require any intervention as many are often latent carriers and do not show signs of disease.
- Animals that test negative for *Salmonella* sp. on a single test may still be positive because intermittent shedding is common.
- Those with salmonellosis are likely to recover and mortalities are typically low.

MISCELLANEOUS

COMMENTS

N/A

ZOONOTIC POTENTIAL

- Crocodilians must be considered a possible source because they serve as reservoirs and latent carriers of *Salmonella* spp.
- To minimize the zoonotic potential, it is important to practice strict hygiene and biosecurity.

SYNONYMS

- Salmonellosis
- Typhoid fever

ABBREVIATIONS

- PCR = polymerase chain reaction
- XLD = xylose lysine deoxycholate
- XLT-4 = xylose-lysine Tergitol 4

INTERNET RESOURCES

Center for Food Security and Public Health. Reptile Associated Salmonellosis. January 2013. http://www.cfsph.iastate.edu/Factsheets/pdfs/reptile_associated_salmonellosis.pdf

Suggested Reading

Mannolis SC, Webb GJ, Pinch D, et al. Salmonella in captive crocodiles (*Crocodylus johnstoni* and *C. porosus*). *Aust Vet J* 1991;20(3):377–378.

Ocholi RA, Enurah LU. Salmonellosis in a captive crocodile (*Crocodylus niloticus*) due to *Salmonella choleraesuis*. *J Zoo Wildl Med* 1989;20(3):377–378.

Sakaguchi K, Nevarez JG, Del Piero F. *Salmonella enterica* serovar Pomona infection in farmed juvenile American alligators (*Alligator mississippiensis*). *Vet Pathol* 2017;54(2):316–319.

Scott T, Foster BG. *Salmonella* spp. in free-ranging and farmed alligators (*Alligator mississippiensis*) from Texas and Louisiana U.S.A. *Aquaculture* 1997;156(1–2):179–181.

Authors Sean M. Perry, DVM, Mark A. Mitchell, DVM, MS, PhD, DECZM (Herpetology), and Javier G. Nevarez, DVM, PhD, DACZM, DECZM (Herpetology)

SQUAMOUS CELL CARCINOMA

BASICS

DEFINITION/OVERVIEW

SCCs are malignant epithelial cell tumors, most commonly associated with cutaneous or mucocutaneous regions of the body. SCCs are most commonly found on the skin or associated with oropharyngeal tissues. They tend to be well differentiated, with some evidence of local infiltration of adjacent tissues, and limited evidence of metastatic behavior. SCCs are not uncommon in reptile species, and have been identified in one crocodile in which the tumor metastasized to the liver.

ETIOLOGY/PATHOPHYSIOLOGY

- An underlying cause of SCCs in reptiles is unknown.
- Published hypotheses with respect to risk factors and etiology include those based on mammalian or avian examples: overexposure to ultraviolet radiation, including exposure at higher altitudes, light skin color, chronic hypovitaminosis A, and possibly chronic viral infections.
- There is no evidence that any of these risk factors are associated with reptile SCCs.
- No viruses have been associated with SCCs in reptiles.
- Most reptile SCCs are locally invasive, but not associated with metastatic behavior.
- A wild-caught Australian saltwater crocodile was found to have a locally invasive SCC on the toes of one hind limb, with metastasis in the liver.

SIGNALMENT/HISTORY

- There is no clear predisposition with respect to species or sex.
- There may be an association between the presence of SCCs and increasing age of the reptile, but this has not been evaluated systematically.
- Historically, reptiles diagnosed with SCC are observed to have a focal mass or masses anywhere on the skin, within the oral cavity or at other mucocutaneous junctions.
- The raised tissue may become hemorrhagic, ulcerative and/or necrotic.
- With chronicity, bacterial abscessation may develop within or in close association with the tumor.
- Most commonly, the neoplastic cells invade adjacent tissues.
- Depending on the site of the tumor, the animal may become hyporexic/anorexic, exhibit a depressed attitude, and/or favor a limb/eye or other anatomical sites that may be involved.
- If the eyes are involved, vision may become impaired and the animal may, uncharacteristically, fall from cage furniture or not be able to find food.

CLINICAL PRESENTATION

- The clinical signs may be somewhat variable depending on the anatomic locations of the mass.
- Discrete skin lesions tend to appear raised, with erythema, hemorrhage, and/or ulceration, or appear as chronic nonhealing wounds.
- If the lesions involve the digits, there may be more diffuse swelling and some degree of lameness.
- With SCCs of the oropharynx, hyporexia or anorexia may be present, in addition to masticatory dysfunction and mild oral hemorrhage.

RISK FACTORS

Husbandry

- Purely hypothetical risk factors in reptiles are based on mammalian or avian risk factors.
- In the case of husbandry, hypovitaminosis A or excessive ultraviolet light exposure could be predisposing risk factors but there is no evidence documenting a link between these factors and SCCs.

Others

N/A

DIAGNOSIS

DIFFERENTIAL DIAGNOSIS

- Bacterial abscesses
- Fungal granulomas (especially *Chrysosporium* species)
- Viral papillomatous lesions
- Chronic traumatic wounds with fibrosis.
- Cloacal prolapse
- Other neoplastic diseases (e.g., melanoma, fibrosarcoma, cutaneous papilloma, fibropapilloma, lipoma, spindle cell sarcoma, and chromatophorma)

DIAGNOSTICS

- Histopathology of the lesion is the gold standard for diagnosis, through complete surgical excision or biopsy of the mass.
- A fine-needle aspirate with cytologic evaluation may or may not be diagnostic.
- Imaging modalities, such as radiography or CT may be helpful in detecting local soft tissue or bone involvement.
- Contrast CT may be useful when trying to evaluate for metastases.

PATHOLOGICAL FINDINGS

- In domestic mammals, histologic subtypes of SCCs are typically described as poorly, moderately, or well differentiated.
- In general, SCCs are histopathologically characterized as round to polygonal-shaped cells with varying amounts of basophilic cytoplasm, and keratinization.
- The nuclei tend to be round, with significant variation in size and chromatin pattern, from coarsely stippled to pyknotic, and commonly with perinuclear vacuoles.
- Frequently, there is marked variation in nucleus to cytoplasmic ratio because the cells vary in degree of differentiation.
- In reptiles, the histologic description of SCC is similar. Typically, there are anastomosing cords and nests of polygonal cells with abundant eosinophilic cytoplasm, distinct intercellular bridges, and round to oval nuclei with finely stippled chromatin and multiple nucleoli, with occasional mitotic figures.
- Neoplastic cells are described as having differing levels of anisokaryosis, and frequently form circular keratinized foci consistent with keratin pearls, and usually invade and/or replace adjacent tissues.

TREATMENT

APPROPRIATE HEALTH CARE

N/A

NUTRITIONAL SUPPORT

- Nonspecific nutritional support may include regular force-feeding of an appropriate commercial diet and/or placement of an esophagostomy tube to facilitate administering nutritional supplements.
- The directions on the label of the commercial diet can be followed for appropriate volume per feeding and frequency.

CLIENT EDUCATION/HUSBANDRY RECOMMENDATIONS

N/A

MEDICATIONS

DRUG(S) OF CHOICE

- Besides surgical excision, no other treatments have been reported in crocodilians.
- Radiation therapy, intratumoral therapy and cisplatin or carboplatin-impregnated beads have been performed in other reptile species with limited success.
- Antimicrobial drugs may be used as needed for secondary bacterial infections.
- NSAIDs may help with any discomfort, but there are no systematically derived data with respect to efficacy of NSAIDs in any reptile species.

• Surgical excision with histopathologic evidence of clean margins is the treatment of choice.
• In birds and mammals, focal SCCs have been treated with surgical debulking and intralesional platinum-based chemotherapeutic agents (e.g., cisplatin or carboplatin-impregnated beads).
• Depending on the species, meloxicam may be administered orally or subcutaneously 0.2–0.5 mg/kg.

PRECAUTIONS/INTERACTIONS

• Should the owner elect intralesional chemotherapy, the possible outcomes include lack of therapeutic response, systemic absorption of the chemotherapeutic agent causing hyporexia/anorexia, depressed attitude, anemia or other blood cell changes, and necrosis of surrounding healthy tissues.
• With surgical excision of a SCC, recurrence should be considered and discussed with the owner.

FOLLOW-UP

PATIENT MONITORING

• SCCs are likely to recur with incomplete surgical excision, and may recur regardless of complete surgical excision.
• There are a few documented cases of local tissue invasion and/or metastasis.
• The patient should be monitored for recurrence of the tumor, and contrast CT may be of some use in monitoring for local invasion or metastatic disease.
• If treatment is recommended and accepted by the owner (partial excision and intralesional chemotherapy or electrochemotherapy), the treatment site should be monitored for secondary microbial infection or self-trauma.
• The owner should be instructed to report any signs of skin discoloration, discharge, or dysfunction of the anatomical region of the original tumor.
• Because of possible systemic absorption of locally administered chemotherapeutic agents, a complete blood count and biochemical profile should be evaluated prior to the start of chemotherapy, and serially evaluated during and after the course of chemotherapy.

EXPECTED COURSE AND PROGNOSIS

• With complete surgical excision and clean tissue margins as evidenced by histopathology, the prognosis is good-to-guarded, with the possibility of recurrence.
• With recent published cases documenting metastatic disease, a guarded prognosis is wise until we know more about the behavior of SCCs across multiple reptile species.
• There may be some promising new intralesional chemotherapeutic techniques or refined radiation therapy techniques applied to future cases of SCCs in reptiles, which may improve prognostic factors.

MISCELLANEOUS

COMMENTS

N/A

ZOONOTIC POTENTIAL

N/A

SYNONYMS

N/A

ABBREVIATIONS

• CT = computed tomography
• SCC = squamous cell carcinoma
• NSAIDs = nonsteroidal anti-inflammatory drug

Suggested Reading

Christman J, Devau M, Wilson-Robles H, et al. Oncology of reptiles: Diseases, diagnosis, *and treatment. Vet Clin North Am Exot Anim Pract* 2017;20(1):87–110.
Hill AG, Dennis MM, Pynea M. Squamous cell carcinoma with hepatic metastasis in a saltwater crocodile (*Crocodylus porosus*). *Aust Vet J* 2016;94(3):83–86.
Johnson J, Naples LM, Chu C, et al. Cutaneous squamous cell carcinoma in a panther chameleon (*Furcifer pardalis*) and treatment with carboplatin implantable beads. *J Zoo Wildl Med* 2016;47(3):931–934.
Lanza A, Baldi A, Spugnini EP. Surgery and electrochemotherapy for the treatment of cutaneous squamous cell carcinoma in a yellow-bellied slider (*Trachemys scripta scripta*). *J Am Vet Med Assoc* 2015;246(4):455–457.
Sykes JM, Trupkiewicz JG. Reptile neoplasia at the Philadelphia Zoological Garden, 1901–2002. *J Zoo Wildl Med* 2006;37(1):11–19.

Author Kurt K. Sladky, MS, DVM, DACZM, DECZM (Zoo Health Management & Herpetology)

WEST NILE VIRUS

BASICS

DEFINITION/OVERVIEW

WNV is a single-stranded RNA arbovirus in the genus *Flavivirus*. First reported in Africa in 1937, it is now endemic in the United States. It has been reported in all states and the District of Columbia but not Hawaii. It is also present in Central America, South America, the Caribbean, West Asia, and parts of Africa, the Middle East, and Europe. The majority of WNV infections leading to clinical signs have been reported from captive reared American alligators (*Alligator mississippiensis*). There are serological reports from Nile crocodiles and Morelet's crocodile.

ETIOLOGY/PATHOPHYSIOLOGY

- The enzootic cycle is maintained primarily between birds and mosquitoes but direct transmission through contact with infected tissues and/or blood is also possible.
- The incidence of WNV infection resulting in clinical signs is higher for captive-reared crocodilians in commercial operations.
- It is believed that the higher, constant temperatures (average of 29 degrees C/85 degrees F) at which these animals are maintained year round allow viral replication and hence clinical signs.
- While a number of crocodilian species are known to have antibodies to WNV, clinical signs or pathologic findings associated with WNV infection have not been reported from free-ranging crocodilians.

SIGNALMENT/HISTORY

- WNV can affect crocodilians of any age and sex.
- Infections typically occur in captive reared animals housed indoors and maintained above 27 degrees C (80 degrees F).
- Infections are more prevalent in the fall and winter when mosquitoes enter buildings seeking warmth.

CLINICAL PRESENTATION

- There are two classic presentations for WNV in American alligators.
- One is per acute to acute onset of mortality associated with neurologic signs. Signs include weakness, lethargy, anorexia, head tilt, muscle tremors and abnormal swimming or flotation.
- The second presentation is the appearance of lesions on the skin of animals that survive infection.

RISK FACTORS

- Captive reared, kept above 27 degrees C (80 degrees F).
- Fall and wintertime in the United States.

Husbandry

- Structural deficits in buildings provide enough air gaps for mosquitoes to enter the building.
- Keep the doors open during feeding and cleaning.

Others

Increased mosquito populations

DIAGNOSIS

DIFFERENTIAL DIAGNOSIS

- For acute presentation: oxygen depletion/ammonia toxicity, pneumonia.
- For chronic presentation: skin blemishes caused by tooth marks, nails, other skin defects.
- Must confirm lesions via histology.

DIAGNOSTICS

- RT-PCR is the most sensitive diagnostic test. Liver and brain tissue (pooled samples) can be used for fast diagnosis. RT-PCR of colon biopsies from live animals can also be used for antemortem diagnosis if the virus is present in the intestinal tract. RT-PCR can also be used to tests the skin lesions. Vaccine status and timing must be known, as the PCR may detect the vaccine in the liver of vaccinated animals for up to 30 days.
- Culture: because they can serve as amplifiers, growth in culture is fairly easily achieved from liver, brain, or colon of infected animals.
- Serology: plaque reduction neutralization can be used for detection of antibodies. A competitive ELISA has also been validated for use in American alligators.
- Histopathologic evaluation provides supportive evidence for other diagnostics. It is also essential for confirmation of the skin lesions.
- Immunohistochemistry: positive staining is commonly observed in the brain and intestines but not in the skin lesions.

PATHOLOGICAL FINDINGS

- Acute: light microscopy of tissues from infected animals may reveal diffuse severe heterophilic, histiocytic, and necrotizing enterocolitis, heterophilic meningoencephalitis, necrotizing and heterophilic hepatitis, heterophilic and histiocytic splenitis, generalized heterophilic and histiocytic lymphoid folliculitis, and necrotizing and heterophilic pancreatitis. Mild multifocal heterophilic and lymphohistiocytic interstitial nephritis, gastritis, and mild pulmonary congestion and edema may also be present.
- Chronic: lymphohistiocytic infiltration of the dermis.

TREATMENT

APPROPRIATE HEALTH CARE

- There is no treatment for WNV in crocodilians.
- Animals will either die from initial infection or will recover without any appreciable long-term effects other than development of skin lesions.
- While these lesions have a negative impact on the commercialization of the hides, they do not affect the health of the animals.
- Mosquito control, strict quarantine, biosecurity, and hygiene are essential for the prevention of WNV.

NUTRITIONAL SUPPORT

N/A

CLIENT EDUCATION/HUSBANDRY RECOMMENDATIONS

- Mosquito control measures and vaccination against WNV is critical for prevention in commercial alligator farms.
- Once WNV is present in any operation, it is critical to maintain strict isolation of affected animals and those contained within the same building.
- Animals must not be moved to other areas or buildings.
- Failure to isolate the animals may result in the spread of the virus.
- Strict biosecurity measures, especially in the affected buildings, are essential to stop the spread of the virus.
- Tools, such as nets, feeding utensils, and boots, should be left in the affected area and not introduced to other areas or buildings.
- Once the infection runs its course, the surviving animals will continue to thrive; however, the duration of viral shedding is unknown.
- Mosquito control, strict quarantine, and biosecurity have significantly decreased the prevalence of WNV in commercial operations.
- An alligator specific WNV vaccine has been available since 2012.

MEDICATIONS

DRUG(S) OF CHOICE

- WNV vaccine is an effective commercial WNV vaccine available from Boehringer Ingelheim Vetmedica for use in American alligators.
- For hatchlings, an initial 0.25 ml injection IM is followed by a second injection in 2–4 weeks later. A yearly booster is required.

PRECAUTIONS/INTERACTIONS

N/A

FOLLOW-UP

PATIENT MONITORING

Skin lesions may develop within 4 weeks of infection.

EXPECTED COURSE AND PROGNOSIS

- Mortality can be as high as 60% and morbidity can reach 100% of animals within an enclosure.
- Those that recover from infection have an excellent long-term prognosis but are likely to develop skin lesions.

MISCELLANEOUS

COMMENTS

N/A

ZOONOTIC POTENTIAL

- Alligators have been shown to be good amplifiers of the virus, which can be found in the blood, tissues, and feces.
- Transmission form an alligator carcass to humans has been documented.
- All necessary precautions must be taken when working with crocodilians infected with WNV.

SYNONYMS

PIX disease and LPSA have been used to describe the dermatitis that occurs in animals that survive WNV infection.

ABBREVIATIONS

- ELISA = enzyme-linked immunosorbent assay
- IM = intramuscular
- LPSA = lymphohistiocytic proliferative syndrome of alligators
- RT-PCR = reverse transcriptase polymerase chain reaction
- WNV = West Nile virus

INTERNET RESOURCES

Nevarez J. Lymphohistiocytic Proliferative Syndrome of Alligators (Alligator mississippiensis): a cutaneous manifestation of West Nile virus. PhD dissertation, Louisiana State University, 2007. https://digitalcommons.lsu.edu/gradschool_dissertations/3521

Suggested Reading

Higbie CT, Nevarez JG, Roy AF, Del Piero F. Presence of West Nile virus RNA in tissues of American alligators (*Alligator mississippiensis*) vaccinated with a killed West Nile virus vaccine. *J Herp Med Surg* 2017;27(1–2):18–21.

Jacobson ER, Ginn PE, Troutman JM, et al. West Nile virus infection in farmed American alligators (*Alligator mississippiensis*) in Florida. *J Wildl Dis* 2005;41(1):96–106.

Miller DL, Mauel MJ, Baldwin C, et al. West Nile virus in farmed alligators. *Emerg Infect Dis* 2003;9(7):794–799.

Nevarez JG, Mitchell MA, Kim DY, et al. West Nile virus in alligator ranches from Louisiana. *J Herp Med Surg* 2005;15(3):4–9.

Nevarez JG, Mitchell MA, Morgan TW, et al. Association of West Nile virus with lymphohistiocytic proliferative cutaneous lesions in American alligators (*Alligator mississippiensis*) detected by RT-PCR. *J Zoo Wildl Med Surg* 2008;39(4):562–566.

Author Javier G. Nevarez, DVM, PhD, DACZM, DECZM (Herpetology)

SECTION VI

AMPHIBIANS

ABSCESSES

BASICS

DEFINITION/OVERVIEW

Abscesses are firm, sometimes painful, masses of different shape and diameter that occur within the integumentary tissue, the body cavity, or internal organs. Bacterial abscesses are common, but some may be fungal or sterile. Local inflammatory necrotizing changes are often present.

ETIOLOGY/PATHOPHYSIOLOGY

- Several bacteria have been described in association with abscesses. Most of them are opportunistic microbiota in immunocompromised amphibians: *Pseudomonas* spp., *Salmonella* spp., *Vibrio* spp., *Mycobacterium* spp., etc.
- Isolation of *Mycobacterium* spp. is common in certain groups of amphibians, due in part to the ubiquity of this microorganism in the environment.
- The route of infection is usually ingestion, although invasion of skin lesions is possible.

SIGNALMENT/HISTORY

- Cutaneous abscesses in amphibians have a very evident appearance, and are well-described in the literature.
- There is no specific predisposing signalment but animals maintained in poor husbandry conditions are more likely to be exposed to a higher environmental bacterial load and thus more predisposed to infections. These animals may also be immunocompromised and more prone to secondary opportunistic infections.

CLINICAL PRESENTATION

- Abscesses may be found in the skin, heart, liver, spleen, kidneys, and gastrointestinal tract.
- They may also be observed in the coelomic cavity during endoscopic examination.

RISK FACTORS

Husbandry

Poor husbandry leading to poor soil, water, or air quality.

Others

- Immunocompromised individuals
- Stress

DIAGNOSIS

DIFFERENTIAL DIAGNOSIS

- Parasitic cysts
- Dermatosepticemia
- Changes in color or ulcerative lesions of the skin caused by *Pseudocapillaroides*.
- Neoplasms
- Mineral deposits

DIAGNOSTICS

Cytology

- All skin lesions require cytological evaluation using RAL Diff-Quik™ (Siemens Healthineers, Erlangen, Germany) and Ziehl–Neelsen stains. Through imprinting of the affected area, we can see a large number of leukocytes, a multitude of bacteria or fungi and cellular detritus.
- Culture and sensitivity: to discover the true etiology and best therapeutic approach, the organism must be cultured.
- PCR/gene sequencing: as they become more readily available, these techniques may provide a more precise identification of the organism.

Hematology

A hematological examination reveals leukocytosis. Heterophiles are reactive (toxic granulation). Mitosis is observed in many leukocytes.

Imaging

- Radiology: look for bony lesions that may be associated or suggestive of an infectious process (skull, long bones).
- Ultrasound: abscesses may appear hypoechoic to more hyperechoic, depending on the thickness of the material within. In advanced stages, there is a thin layer of fibrin that surrounds the abscess and under it the inflammatory liquid that forms the internal caseum. Ultrasound guided aspirates can be used to obtain cytological samples.

PATHOLOGICAL FINDINGS

- Histopathology of the excised tissues usually shows septic heterophilic inflammation with necrosis and granulation tissue, bacteria, and sometimes fungal elements.
- Variably thick bands of dense collagenous tissue partially surround the affected areas, which can impede drug penetration (antibiotics) into the tissue.

TREATMENT

APPROPRIATE HEALTH CARE

- Masses must be surgically opened and the contents removed, including the external layer (capsule), to avoid relapse.
- Appropriate therapy must be instituted according to etiology.

NUTRITIONAL SUPPORT

- There are no specific nutritional recommendations for avoiding abscesses in amphibians.
- Poor feeding may be a predisposing cause for the animal to undergo local infections due to immunosuppression linked to malnutrition.
- Diet should always be as varied as possible and adapted to each species (combine commercial insects or worms such as *Drosophila, Grillus, Locusta, Tenebrio, Galleria*) and try not to fall into the monotony of feeding a single prey item. Nutritional support via gavage feeding should be implemented for anorectic animals.

CLIENT EDUCATION/HUSBANDRY RECOMMENDATIONS

- Proper husbandry is essential for the health of captive amphibians.
- The enclosure, substrate, and associated materials (bowls, cage furniture, accessories, etc.) must be cleaned and disinfected on a regular basis.
- Do not use wild-collected soil, plants, rocks, or other materials without first cleaning and disinfecting them.
- Do not use disinfectants or cleaners that may be toxic or are known to be toxic to other animals.
- Quarantine of recently acquired amphibians for 60–90 days is essential to minimize disease transfer.
- Open wounds can become easily infected, especially in an environment which has not been kept clean.
- Wounds are most likely to occur during the first few weeks when the animal is becoming acclimated; leave it alone as much as possible during this time.

SURGICAL CONSIDERATIONS

- Before performing surgery, consider whether it is possible to close the skin and provide adequate postoperative care.
- Postoperatively considerations include keeping the animal in a separate clean container until healing has occurred to minimize environmental contamination.
- Maintaining clean water for aquatic species is critical for proper healing.

MEDICATIONS

DRUG(S) OF CHOICE

- Amikacin 5 mg/kg IM q48h for 5–14 treatments
- Ceftazidime 20 mg/kg IM or ICe q24–48h
- Ciprofloxacin 10 mg/kg PO q24h, or 500 mg/75 liters of water in baths daily for 6–8 hours.
- Enrofloxacin 5–10 mg/kg SC, IM, ICe, topically, or PO q24h for 7–21 days
- Piperacillin 100 mg/kg SC, IM, ICe once daily
- Metronidazole 50 mg/kg PO q24h for 3 days for anaerobic infections, increasing the dose by 20% if used topically.

• Metronidazole can also be used at a rate of 50 mg/liter of water in baths for up to 24 hours.
• Metronidazole can also be given by bioencapsulation in *Artemia salina* (after Artemia baths for 24 hours in solution of metronidazole at 10 g/l, *Artemia* becomes a "rich" live prey in metronidazole for 30 minutes). It can be used in fish and small amphibians.

PRECAUTIONS/INTERACTIONS

• Water baths containing antibiotics or topical applications may not provide as consistent distribution as parenteral administration.
• White blood cell changes were observed in Egyptian toads exposed to chloramphenicol at 5 mg/40 g of body weight for 12 weeks. While this would be a longer treatment period than in most clinical cases, its secondary toxic effects should be considered.
• Shorter-term therapy has been used for treatment of chytridiomycosis in other amphibian species.

FOLLMOW-UP

PATIENT MONITORING

• A positive response to therapy consists of the disappearance of abscesses without reoccurrence.
• To confirm this, a weekly visual check of affected animals should be carried out when lesions are external.

EXPECTED COURSE AND PROGNOSIS

• The prognosis will depend on the location and number of abscesses and the etiologic agent.
• In general, after antibiotic treatment and/or surgical excision, the prognosis is good with a complete cure after 4 weeks of therapy.
• Euthanasia of the animals infected with *Mycobacterium* sp. and strict quarantine (minimum of 180 days) of any tank mates is recommended.

MISCELLANEOUS

COMMENTS

N/A

ZOONOTIC POTENTIAL

• Many of the aforementioned bacterial species have zoonotic potential.
• Care must always be exercised when working with amphibians.
• In 2011, an outbreak of *Salmonella typhimurium* associated with African dwarf frogs was reported in the United States.
• Despite being rarely described, we can consider that *Mycobacterium* microorganisms recovered from amphibians are also potential cause of zoonoses.
• A *Brucella inopinata*-like bacterium was obtained in pure culture from a big-eyed tree frog (*Leptopelis vermiculatus*). Although a very rare case, the organism is a potential human pathogen and may present a risk for people handling amphibians.
• Preventive prophylaxis (handling using gloves, disinfection of materials, avoiding contact with children) should be used when working with abscesses in amphibians.

SYNONYMS

• Dermatitis
• Granuloma

ABBREVIATIONS

• ICe = intracoelomic
• IM = intramuscular
• PCR = polymerase chain reaction
• PO = per os
• SC = subcutaneous

INTERNET RESOURCES

• Amphibian Ark. Husbandry documents. http://www.amphibianark.org/husbandry-documents
• Kaplan M. Salamanders and newts. Melissa Kaplan's Herp Care Collection, 1993, updated January 1, 2014. http://www.anapsid.org/sallies.html

Suggested Reading

Allender MC, Kastura M, George R, et al. Bioencapsulation of metronidazole in adult brine shrimp (*Artemia* sp.). *J Zoo Wildl Med* 2011;42(2):241–246.

Clayton L, Manharth A, Pessier AP. Systemic mycobacteriosis due to *Mycobacterium avium* complex in a marine toad (*Bufo marinus*). *Proc ARAV* 2004;11:159.

Fischer DC, Lorenz N, Heuser W, et al. Abscesses associated with a brucella inopinata–like bacterium in a big-eyed tree frog (*Leptopelis vermiculatus*). *J Zoo Wildl Med* 2012;43(3):625–628.

Martinho F, Heatley JJ. Amphibian mycobacteriosis. *Vet Clin North Am Exot Anim Pract* 2012;15:113–119.

Author Albert Martínez-Silvestre, DVM, MSc, PhD, DECZM (Herpetology), EBVS European Veterinary Specialist in Herpetological Medicine and Surgery, Acred. AVEPA (Exotic Animals)

AMMONIA TOXICOSIS

BASICS

DEFINITION/OVERVIEW

Environmental ammonia toxicosis in amphibians is generally associated with industrial agricultural fertilizer runoff. These contaminants flow and concentrate into bodies of water where amphibians can congregate. This causes increased levels of inorganic nitrogenous compounds (ammonia/ammonium, nitrites, nitrates), which occurs more commonly in North America and Europe due to more intensive agricultural practices in these areas. In the captive setting, nitrogenous compounds build up in foul, stagnate bodies of water, or aquariums with a lack and/or break in adequate biological filtration. Ammonia, ammonium and nitrites are more transient in nature. Nitrate is more persistent in the environment and therefore more studied.

ETIOLOGY/PATHOPHYSIOLOGY

Ammonia/Ammonium

- Ammonia (NH_3) is more toxic than ammonium (NH_4^+) and is driven by pH.
- There appear to be species-specific toxicity levels.
- Ammonia levels of 0.42 mg/l and 0.46 mg/l proved toxic, and caused mortality and deformities for embryonic and larval *Rana pipiens* and *Hyla crucifer* (*Pseudacris crucifer*) at 12 degrees C.
- Increased temperature to 20 degrees C increased the LC50 to 1.9 mg ammonia/liter in the same study.
- Ammonium is volatile and toxicity is dependent on rate of off gassing of ammonia to the atmosphere, pH, temperature, and rate of conversion of ammonium to nitrite and nitrate by the nitrifying bacteria *Nitrosomonas* and *Nitrobacter* sp. respectively.

Nitrite

- Nitrite (NO_2^-) can be transient within the water column but becomes toxic within the blood by converting hemoglobin into methemoglobin, making it unable to bind to oxygen.
- Nitrite has been reported to cause mortality, developmental abnormalities, and delayed developmental growth in amphibians.

Nitrate

- Nitrate (NO_3^-) is the most persistent nitrogenous compound within the aquatic environment.
- The mechanism of toxicity is not fully understood currently.
- While nitrite is actively transported into the body, nitrate is not. It only enters the extracellular space by passive diffusion, so it is considered less toxic.
- Studies have been inconsistent in demonstrating the toxic effects of nitrate, which is believed to be due to the specific type of nitrate used within the study.
- Species-specific tolerance and sensitivities do seem to occur.
- Nitrate toxicity may cause disruption in osmoregulation.
- It has been reported that increased nitrate levels interfere with iodine uptake and so decrease thyroxine production, a key hormone in metamorphosis and development.
- It has been reported in *Rana pipiens* and *Xenopus laevis* that the combined effect of the herbicide atrazine and nitrate can be an endocrine disruptor, and causes an increased skew in females in larval development, altered follicular morphology, and steroidogenesis.
- Excess nitrates in the natural ecosystem can lead to eutrophication and anoxic conditions in the water column, which are sequelae to toxic levels of ammonia and nitrite.
- In North America, there is an indirect correlation between increased nitrates and increased numbers the trematode *Ribeiroia*, which is known to cause limb malformations in amphibians.

SIGNALMENT/HISTORY

- All ages can be affected
- Free-ranging amphibians will be affected in areas where there is large amount of land used for agricultural, use of fertilizers, and areas of stagnated water.
- Captive amphibians will be affected with poor aeration and water quality.

CLINICAL PRESENTATION

- Neurological dysfunction
- Lethargy
- Dyspnea
- Color change
- Increased mucus production
- Sudden death

RISK FACTORS

Husbandry

Poor aeration and water quality.

Others

Close proximity to areas where there is a large presence of fertilizer use, especially in an agricultural setting.

DIAGNOSIS

DIFFERENTIAL DIAGNOSIS

Other toxins

DIAGNOSTICS

- Clinical signs depend widely on the length and intensity of exposure.
- Measurement of nitrogenous compounds in the water.

PATHOLOGICAL FINDINGS

- Color change
- Increased mucus production
- Developmental abnormalities
- Mass concentrated mortality

TREATMENT

APPROPRIATE HEALTH CARE

Amphibians produce ammonia as their main nitrogenous excretion and therefore rely on their aquatic environment to dilute and remove this toxic byproduct.

NUTRITIONAL SUPPORT

Supportive care with addition of clean well oxygenated water.

CLIENT EDUCATION/HUSBANDRY RECOMMENDATIONS

- Practice proper hygiene with clean well oxygenated water sources.
- Proper biofiltration is essential in the tank setting.

MEDICATIONS

DRUG(S) OF CHOICE

- Calcium if tetany is present
- Methylene blue baths at 2 mg/l or 9 mg/kg ICe, IV for methemoglobinemia
- In a captive setting, sodium formaldehyde bisulfate (Amquel®, Kordon LLC, Hayward, CA) can be added to reduce nitrogenous products.

PRECAUTIONS/INTERACTIONS

N/A

FOLLOW-UP

PATIENT MONITORING

N/A

EXPECTED COURSE AND PROGNOSIS

Fair to poor

MISCELLANEOUS

COMMENTS

N/A

ZOONOTIC POTENTIAL

N/A

SYNONYMS

Amphibian poisoning

ABBREVIATIONS

- ICe = intracoelomic
- IV = intravenous
- LC50 = lethal dose 50%

INTERNET RESOURCES

Poole VA, ed. Amphibian Husbandry Resource Guide. Association of Zoos and Aquariums, Edition 2.0, 2012. https://www.speakcdn.com/assets/2332/amphibianhusbandryresourceguide.pdf

Suggested Reading

Mann RM, Hyne RV, Choung CB, Wilson SP. Amphibians and Agricultural Chemicals: Review of the Risks in a Complex Environment. *Environ Pollut* 2009;157(11):2903–2927.

Whitaker BR. Water quality. In: *Wright KM, Whitaker BR. Amphibian Medicine and Captive Husbandry*. Malabar, FL: Krieger; 2001:147–157.

Author Elsburgh O. Clarke III, DVM, DACZM

ANEMIA

BASICS

DEFINITION/OVERVIEW

Anemia is a reduction in the number of red blood cells as measured by a decrease in PCV or hematocrit. Anemia can occur from one of four main causes: decreased erythropoietic activity, hemorrhage, destruction of red blood cells, or sequestration. In amphibians, the first two are more common.

ETIOLOGY/PATHOPHYSIOLOGY

- Trauma
- Hemorrhage
- Maladaptation syndrome
- Infectious diseases (blood parasites/ ranavirus, etc.).
- Toxicity: metals can produce anemia in amphibians due to their blood toxicity. In the Indian tree frog (*Polypedates maculatus*), a decrease of red blood cells, hemoglobin, PCV and MCV has been demonstrated due to hemolysis after exposure to lead acetate.
- Toads respond to hypoxia and anemia by an increasing heart rate and pulmocutaneous blood flow and reducing the net cardiac right-to-left-shunt. However, anemia does not alter arterial CO_2 partial pressure in toads. As a collateral effect, experimentally induced anemia in *Bufo (Duttaphrynus) melanostictus*, either by administration of phenylhydrazine or by splenectomy stimulated spermatogenic and steroidogenic activities in the testes.

SIGNALMENT/HISTORY

- No specific signalment or history.
- Wild-caught amphibians may be more predisposed.

CLINICAL PRESENTATION

- Non-specific clinical signs including lethargy, anorexia, and light changes in color intensity have been observed in amphibians with anemia.
- Behavioral changes may also be observed.

RISK FACTORS

Husbandry

- Insufficient facilities
- Inadequate food
- Not meeting needs at specific stages of life (growth, gestation, hibernation, etc.).

Others

- Axolotls (*Ambystoma* sp.) prefer somewhat hard water, and those housed in soft water will often suffer from temporary anemia. The animal becomes pale and its gills lose their coloration for a few minutes or hours.
- This is not a dangerous condition but supplementing the hardness of the water with added salts can prevent it.

DIAGNOSIS

DIFFERENTIAL DIAGNOSIS

- Trauma leading to external or internal hemorrhage.
- Maladaptation syndrome associated anemia: reported in stressed frogs and toads, associated with captivity or catching wild amphibians.
- Bone marrow toxicity
- Decreased hormonal stimulation
- Underlying inflammatory disease
- Neoplasia
- Malnutrition
- Parasites: anemia in apparently healthy frogs may be due to infection with the lung parasite *Distomum cylindraceum*, which, when present in sufficiently large numbers, can diminish the available supply of red blood cells.
- Trypanosomiasis may cause anorexia, lethargy, pallor, splenomegaly, and splenic necrosis.

DIAGNOSTICS

Physical exam

- Examination of mucous membranes and general pallor.

Blood analysis

- EDTA can cause hemolysis in some amphibian species; lithium heparin is recommended for blood collections.
- Collection of blood from anurans (frogs and toads) can be achieved through venipuncture of the femoral vein, ventral abdominal vein, or lingual venous plexus, puncture of the facial (maxillary) or musculocutaneous vein or cardiac puncture.
- Peripheral venipuncture in Urodela (newts and salamanders) may not require chemical restraint and may be performed in a manner similar to that used in lizard species for the ventral coccygeal vein.
- The use of heparinized hematocrit tubes may facilitate collection of the small volumes needed for centrifugation and evaluation of PCV.
- Evaluation of a blood smear may reveal increased number of reticulocytes, erythrocytes with anisocytosis, polychromasia, hypochromasia or poikilocytosis.

Hemoglobin

- Normal hemoglobin values range from 0.8 mml/l to 1.4 mmol/l according to species. Lower values should suggest anemia.

Hematocrit/PCV

- The mean PCV of most healthy amphibians is 30%, with a range of 20–45%; a PCV of less than 20% is suggestive of anemia.

PATHOLOGICAL FINDINGS

- In *Rana pipiens*, maximal rates of oxygen consumption declined with anemia. Anemic frogs accumulated lactate faster than control frogs during exercise.
- The erythrocytes of amphibians are large (high MCV) compared with those of other vertebrates, including reptiles.
- Normal amphibian erythrocytes do exhibit slight anisocytosis; however, increased anisocytosis suggests an increased concentration of large red cells due to erythroid regeneration or erythroid dyscrasia (e.g., nutritional deficiency or toxicity). This may be seen in association with a regenerative response to a hemolytic or hemorrhagic anemia.
- The presence of numerous isolated red-cell nuclei and decrease in the number or almost total absence of red cells in amphibians are in proportion to the severity of the underlying disease.
- An increased concentration of reticulocytes indicates increased erythropoiesis as a compensatory regenerative response. How rapidly anemia develops in cases of decreased erythropoiesis depends on red blood cell life span, which can be greater than 100 days in some species.

TREATMENT

APPROPRIATE HEALTH CARE

- Often, anemia is a chronic condition in amphibians.
- Successful treatment is dependent on knowledge of the underlying etiology and should aim to treat that cause in addition to supportive therapy.

NUTRITIONAL SUPPORT

- Proper nutrition is key for the prevention and treatment of anemia.
- The diet should be as varied as possible and adapted to each species (combination of commercial invertebrates such as *Drosophila*, *Grillus*, *Locusta*, *Tenebrio*, *Galleria*, etc.) and the owner should try not to fall into the monotony of feeding a single prey item.
- Nutritional support via gavage feeding should be implemented in very ill and/or anorectic animals.

CLIENT EDUCATION/HUSBANDRY RECOMMENDATIONS

- It is recommended to perform annual health evaluations of the animals at risk. These evaluations should include blood tests and fecal exams.
- Any treatments must be performed based on the results of the exams and the historical data for the collection. Newly acquired and quarantined animals should also be tested.
- Generally, it is wise to assume that any cleaning agent applied to enclosures or equipment to be used for amphibian husbandry is a potential toxin and can produce anemia, as well as other symptoms, therefore vigorous and thorough rinsing before use is essential.

MEDICATIONS

DRUG(S) OF CHOICE

- Hemorrhagic anemia: control of bleeding by applying pressure. The use of hemostatic agents such as D-aminocaproic acid or ethamsylate has not been reported in amphibians; thus the doses are empirical (0.1 ml/kg). The efficacy of blood replacers or transfusions has not been well studied at this time.
- Maladaptation syndrome: the first aspect of treatment consists of providing an appropriate environment for the species followed by fluid therapy and nutritional support.
- Iron dextran (12 mg/kg, IM every 7 days) and cyanocobalamin (vitamin B12 10–2000 iu according to the animal weight as single IM or SC dose.
- Fluid therapy: fluid selection should match the physiologic state of the animal. For dehydrate patients, an isotonic amphibian Ringer solution or a hypotonic solution can be used to ensure fluid absorption, especially when administered via a bath. For edematous patients, short baths with hypertonic solution may be used to help to resolve the edema.

PRECAUTIONS/INTERACTIONS

- Some drugs can produce anemia in amphibians.
- While there are no clear links between clinically used drugs and anemia, an investigation with newts and frogs reported that anemia was pharmacologically induced with intracoelomic injections of 1-acetyl-2-phenylhydrazine dissolved in 10% ethanol.

FOLLOW-UP

PATIENT MONITORING

- Because of the small size of many amphibians, monitoring should rely on assessment of the behavior and clinical signs of the affected animal, not just on blood sampling.
- If the treatment is appropriate, the amphibian should become progressively more active and alert, with interest in hunting, shelter or mating behaviors.

EXPECTED COURSE AND PROGNOSIS

- Repeated blood samplings after 1 week and 1 month may show early signs of regeneration.
- Repeated blood sampling may be contraindicated, especially in cases of non-regenerative anemia, when working with small patients, or if the underlying etiology is not being treated.
- If the underlying cause of anemia is properly diagnosed and can be effectively treated, prognosis is good.

MISCELLANEOUS

COMMENTS

N/A

ZOONOTIC POTENTIAL

N/A

SYNONYMS

N/A

ABBREVIATIONS

- EDTA = ethylenediaminetetraacetic acid
- IM = intramuscular
- MCV = mean corpuscular volume
- PCV = packed cell volume
- SC = subcutaneous

INTERNET RESOURCES

Clare JP. Requirements and water conditions. Axolotls. http://www.axolotl.org/requirements.htm

Suggested Reading

Allender M, Fry MM. Amphibian hematology. *Vet Clin North Am Exot Anim Pract.* 2008;11:463-480.

Cital S, Goodnight A. Reptile and amphibian transfusion medicine. In: Yagi K, Holowaychuk M, eds. Manual of Veterinary Transfusion Medicine and Blood Banking. Aimes, IA: John Wiley & Sons, Inc; 2016:359–364.

Emerson H, Norris C. “Red-leg:” An infectious disease of frogs. *J Exp Med* 1905;7(1):32–58.

Forzan MJ, Vanderstichel RV, Ogbuah CT, et al. Blood collection from the facial (maxillary)/musculo-cutaneous vein in true frogs (family Ranidae). *J Wildl Dis* 2012;48:176–180.

Heatley JJ, Johnson ME. Clinical Technique: Amphibian Hematology: A Practitioner's Guide. *J Exot Pet Med* 2009;18:14–19.

Author Albert Martínez-Silvestre, DVM, MSc, PhD, DECZM (Herpetology), EBVS European Veterinary Specialist in Herpetological Medicine and Surgery, Acred. AVEPA (Exotic Animals)

ANOREXIA

BASICS

DEFINITION/OVERVIEW

Anorexia is the lack of appetite or intake of food, and does not define an underlying cause. Many pathological and even physiological conditions can result in decreased food intake. Anorexia must be distinguished from decreased appetite, which is also known as hypophagia.

ETIOLOGY/PATHOPHYSIOLOGY

- Anorexia may be a normal physiologic process during certain times of the year (e.g., hibernation, estivation, reproductive season).
- Pathologic causes of anorexia may stem from either GI or extra-GI disease (e.g., any painful condition or systemic illness).
- Prolonged anorexia may lead to hepatic lipidosis, which may result in nausea, leading to continued lack of food intake.
- Nutritional imbalances and metabolic derangements can occur with chronic anorexia and cachexia may ensue.
- Primarily, the gastrointestinal and musculoskeletal systems are affected with anorexia.
- Animals that are not consuming food for prolonged periods of time may not defecate significant amounts.
- As the body begins to break down adipose tissue stores and muscle, bony prominences become more obvious as body condition decreases.
- The coelomic cavity may be small and lean in cachectic amphibians.

SIGNALMENT/HISTORY

- Anorexia may be encountered in both young and old animals and shows no sex predilection.
- Lack of appetite is a normal finding in estivating or hibernating animals.

CLINICAL PRESENTATION

- An isolated incident or occasional episodes of anorexia in otherwise healthy animals may be inconsequential.
- A lack of food intake over an extended period outside of normal physiological processes should be a cause for concern.
- May be preceded by hypophagia
- Clients may report repeated attempts at feeding.
- Clinical signs in chronic cases may include a decreased BCS with prominent bony protuberances, dehydration, and muscle wasting.

RISK FACTORS

Husbandry

- In newly acquired amphibians, a period of acclimatization may be necessary prior to an animal feeling secure enough to start eating on its own.
- Inappropriate environmental temperature or humidity level for the species, malnutrition, poor water quality, overcrowding, rapid change of diet, lack of provision of hiding areas, and improper lighting are all factors that may serve as a stressor for the animal and contribute to anorexia.

Others

- Physiologic
- Cardiovascular disease: cardiomyopathy, congestive heart failure.
- Reproductive season: gravid females, breeding males.
- Reproductive disease: pre- or postovulatory dystocia.
- Respiratory infections: mycobacteriosis
- Viral infections: ranaviral infections
- Fungal infections: chytridiomycosis
- Systemic illness: septicemia
- GI disease: stomatitis, foreign bodies, neoplasia, constipation, intussusception, gastroenteritis, prolapses.
- Parasitic disease: ectoparasites and endoparasites.
- Neurologic disease
- Toxic diseases
- Metabolic: nutritional secondary hyperparathyroidism.
- Any potentially painful condition: ophthalmic disease, orthopedic conditions, cellulitis, trauma.

DIAGNOSIS

DIFFERENTIAL DIAGNOSIS

- Conditions that result in failed food prehension (disorders of the tongue or oral cavity) or processing may result in animals that attempt to eat (have an appetite) but are unable to do so successfully.
- It is essential to distinguish between hypophagia and anorexia.
- When evaluating an anorexic amphibian, it is important to differentiate between physiologic and non-physiologic causes.

DIAGNOSTICS

- Baseline blood work: findings on complete blood count and biochemistry panels are usually non-specific or may underline the disease process(es) resulting in the observed anorexia. Bile acids and liver leakage enzymes may be increased if hepatic lipidosis is present secondary to prolonged anorexia.
- Additional diagnostics, including infectious or parasitic disease testing, may be warranted, based on patient history and physical exam findings. Presumed underlying causes should be thoroughly investigated.
- Diagnostic imaging should be part of the diagnostic evaluation for amphibians that are presented for anorexia.
- Evidence of hepatic lipidosis or a generalized decrease in the size of the GI tract may be observed with diagnostic imaging in animals undergoing prolonged periods of anorexia.
- Ultrasound, coelioscopy, and CT are more helpful for diagnosing hepatic lipidosis than survey radiography.
- Radiography may be beneficial to look for evidence of impaction, especially if the animal is housed on a gravel substrate.

PATHOLOGICAL FINDINGS

- Findings depend on underlying cause of the anorexia.
- Hepatic lipidosis may be supported by advanced imaging and biochemistry evaluation.

TREATMENT

APPROPRIATE HEALTH CARE

- Simply providing appropriate husbandry will help to prevent many causes of anorexia in amphibians.
- Prompt diagnosis of true anorexia enables initiation of proper nutritional support and may prevent development of hepatic lipidosis.
- Supportive care is continued while an underlying cause for the anorexia is identified.
- Gravid individuals may decrease their amount of food consumption due to a lack of coelomic space from the eggs.
- Animals that are anorectic from an underlying pathologic condition may cease or abort reproductive activity due to preferential allotment of energy for other physiologic functions.
- Male amphibians may drop substantial body weight during the active breeding season due to time and energy spent on breeding over feeding.

NUTRITIONAL SUPPORT

- The decision to provide nutritional support should be based on BCS and percentage of body weight loss over time, as tube feeding can be stressful to the patient.
- Before starting any therapeutics, it is essential to ensure that animals are housed in appropriate environments maintained at their preferred optimum temperature zone, to maintain proper metabolism for takeup of the provided nourishment.
- Commercial, high-calorie critical care formulations may be provided orally via syringe or directly into the stomach by gavage.
- For more stable patients, assist-feeding may be attempted by gently placing killed prey items in the back of the oral cavity to promote swallowing.

- Esophagostomy tubes are not routinely placed in amphibians, but may be considered in some species, especially when gavage feeding proves to be too stressful.
- It is recommended to start feeding anorectic animals half of their calculated energy requirements initially, then slowly over 5–7 days increasing the amount up to the full energy requirement.
- Husbandry and dietary deficiencies must be corrected as part of the treatment protocol.

CLIENT EDUCATION/HUSBANDRY RECOMMENDATIONS

- A thorough review of the current husbandry practices must be carried out.
- Temperature, humidity, light type and cycle, diet type, and feeding frequency are specific husbandry factors that can commonly contribute to anorexia if not applied properly to the species.
- Husbandry and dietary deficiencies must be corrected as part of the treatment protocol.
- Live prey (e.g., crickets, mealworms) should only be offered in small amounts.
- It is best to offer small meals frequently rather than one single large meal.
- Any uneaten prey items must be removed from the enclosure after feeding has stopped to ensure that they do not attack a debilitated amphibian.

MEDICATIONS

DRUG(S) OF CHOICE

According to diagnosed underlying etiology. In absence of a definitive diagnosis, supportive therapy can be instituted.

PRECAUTIONS/INTERACTIONS

- Exercise caution when force-feeding to prevent dental, mandibular and/or GI trauma.
- Be careful not to administer too large a volume of nutritional formula in small patients.
- A maximum of 3–6% of body weight should be administered in a single feeding.

FOLLOW-UP

PATIENT MONITORING

- Individuals should be monitored for resolution of anorexia following correction of husbandry or initiation of treatment.
- Body weight should be monitored at least twice weekly as an objective measure of response to therapy.
- Defecation should also be monitored to ensure that the GI is functional and the animal is able to digest the food properly.
- Weight gains in the absence of defecation may indicate lack of digestion and should prompt re-evaluation of the patient.
- Fluid retention must also be ruled out as a cause of weight gain.
- Serial imaging and blood chemistry evaluation may be considered to monitor for development or resolution of secondary hepatic lipidosis.

EXPECTED COURSE AND PROGNOSIS

- Physiologic anorexia should resolve once the animal has finished hibernation or reproductive cues have subsided.
- Non-physiologic anorexia may continue until the underlying etiology is identified and treated.
- Prognosis for resolution of anorexia depends on the type and severity of the underlying etiology.

MISCELLANEOUS

COMMENTS

N/A

ZOONOTIC POTENTIAL

N/A

SYNONYMS

- Anophagia
- Aphagia
- Inappetence

ABBREVIATIONS

- BCS = body condition score
- CT = computed tomography
- GI = gastrointestinal

Suggested Reading

Hadfield CA, Clayton LA, Barnett SL. Nutritional support of amphibians. J Exot Pet Med 2006;15:255–263.

Wright KM, Whitaker BR. Amphibian Medicine and Captive Husbandry. Malabar, FL: Krieger; 2001.

Author Grayson Doss, DVM, DACZM

BUPHTHALMOS

BASICS

DEFINITION/OVERVIEW
Buphthalmos is an enlarged globe that is positioned normally in the socket.

ETIOLOGY/PATHOPHYSIOLOGY
An increase in IOP causing enlargement and distention of the globe secondary to chronic glaucoma.

SIGNALMENT/HISTORY
- There is no standard signalment for this disease.
- Common findings in the history may include tearing and squinting noted by the owners, as well as an asymmetry of the globes, and loss of vision on the affected side(s).

CLINICAL PRESENTATION
- While it can be bilateral, most cases in amphibians are unilateral.
- The corneal diameter of the affected eye is increased due to globe stretching.
- Blepharospasm and epiphora
- Unlike exophthalmia, the conjunctiva and position of the nictitans is usually normal.
- Red ciliary flush (red ring around the cornea) and congested episcleral vessels.
- Lens luxation and/or cataracts in the affected eye(s).
- Retropulsion of the globe is normal but the globe itself may feel more firm than normal.

RISK FACTORS

Husbandry
Diet and environmental factors are likely to have an effect on the development of cataracts, including toxin exposure, excessive sunlight, and cold temperatures.

Others
- Trauma, especially if there is corneal penetration can induce uveitis and cataract formation.
- The presence of a cataract may increase the chance of lens luxation and/or lens induced uveitis, both of which can lead to glaucoma.

DIAGNOSIS

DIFFERENTIAL DIAGNOSIS
- It is important to first differentiate between exophthalmia and buphthalmos.
- Glaucoma in amphibians is usually secondary to outflow obstruction of the aqueous humor, which is most often caused by uveitis, lens luxation, intraocular parasites, or intraocular neoplasia.

DIAGNOSTICS
- Physical examination findings should raise suspicion of buphthalmos, which is confirmed by finding elevated IOP.
- Normal IOP has not been reported in amphibians but, since most cases are unilateral, a significant difference in IOP between the eyes may be most indicative of a problem.
- Ocular examination and ultrasound are helpful in further evaluating the root cause, although scleral ossicles, if present, can limit visualization.

PATHOLOGICAL FINDINGS
Chronically elevated IOP will lead to pain and blindness.

TREATMENT

APPROPRIATE HEALTH CARE
As most of these cases present in a chronic state, vision is often already lost and medications are used to control pain and slow the disease process during diagnostic evaluation.

NUTRITIONAL SUPPORT
- Additional nutritional support is not necessary in most cases if the IOP can be brought down.
- If needed, tube feeding can be used to provide nutritional support.

CLIENT EDUCATION/HUSBANDRY RECOMMENDATIONS
- While buphthalmos can occur in any animal, those with husbandry deficiencies may be at increased risk.
- Maximizing the husbandry of the animal will improve the chance for a successful outcome.

SURGICAL CONSIDERATIONS
Enucleation as a salvage procedure is usually indicated.

MEDICATIONS

DRUG(S) OF CHOICE
- If acute glaucoma is suspected, it is important to start treatment immediately with topical beta-adrenergic blockers (such as timolol) and CAIs (such as dorzolamide) two or three times daily to reduce IOP and preserve vision.
- If uveitis is suspected, systemic and topical antibiotics (such as ceftazadime 20 mg/kg IM or SC q48–72h) and steroids (prednisolone 0.25–0.5 mg/kg daily, or dexamethasone 0.04–0.08 mg/kg daily) should also be instituted.

PRECAUTIONS/INTERACTIONS
N/A

FOLLOW-UP

PATIENT MONITORING
Serial IOPs are useful to determine whether there is a response to therapy.

EXPECTED COURSE AND PROGNOSIS
- Prognosis is related to the underlying cause of the glaucoma, which is not always readily identifiable.
- Enucleation of the diseased globe will resolve the issue in most cases.

MISCELLANEOUS

COMMENTS
N/A

ZOONOTIC POTENTIAL
Depends on the cause of the buphthalmos, but low to most often no zoonotic potential.

SYNONYMS
N/A

ABBREVIATIONS
- CAI = carbonic anhydrase inhibitor
- IM = intramuscular
- IOP = intraocular pressure
- SC = subcutaneous

Suggested Reading

Whitaker BR, Wright KM. Clinical techniques. In: Wright KM, Whitaker BR. *Amphibian Medicine and Captive Husbandry*. Malabar, FL: Krieger; 2001:89–110.

Whitaker BR, Wright KM. The amphibian eye. In: Wright KM, Whitaker BR. *Amphibian Medicine and Captive Husbandry*. Malabar, FL: Krieger; 2001:245–252.

Wright KM. Overview of amphibian medicine. In: Mader DR, ed. *Reptile Medicine and Surgery*. 2nd ed. St. Louis, MO: Elsevier Saunders; 2006:941–971.

Author Christopher S. Hanley, DVM DACZM

CARDIAC DISEASE

BASICS

DEFINITION/OVERVIEW

Primary cardiovascular diseases have not been extensively studied in amphibians but seem to be rare. Diseases include myocarditis, epicarditis and cardiac granulomas, atherosclerosis, parasitic infestations, congenital heart defects, and tumors.

ETIOLOGY/PATHOPHYSIOLOGY

Infectious

Unlike in reptiles, extension of systemic infection to the heart is rare in amphibians, despite their relatively high prevalence of septicemia.

Bacterial, Parasitic, Fungal and Viral

- *Mycobacterium* spp., *Chlamydophila* spp., candidiasis, zygomycosis, geotrichosis, chromomycosis, phaeohyphomycosis, and ranaviruses (Frog virus 3, tadpole edema virus): myocarditis, epicarditis, and cardiac granulomas.
- Chytridiomycosis (*Batrachochytrium dendrobatidis*): skin lesions can cause electrolytic imbalances and alter cardiac conduction.
- Parasitic: trematodes (ex: *Clinostomum*): pericardial effusion and respiratory compromise.

Non-Infectious

- Atherosclerosis: associated with hypercholesterolemia in some but not all cases and nutritional causes may have been implicated. Can be associated with myocarditis.
- Congenital heart defects: non-functional lymph hearts resulting in edema (sporadically found in laboratory *Xenopus laevis*), "cardiac nonfunction" mutation in the Mexican axolotl (*Ambystoma mexicanum*) resulting in a non-beating heart and edema in homozygous animals.
- Tumors: cardiovascular neoplasms appear to be extremely rare in amphibians.

SIGNALMENT/HISTORY

Owners usually report weakness and/or edema (abnormal shape), which can be the consequence of heart failure.

CLINICAL PRESENTATION

- Often asymptomatic
- As generalized congestive heart failure is to be expected in species possessing only one ventricle, the hands-on examination may reveal the presence of subcutaneous, lymphatic, and coelomic edema (together referred to as hydrops).

RISK FACTORS

Husbandry

Inadequate husbandry, resulting in chronic stress, immune suppression and malnutrition, is the most likely predisposing factor for the development of cardiovascular conditions in captive amphibians.

Others

- Atherosclerosis
- Bacterial infections
- Viral diseases

DIAGNOSIS

DIFFERENTIAL DIAGNOSIS

- All other diseases that induce weakness and/or hydrops (such as sepsis, viral infection, renal disease, hepatic disease, hypocalcemia, hypoproteinemia, skin diseases, parasites, toxins, traumatic handling).
- Some frogs may inflate themselves as a defensive measure, which should not be interpreted as abnormal.

DIAGNOSTICS

- As for other organ systems, check history, water quality, and osmolality.
- Cardiologic evaluation: very limited in amphibians.
- Hands-off examination: abnormal shape, coelomic distention, localized edema, and cutaneous abnormalities.
- Fluid sample should be collected for analysis at this time for cytology and culture.
- Auscultation: use a Doppler probe placed on the cranioventral aspect of the animal. In large frogs, cardiac auscultation is possible, but care should be taken not to damage the fragile skin with the diaphragm or the bell of the stethoscope. In some species, the heart may be seen beating on the ventral aspect in the area of the xiphoid.
- Clinical pathology: non-specific—changes in plasma/lymph osmolality and electrolyte concentrations may be seen with various causes of hydrops. Hypercholesterolemia can be associated with atherosclerosis and lipid disorders. Hypochloremia, hyponatremia and hypokaliemia can be seen in case of chytridiomycosis.
- Electrocardiography: minimal use, even though ECG has been extensively used in the frog to study cardiac electrophysiology. Anesthesia required for a proper recording. ECG parameter measurements may vary with temperature. SV (sinus venosus) and B (bulbus cordis) waves are usually present.

Imaging

- Radiography is of limited utility
- Ultrasound: described in anurans, by placing the probe ventrally directly on the skin on the xyphoid area. Three views, the parasternal long axis, the subcostal three-chamber, and the high sternal views were described in two *Xenopus* spp. of different size. Intracardiac anatomy, truncus arteriosus, and major vascular trunks can be visualized.
- Doppler can also be performed. Lymph hearts ultrasound measurements were performed in two anuran species using a high-frequency sonographic probe.
- When using ultrasound, ascites can also be visualized to differentiate coelomic effusion from other causes of cœlomic enlargement.
- Coelioscopy may allow the visualization of the pericardium in the coelomic cavity.

PATHOLOGICAL FINDINGS

Gross and histopathologic findings depend on the type of heart disease (myocardial granulomas, myocarditis, epicarditis, atherosclerosis, etc.).

TREATMENT

APPROPRIATE HEALTH CARE

- No specific treatments have been reported in amphibians other than physiological experiments.
- Treatment of infectious and cutaneous diseases must be considered if needed.

NUTRITIONAL SUPPORT

No specific nutritional support considerations and/or recommendations.

CLIENT EDUCATION/HUSBANDRY RECOMMENDATIONS

- Reduce stress and handling
- Regularly control water quality and osmolality.

MEDICATIONS

DRUG(S) OF CHOICE

N/A

PRECAUTIONS/INTERACTIONS

N/A

FOLLOW-UP

PATIENT MONITORING

Repeated ultrasound examinations to monitor heart function and hydrops when present.

EXPECTED COURSE AND PROGNOSIS

As no specific treatment is available, fast deterioration can be expected.

CARDIAC DISEASE (CONTINUED)

MISCELLANEOUS

COMMENTS

N/A

ZOONOTIC POTENTIAL

- No reported case of zoonotic cardiovascular disease transmitted by these animals.
- Some of the infectious causes could be potentially zoonotic.

SYNONYMS

- Cardiovascular disease
- Heart disease

ABBREVIATIONS

ECG = electrocardiogram

Suggested Reading

Beaufrère H, Schilliger L, Pariaut R. Cardiovascular system. In: Mitchell MA, Tully TN, eds. *Current Therapy of Exotic Animal Practice*. St. Louis, MO: Elsevier; 2016:151–220.

Green DE. Pathology of amphibia. In: *Wright KM, Whitaker BR. Amphibian Medicine and Captive Husbandry. Malabar, FL*: Krieger; 2001:401–485.

Whitaker BR, Wright KM. Clinical techniques. In: Wright KM, Whitaker BR. *Amphibian Medicine and Captive Husbandry*. Malabar, FL: Krieger; 2001:89–110.

Author Lionel Schilliger, DVM, DECZM (Herpetology), DABVP (Reptile & Amphibian Practice)

CHLAMYDIOSIS

BASICS

DEFINITION/OVERVIEW

Chlamydia spp. are obligate intracellular, Gram-negative, coccoid organisms of the family Chlamydiaceae. Chlamydiosis is a systemic disease in amphibians, usually leading to debilitation and death. Although only a handful of reports exist, disease has been reported in several frog species, toads and newts. Most information on chlamydiosis infections in amphibians originates from reports in the African clawed frog (*Xenopus* spp.). Newer reports of infections in amphibians have speciated *Chlamydia pneumoniae*, while older outbreaks in African clawed frogs were attributed to *C. psittaci*. Analysis of tissues from frogs that died in distinct mass mortality events revealed the presence of *C. pneumoniae*, *C. abortus*, and *C. suis* in some animals. In this same study, three clinically healthy clawed frogs were PCR positive for *C. suis*. Taxonomic classification of chlamydial organisms has historically been controversial. The family Chlamydiaceae was, until recently, divided into the two genera, *Chlamydia* and *Chlamydophila*; current recommendations, however, have assigned all species under the single genus *Chlamydia*.

ETIOLOGY/PATHOPHYSIOLOGY

- The chlamydial organism exists in two separate forms, and sometimes an intermediate form. The elementary body is the metabolically inactive, infective stage that can persist in the environment. Once inside the host cell, the organism differentiates into an active, replicating form known as the reticulate body; this form is metabolically active, but non-infective.
- While transmission in amphibians is not well described, it is suspected to occur through ingestion of or inhalation of elementary bodies as in other animals. Elementary bodies are able to fuse to cell membranes (mainly epithelial cells of mucous membranes and macrophages) for transport into the cell via endocytosis.
- Although the mechanism is poorly understood, environmental stress, including antibiotic therapy, can push the chlamydial organism into a quiescent form known as the aberrant body, making eradication difficult.
- Chlamydiosis can affect multiple systems in amphibians.
- Alimentary and hematolymphopoietic: the liver and spleen are the most commonly affected organs and collection of these tissues is highly recommended for diagnostic testing.
- Cardiorespiratory: significant cardiac pathology, including epicarditis and myocarditis, has been reported.
- Integumentary: generalized subcutaneous edema may be present.
- Urinary: glomerulonephritis and interstitial nephritis have been reported in African clawed frogs.

SIGNALMENT/HISTORY

Incidence appears to be high in certain captive colonies of frogs, with only sporadic outbreaks in wild amphibians.

CLINICAL PRESENTATION

- Lethargy
- Anorexia
- Generalized edema or anasarca
- Sloughing of the skin
- Depigmentation of the skin
- Petechiation of the skin
- Poor body condition
- Abnormal mentation
- Sudden death
- Vomiting

RISK FACTORS

Husbandry

- Lack of adequate quarantine procedures may result in introducing the organism into a stable population.
- Feeding a contaminated meat product was presumed to be the cause of one major outbreak in clawed frogs.

Others

N/A

DIAGNOSIS

DIFFERENTIAL DIAGNOSIS

- Cutaneous changes occasionally observed with chlamydiosis can resemble other diseases. Disorders (both infectious and non-infectious) causing generalized edema or "hydrops" should be ruled out.
- Bacterial dermatosepticemia
- Mycobacteriosis
- Cutaneous fungal disease
- Systemic bacterial infections
- Chytridiomycosis
- *Ranavirus* infection
- *Iridovirus* infection
- Cutaneous parasites
- Cutaneous neoplasia

DIAGNOSTICS

- A wild giant barred frog (*Mixophyes iteratus*) infected with *C. pneumoniae* had a nonregenerative anemia, leukopenia, and hypoproteinemia; aspartate aminotransferase was also markedly elevated. However, there are no characteristic hematologic changes associated with chlamydiosis.
- Histopathology: intracytoplasmic chlamydial inclusions may be identified on histopathologic examination of infected tissues with hepatocytes being of primary interest.
- Immunohistochemistry and PCR can be used to diagnose clinical and subclinical infections.
- Electron microscopy: the two forms of the organism—elementary and reticulate bodies—may be identified within affected cells. Intermediate stages may also be observed.
- Culture

PATHOLOGICAL FINDINGS

- During gross examination, the liver is often enlarged and mottled or discolored.
- The spleen and gallbladder may also be enlarged.
- Generalized subcutaneous edema is another common finding.
- Skin ulceration, sloughing, depigmentation, or petechiation may be observed.
- On histopathology, basophilic intracytoplasmic inclusions are often identified in affected tissue sections.
- Hepatitis or hepatic necrosis is a common finding.
- Coelomic effusion may be present in affected animals.
- Chronic, severe, mononuclear pneumonia, and splenic and bone marrow hemopoietic cell depletion were found in a giant barred frog infected with *C. pneumoniae.*
- Splenic reticuloendothelial cell hyperplasia may also be seen.
- Interstitial nephritis, glomerulonephritis, and granulomatous endomyocarditis have been reported in African clawed frogs.

TREATMENT

APPROPRIATE HEALTH CARE

N/A

NUTRITIONAL SUPPORT

Infected amphibians may need nutritional support and hydration therapy during treatment.

CLIENT EDUCATION/HUSBANDRY RECOMMENDATIONS

- Because of the potential for zoonosis, clients should exercise appropriate caution when interacting with or cleaning enclosures of *Chlamydia* spp. positive animals.
- There are no reports of chlamydial infections in humans linked to exposure with infected amphibians.
- Because *C. pneumoniae* is a well-described cause of pneumonia in humans, infected humans should limit contact with amphibians

in order to minimize the risk of potential anthropozoonotic infections.
• If chlamydial disease is suspected, a postmortem examination should be performed using appropriate personal protective equipment to minimize the risk of zoonotic infection.

MEDICATIONS

DRUG(S) OF CHOICE

• Tetracyclines are the treatment of choice for chlamydiosis.
• Doxycycline 5–10 mg/kg PO q12–24h; 10–50 mg/kg PO q24h reported for African clawed frogs; 50 mg/kg IM q7d
• Oxytetracycline 50 mg/kg PO q24h; 50–100 mg/kg IM q48h; 100 mg/l, 60-minute bath, q24h
• Tetracycline 50 mg/kg PO q12h

PRECAUTIONS/INTERACTIONS

Be mindful when administering oral calcium in foods or as supplements, as the gastrointestinal absorption of tetracyclines is inhibited by calcium.

FOLLOW-UP

PATIENT MONITORING

• Affected animals should be monitored for progression of clinical signs and treated for secondary bacterial infections or dehydration as needed.
• Septicemia or bacterial infections are common in amphibians with chlamydiosis; consider treating affected individuals or cohoused animals prophylactically for Gramnegative bacterial infections.
• Affected individuals should be separated from non-affected animals.
• Euthanasia is recommended for animals with a poor quality of life.

EXPECTED COURSE AND PROGNOSIS

• There is little information regarding treatment success in amphibians infected with *Chlamydia* spp.
• The prognosis for animals that present debilitated or with secondary septicemia is poor.

MISCELLANEOUS

COMMENTS

N/A

ZOONOTIC POTENTIAL

Although zoonotic transmission has not been reported, *C. pneumoniae* is a known pathogen in humans.

SYNONYMS

Chlamydophilosis

ABBREVIATIONS

PCR = polymerase chain reaction

Suggested Reading

AbdelRahman YM, Belland RJ. The chlamydial developmental cycle. *FEMS Microbiol Rev* 2005;29:949–959.

Blumer C, Zimmermann DR, Weilenmann R, et al. Chlamydiae in free-ranging and captive frogs in Switzerland. *Vet Path* 2007;44:144–150.

Hammerschlag MR. The intracellular life of Chlamydiae. *Semin Pediatr Infect Dis* 2002;13:239–248.

Howerth EW. Pathology of naturally occurring chlamydiosis in African clawed frogs (*Xenopus laevis*). *Vet Path* 1984;21:28–32.

Pessier AP. An overview of amphibian skin disease. *Semin Avian Exot Pet Med* 2002;11:162–174.

Pessier AP. Diseases of amphibians: it isn't just redleg anymore. In: Mader DR, Divers SJ, eds. *Current Therapy in Reptile Medicine and Surgery*. Saint Louis, MO: Elsevier Saunders; 2014: 247–254.

Reed KD, Ruth GR, Meyer JA, Shukl SK. *Chlamydia pneumoniae* infection in a breeding colony of African clawed frogs (*Xenopus tropicalis*). *Emerg Infect Dis* 2000;6:196.

Wright KM, Whitaker BR. *Amphibian Medicine and Captive Husbandry*. Malabar, FL: Krieger; 2001.

Author Grayson Doss, DVM, DACZM

CHYTRIDIOMYCOSIS

BASICS

DEFINITION/OVERVIEW

Chytridiomycosis is a highly contagious and lethal skin infection of amphibians, with two species of primitive, mostly aquatic fungi in the order Chytridiales, class Chytridiomycota. Chytridiomycosis is a disease that has had significant impact on populations of wild amphibians, leading to rapid global decline and extinction of at least 200 species. Devastating outbreaks have also occurred in captive amphibians. Anurans, caudates, and caecilians are all susceptible. The other 750+ known chytrid fungal species are ubiquitous plant or algae parasites, or decomposers.

ETIOLOGY/PATHOPHYSIOLOGY

- Chytridiomycosis in amphibians is caused by *Batrachochytrium dendrobatidis* and *B. salamandrivorans*.
- *B. dendrobatidis* has been found to infect over 500 species of wild and captive amphibians belonging to all three orders: anurans (frogs, toads), caudates (or urodeles: salamanders, newts), and caecilians.
- Motile, free-swimming, flagellated, zoospores attach to the skin, encyst, and invade epithelial cells to form thalli that become zoosporangia in which asexual zoospores develop.
- Zoospores exit the zoosporangia through a discharge tube and the cycle resumes.
- Disease is a result of breaches in integument integrity, epidermal hyperplasia causing interference with oxygen and CO_2 cutaneous exchange, and with fluid and electrolyte osmoregulation, and secondary infections.
- Infection with *B. salamandrivorans* is a more recent event reported in salamanders in Europe.
- Pathophysiology is likely similar to that of *B. dendrobatidis*.

SIGNALMENT/HISTORY

- For *B. dendrobatidis*, any post-metamorphic anuran, caudate, or caecilian, both sexes.
- Infection in tadpoles also, but targets the oral disk, which is keratinized, affecting feeding ability.
- Wild or captive animals. *B. salamandrivorans* is reported from wild and captive fire salamanders in Europe.
- Some species may be asymptomatic carriers, like African clawed frogs, which are used in laboratories, and North American bullfrogs farmed for meat, so that the global trade in these frogs might have helped spread the disease worldwide.

CLINICAL PRESENTATION

- Can present as an acute, severe mortality event, in wild or captive amphibian populations.
- Animals may be dead, dying, depressed, or weak and unwilling to move.
- Excess, hyperplastic skin, or skin sloughing, and erythema often over the ventrum and feet are particularly suggestive.
- Sick frogs may seek immersion in water.
- Weight loss, anorexia, and central nervous system signs such as ataxia, loss of righting reflex, convulsions, or any combination of the above.
- May progress quickly to affect all animals within a captive population. Signs may be subtle to absent in some frog species, such as African clawed frogs, North American bullfrogs, or fire-bellied toads.
- Infection with *B. salamandrivorans* usually results in a severe ulcerative dermatitis in susceptible caudates.

RISK FACTORS

Husbandry

- Prevention is key
- Repeated PCR testing of all animals, prior to acquisition and/or during quarantine, is ideal.
- Optimal husbandry is critical in captive amphibians.
- Overcrowding, inadequate temperature and humidity and, in aquatic species, fluctuant water quality parameters may compound disease.
- Isolate sick animals as soon as clinical signs are noted.
- Using proper biosecurity measures is also essential.

Others

N/A

DIAGNOSIS

DIFFERENTIAL DIAGNOSIS

- Viral infection, especially ranavirus infections.
- Septicemia with coliforms, *Chlamydia*, or *Bordetella* may present similarly.
- Amphibians also easily absorb environmental toxins through skin.

DIAGNOSTICS

- Clinical signs may lead to presumptive diagnosis of chytridiomycosis.
- Cytology with Congo red or histology on shed skin may reveal zoosporangia.
- PCR on skin or other sample/material probably quickest and surest way to diagnose.

PATHOLOGICAL FINDINGS

- Epidermal hyperplasia and hyperkeratosis with intralesional zoosporangia.
- Variable mixed inflammatory cell influx, edema, vascular congestion.

TREATMENT

APPROPRIATE HEALTH CARE

- Strict standard biosecurity measures should be followed whenever treating amphibians with confirmed or suspected chytridiomycosis.
- Tanks and tools should be disinfected as should water before being discarded.
- Many drug protocols have been described, with variable results.

NUTRITIONAL SUPPORT

- Supportive fluid therapy with electrolyte solutions may help individual animals.
- Thermal support, and other supportive measures such as assist-feeding, probably indicated in most cases.

CLIENT EDUCATION/HUSBANDRY RECOMMENDATIONS

- Strict 6–8 weeks of quarantine, with animals tested for *B. dendrobatidis* and/or *B. salamandrivorans* at least twice using PCR and skin swabs.
- Isolation of sick animals and thorough hygiene.
- Critical review of husbandry

MEDICATIONS

DRUG(S) OF CHOICE

Itraconazole

- Soak 0.00025–0.01% for 5–15 minutes/day for 7–11 days
- Oral 0.1 mg/kg once daily for 5 days

Terbinafine

Soak 0.01% or 0.005% (terbinafine in alcohol) for 5 minutes for 5 consecutive days or every other day for 12 days proved efficacious and safe for five different species of amphibians.

Voriconazole

- Topical spray: midwife toads sprayed once daily for 7 days with a 1.25 µg/ml aqueous solution of voriconazole cleared infection.
- Fire salamanders with *B. salamandrivorans* treated topically with a combination of polymyxin E (2000 iu/ml) and voriconazole (12.5 µg/ml) at an ambient temperature of 20 degrees C cleared infection.

CHYTRIDIOMYCOSIS (CONTINUED)

Others

- Bath with malachite green or new methylene blue (0.1 mg/l) and formalin (25 ppm) daily for 5 days or bath with chloramphenicol (0.002%) for 2–4 weeks.
- Treatment should be selected based on the species, the number of animals involved, the size of the animals, and should rely on published studies that document both efficacy and safety.

PRECAUTIONS/INTERACTIONS

- Follow suggested treatment protocols carefully.
- Amphibians are easily overdosed and do not tolerate handling and stressful events well.
- Skin is easily traumatized when restrained.

FOLLOW-UP

PATIENT MONITORING

Swabs can be submitted at intervals to maximize chances of early detection of *B. dendrobatidis* in a captive set up.

EXPECTED COURSE AND PROGNOSIS

- Prognosis is poor in clinically ill animals.
- Early diagnosis improves the prognosis.

MISCELLANEOUS

COMMENTS

N/A

ZOONOTIC POTENTIAL

N/A

SYNONYMS

N/A

ABBREVIATIONS

PCR = polymerase chain reaction

Suggested Reading

Forzan MJ, Gunn H, Scott P. Chytridiomycosis in an aquarium collection of frogs: Diagnosis, treatment, and control. *J Zoo Wildl Med* 2008;39:406–411.

Gray MJ, Lewis JP, Nanjappa P, et al. *Batrachochytrium salamandrivorans*: The North American response and a call for action. *PLoS Pathog* 2015;11(12):e1005251.

Martel A, Van Rooij P, Vercauteren G, et al. Developing a safe antifungal treatment protocol to eliminate *Batrachochytrium dendrobatidis* from amphibians. *Med Mycol* 2010;49:143–149.

Mutschman F. Chytridiomycosis in amphibians. *J Exotic Pet Med* 2015;24:276–282.

Pessier AP, Mendelson JR, III. *A Manual for Control of Infectious Diseases in Amphibian Survival Assurance Colonies and Reintroduction Programs*. Apple Valley, MN: IUCN/SSC Conservation Breeding Specialist Group; 2009.

Van Rooij P, Martel A, Haesebrouck F, Pasmans F. Amphibian chytridiomycosis: A review with focus on fungus-host interactions. *Vet Res* 2015;46:137–159.

Author Jean A. Paré, DMV, DVSc, DACZM, DECZM (Zoo Health Management)

CRYPTOSPORIDIUM

BASICS

DEFINITION/OVERVIEW

Cryptosporidium spp. are apicomplexan parasites typified by possessing an apical complex, and with four naked sporozoites within each oocyte. *Cryptosporidium* spp. can be distinguished from other coccidian parasites by the location they occupy within the host cell membrane, their capacity for autoinfection, and their resistance to anti-parasitic medications. Possessing a durable oocyst wall consisting of a double layer of a protein–lipid–carbohydrate matrix, Cryptosporidium is highly resistant to environmental degradation and chemical disinfection. Historically, oocyst morphology has been used for species identification, but this is considered unreliable and species assignment is now determined by molecular characteristics. *Cryptosporidium* is ubiquitous in the environment and are globally distributed. There is scant information on cryptosporidiosis in amphibian species.

ETIOLOGY/PATHOPHYSIOLOGY

- Reports of *Cryptosporidium* infections in amphibians are very rare.
- To date, there have only been three reports of clinical disease from unspecified *Cryptosporidium* sp., all of which have been in frogs.
- *Cryptosporidium fragile* was isolated from subclinical black-spined toads (*Duttaphrynus melanostictus*).
- *Cryptosporidium* has been identified in the feces of apparently healthy wild amphibians.
- Transmission is likely to be direct, with amphibians probably becoming infected after ingesting oocysts that have been shed in feces.
- It is not known if autoinfection occurs in amphibians, and parasitism appears to be limited to the stomach.

SIGNALMENT/HISTORY

A history of chronic ill thrift.

CLINICAL PRESENTATION

The most common clinical signs are lethargy and chronic wasting.

RISK FACTORS

Husbandry

The greatest risk factor for developing infection is poor quarantine of new animals entering a collection.

Others

N/A

DIAGNOSIS

DIFFERENTIAL DIAGNOSIS

- Gastritis: bacterial or other protozoal disease.
- Wasting: husbandry-related inappetence, other disease causing weight loss.

DIAGNOSTICS

- Examination of feces with acid-fast stain.
- PCR can be used to test either feces or gastric lavage samples. Can also differentiate between *Cryptosporidium* species.
- Gastric biopsy may be possible in large individuals.

PATHOLOGICAL FINDINGS

- Hyperplasic gastric mucosa with frond-like folds lined by numerous epithelial cells.
- *Cryptosporidium* organisms may be seen lining the superficial mucosa and glands within the stomach.

TREATMENT

APPROPRIATE HEALTH CARE

N/A

NUTRITIONAL SUPPORT

Stomach tubing with easily digestible proteins and supportive fluid therapy are important for case management.

CLIENT EDUCATION/HUSBANDRY RECOMMENDATIONS

Clients should be made aware of the insidious nature of infection, the unlikelihood of successful treatment, and the risks that affected animals pose to the remaining collection.

MEDICATIONS

DRUG(S) OF CHOICE

N/A

PRECAUTIONS/INTERACTIONS

- Elimination of *Cryptosporidium* from amphibians has not been attempted.
- Euthanasia should be strongly considered for affected animals to limit spread.
- If euthanasia is not an option, diseased amphibians should be separated from the remaining collection, and strict barrier nursing protocols enacted to prevent spread.

FOLLOW-UP

PATIENT MONITORING

Repeat fecal examination at monthly intervals.

EXPECTED COURSE AND PROGNOSIS

Grave prognosis, likely chronic wasting and death.

MISCELLANEOUS

COMMENTS

N/A

ZOONOTIC POTENTIAL

- The zoonotic potential of *Cryptosporidium* spp. infecting amphibians is unknown.
- It is prudent that people exercise caution with suspected cases, especially individuals that may be immunocompromised.

SYNONYMS

N/A

ABBREVIATIONS

PCR = polymerase chain reaction

Suggested Reading

Green SL, Bouley DM, Josling CA, Fayer R. Cryptosporidiosis associated with emaciation and proliferative gastritis in a laboratory-reared South African clawed frog (*Xenopus laevis*). *Comp Med* 2003;53(1):81–84.

Jirku M, Valigurova A, Koudela B, et al. New species of *Cryptosporidium tyzzer*, 1907 (Apicomplexa) from amphibian host: morphology, biology and phylogeny. *Folia Parasitol* 2008;55:81–94.

Kyzy MSO. Intestinal coccidia (Eucoccidia, Sporozoa, Apicomplexa) of some amphibia in Azerbaijan. *Protistology* 2010;6(3):218–222.

Plutzer J, Karanis P. Genetic polymorphism in *Cryptosporidium* species: an update. *Vet Parasitol* 2009;165(3–4):187–199.

Author T. Franciscus Scheelings, BVSc, MVSc, PhD, MANCVSc (Wildlife Health), DECZM (Herpetology)

DERMATOSEPTICEMIA

BASICS

DEFINITION/OVERVIEW

Dermatosepticemia is a generalized infection of the skin leading to septicemia, usually caused by Gram-negative bacteria. Often predisposed by an imbalance between the immunological state of the amphibian and environmental bacterial overgrowth. The causative agents are often opportunistic, and mixed infections (several bacteria and fungi) are not uncommon.

ETIOLOGY/PATHOPHYSIOLOGY

- Historically, the most frequently implicated etiological agent has been *Aeromonas hydrophila*.
- Current taxonomic changes of the *Aeromonas* group and new case descriptions have revealed a wide range of bacteria causing dermatosepticemia.
- Many of these bacteria are frequently isolated from aquatic environments, including species of *Flavobacterium*, *Pseudomonas*, *Citrobacter*, *Alcaligenes* and *Enterobacter*.
- *Salmonella* may also be involved. In addition, some Gram-positive bacteria (e.g., *Streptococcus* and *Staphylococcus*) have also been reported.
- If a specific bacterial species is not isolated in pure culture during a septic outbreak, another cause, such as iridovirus, chlamydiosis, fungi, malnutrition, intoxication, or other lethal stressors, should be considered.

SIGNALMENT/HISTORY

- No species, age or sex predilection.
- May be associated with mass mortality events.

CLINICAL PRESENTATION

- Clinicals signs are associated with the cutaneous infection and consequent septicemia.
- Erythema, primarily on the ventrum (coelom, thighs, digital membranes, etc.) is due to vasodilation, congestion, and petechial, paintbrush, or ecchymotic hemorrhages.
- Other clinical signs may include anorexia, swelling, edema (generalized or localized to extremities or the lymphatic sacs), coelomic effusion, blood blisters, and epidermal erosions, ulcers, sloughing, or necrosis.
- Animals may also present lethargic and anorexic.
- There may be cases of mortality without previous signs.
- In the final phases of the disease, convulsions, hemoptysis, and/or gastric prolapse may be observed.

RISK FACTORS

Husbandry

Review maintenance measures to rule out stressors, such as inappropriate temperature and humidity, water quality, or presence of toxins (e.g., ammonia, chlorine, salt, environmental insecticides, algaecide, nicotine, or household chemicals).

Others

- Trauma due to attacks from conspecifics or bites from prey items may aid in bacterial colonization.
- Check for water quality and substrate conditions, ensuring pH is appropriate for the species.
- Gas bubble disease or supersaturation may also be an important predisposing factor.

DIAGNOSIS

DIFFERENTIAL DIAGNOSIS

- Other non-bacterial pathogens that may present with similar clinical signs include viral disease (*Ranavirus*), *Batrachochytrium spp.*, *Chlamydia* or *Chlamydia*-like organisms.
- The parasite *Pseudocapillaroides* may cause changes of color or ulcerative lesions of the skin.

DIAGNOSTICS

- A full diagnostic workup including gross pathology and histopathology, bacterial and fungal culture is essential for definitive diagnosis.
- The results of microbiological cultures are best interpreted in correlation with cytology and histopathology.
- *Ranavirus* infection, chytridiomycosis and chlamydiosis can be ruled out via PCR as needed.

PATHOLOGICAL FINDINGS

Cytology

- It is typical to find phagocytic leukocytes in amphibians with septicemia.
- Leukocyte morphology can be a good diagnostic and prognostic indicator of the disease.

Histopathology

- Skin lesions are usually characterized by multifocal, variably extensive, grey patches that are consistent with areas of severe epidermal hyperplasia and necrosis.
- Intranuclear eosinophilic to amphophilic inclusions associated with minimal inflammatory response may also be observed.
- These lesions are compatible not only with bacteria but also with viral infections.

TREATMENT

APPROPRIATE HEALTH CARE

- Stabilize electrolyte imbalances and dehydration by bathing in a solution of amphibian ringers or modified saline solution (0.6%).
- Antibiotic treatment should be broad spectrum and supported by results of culture and sensitivity.
- Parenteral administration is preferred to provide more consistent drug levels, but bath administration may also be considered.
- Oxygen therapy should be considered in very debilitated or lethargic patients.

NUTRITIONAL SUPPORT

- Gavage feeding of carnivore diets should be carried out in anorexic animals to help support recovery.
- For small patients, food may be administered using pipettes rather than gavage needles.

CLIENT EDUCATION/HUSBANDRY RECOMMENDATIONS

- In captive populations, correction of poor husbandry practices to reduce stress and self-inflicted injury and to improve sanitation and other environmental conditions is essential.
- Proper husbandry considerations for captive amphibians must include nutritional needs, as well as space, temperature, humidity, water quality, and light requirements, all of which will vary considerably among given species and life stages.
- Proper oxygenation of the water is also essential for aquatic and semiaquatic amphibians.

MEDICATIONS

DRUG(S) OF CHOICE

- Some preferred drugs include amikacin combined with metronidazole or piperacillin, fluoroquinolones, and potentiated sulfas.
- With long-term broad-spectrum antibiotic use, concurrent therapy with an antifungals can be considered to avoid overgrowth or opportunistic fungal infections.

PRECAUTIONS/INTERACTIONS

N/A

FOLLOW-UP

PATIENT MONITORING

N/A

EXPECTED COURSE AND PROGNOSIS

Treatment often may be impractical or unsuccessful, depending on the causative agent, chronicity of the disease, efficacy of antimicrobial treatment regimes, and presence of concurrent pathogens.

MISCELLANEOUS

COMMENTS

- Postmortem bacterial invasion of organs is a common phenomenon among aquatic vertebrates, including amphibians, and it occurs much more rapidly than in terrestrial, endothermic vertebrates.
- Diagnosis of this syndrome is unreliable when it is based solely on bacterial isolation from tissues of an amphibian that died more than1–3 hours before the necropsy.
- It is highly likely that this practice has historically led to considerable overdiagnosis of dermatosepticemia as the etiology of epizootics among diseased amphibian populations.

ZOONOTIC POTENTIAL

There is a zoonotic risk depending on the organism associated with the dermatosepticemia (i.e., *Chlamydia* spp.).

SYNONYMS

- Bacterial dermatosepticemia
- Peracute/acute bacterial septicemia
- Red-leg
- Red-leg syndrome
- Sepsis

ABBREVIATIONS

PCR = polymerase chain reaction

INTERNET RESOURCES

- PetMD Editorial. "Red-leg" syndrome in amphibians. PetMD, September 23, 2008. http://www.petmd.com/reptile/conditions/skin/c_rp_am_red_leg
- PetMD Editorial. Bacterial Infection in Amphibians: Mycobacteriosis. PetMD, September 23, 2008. https://www.petmd.com/reptile/conditions/skin/c_rp_am_mycobacteria

Suggested Reading

Densmore CL, Green DE. Diseases of amphibians. *ILAR J* 2007;48(3):235–254.

Garner MM. Master class: Diseases of amphibians. *Proc ARAV.* 2009;16:16–32.

Taylor SK, Green E, Wright KM, Whitaker BR. Bacterial diseases. In: Wright KM, Whitaker BR. *Amphibian Medicine and Captive Husbandry*. Malabar, FL: Krieger; 2001:161–166.

Author Albert Martínez-Silvestre, DVM, MSc, PhD, DECZM (Herpetology), EBVS European Veterinary Specialist in Herpetological Medicine and Surgery, Acred. AVEPA (Exotic Animals)

DIARRHEA

BASICS

DEFINITION/OVERVIEW

Diarrhea is the production of unformed or liquid fecal matter. It is often associated with increased fecal volume and frequency of defection.

ETIOLOGY/PATHOPHYSIOLOGY

- Diarrhea is usually associated with enteritis due to parasitic or bacterial infections.
- Salmonellosis should always be a differential in amphibians with diarrhea.
- Environmental factors, such as low temperatures, can lead to decreased gastrointestinal motility, dysbacteriosis, and diarrhea, due to overgrowth of opportunistic pathogens.
- Nematodes: *Strongyloides* spp
- Amoebiasis: *Entamoeba ranarum* can cause diarrhea with frank blood.

SIGNALMENT/HISTORY

- Inappropriate husbandry
- Low environmental temperatures and overcrowding (stress) can lead to enteritis and diarrhea.
- New amphibian introductions into the collection without proper quarantine.

CLINICAL PRESENTATION

- Depending on duration (acute vs. chronic), severity, and etiology of diarrhea.
- Presence of abnormally soft or liquid fecal matter in transport container.
- Chronic diarrhea can lead to weight loss and cachexia due to malabsorption of nutrients.
- Cloacal prolapse

RISK FACTORS

Husbandry

- Change in diet
- Poor sanitation often leads to high endoparasite load because of the direct life cycle of many intestinal parasites.
- Overcrowding resulting in stress
- Inappropriate (too low or to high) environmental temperatures.

Others

Lack of fecal parasitology screening after acquisition of new amphibians.

DIAGNOSIS

DIFFERENTIAL DIAGNOSIS

Polyuria

DIAGNOSTICS

- Fecal direct wet mount to evaluate for motile protozoa. Use fresh, non-refrigerated fecal sample to avoid stimulating protozoa to encyst.
- Fecal flotation to evaluate for helminths and protozoa (coccidian, amoeba cysts).
- Cytology of feces with routine stains. The presence of blood or inflammatory cells is associated with pathology and should prompt appropriate therapy.
- It is important to rule out the presence of parasites originating from prey items.

PATHOLOGICAL FINDINGS

- Enteritis
- Liquid intestinal content
- Emaciation

TREATMENT

APPROPRIATE HEALTH CARE

- Identification of the underlying cause is necessary to improve outcome and reduce the risk of reoccurrence.
- Keep on moist paper towels until treatment is completed and recheck fecal exams.
- Frequent removal of feces to prevent reinfection is needed.

NUTRITIONAL SUPPORT

- Provide nutritional support to emaciated and/or anorexic animals.
- Provide fluid therapy to dehydrated animals.

CLIENT EDUCATION/HUSBANDRY RECOMMENDATIONS

- Diarrhea is a clinical sign associated with an underlying disease, improper husbandry, or nutrition.
- Correction of husbandry is always recommended to in help improve the outcome.

MEDICATIONS

DRUG(S) OF CHOICE

For Parasitic Infections

- Fenbendazole 50 mg/kg PO, repeat in 14 days
- Oxfendazole 5 mg/kg PO once
- Pyrantel pamoate 5-10 mg/kg PO q24h for 3 days, repeat in 3 weeks.
- Ivermectin 0.2 mg/kg topically, PO, repeat in 2 weeks.
- Metronidazole 100 mg/kg PO once then repeated in 14 days; 50 mg/kg PO q24h for 5 days.
- Metronidazole baths at 500 mg/l for 15–30 minutes every 5 days or 6.6 mg/l for 8 hours for more sensitive species.

For Bacterial Enteritis

- Amikacin 5 mg/kg IM, SC, ICe q24–48h
- Chloramphenicol 50 mg/kg PO, IM, SC q12–24h; 20 mg/l continuous bath changed daily.
- Ceftazidime 20 mg/kg IM q48–72h
- Ciprofloxacin 10 mg/kg PO q24h; 10 mg/l bath for 6–8hours daily.
- Enrofloxacin 10 mg/kg PO, SC q24h
- Metronidazole 10–20 mg/kg PO q24h; 50 mg/l continuous bath changed daily.
- Trimethoprim/sulfa 20 mg/kg PO q24h

PRECAUTIONS/INTERACTIONS

- Fenbendazole has been shown in other reptiles to cause bone marrow suppression and temporary pancytopenia. Avoid dosages greater than 20 mg/kg.
- Ivermectin may cause flaccid paralysis in some species.

FOLLOW-UP

PATIENT MONITORING

- Return to normal fecal consistency.
- Weight gain and maintenance of hydration.
- Repeat fecal exams to ensure treatment is effective.
- Prevention of reinfection is critically important during and following treatment against parasites with a direct life cycle.

EXPECTED COURSE AND PROGNOSIS

- If dietary causes are responsible for the diarrhea, then prognosis is excellent to good.
- Animals in good body condition and no concurrent morbidities have an excellent to good prognosis.
- Animals in poor body condition with signs of systemic illness (dehydration, lethargy, etc.) have a guarded to poor prognosis.
- There is currently no effective treatment against *Cryptosporidium* spp.

MISCELLANEOUS

COMMENTS

N/A

ZOONOTIC POTENTIAL

Salmonella spp. may be commonly shed by amphibians with and without diarrhea.

SYNONYMS

N/A

ABBREVIATIONS

- ICe = intracoelemic
- IM = intramuscular
- PO = per os
- SC = subcutaneous

Authors Javier G. Nevarez, DVM, PhD, DACZM, DECZM (Herpetology), and Christoph Mans, Dr. med. vet., DACZM

EIMERIA

BASICS

DEFINITION/OVERVIEW

Eimeria is an apicomplexan parasite characterized by oocytes having four sporocysts that each contain two sporozoites. *Eimeria* spp. are commonly reported in amphibians and form a normal component of the gastrointestinal flora without causing disease.

ETIOLOGY/PATHOPHYSIOLOGY

- Numerous *Eimeria* spp. have been reported from amphibians and all appear to be commensal organisms.
- Transmission is likely direct, with animals becoming infected by ingested oocyts shed in the feces.

SIGNALMENT/HISTORY

N/A

CLINICAL PRESENTATION

- Clinical disease due to *Eimeria* infection has not been reported.
- Amphibians appear to be asymptomatic carriers.

RISK FACTORS

Husbandry

- New (captive or wild) animals entering a collection with poor hygiene and high stocking densities.
- Juvenile or larval stages may potentially be at higher risk.

Others

Concurrent disease or excessive stress may cause immunosuppression, increasing risks of disease expression.

DIAGNOSIS

DIFFERENTIAL DIAGNOSIS

Other gastrointestinal disease such as bacterial or protozoal infections (i.e., *Isospora*).

DIAGNOSTICS

- Examination of feces for presence of oocysts using light microscopy is the most reliable test.
- Molecular techniques such as PCR may aid in species delineation but are unlikely to improve treatment efficacy or prognosis.
- Protozoa may also be seen in biopsy or necropsy samples.
- For preservation of coccidia for future diagnostics, fecal samples should be stored in 2–3% aqueous (w/v) potassium dichromate ($K_2Cr_2O_7$).

PATHOLOGICAL FINDINGS

N/A

TREATMENT

APPROPRIATE HEALTH CARE

N/A

NUTRITIONAL SUPPORT

N/A

CLIENT EDUCATION/HUSBANDRY RECOMMENDATIONS

- Remove and isolate sick individuals and reduce stress by providing optimal living conditions, and hygiene.
- Thorough cleaning of cage to reduce environmental contamination of oocysts.
- Ensure quarantine protocols have been adopted for all new arrivals.
- During quarantine, all animals should be subjected to repeated clinical and fecal examinations.

MEDICATIONS

DRUG(S) OF CHOICE

- Must only be performed if clinical disease has been confirmed since amphibians appear to be asymptomatic carriers.
- Ponazuril 30 mg/kg PO q12h for 3 days, repeat in 3 weeks.

PRECAUTIONS/INTERACTIONS

N/A

FOLLOW-UP

PATIENT MONITORING

Repeat fecal examination at monthly intervals.

EXPECTED COURSE AND PROGNOSIS

Prognosis likely to be good provided adequate husbandry and concurrent disease are not complicating factors.

MISCELLANEOUS

COMMENTS

N/A

ZOONOTIC POTENTIAL

Due to their high host specificity, there is no known zoonotic risk with any *Eimeria* species.

SYNONYMS

N/A

ABBREVIATIONS

PCR = polymerase chain reaction

Author T. Franciscus Scheelings, BVSc, MVSc, PhD, MANCVSc (Wildlife Health), DECZM (Herpetology)

ENTAMOEBA

BASICS

DEFINITION/OVERVIEW

Entamoeba is considered to be a significant parasite of amphibians. *Entamoeba* spp. are capable of forming pseudopodia. *Entamoeba* is characterized into two groupings based on the number of nuclei present. Those species in the group containing four nuclei are considered to be pathogenic and are the main concern for amphibians; those in the group containing eight nuclei are considered to be noninvasive. *Entamoeba ranae* has been reported to cause significant mortality in amphibians. Virulence can differ between strains of *Entamoeba. Copramoeba, Hartmanella, Mastigamoeba,* and *Vahlkampfia* are other genera of amoeba reported in amphibians.

ETIOLOGY/PATHOPHYSIOLOGY

- *Entamoeba* has a direct life cycle and transmission is the through fecal–oral route.
- Cysts are ingested and then undergo excystation in the intestinal tract.
- The motile feeding trophozoite can also encyst and then be passed through the host's GI tract and in the feces.
- Trophozoites undergo encystation, in which infective cysts are formed and then excreted in feces.
- Cysts can remain infective for 14+ days at temperatures of 8 degrees C and several days at 37 degrees C.
- Secondary bacterial infections are a common occurrence.

SIGNALMENT/HISTORY

- All ages can be affected.
- Animals consistently kept in temperatures 25–33 degrees C.
- Stressed animals or animals with concurrent infections, emaciation, or inadequate ingesta.

CLINICAL PRESENTATION

- Diffuse necrotizing enterohepatitis, enteritis, and renal amoebiasis are the most common clinical presentation in afflicted amphibians.
- Activity at abnormal times of the day, anorexia, diarrhea, dehydration, weight loss, bloody and mucoid stools, hardening of the large intestinal tract that can be palpated, intussusception, vomiting, convulsions, listlessness, renal failure, ascites, and sudden death.

RISK FACTORS

Husbandry

- Improper husbandry, hygiene, and nutrition.
- Housed with infected animals, decreased immune status, temperatures held between 25 and 33 degrees C.
- Invertebrates (i.e., roaches and flies) act as mechanical vectors.
- Being housed with chelonian species can lead to exposure and disease from their *Entamoeba* spp.

Others

N/A

DIAGNOSIS

DIFFERENTIAL DIAGNOSIS

- Salmonellosis
- GI helminths

DIAGNOSTICS

- Microscopic evaluation (wet mount) of fresh fecal material to visualize trophozoites and cysts.
- Trophozoites may be seen in fresh fecal but die rapidly within 20–30 minutes once outside the host.
- SAF technique can be used for better visualization.
- Fecal/cysts can be placed within a petri dish with water and trophozoites will emerge from the dissolved envelope within several hours.
- PCR assays can be used to distinguish species of entamoeba.
- Leukocyte and erythrocytes presence within fecal material should indicate pathogenicity or nonpathogenic commensals.

PATHOLOGICAL FINDINGS

- Diarrhea
- Dehydration
- Weight loss
- Marked intestinal lymphoplasmacytic infiltration with ulcerations.
- Necrotizing enterohepatitis
- Enteritis
- Nephritis

TREATMENT

APPROPRIATE HEALTH CARE

N/A

NUTRITIONAL SUPPORT

Vitamin supplementation may be indicated if diarrhea and dehydration are severe.

CLIENT EDUCATION/HUSBANDRY RECOMMENDATIONS

- Practice proper hygiene and biofiltration.
- Do not house with chelonians.

MEDICATIONS

DRUG(S) OF CHOICE

- Metronidazole 100 mg/kg PO once, then repeated in 14 days.
- Larval stages: metronidazole baths at 500 mg/l for 15–30 minutes every 5 days; 6.6 mg/l for 8 hours for more sensitive species.
- Electrolyte baths
- Supportive care

PRECAUTIONS/INTERACTIONS

N/A

FOLLOW-UP

PATIENT MONITORING

Repeat fecal examinations and weight monitoring to determine response to therapy.

EXPECTED COURSE AND PROGNOSIS

Fair

MISCELLANEOUS

COMMENTS

N/A

ZOONOTIC POTENTIAL

E. histolytica and *E. dispar*, species found in humans, are morphologically similar to *E. invadens* but are considered to be nonpathogenic.

SYNONYMS

N/A

ABBREVIATIONS

- GI = gastrointestinal
- PCV = packed cell volume
- PO = per os
- SAF = sodium acetate acetic acid formalin

INTERNET RESOURCES

Poole VA, ed. Amphibian Husbandry Resource Guide. Association of Zoos and Aquariums, Edition 2.0, 2012. https://www.speakcdn.com/assets/2332/amphibianhusbandryresourceguide.pdf

Suggested Reading

Poynton SL, Whitaker BR. Protozoa and metazoa infecting amphibians. In: Wright KM, Whitaker BR. *Amphibian Medicine and Captive Husbandry*. Malabar, FL: Krieger; 2001:193–221.

Author Elsburgh O. Clarke III, DVM, DACZM

EXOPHTHALMIA

BASICS

DEFINITION/OVERVIEW

Exophthalmia is the anterior protrusion of a normal-sized globe.

ETIOLOGY/PATHOPHYSIOLOGY

Space-occupying swelling or mass in the orbit placing pressure on the globe, displacing it anteriorly.

SIGNALMENT/HISTORY

- There is no standard signalment for this disease.
- Gradual protrusion of the eye, possibly preventing blinking.
- Potentially, anorexia

CLINICAL PRESENTATION

- While it can be bilateral, exophthalmia is more commonly unilateral.
- The displacement of the globe will often push the eyelids forward, cause protrusion of the nictitans, and excessive conjunctiva may be visible.
- Retropulsion of the globe is met with resistance due to the presence of the retrobulbar swelling.

RISK FACTORS

Husbandry

- Inadequate husbandry, especially hypothermia, may predispose animals to this condition due to decreased immune function leading to retrobulbar cellulitis and/or abscessation.
- Hypovitaminosis A in some species of amphibians causes squamous metaplasia of the orbital glands and ducts, as well as decreased immune function, and may present as bilateral exophthalmia.

Others

N/A

DIAGNOSIS

DIFFERENTIAL DIAGNOSIS

- It is important to first differentiate between exophthalmia and buphthalmos.
- The most common cause for exophthalmia in amphibians is trauma.
- Other differentials include cellulitis, retrobulbar abscessation, granulomas, neoplasia, mucoceles, and sialoadenitis.
- Generalized edema may also cause bilateral exophthalmia.

DIAGNOSTICS

- Physical examination will confirm exophthalmia is present.
- A thorough oral examination is useful, as the eyes are separated from the buccal cavity only by a thin membrane.
- Additional diagnostics are often necessary to determine the cause of exophthalmia.
- Radiography of the head can be of diagnostic value if the animal is large enough to provide a good level of detail on the films.
- For larger species, ocular ultrasound can be helpful in evaluating the problem, although some species have scleral ossicles that can limit imaging.
- Advanced imaging, such as CT or MRI, is helpful in determining the extent of the mass and if resection is possible.
- If size permits, a CBC may provide information on the cause and severity of the condition.
- Surgical exploratory of the retrobulbar space to collect biopsies and resect any masses present is the most definitive way to achieve a diagnosis, but in many cases this requires enucleation to reach the retrobulbar space.
- For some species, it may be possible to enter the retrobulbar space through the oral cavity to at least collect samples for FNA or biopsy.

PATHOLOGICAL FINDINGS

Histology and culture are most useful to diagnose the cause of the exophthalmia and allow the clinician to form an appropriate treatment plan.

TREATMENT

APPROPRIATE HEALTH CARE

N/A

NUTRITIONAL SUPPORT

- Additional nutritional support is not necessary if the animal is eating, but it may be necessary to tube feed if anorexia is occurring.
- Assessment of the diet for adequate vitamin A levels is important and should be done to rule out hypovitaminosis A as a potential cause or contributor to this condition in amphibians.

CLIENT EDUCATION/HUSBANDRY RECOMMENDATIONS

- While exophthalmia can occur in any animal, those with husbandry deficiencies may be at increased risk.
- In addition to medical and surgical therapy, maximizing the husbandry of the animal will improve the chance for a successful outcome.

MEDICATIONS

DRUG(S) OF CHOICE

- Treatment should be based on results of culture, histology, and/or FNA.
- Starting an appropriate broad-spectrum antibiotic with a good Gram-negative spectrum (such as ceftazadime 20 mg/kg IM or SC q48–72h) and anti-inflammatory (such as meloxicam 0.2–0.3 mg/kg IM or SC q24–48h) can be helpful while test results are pending.

PRECAUTIONS/INTERACTIONS

N/A

FOLLOW-UP

PATIENT MONITORING

If size permits, serial CBCs, especially if the first one was abnormal, may provide an indication of response to treatment.

EXPECTED COURSE AND PROGNOSIS

- Prognosis is related to the underlying cause of the exophthalmia.
- Cellulitis and trauma have the most favorable outcomes.
- Retrobulbar abscesses can be extensive and therefore carry a more guarded prognosis.
- Retrobulbar neoplasia usually carries a poor prognosis because of location and inability to get clean margins.

MISCELLANEOUS

COMMENTS

N/A

ZOONOTIC POTENTIAL

Depends on the cause of the retrobulbar swelling but generally low to no zoonotic potential.

SYNONYMS

- Exophthalmos
- Proptosis—severe case of exophthalmia

ABBREVIATIONS

- CBC = complete blood count
- CT = computed tomography
- FNA = fine needle aspiration
- IM = intramuscular
- MRI = magnetic resonance imaging
- SC = subcutaneous

EXOPHTHALMIA (CONTINUED)

Suggested Reading

Whitaker BR, Wright KM. Clinical techniques. In: Wright KM, Whitaker BR. *Amphibian Medicine and Captive Husbandry*. Malabar, FL: Krieger; 2001:89–110.

Whitaker BR, Wright KM. The amphibian eye. In: Wright KM, Whitaker BR. *Amphibian Medicine and Captive Husbandry*. Malabar, FL: Krieger; 2001: 245–252.

Wright KM. Overview of amphibian medicine. In: Mader DR, ed. *Reptile Medicine and Surgery*. 2nd ed. St. Louis, MO: Elsevier Saunders; 2006:941–971.

Author Christopher S. Hanley, DVM, DACZM

GIARDIA

BASICS

DEFINITION/OVERVIEW

The parasitic organism *Giardia* can be carried by pet amphibians, especially wild-caught animals, in the intestinal tract. Unlike in mammalian species, it is rare to see clinical disease other than in stressed or debilitated animals.

ETIOLOGY/PATHOPHYSIOLOGY

- *Giardia agilis* is the species that may affect amphibians.
- Infection occurs by the fecal–oral route through ingestion of cysts in contaminated water or food.
- In the small intestine, the cysts release trophozoites, which multiply in the lumen of the proximal small intestine, where they can be free or attached to the mucosa by a ventral sucking disk.
- Encystation occurs as the parasites move toward the colon.
- Cysts are shed in the feces and are infectious immediately when passed.

SIGNALMENT/HISTORY

- *Giardia* can be present in animals of any age and sex.
- It is far more commonly seen in wild-caught animals.
- It may present more commonly in animals who are stressed due to poor husbandry, shipping, or other underlying disease.

CLINICAL PRESENTATION

- Typically, the animal will have no clinical signs, but the organism is found incidentally on a fecal exam.
- Alternatively, the animal can have signs of enteritis including diarrhea, hematochezia, foul odor to the feces, and/or decreased appetite.

RISK FACTORS

Husbandry

- Clinical disease is more likely to be seen in any stressed animals, which can occur with any deficiencies in husbandry.
- These can include poor water quality, improper temperatures, lighting, diet or feeding regimen, failure to clean the cage regularly or thoroughly.
- The organism can survive longer in moist conditions, so proper water quality and cage cleaning are essential.

Others

N/A

DIAGNOSIS

DIFFERENTIAL DIAGNOSIS

Other protozoal organisms, both identified incidentally on fecal exam and/or as cause of clinical disease and similar symptoms:

- Proteromonads
- Retortamonads
- Diplomonads
- Oxymonads
- Trichomonads

Infectious enteritis:

- Bacterial
- Fungal
- Viral
- Parasitic

DIAGNOSTICS

- Fecal flotation and saline direct wet mount (include both plain saline and Lugol's iodine stain).
- Zinc sulfate flotation
- ELISA is typically species specific, so may not be reliable for *G. agilis*.

PATHOLOGICAL FINDINGS

- This condition typically does not have clinical disease associated with it.
- *Giardia* in other species can cause loss of intestinal brush border surface area, villous flattening and atrophy.
- There is also an increase in crypt length and crypt cell proliferation.
- Edema or ascites may be present with fluid disturbances.

TREATMENT

APPROPRIATE HEALTH CARE

N/A

NUTRITIONAL SUPPORT

- If clinical disease is present, and patient is not eating, weak, or lethargic, then supportive feeding may be indicated.
- Most can be fed at 1–2% of body weight once daily using a liquid carnivore diet.
- Fluid baths with electrolytes should be used if patient is dehydrated.

CLIENT EDUCATION/HUSBANDRY RECOMMENDATIONS

- *Giardia* cysts are infective immediately when shed in the feces, therefore proper hygiene is necessary to prevent reinfection.
- At the initiation of treatment, the entire enclosure and its contents should be cleaned with hot soapy water, rinsed, then disinfected with dilute bleach or an ammonia-based cleaner.
- Any cleaners need to be rinsed thoroughly as they will be absorbed through amphibian skin and cause toxicity.
- Use minimal cage furnishings and non-particulate substrate such as paper towels for the duration of treatment.
- Alternatively place the animal in a clean environment free of cysts for 24 hours after each treatment.
- Each time the animal defecates, the feces need to be removed as soon as possible and the cage disinfected again, especially before feeding as prey items may walk through fecal material before being ingested.
- Because *Giardia* is often secondary, it is important to optimize husbandry and care for the animal to recover.

MEDICATIONS

DRUG(S) OF CHOICE

- Metronidazole —many dosing regimens exist—consider each animal on a case by case basis.
- Use lower dose for unfamiliar or sensitive species.
- PO doses can also be applied topically (see Precautions/Interactions).
- Metronidazole 10 mg/kg PO q24h for 5–10 days; 50mg/kg PO q24h for 3–5 days; 100 mg/kg PO q24h for 3 days; 50 mg/l 24-hour bath.

PRECAUTIONS/INTERACTIONS

- Injectable forms of metronidazole are acidic in nature and should be used as baths, not applied directly topically unless diluted.
- Use lower doses for unfamiliar species to prevent toxicity or deaths.

FOLLOW-UP

PATIENT MONITORING

- Repeat fecal exam at the end of treatment to confirm the organism has been cleared.
- If clinical signs were present, those should be resolved as well.

EXPECTED COURSE AND PROGNOSIS

- If *Giardia* is found on a fecal exam, treatment, together with good hygiene, will typically clear the organism, or at least reduce the parasite load.
- *Giardia* is most often identified in animals that are otherwise sick or stressed, so the underlying disease process also needs to be addressed for the animal to recover.

GIARDIA (CONTINUED)

MISCELLANEOUS

COMMENTS

N/A

ZOONOTIC POTENTIAL

- While *G. agilis* has not been known to affect humans, other species of *Giardia* can, so zoonotic potential can be assumed.
- Since transmission is via fecal–oral route, prevention relies on washing hands after handling an amphibian or cleaning the cage and practicing good overall hygiene measures.
- The animal should never come in contact with areas where human food is prepared or eaten.
- In the case of an active infection, the owner should wear gloves and the cage should be thoroughly cleaned and disinfected after each time the animal defecates to help avoid infection or reinfection of the animal.

SYNONYMS

N/A

ABBREVIATIONS

- ELISA = enzyme-linked immunosorbent assay
- PO = per os

INTERNET RESOURCES

- Centers for Disease Control and Prevention. Giardia and pets. July 21, 2015. https://www.cdc.gov/parasites/giardia/prevention-control-pets.html
- Center for Food Security and Public Health. Giardiasis. December 2012. http://www.cfsph.iastate.edu/Factsheets/pdfs/giardiasis.pdf

Suggested Reading

Poynton SL, Whitaker BR. Protozoa and metazoa infecting amphibians. In: Wright KM, Whitaker BR. *Amphibian Medicine and Captive Husbandry*. Malabar, FL: Krieger; 2001:196–222.

Sogayar ML, Gregório EA. *Giardia agilis*: Ultrastructure of the trophozoites in the frog intestine. *Mem Inst Oswaldo Cruz* 1998;93:357–361.

Author Stacey Leonatti Wilkinson, DVM, DABVP (Reptile and Amphibian)

GOUT

BASICS

DEFINITION/OVERVIEW

Gout may be seen in amphibians due to the buildup of uric acid crystals deposited in or around the joints or throughout visceral organs.

ETIOLOGY/PATHOPHYSIOLOGY

- Protein is broken down in the body into purines and pyrimidines.
- In certain amphibian species, the end-product of purine degradation is uric acid. This is excreted via the renal tubules.
- Increased production of uric acid may occur due to excessive levels of dietary proteins or potentially an inherited enzyme defect, as occurs in humans.
- Alternatively, excretion may be compromised, for example by dehydration, starvation, nephrotoxic drugs, or renal pathology.
- Uric acid is a relatively insoluble substance so when levels are elevated in the blood or in other body fluids, crystallization will occur and deposits will form.
- These uric acid crystals may deposit in the joints (articular gout), around the joints (periarticular gout) or throughout the kidneys (renal gout).
- Potentially, deposits may also be seen within other internal organs.

SIGNALMENT/HISTORY

- More likely to be seen in terrestrial amphibians with a history of husbandry deficits such as prolonged periods of dehydration.
- May potentially have been previously treated with potentially nephrotoxic drugs.

CLINICAL PRESENTATION

- Animals with articular or periarticular gout usually present with obvious joint swellings.
- One or more joints may be affected and the animal may be lame.
- Animals with renal gout may be asymptomatic or have non-specific signs such as lethargy and reduced appetite.

RISK FACTORS

Husbandry

- Inappropriately high environmental temperatures.
- Inappropriate water provision (e.g., low humidity or lack of fresh water).

Others

Administration of potentially nephrotoxic drugs (e.g., aminoglycosides), especially to dehydrated patients.

DIAGNOSIS

DIFFERENTIAL DIAGNOSIS

- Pseudogout
- Septic arthritis
- Trauma
- Metabolic bone diseases

DIAGNOSTICS

- Gout may be suspected on history and clinical examination, but diagnostic testing will be necessary for definitive diagnosis.
- Cytologic examination of aspirates from affected joints for articular or periarticular gout.
- For visceral gout, biopsies need to be taken for histopathology.
- Demonstration of uric acid (usually monosodium urate) crystals is necessary for definitive diagnosis.
- Blood uric acid levels may be elevated, but this will depend on the stage in the disease process.
- On radiography of affected limbs, lytic lesions may be seen in and around joints. Crystals are radiolucent so will not be detected.
- Surgical removal of tophi may be considered if only one joint is affected, but permanent damage to the joint may already have occurred.
- Amputation of the affected bones or even euthanasia may be considered in severe cases.

PATHOLOGICAL FINDINGS

- On gross postmortem examination, small white nodules (tophi) can be seen scattered throughout visceral organs, within or around joints.
- On histopathological examination, tophi are often surrounded by granulomatous inflammation.

TREATMENT

APPROPRIATE HEALTH CARE

- Treatment aims to lower blood uric acid levels and promote uric acid excretion.
- Supportive treatment should always include appropriate analgesia, as in other species this is known to be a painful condition.

NUTRITIONAL SUPPORT

- Some patients may be anorexic and severely dehydrated on presentation.
- Fluid deficits should always be corrected and nutritional support provided.
- Care should be taken to provide an appropriate diet low in dietary purines to minimize further uric acid production.

CLIENT EDUCATION/HUSBANDRY RECOMMENDATIONS

- Husbandry should be reviewed to identify any predisposing factors, such as inappropriate temperatures or low humidity, and these should be corrected.
- Clean fresh water should always be available in a recognizable form for the species.
- Diet should be reviewed to ensure that it is appropriate for the species and not too high in proteins.
- Clients should be advised that this is a condition that will require long-term management and can potentially be very painful if allowed to progress.

MEDICATIONS

DRUG(S) OF CHOICE

- Allopurinol is the most common choice for treating gout. It is a xanthine oxidase-inhibiting drug which works by inhibiting the conversion of hypoxanthine and xanthine to uric acid in the liver, consequently reducing blood uric acid levels.
- If blood uric acid levels remain consistently low, existing deposits may potentially dissolve.
- Doses of 10–20 mg/kg PO q24h are recommended based on doses that appear effective in reptiles.

PRECAUTIONS/INTERACTIONS

Patients should always be hydrated prior to allopurinol administration.

FOLLOW-UP

PATIENT MONITORING

- Response to therapy is usually monitored by physical examination findings (e.g., increase in activity levels or no progression in joint swellings).
- Repeat blood samples can also be taken to recheck uric acid levels which would be expected to start reducing within 7 days of allopurinol treatment, based on other species.

EXPECTED COURSE AND PROGNOSIS

- The prognosis for patients with severe widespread disease is poor, but if diagnosed early the condition could be managed successfully.
- If left untreated, the disease will progress with widespread uric acid deposition, ultimately resulting in organ failure and death.

GOUT (CONTINUED)

MISCELLANEOUS

COMMENTS
N/A

ZOONOTIC POTENTIAL
N/A

SYNONYMS
N/A

ABBREVIATIONS
PO = per os

INTERNET RESOURCES
Veterinary Information Network: www.vin.com

Suggested Reading

Duncan M. Gout in exotic animals. In: Miller RE, Fowler ME, eds. *Fowler's Zoo and Wild Animal Medicine Volume 8.* St Louis, MO: Elsevier Saunders; 2015:667–670.

Wright KM. Idiopathic syndromes. In: Wright KM, Whitaker BR. *Amphibian Medicine and Captive Husbandry.* Malabar, FL: Krieger; 2001:239–244.

Author Joanna Hedley BVM&S, DZooMed (Reptilian), DECZM (Herpetology), MRCVS

HEXAMITA

BASICS

DEFINITION/OVERVIEW
Hexamita is a small flagellate parasite which can be found in the intestinal tract of amphibians.

ETIOLOGY/PATHOPHYSIOLOGY
- *Hexamita intestinalis* is the usual cause of disease in captive animals.
- *H. batrachorum* has also been isolated from laboratory amphibians.
- Infection is thought to occur by ingestion of an infective cyst, which passes into the gastrointestinal tract.
- Reproduction is by simple binary fission, usually in the large intestine.
- In low numbers, infection does not appear to cause a problem, but heavy burdens may lead to inflammation of the intestines, often with secondary bacterial infection.
- The parasite may also potentially ascend via the bile ducts to the gall bladder.
- Transmission can occur via urine or feces.

SIGNALMENT/HISTORY
- Disease has been described in a wide variety of amphibian species, including frogs, toads, salamanders, and newts, with no typical signalment.
- Signs may be seen following a stressful episode such as the introduction of new animals or recent transport.

CLINICAL PRESENTATION
- Animals with *Hexamita* infection may be asymptomatic or may have non-specific signs such as lethargy and reduced appetite.
- In severe infections, diarrhea may be seen.

RISK FACTORS

Husbandry
- Suboptimal husbandry may lead to chronic stress and a subsequent increase in parasite numbers.
- Poor hygiene will increase the risk of disease transmission.

Others
- Concurrent parasite infection
- Other intestinal disease

DIAGNOSIS

DIFFERENTIAL DIAGNOSIS
- Amoebiasis
- Coccidiosis
- Bacterial enteritis
- Other commensal intestinal flagellates

DIAGNOSTICS
- Diagnosis in a live animal is usually presumptive based on history, clinical examination, and the identification of *Hexamita* flagellates in a fecal sample.
- Analysis of a fresh fecal sample may reveal small fast-moving flagellates (10–16 microns) characterized by six anterior flagella.
- In small samples, the parasite will rapidly desiccate and die.

PATHOLOGICAL FINDINGS
- No specific postmortem findings have been attributed to *Hexamita* infection.
- Inflammation of the intestines, and potentially bile ducts, in association with high levels of the flagellated parasite would be highly suspicious.

TREATMENT

APPROPRIATE HEALTH CARE
- Treatment involves both reducing the level of parasite present in the intestines and symptomatic treatment of diarrhea.
- Concurrent parasite infection and secondary bacterial infections should also be treated.

NUTRITIONAL SUPPORT
- Some patients may be anorexic and severely dehydrated on presentation.
- Fluid deficits should always be corrected, and nutritional support provided as needed.

CLIENT EDUCATION/HUSBANDRY RECOMMENDATIONS
- Hygiene measures should be reviewed to minimize the risk of disease transmission and any husbandry deficits should be improved.
- Any potential causes of stress should also be considered and minimized.

MEDICATIONS

DRUG(S) OF CHOICE
- Metronidazole is the most common choice for treating *Hexamita*.
- Various treatment regimens have been recommended based on those effective in reptiles.
- Doses range from 100–125 mg/kg PO once, then repeated after 14 days, to 50 mg/kg PO q24h for 3–5 days for severe infections.

PRECAUTIONS/INTERACTIONS
Hepatotoxicity and central nervous system toxicity have occasionally been reported in other species following metronidazole use, so care should be taken if pre-existing hepatic dysfunction is suspected.

FOLLOW-UP

PATIENT MONITORING
- Response to therapy is usually monitored by a reduction in clinical signs (e.g., improved appetite).
- Repeat fecal samples should also be checked following treatment.

EXPECTED COURSE AND PROGNOSIS
- The prognosis for patients with extensive intestinal damage is poor.
- If diagnosed early the condition can be managed successfully.

MISCELLANEOUS

COMMENTS
N/A

ZOONOTIC POTENTIAL
N/A

SYNONYMS
N/A

ABBREVIATIONS
PO = per os

INTERNET RESOURCES
Veterinary Information Network
www.vin.com

Suggested Reading

Green DE. Pathology of Amphibia. In: Wright KM, Whitaker BR. *Amphibian Medicine and Captive Husbandry*. Malabar, FL: Krieger; 2001:401–486.
Mitchell MA. Parasites of amphibians. In: Baker DG, ed. *Flynn's Parasites of Laboratory Animals*, 2nd ed. Ames, IA: Blackwell; 2007:118–171.

Author Joanna Hedley BVM&S, DZooMed (Reptilian), DECZM (Herpetology), MRCVS

HYPERVITAMINOSIS A

BASICS

DEFINITION/OVERVIEW

Hypervitaminosis A is well recognized as a health concern in captive adult anurans. It can occur due to administration of OTC supplements provided by well-meaning owners, parenteral overdosing by veterinarians, or feeding diets with high animal rather than plant-based (beta carotene) vitamin A levels. Oversupplementation to manage a perceived or real deficiency leads to hypervitaminosis A.

ETIOLOGY/PATHOPHYSIOLOGY

- In vertebrates, vitamin A forms are trans-retinyl esters, trans-retinol, -retinal and -retinoic acid (99% of all vitamin A present in body), while the major dietary provitamin A carotenoid is beta carotene.
- The all-trans-vitamin A isomers are the only forms used physiologically.
- The liver absorbs and stores preformed vitamin A; at a certain point, storage capacity is reached and toxicity occurs.
- Other storage sites include adipose, lung, and kidney.
- In humans, retinoid delivery pathway to tissues involves primarily retinol bound to retinol-binding protein; chylomicrons, very low density lipoprotein and low density lipoprotein, and albumin, also provide transport.
- Adverse effects in humans include increased bone turnover by suppressing osteoblast activity and stimulating osteoclast formation. This can lead to hypercalcemia, osteoporosis, pathologic fractures, altered skeletal development in children, and skeletal pain.
- Vitamin A is fat-soluble and high levels can affect metabolism of other fat-soluble vitamins (D, E, and K); with the effects on vitamin D contributing to bone pathology, although stimulation of bone resorption by vitamin A is reported independent of effects on vitamin D.
- Vitamin A can have a toxic effect on mitochondrial function. It can also cause hypothyroidism in mice.

SIGNALMENT/HISTORY

- First time owner of amphibians/species, tadpole or metamorph.
- Owner using OTC vitamin A drops or multivitamins with vitamin A in formulation other than beta carotene, using cod liver oil, or feeding liver/vertebrate prey too frequently.

CLINICAL PRESENTATION

- Vague signs, such as anorexia, dehydration, lethargy, weight loss.
- Usually has a dermatological component including dysecdysis, excess ecdysis, ulceration, and sloughing.
- Secondary bacterial and fungal infections can occur.
- Based on pathophysiology, suspect that metabolic bone diseases may have interplay with hypervitaminosis A.
- In tadpoles, the loss of rostral tentacles, tail resorption, accelerated or delayed development, chronic diarrhea, hyperpigmented and hemorrhagic skin, developmental abnormalities of the limbs and eyes, and abnormal development of the keratinized epidermis of the jaws may occur.

RISK FACTORS

Husbandry

N/A

Others

- Tadpole
- Reproductively active female
- Liver disease
- Iatrogenic dietary or parenteral oversupplementation of non-beta carotene vitamin A.

DIAGNOSIS

DIFFERENTIAL DIAGNOSIS

- Hypovitaminosis A
- Infection
- Hepatic/renal disease
- UVB/thermal burns
- Poor overall husbandry/diet
- Improper conspecific arrangement
- Metabolic bone diseases
- Water-based toxins

DIAGNOSTICS

- Liver biopsy for histopathology and testing vitamin A levels (normal values for the species not readily available).
- Presumptive diagnosis based upon history/clinical presentation.

PATHOLOGICAL FINDINGS

- Hepatic fibrosis
- Hepatocellular degeneration
- Osteoporosis
- Decreased/abnormal bony growth and development in tadpoles/metamorphs.
- Epidermal ulceration

TREATMENT

APPROPRIATE HEALTH CARE

N/A

NUTRITIONAL SUPPORT

Unknown

CLIENT EDUCATION/HUSBANDRY RECOMMENDATIONS

- Proper education about correct diet for the species, discussing correct formulation of vitamin A for the species.
- Clear explanation of differences between water-soluble and fat-soluble vitamins.

MEDICATIONS

DRUG(S) OF CHOICE

- Discontinuing supplementation of non-beta carotene vitamin A.
- Other treatment focuses on managing with systemic antibiotics/antifungals.
- Judicious topical use of silver sulfadiazine cream for epidermal ulcers can help.
- Pain management should be considered.
- Systemic fluid therapy via passive soaking. Anurans with developmental abnormalities may need to be euthanized for humane reasons.

PRECAUTIONS/INTERACTIONS

Oversupplementation of vitamin A can have negative interactions with other fat-soluble vitamins (D, E, K) leading to either decreased absorption or excess accumulation.

FOLLOW-UP

PATIENT MONITORING

- Reassessment of clinical manifestation
- Re-evaluation of current diet plan.
- Repeat liver biopsy if feasible.

EXPECTED COURSE AND PROGNOSIS

- In adults, clinical resolution can take many months, with most dermatological manifestations resolving, although skeletal and hepatic damage may be permanent.
- For tadpoles, abnormalities are likely irreversible, and euthanasia may be warranted.

MISCELLANEOUS

COMMENTS

N/A

ZOONOTIC POTENTIAL

N/A

SYNONYMS

N/A

ABBREVIATIONS

- OTC = over the counter
- UVB = ultraviolet B

Suggested Reading

Clugston RD, Blaner WS. Vitamin A (retinoid) metabolism and actions: What we know and what we need to know about amphibians. *Zoo Biol* 2014;33(6):527–535.

Author Eric Klaphake, DVM, DACZM

HYPOVITAMINOSIS A

BASICS

DEFINITION/OVERVIEW

Hypovitaminosis A is well-recognized health concern in captive anurans, especially those being fed captive-raised invertebrates.

ETIOLOGY/PATHOPHYSIOLOGY

- In vertebrates, vitamin A forms are trans-retinyl esters, trans-retinol, -retinal and -retinoic acid (99% of all vitamin A present in body), while the major dietary provitamin A carotenoid is beta carotene.
- The all-trans-vitamin A isomers are only forms used physiologically. Adult amphibians need these forms in their diet, while tadpoles can convert carotenoids. The liver absorbs and stores preformed vitamin A.
- Other storage sites include adipose, lung, and kidney.
- In humans, retinoid delivery pathway to tissues involves primarily retinol bound to retinol-binding protein; chylomicrons, very low density lipoprotein and low density lipoprotein, and albumin, also provide transport.
- Adverse effects in humans include night blindness, impaired immune function, cancer, and birth defects.

SIGNALMENT/HISTORY

- First-time owner of amphibians/species, tadpole, or metamorph.
- Supplementing with beta carotene-based vitamin A or no supplementation.
- Feeding invertebrates without eyes.

CLINICAL PRESENTATION

- Present with vague signs such as anorexia, dehydration, lethargy, weight loss.
- The anuran may also have dull coloration for its species/sex/season/age.
- Squamous metaplasia of mucus-secreting epithelia underlies most clinical manifestations—especially lingual squamous metaplasia (short tongue syndrome)—also conjunctiva and reproductive organs.
- In short-tongue syndrome, the anuran cannot capture prey.
- Periorbital edema may be noted in both eyes.
- Increased ecdysis frequency may occur.

RISK FACTORS

Husbandry

Feeding invertebrates without eyes (e.g., mealworms, superworms; adult beetle form OK)

Others

N/A

DIAGNOSIS

DIFFERENTIAL DIAGNOSIS

- Infection
- Hepatic/renal disease
- Poor overall husbandry/diet
- Improper conspecific arrangement
- Metabolic bone diseases
- Water-based toxins
- Tongue trauma

DIAGNOSTICS

- Presumptive diagnosis based upon history/clinical presentation.
- Liver biopsy for histopathology and testing vitamin A levels can be performed but there is a lack of normal values.
- Sex of animal, species, testing methodology, and reported units can affect results.
- In Wyoming toads, liver retinol with short tongue syndrome was ten-fold lower than wild conspecifics.

PATHOLOGICAL FINDINGS

Squamous metaplasia; need pathologist familiar with normal amphibian histology or can be missed.

TREATMENT

APPROPRIATE HEALTH CARE

- Parenteral vitamin A
- Other treatment focuses on managing with systemic antibiotics/antifungals for secondary infections.
- Judicious topical use of silver sulfadiazine cream for epidermal ulcers can help.

NUTRITIONAL SUPPORT

- Large anurans and salamanders can be fed whole prey still containing the liver.
- Supportive feeding may be needed until the amphibian feels better.
- Invertebrates store retinols in the retina only, so invertebrates (or juvenile forms) without eyes have no vitamin A.
- Invertebrates must be dusted immediately before feeding, as the vitamin powder is usually self-groomed off the invertebrate before the reptile has ingested it.
- Gut-loading guidelines are still controversial but seem to still be the best option—especially consider the Li diet (see Suggested Reading).
- Consider feeding non-toxic, wild-caught invertebrates, as they generally have much higher levels of vitamin A than captive-raised invertebrates.

CLIENT EDUCATION/HUSBANDRY RECOMMENDATIONS

- Proper education about correct diet for the species, discussing correct formulation of vitamin A for the species.
- Clear explanation of differences between water-soluble and fat-soluble vitamins.

MEDICATIONS

DRUG(S) OF CHOICE

- Parenteral vitamin A (usually has vitamin D3 as well) 500–5000 iu/kg IM every 7–14 days for up to 4 treatments.
- Topical administration of a water-soluble emulsion of retinyl palmitate (AQUASOL A® Parenteral, AstraZeneca LP, Westborough, MA) 50 iu q48h or once a week achieves levels 4.5- and 2.5-fold higher than standard nutrition.
- Dose with care to avoid oversupplementation with vitamin A in the retinol form.

PRECAUTIONS/INTERACTIONS

Oversupplementation of vitamin A can have negative interactions with other fat-soluble vitamins (D, E, K) leading to either decreased absorption or excess accumulation.

FOLLOW-UP

PATIENT MONITORING

- Reassessment of clinical manifestation
- Check on current diet plan by owner (to avoid recurrence).
- Repeat liver biopsy if financially and situationally feasible.

EXPECTED COURSE AND PROGNOSIS

- Usually chronic; clinical resolution can take several months, with most manifestations resolving, although renal damage may be permanent.
- Ocular and short-tongue syndrome manifestations have been reported to improve with correct supplementation.

MISCELLANEOUS

COMMENTS

N/A

ZOONOTIC POTENTIAL

N/A

SYNONYMS

N/A

ABBREVIATIONS

IM = intramuscular

HYPOVITAMINOSIS A (CONTINUED)

INTERNET RESOURCES

Zoo Biology Special Issue: Amphibian Nutrition and Health. 2014;33(6):483–592. http://onlinelibrary.wiley.com/doi/10.1002/zoo.v33.6/issuetoc

Suggested Reading

Clugston RD, Blaner WS. Vitamin A (retinoid) metabolism and actions: What we know and what we need to know about amphibians. *Zoo Biol* 2014;33(6):527–535.

Ferrie GM, Alford VC, Atkinson J, et al. Nutrition and health in amphibian husbandry. *Zoo Biol* 2014;33(6):485–501.

Li H, Vaughan MJ, Browne RK. A complex enrichment diet improves growth and health in the endangered Wyoming toad (*Bufo baxteri*). *Zoo Biol* 2009;28:197–213.

Author Eric Klaphake, DVM, DACZM

HYPOVITAMINOSIS B

BASICS

DEFINITION/OVERVIEW

Hypovitaminosis B generally refers to hypothiaminosis. It is a health concern in amphibians that are fed fish, whether live or frozen thawed. Other cases have been reported in reptiles fed vitamin supplements lacking thiamine and so may apply to amphibians as well.

ETIOLOGY/PATHOPHYSIOLOGY

- In humans, thiamine deficiency can occur rapidly and can advance to metabolic coma and death.
- Causes include malnutrition, a diet high in thiaminase-rich foods (raw freshwater fish, raw shellfish, ferns), chronic gastrointestinal diseases, and diabetes mellitus.
- Thiamine derivatives and thiamine-dependent enzymes are present in all cells, but the nervous system is very sensitive, leading to nerve fiber myelin sheath degeneration, causing necrotizing encephalopathy and peripheral neuritis.
- Bilateral vision loss due to optic neuropathy can occur.
- Thiamine is a water-soluble vitamin synthesized by bacteria, fungi, and plants.
- Captive amphibians being fed fish as only or significant portion of diet can be affected.
- Feeding fish high in thiaminase, such as goldfish and fathead minnow, improperly thawed fish (thawing too slowly), or fish that has been frozen a long time can all be factors.
- Thiamine is a rapidly deteriorating vitamin so it is important to ensure that supplements are stored and used properly.

SIGNALMENT/HISTORY

- Fish as primary diet
- Using an expired vitamin supplement.

CLINICAL PRESENTATION

B vitamin deficiencies in amphibians have been associated with neurological and musculoskeletal abnormalities including hindlimb paresis, paralysis, scoliosis, and spindly leg syndrome.

RISK FACTORS

Husbandry

N/A

Others

Exclusive to predominant piscivores

DIAGNOSIS

DIFFERENTIAL DIAGNOSIS

- Trauma
- Infectious encephalitis
- Toxins
- Metabolic bone diseases
- Hepatoencephalopathy
- Neoplasia
- Cardiac disease
- Renal disease

DIAGNOSTICS

Usually based on history, clinical signs, and response to thiamine (B-complex vitamins) treatment.

PATHOLOGICAL FINDINGS

- Cerebral cortical necrosis
- Peripheral neuritis
- Peripheral nerve demyelination

TREATMENT

APPROPRIATE HEALTH CARE

N/A

NUTRITIONAL SUPPORT

- Avoid feeding fish known to have high thiaminase levels, such as goldfish and fathead minnows.
- Proper storage of frozen fish by not keeping beyond 6 months of death/freezing.
- Rapid thawing for 5 minutes in water at 80 degrees C (175 degrees F) denatures thiaminase.
- Thawing in a refrigerator also avoids thiaminase activation.
- An added level of protection would be to add 25 mg thiamine/kg fish.
- Do not use vitamin supplements beyond expiration date or 6 months after opened.

CLIENT EDUCATION/HUSBANDRY RECOMMENDATIONS

- Proper education about expiration dates/opening dates of vitamin supplements.
- Avoiding certain live fish species.
- Proper thawing techniques for frozen fish.

MEDICATIONS

DRUG(S) OF CHOICE

- Thiamine administered at 50–100 mg/kg IM, SC, or PO q24h until resolution of clinical signs.
- A vitamin B complex formulation is less ideal but can be used if thiamine only supplement is not available.
- Supplementation with thiamine

PRECAUTIONS/INTERACTIONS

N/A

FOLLOW-UP

PATIENT MONITORING

- Reassess diet
- Diet processing/handling
- Supplementation at every visit

EXPECTED COURSE AND PROGNOSIS

- If thiamine deficiency without concurrent issues, should have immediate response to therapy, although repeated treatments may be needed.
- In non-piscivores, often not considered and diagnosed postmortem on histopathology.
- Spindly leg syndrome will not correct; euthanasia is recommended.

MISCELLANEOUS

COMMENTS

N/A

ZOONOTIC POTENTIAL

N/A

SYNONYMS

N/A

ABBREVIATIONS

- IM = intramuscular
- PO = per os
- SC = subcutaneous

Suggested Reading

Densmore CL, Green DE. Diseases of amphibians. *ILAR J* 2007;48(3):235–254.

Author Eric Klaphake, DVM, DACZM

ICHTHYOPHONUS

BASICS

DEFINITION/OVERVIEW

The genus *Ichthyophonus* encompasses protozoal organisms of the class Mesomycetozoea, which are also closely related to fungi. *Ichthyophonus* is a pathogen of freshwater and saltwater fish, and similar parasites, described as *Ichthyophonus*-like organisms, have been known to infect and cause mass morbidity and mortality in wild amphibians, particularly newts and ranids. These organisms bear similarities with the fish pathogen, *Ichthyophonus hoferi*, although obvious differences exist. Ichthyophonosis in amphibians is infection with these *Ichthyophonus*-like organisms, as further taxonomic classification has not been performed. A survey conducted in wild amphibians concluded that ichthyophonosis appears to be enzootic in Quebec.

ETIOLOGY/PATHOPHYSIOLOGY

- The life cycle is currently unknown.
- *Ichthyophonus*-like organisms usually form spores in skeletal muscle, resulting in a granulomatous myositis.
- Grossly visible body swellings may be present associated with areas containing a large number of spores.
- Transmission is believed to occur through the amphibian leech (*Placobdella picta*) rather than through a tropic mechanism, as happens in fish, but definitive evidence is lacking.
- Affected animals may be subclinical or noticeably debilitated.
- *Ichthyophonus* usually affects the musculoskeletal and occasionally the dermatologic systems.
- Unlike in fish, where *Ichthyophonus* can spread systemically, infections in amphibians appear to be localized only to skeletal muscle tissue and, rarely, the subcutis.

SIGNALMENT/HISTORY

- Ichthyophonosis has been reported in both juvenile and adult amphibian of numerous species with no apparent age predilection.
- In one study of wild red-spotted newts (*Notophthalmus viridescens*), both male animals and larger individuals had a higher risk of infection with *Ichthyophonus*-like organisms.

CLINICAL PRESENTATION

- The severity of clinical signs may vary between individuals, and infections may be subclinical.
- Lethargy, anorexia, weight loss, cutaneous swellings, epaxial muscle swelling, and muscle wasting have been reported in infected amphibians.
- Animals may not respond in a normal vigorous fashion when handled or touched.
- Ventral cervical swelling was reported in one affected salamander.
- In animals with translucent skin, intramuscular cysts may be visible.

RISK FACTORS

Husbandry

N/A

Others

- Wild-caught amphibians from areas know to harbor the organism are at an increased risk of being infected.
- A wild-caught leopard frog (*Rana pipens*) housed in a captive research colony that was found dead was infected with an *Ichthyophonus*-like organism.
- While not proven, exposure to the potential amphibian leech vector *P. picta* may greatly increase risk of infection.

DIAGNOSIS

DIFFERENTIAL DIAGNOSIS

- Because of the often non-specific clinical signs, ichthyophonosis may resemble other disorders resulting in cutaneous abnormalities or red-leg syndrome (dermatosepticemia).
- Differentials include other parasitic diseases that can result in gross body swellings (e.g., trematodiasis) or disorders that affect skeletal muscle.
- Mycobacteriosis should also be considered.

DIAGNOSTICS

Diagnosis is typically performed through histopathology and histochemical examination of affected muscle tissue.

PATHOLOGICAL FINDINGS

- Granulomatous inflammation is usually present surrounding the spores.
- Granulomatous myositis is a common finding.
- Eosinophilic myositis has also been reported.
- The organism does not appear to have a predilection for specific muscles.
- Both smaller passive or resting spores (40–100 µm) and larger active spores (100–240 µm) may be appreciated within affected tissues; passive spores have a noticeably thicker wall.
- In one tree frog, spores extended underneath muscle into the adjacent wall of the coelomic cavity.
- Cachexia or signs of secondary bacterial infections may be present in debilitated animals.

TREATMENT

APPROPRIATE HEALTH CARE

N/A

NUTRITIONAL SUPPORT

Nutritional support with critical care diets may be required once animals become anorexic.

CLIENT EDUCATION/HUSBANDRY RECOMMENDATIONS

N/A

MEDICATIONS

DRUG(S) OF CHOICE

- There is currently no known treatment for ichthyophonosis in amphibians.
- Supportive care (thermal and nutritional support, hydration) and prophylactic antimicrobial therapy or euthanasia is recommended for debilitated animals.

PRECAUTIONS/INTERACTIONS

Treatment for secondary infections may be considered to prevent increasing morbidity or mortality.

FOLLOW-UP

PATIENT MONITORING

- Affected animals should be monitored for progression of clinical signs and treated for secondary bacterial infections or dehydration as needed.
- Affected individuals should be separated from non-affected animals.
- Euthanasia is recommended for animals with a poor quality of life.

EXPECTED COURSE AND PROGNOSIS

- Once infected and spores are present within the skeletal muscle, prognosis for resolution is poor.
- Secondary bacterial infections may occur following immunosuppression or ulceration of skin.
- Sudden death has been reported with heavy infections.
- Increased risk of predation in wild animals is likely.
- In all reports of amphibians infected with *Ichthyophonus*-like organisms, all animals died or were euthanized.

MISCELLANEOUS

COMMENTS
N/A

ZOONOTIC POTENTIAL
None reported

SYNONYMS
N/A

Suggested Reading

Mendoza L, Taylor JW, Ajello L. The class Mesomycetozoea: a heterogeneous group of microorganisms at the animal-fungal boundary. *Annu Rev Microbiol* 2002;56:315–344.

Mikaelian I, Ouellet M, Pauli B, et al. *Ichthyophonus*-like infection in wild amphibians from Quebec, Canada. *Dis Aquat Organ* 2000;40:195–201.

Raffel TR, Dillard JR, Hudson PJ. Field evidence for leech-borne transmission of amphibian *Ichthyophonus* sp. *J Parasitol* 2006;92:1256–1264.

Author Grayson Doss, DVM, DACZM

ISOSPORA

BASICS

DEFINITION/OVERVIEW

Isospora is an apicomplexan parasite characterized by oocytes having two sporocysts that each contain four sporozoites. Like *Eimeria*, *Isospora* is typically an intracytoplasmic parasite, although some species have been described as having intranuclear development.

ETIOLOGY/PATHOPHYSIOLOGY

- Numerous *Isospora* spp. have been reported from amphibians and all appear to be commensal organisms.
- Transmission is likely direct, with animals becoming infected by ingested oocyts shed in the feces.

SIGNALMENT/HISTORY

N/A

CLINICAL PRESENTATION

- Clinical disease due to *Isospora* infection has not been reported in amphibians.
- Amphibians appear to be asymptomatic carriers.

RISK FACTORS

Husbandry

- New (captive or wild) animals entering a collection with poor hygiene and high stocking densities.
- Juvenile or larval stages may potentially be at higher risk.

Others

Concurrent disease or excessive stress may cause immunosuppression thus increasing risks of disease expression.

DIAGNOSIS

DIFFERENTIAL DIAGNOSIS

Other gastrointestinal disease such as bacterial or protozoal infections (i.e., *Eimeria*).

DIAGNOSTICS

- Examination of feces for presence of oocysts using light microscopy is the most reliable test.
- Molecular techniques such as PCR may aid in species delineation but are unlikely to improve treatment efficacy or prognosis.
- Protozoa may also be seen in biopsy or necropsy samples.
- For preservation of coccidia for future diagnostics, fecal samples should be stored in 2–3% aqueous (w/v) potassium dichromate ($K_2Cr_2O_7$).

PATHOLOGICAL FINDINGS

N/A

TREATMENT

APPROPRIATE HEALTH CARE

N/A

NUTRITIONAL SUPPORT

N/A

CLIENT EDUCATION/HUSBANDRY RECOMMENDATIONS

- Remove and isolate sick individuals and reduce stress by providing optimal living conditions and hygiene.
- Thoroughly clean the cage to reduce environmental contamination of oocysts.
- Ensure that quarantine protocols have been adopted for all new arrivals.
- During quarantine, all animals should be subjected to repeated clinical and fecal examinations.

MEDICATIONS

DRUG(S) OF CHOICE

- Treatment must only be given if clinical disease has been confirmed, since amphibians appear to be asymptomatic carriers.
- Ponazuril 30 mg/kg PO q12h for 3 days; repeat in 3 weeks.

PRECAUTIONS/INTERACTIONS

N/A

FOLLOW-UP

PATIENT MONITORING

Repeat fecal examination at monthly intervals.

EXPECTED COURSE AND PROGNOSIS

Prognosis likely to be good provided adequate husbandry and concurrent disease are not complicating factors.

MISCELLANEOUS

COMMENTS

N/A

ZOONOTIC POTENTIAL

Due to their high host specificity, there is no known zoonotic risk with any *Isospora* species.

SYNONYMS

N/A

ABBREVIATIONS

- PCR = polymerase chain reaction
- PO = per os

Author T. Franciscus Scheelings, BVSc, MVSc, PhD, MANCVSc (Wildlife Health), DECZM (Herpetology)

LOWER RESPIRATORY TRACT DISEASE

BASICS

DEFINITION/OVERVIEW

In amphibians, diseases of the respiratory tract can occur for various reasons. A wide variety of signs can be shown due to the different modes of respiration in larval and adult forms, and across species. Moist skin can be responsible for up to 70% of the gas exchange in some species. Larva and neotenic species also rely on gills, while adult amphibians use lungs. Some species lack lungs. Caecilians and anurans have three modes of respiration: pulmonic, buccopharyngeal, or cutaneous respiration, while adult neotenic anurans have branchial respiration from retained gill structures. In most post-metamorphic amphibians, buccopharyngeal and pulmonary respiration take place, as well as cutaneous gas exchange. The glottis is located on the floor of the pharynx and leads into the larynx, which is a narrow triangular chamber in amphibians and is supported by lateral cartilage. In general, the trachea (if it exists, as it does in caecilians, salamanders, and pipid frogs) is composed of complete cartilaginous rings, is generally short, and bifurcates quickly into the main bronchi. The lungs of amphibians lack true alveoli. In many amphibians, reticulate folds of pulmonic tissue in the mostly sac-like lungs increase the surface for gas exchange. In general, the distinction between URTD and LRTD is not always easy to define. Clinical signs of LRTD in amphibians are usually hard to determine. In many cases, diagnosis can only be made after death.

ETIOLOGY/PATHOPHYSIOLOGY

- Dependent on the amphibian species.
- Bacteria: including *Mycobacteria*, mostly Gram-negatives; pneumococcal pneumonia is described in tadpoles.
- Fungi: (e.g., *Mucor* spp., *Candida* spp., and molds such as *Basidiobolus*, *Hormodendrum dermatitidis* or *Fonsecaea*).
- Parasites: nematodes (*Rhabdias* spp., *Cosmocerca* spp. in the lungs of amphibians), trematodes (*Haematoloechus* spp.), digenea and cestode larvae, pentastomids.
- Viral infection: *Ranavirus* causing hemorrhage and necrosis throughout the body, including the respiratory tract (trachea and URT).
- Neoplasia (multicentric adenocarcinoma, pulmonary carcinoma).
- Foreign bodies within the oral cavity, trachea, bronchus or lung. or perforating foreign bodies of adjacent organs (e.g., gastrointestinal tract).
- Trauma
- Intoxication through absorption or inhalation of dust, smoke, aerosols, disinfectants, or other environmental toxins (algicidals, chlorine, ammonia, etc.).
- Immunosuppression or husbandry deficiencies as predisposing factors.

SIGNALMENT/HISTORY

No age, sex, or species predisposition.

CLINICAL PRESENTATION

- Dependent on the underlying cause and amphibian species.
- In most if not all cases, signs are not apparent until advanced state of disease.
- Non-specific signs such as anorexia, lethargy, inactivity.
- Tachypnea or dyspnea (inspiratory or inspiratory and expiratory).
- Respiratory distress (intermittent or persistent).
- Gaping of the mouth
- Gurgling
- Acute death
- In special cases of pneumococcal pneumonia, normal movement of tadpoles is disturbed because of emphysematous lungs.

RISK FACTORS

Husbandry

- Dependent on the underlying cause and amphibian species.
- Stressors and inappropriate husbandry
- Improper transport conditions
- Inadequate cage set up
- Ponds, tanks, or enclosures polluted. with sewage
- Inappropriate temperatures
- Poor hygiene
- Oxygen imbalances
- High levels of ammonia and chlorine.
- Incorrect pH
- Nitrogen oversaturation

Others

- Immunosuppression, which may be caused by stress, importation, overcrowding, relocation, concurrent disease or inappropriate husbandry, malnutrition and inadequate temperatures.
- Severe endoparasitism may be a predisposing factor or even cause of the disease.

DIAGNOSIS

DIFFERENTIAL DIAGNOSIS

- Infectious diseases (bacterial, viral, fungal, parasitic)
- Neoplasia
- Foreign bodies
- Perforating foreign bodies
- Trauma
- Improper husbandry, with focus on water quality.

DIAGNOSTICS

- Physical exam, including thorough exam of the oral cavity and choana. The use of magnification may aid in identifying subtle lesions.
- Bacterial culture and sensitivity (aerobic and anaerobic) of oral swab.
- Fungal culture of swabs of the oral cavity.
- Cytology of oral swab
- PCR for the diagnosis of *Ranavirus*.
- Parasites: microscopy of oral or cloacal swab or oropharyngeal mucus examination and fecal exam.
- Diagnostic imaging (radiography, ultrasound, CT, MRI)
- Endoscopy

PATHOLOGICAL FINDINGS

- Pathologic findings will vary according to the underlying cause and may range from mild to severe.
- Infiltrates of phagocytic cells laden with bacteria may be visible in cases of pneumococcal pneumonia in tadpoles.
- Mycobacterial infection of the viscera does not usually spread to the lungs, but if it does, it usually leads to the death of the animal before other organs are affected.
- Gradually, both lungs become infected from the bifurcation to the main bronchus and become completely solidified, and the number of acid-fast bacilli is very high.

TREATMENT

APPROPRIATE HEALTH CARE

N/A

NUTRITIONAL SUPPORT

- Nutritional supplementation for anorexic animals is essential for recovery.
- Carnivore critical care diets can be fed until the amphibian starts eating on its own.

CLIENT EDUCATION/HUSBANDRY RECOMMENDATIONS

- Correct any husbandry deficiencies, with special attention to temperature, humidity, and ventilation.
- Isolate animal from others in collection, especially when viral etiology is suspected.
- It is important to ensure a full course of treatment to avoid recurrence of disease.

LOWER RESPIRATORY TRACT DISEASE (CONTINUED)

MEDICATIONS

DRUG(S) OF CHOICE

- Treatment depends on the underlying cause and the affected snake species.
- Bacterial – systemic or nebulized antibiotics (e.g. amikacin, doxycycline, gentamycin, enrofloxacin, oxytetracycline), preferably according to sensitivity panel.
- Local instillation of antibiotics (injectable or ophthalmic solutions) in the nasal passage may also be effective.
- Fungi – systemic, local, nebulized antifungals (e.g. terbinafine, voriconazole, amphotericin B).
- Viral – separation, strict quarantine, and intensive supportive therapy.
- Antiviral therapy has had low success.
- Euthanasia is often required, depending on the state of the animal and the disease.
- Parasitic – antiparasitic treatment according the species.
- In some cases, physical removal of the parasites via surgery or endoscopy may be tried.
- In case of confirmed mycobacterial infection, no treatment is possible, and euthanasia is necessary.
- Neoplasia – surgical removal is not feasible in most cases.
- Optimize husbandry conditions

PRECAUTIONS/INTERACTIONS

- Many systemic antibiotics (e.g., aminoglycosides, fluoroquinolones) are excreted through the kidney or show renal toxicity, thus avoidance of those or supplemental fluid administration is recommended.
- Systemic use of itraconazole may cause severe side effects in some snakes.

FOLLOW-UP

PATIENT MONITORING

- Improvement of clinical signs should be expected within 1–2 weeks for bacterial and fungal infections when definitive diagnosis and treatment are employed.
- It is critical to continue treatment until clinical signs are fully resolved and repeating cultures to confirm resolution of infection if unsure.
- In cases that do not show any improvement or worsen during the first 1–2 weeks of treatment, it should be considered that the etiology and/or treatment are not accurate.
- Viral infections should also be considered in cases that do not respond to therapy or have chronic, intermittent recurrence of disease.
- Repeat diagnostics may be needed to assess resolution or progression of disease.

EXPECTED COURSE AND PROGNOSIS

- Depending on the etiology
- Bacterial: good prognosis depending on response to antibiotics.
- Fungal: guarded to poor prognosis.
- Viral: poor to grave prognosis, especially when showing clinical signs.
- Parasitic: good to guarded prognosis; *Rhabdias* infections of the lung can carry poor prognosis.
- Neoplastic: grave prognosis
- Others: depend on severity and involvement of other tissues.

MISCELLANEOUS

COMMENTS

The amphibian lung is relatively fragile and is easily ruptured if overinflated.

ZOONOTIC POTENTIAL

- Depending on the causative agent
- *Mycobacterium* spp. and *Chlamydia* spp. should be considered as possibly zoonotic, depending on the species.

SYNONYMS

Pneumonia

ABBREVIATIONS

- CT = computed tomography
- LRT = lower respiratory tract
- LRTD = lower respiratory tract disease
- MRI = magnetic resonance imaging
- PCR = polymerase chain reaction
- URT = upper respiratory tract

Suggested Reading

Mitchell MA. Zoonotic diseases associated with reptiles and amphibians: An update. *Vet Clin North Am Exot Anim Pract* 2011;14(3):439–456.

Noble GK. The respiratory system. In: Noble GK, ed. *The Biology of the Amphibia*. New York, NY: Dover Publications; 1954:158–178.

Wright KM. Overview of amphibian medicine. In: Mader DR, ed. *Reptile Medicine and Surgery*. 2nd ed. St. Louis, MO: Elsevier Saunders; 2006:941–971.

Author Karina A. Mathes, DVM, Dr. med. vet., DECZM (Herpetology), European Veterinary Specialist in Zoological Medicine (Herpetology), Certified Specialist in Reptiles (Fachtieraerztin fuer Reptilien), Certified Specialist in Reptiles and Amphibians (ZB Reptilien und Amphibien)

MYCOBACTERIOSIS

BASICS

DEFINITION/OVERVIEW

Mycobacteriosis is a cosmopolitan disease that infects both humans and animals. Only atypical or non-tuberculosis *Mycobacterium* spp. have been isolated from amphibians. *Mycobacterium* spp. are more fastidious in ectothermic animals, which tends to result in latent or chronic infections. Mycobacteriosis is the oldest known infectious disease of amphibians and remains a significant source of morbidity and mortality.

ETIOLOGY/PATHOPHYSIOLOGY

- Aerobic, Acid-fast positive, Gram-positive rod bacteria: *Mycobacterium marinum*, *M. liflandii*, *M. chelonae*, *M. fortuitum*, *M. xenopi*, *M. avium* intracellulare complex, *M szulgai*, *M. gordonae*, *M. ulcerans*, *M. ranae*, *M. thamnospheos*, *M. abscessus*.
- *M. liflandii* is characterized by the presence of insertion gene sequences IS2404 and IS 2606, in addition to the production of the toxin mycolactone.
- *M. ulcerans* is also characterized as a mycolactone producing *Mycobacterium*.
- *M. marinum* and *M. ulcerans* are ubiquitous within aquatic environments.
- Transmission of *Mycobacterium* spp. in amphibians is through both direct and indirect contact between infected individuals, contaminated water, and fomites.
- Exposure through skin wounds is considered a common route of exposure; minimizing injuries to the skin is important.
- Ingestion of contaminated food or water can also serve as a direct source of infection.
- Water and biofilms provide natural habitats for *Mycobacterium* spp. and can serve as important sources of infection.
- Vectors, such as protozoa, may also serve as a source of infection.
- Vertical transmission in amphibians has not been documented.

SIGNALMENT/HISTORY

- Any amphibian species, including both juvenile and adult life stages.
- Fully aquatic amphibians appear to be associated with a higher exposure risk.
- Acute death or mass mortality event; individuals with chronic granulomatous skin disease and non-healing ulcers.
- Poor husbandry conditions, including inappropriate environmental temperature (chronically low or high temperatures), high organic loads, poor water quality; no quarantine system, high animal density, and high stress production/breeding settings.
- Affected animals may appear clinically normal and serve as reservoirs or emaciated and experience weight loss while having a good appetite.

CLINICAL PRESENTATION

- Clinical signs associated with *Mycobacterium* spp. infections are non-specific and can range from acute death to no obvious clinical signs in apparently healthy animals.
- *Mycobacterium* spp. should be included in a differential for any amphibian with non-specific clinical signs.
- The following clinical signs have been associated with *Mycobacterium* spp. infections: acute death, high mortality rate, weight loss, lethargy, anorexia, bloating, coelomic effusion, ulcerative or nodular dermatitis, pigmentary changes, abnormal behavior, ataxia, ascites, and draining or non-draining abscesses.
- Skin lesions of any type can be caused by *Mycobacterium* spp. in amphibians.

RISK FACTORS

Husbandry

- Any factor that can lead to stress or immunosuppression can increase the susceptibility of an amphibian to this disease.
- Since it is ubiquitous in the environment, the amphibian is (potentially) constantly exposed to the pathogen in a closed system.
- Attempts to mimic the natural environment of the amphibian can minimize these risks.
- Poor husbandry can lead to increased densities of *Mycobacterium* spp., leading to increased risk of exposure and infection (dose based).
- Low or elevated environmental temperatures can lead to immunosuppression, increasing stress and susceptibility.
- High stocking densities in production systems can be stressful and increase the risk of infection.
- Fully aquatic amphibians are naturally at a higher risk for exposure to *Mycobacterium* spp. because it can be in the water column and on surfaces within the environment.
- High organic loads and poor water quality can contribute to the population growth of these bacteria, and thus the risk of exposure to the amphibian.

Others

N/A

DIAGNOSIS

DIFFERENTIAL DIAGNOSIS

- Any chronic disease process
- Infectious: viral, bacterial, parasitic, and fungal disease: chytridiomycosis (*Batrachochytrium dendrobatidis*), *Aeromonas hydrophila*, *Pseudomonas aeruginosa*, *Ranavirus*, *Chlamydophila* spp.
- Renal failure
- Liver failure
- Heart failure
- Malabsorptive gastrointestinal disease
- Neoplasia: lymphosarcoma, histiocytoma, squamous cell carcinoma.
- Reproductive tract disorders

DIAGNOSTICS

Polymerase Chain Reaction

- Currently considered the most sensitive antemortem assay for diagnosing *Mycobacterium* spp. in amphibians.
- The 16s ribosomal RNA primer is commonly used for mycobacterial PCR assays, although a nested PCR targeting a 65-kDA heat shock protein has also been used.
- Other gene targets for detecting mycobacterial infections in amphibians include MPM-associated IS2404 and IS2606. Sensitives and specificities for these PCRs have yet to be determined.
- Sequencing of the PCR results is important to confirm the species of *Mycobacterium*.

Cytology

- Examination of skin lesions can be a useful first-line diagnostic tool for diagnosing mycobacterial infections.
- Cytology can be used to provide direct evidence of chronic inflammation in the lesions and demonstrate the presence of bacteria.
- Gram stain and acid-fast staining can be used to further characterize the presence of the bacteria, directing the clinician to other more sensitive diagnostics such as PCR and histopathology.

Histopathology

- Tissue biopsy and histology are considered the gold standard for diagnosing a *Mycobacterium* spp. infection.
- In addition to the presence of granulomatous lesions, acid fast stains, including Ziehl–Nelsen and the Fite method, can be used to confirm the presence bacteria within the lesions, with organisms staining as red to pink filamentous rods against a blue to green background.
- This type of diagnostic test has a high specificity but a low sensitivity.

Culture

- This has fallen out of favor for clinical samples because of the special media required to culture *Mycobacterium* spp. and the long culture times associated with growing these organisms.
- Speciation can be performed on cultured samples.
- Antibacterial sensitivities can also be performed on cultured *Mycobacterium* spp. if therapy is elected.

Hematology and Biochemistry

These tests can be used to characterize the physiologic (e.g., inflammation, dehydration, anemia) status of the patient and monitor disease progression.

MYCOBACTERIOSIS (CONTINUED)

PATHOLOGICAL FINDINGS

- Gross necropsy findings can range from a single white to gray focal lesion/nodule to multifocal, coalescing white lesions/nodules in any organ system. Organomegaly is commonly observed in the spleen, kidney, and liver.
- Histopathological findings for chronic mycobacteriosis include granulomatous inflammation with multinucleated giant cells. Granulomas can range from localized centers of macrophages containing intracellular acid-fast bacilli to complex granulomas with caseated centers.

TREATMENT

APPROPRIATE HEALTH CARE

N/A

NUTRITIONAL SUPPORT

- Treatment is not recommended; however, if pursued, nutritional support should be considered.
- Mycobacteriosis can lead to weight loss because of the negative energy balance that develops in these patients.
- Nutritional support can be used to supplement calories and improve the likelihood for treatment success.

CLIENT EDUCATION/HUSBANDRY RECOMMENDATIONS

- Disease exposure and dissemination can be limited by quarantine and testing (PCR) of new amphibian arrivals.
- Implementing husbandry practices that reduce organic loads in both aquatic and terrestrial vivariums is highly recommended.
- Regular water quality monitoring and water changes can minimize pathogen buildup in a closed system.
- Separate life support systems for quarantine and established populations is recommended.
- Husbandry recommendations should be species specific to minimize stress and the potential for compromising the immune system of an amphibian.
- Clients and veterinary staff should follow standard hygiene practices to minimize zoonotic potential.

MEDICATIONS

DRUG(S) OF CHOICE

- There are no proven or approved treatments for mycobacteriosis in amphibians.
- Macrolides (azithromycin and clarithromycin) have been used to treat clinical cases, but clinicians should avoid empirical treatment of these pathogens.
- Euthanasia should be considered to mitigate zoonotic potential in both small and large populations.
- Surgical intervention has been used to treat limb infections.
- In human medicine, treatment of mycobacteriosis is based on culture and sensitivity results and a multi drug-treatment protocol used, including macrolides, aminoglycosides, ethambutol, and/or rifamycins.

PRECAUTIONS/INTERACTIONS

N/A

FOLLOW-UP

PATIENT MONITORING

- Humane euthanasia is recommended for these cases.
- If treatment is pursued, regular examinations and blood work (hematology and biochemistry testing) should be done to evaluate the patient's quality of life and physiologic status.

EXPECTED COURSE AND PROGNOSIS

- Amphibians diagnosed with *Mycobacterium* spp. have a grave prognosis and can serve as a reservoir for the pathogen in closed systems.
- The risk of transmission to other amphibians and the zoonotic disease risk can be used to direct decision making for a case, with most electing for humane euthanasia.
- Therapeutic options are long term, unproven, and have not been successful to date.
- Mycobacteriosis is ultimately fatal in amphibians.

MISCELLANEOUS

COMMENTS

N/A

ZOONOTIC POTENTIAL

- Zoonotic transmission of *Mycobacterium* spp. from amphibians to humans is well documented, but rare.
- *M marinum*, *M. szulgai*, *M. fortuitum*, and *M. chelonae* have all been documented to cause disease in humans.
- *M. marinum* is most commonly diagnosed; it produces granulomatous lesions in the skin and peripheral deep tissues. Zoonotic potential for these bacteria can be reduced by wearing gloves while transporting, handling, or managing the environment of amphibians.

SYNONYMS

- Atypical *Mycobacterium*
- Granulomatous disease
- Vivarium granuloma

ABBREVIATIONS

- MPM = mycolactone-producing mycobacteria
- PCR = polymerase chain reaction assay

INTERNET RESOURCES

- Centers for Disease Control and Prevention. Reptiles and Amphibians. October 28, 2019. https://www.cdc.gov/healthypets/pets/reptiles.html
- Whitaker BR. Infectious Diseases of Amphibians. MSD Manual Veterinary Manual, September 2013. https://www.merckvetmanual.com/exotic-and-laboratory-animals/amphibians/infectious-diseases-of-amphibians
- Wagner J. Zoonoses Associated with Fish and Amphibians. Princeton University Environmental Health and Safety. https://ehs.princeton.edu/node/590

Suggested Reading

Chai N. Mycobacteriosis in amphibians. In: Miller RE, Fowler ME., eds. *Fowler's Zoo and Wild Animal Medicine Current Therapy*. St. Louis, MO: Elsevier Saunders; 2012:224–230.

Latney LV, Klaphake E. Selected emerging diseases of amphibia. *Vet Clin N Am Exot Anim Pract* 2013;16(2):283–301.

Martinho F, Heatley JJ. Amphibian mycobacteriosis. *Vet Clin North Am Exot Anim Pract* 2012;15(1):113–119.

Mitchell MA. Zoonotic diseases associated with reptiles and amphibians: An update. *Vet Clin North Am Exot Anim Pract* 2011;14(3):439–456.

Authors Sean M. Perry, DVM, PhD, and Mark A. Mitchell, DVM, MS, PhD, DECZM (Herpetology)

NUTRITIONAL SECONDARY HYPERPARATHROIDISM

BASICS

DEFINITION/OVERVIEW

NSHP is still a common disorder in amphibian populations. The disease is characterized by hypocalcemia caused by deficiency of calcium and/or vitamin D in the diet, or a lack of UVB light exposure. This results in increased PTH production, leading to increased calcium resorption from the bones. Affected amphibians typically present with functional and morphological bone changes including pathological fractures and/or with tetany, seizure-like activity, and muscle tremors.

ETIOLOGY/PATHOPHYSIOLOGY

- The etiology of NSHP is considered multifactorial.
- Low dietary calcium and/or vitamin D levels or inadequate UVB exposure results in low blood calcium concentrations.
- As a result, the parathyroid glands increase production of PTH to raise calcium concentrations.
- PTH stimulates osteoclastic activity, resulting in different degrees of bone depletion.
- It also stimulates calcium reabsorption in the kidneys.

SIGNALMENT/HISTORY

- Amphibians fed only with superworms (*Zophobas* spp.), mealworms (*Tenebrio* spp.), and waxworms (*Galleria* spp. or *Achroia* spp.) are at risk of suffering NSHP because of the poor calcium-to-phosphorus ratios and high lipid content of this diet.
- NSHP is more common in amphibians that have basking behaviors in the wild (e.g., certain frogs) and are kept without UVB in captivity, compared with cryptic nocturnal species.

CLINICAL PRESENTATION

- Clinical signs vary depending on the severity of the disease.
- Clinical signs of NSHP include reduced food intake, deformation of long bones, tetany, seizure-like activity, and muscle tremors.

RISK FACTORS

Husbandry

- Insufficient calcium intake
- Excessive phosphorus intake
- Insufficient vitamin D intake
- Excessive vitamin A intake
- Insufficient exposure to UVB radiation in the range of 280–315 nm (depending on the species).

Others

Concurrent parasitism may exacerbate NSHP.

DIAGNOSIS

DIFFERENTIAL DIAGNOSIS

- Renal secondary hyperparathyroidism
- Primary hyperparathyroidism

DIAGNOSTICS

- In most cases, NSHP is diagnosed based on clinical presentation and history of inappropriate diet and/or management.
- Radiography, blood work and fecal exams are indicated to confirm the clinical suspicion, determine the severity of the disease, and formulate a prognosis.
- Chemistry panel: hypocalcemia is usually observed in the early and late stages of the disease. It is therefore common to have animals with NSHP be normocalcemic or even hypercalcemic, owing to the active resorption of calcium from the bones. Hyperphosphatemia may be observed concurrently, especially when hypocalcemia is present.
- Radiography: decreased bony cortices and pathologic fractures may be observed. Animals with multiple fractures and decreased cortices across the majority of the long bones tend to have a worse prognosis for recovery.

PATHOLOGICAL FINDINGS

- Gross pathologic findings include softening or alterations of bone tissue.
- Histopathology of long bones may show thinned cortices with layers of osteoblasts and unmineralized osteoid on the periosteal surface.

TREATMENT

APPROPRIATE HEALTH CARE

N/A

NUTRITIONAL SUPPORT

- Amphibians with mild chronic NSHP are often anorectic.
- The anorexia is usually transient and improves once the management is corrected.
- Nutritional support in form of periodic syringe feeding or force feeding with whole preys or critical care diets may be needed.
- The exact amount of vitamin A that should be included in an amphibian diet is currently unclear, as vitamin A has been associated with “short tongue syndrome,” while its excess may inhibit vitamin D absorption.

CLIENT EDUCATION/HUSBANDRY RECOMMENDATIONS

- Provision of UVB through a UVB-emitting lamb in species that exhibits basking behaviors in the wild.
- Provision of a diet that is high in calcium and low in phosphorus.
- Provision of a diet that does not have excess vitamin A.

MEDICATIONS

DRUG(S) OF CHOICE

- In amphibians presented with chronic NSHP, the mainstay of the therapy is an improvement in management and diet.
- Exposure to appropriate UVB emitters (usually around 2%) for basking species is critical.
- A change to a diet that contains the appropriate levels of calcium and vitamin D, with low level of phosphorus is required.
- Administration of oral calcium may assist in the recovery but is ineffective as a standalone treatment.
- In amphibians presented with acute hypocalcemic crisis, calcium gluconate can be administered.
- Calcium gluconate 50–200 mg/kg SC, IM q12–24h; 2.3% bath.
- Calcium glubionate 100 mg/kg PO q12–24h.

PRECAUTIONS/INTERACTIONS

- There is some evidence that, in amphibians, hypervitaminosis of other vitamins such as vitamin A may inhibit calcium uptake by antagonizing calcitriol and aggravating NSHP.
- Exposure to excessive ultraviolet radiation may have important adverse effects in certain amphibian species.

FOLLOW-UP

PATIENT MONITORING

- In cases of acute hypocalcemic crisis, the amphibian requires intensive care and frequent monitoring of ionized calcium levels and ECG activity.
- In cases of chronic NSHP, if the amphibian manages to feed alone, a physical exam once every 7–14 days, accompanied by radiography, is usually adequate to assess response to therapy.

EXPECTED COURSE AND PROGNOSIS

N/A

MISCELLANEOUS

COMMENTS

The benefits and side effects of UV radiation in many amphibian species requires further research.

NUTRITIONAL SECONDARY HYPERPARATHROIDISM (CONTINUED)

COMMENTS

N/A

ZOONOTIC POTENTIAL

N/A

SYNONYMS

- Fibrous osteodystrophy.
- Metabolic bone disease
- Nutrition-related metabolic bone disease.

ABBREVIATIONS

- ECG = electrocardiogram
- IM = intramuscular
- NSHP = nutritional secondary hyperparathyroidism
- PO = per os
- PTH = parathyroid hormone
- SC = subcutaneous
- UVB = ultraviolet B

INTERNET RESOURCES

- Stahl Exotic Animal Veterinary Services. Arboreal Frog Husbandry and Preventative Healthcare. 2018. http://www.seavs.com/pet-care-information/aboreal-frog-care
- Information on the disease in humans: Kim L. Hyperparathyroidism. Medscape, August 18, 2020. http://emedicine.medscape.com/article/127351-overview?pa=mcKd1JF66kULHOzxxIxn2fK%2Bx5xE5kE6dUeU7dvJSrcnjyhACchqCtq5rNZR2UhkQPQxex%2Bo7mr5pATtx84gCBXKySxof3ndUJD5aivxmIc%3D#a4

Suggested Reading

Antwis RE, Browne RK. Ultraviolet radiation and vitamin D3 in amphibian health, behaviour, diet and conservation. *Comp Biochem Physiol A Mol Integr Physiol* 2009;154(2):184–190.

Ferrie GM, Alford VC, Atkinson J, et al. Nutrition and health in amphibian husbandry. *Zoo Biol* 2014;33(6):485–501.

Michaels CJ, Antwis RE, Preziosi RF. Impacts of UVB provision and dietary calcium content on serum vitamin D3, growth rates, skeletal structure and coloration in captive oriental fire-bellied toads (*Bombina orientalis*). *J Anim Physiol Anim Nutr (Berl)* 2015;99(2):391–403.

Authors Paolo Selleri, DMV, PhD, SpecPACS, DECZM (Herpetology & Small Mammals), and Nicola Di Girolamo, DMV, MSc (EBHC), PhD, DECZM (Herpetology)

OXYURIDS

BASICS

DEFINITION/OVERVIEW

Oxyurids (pinworms) are nematodes with a direct life cycle; they are host specific. Oxyurid infestation is rare in amphibians and they are considered non-pathogenic in healthy animals.

ETIOLOGY/PATHOPHYSIOLOGY

- Animals are usually asymptomatic
- Parasites inhabit the lower intestinal tract.
- Severe infestations may cause secondary problems, especially in debilitated and dehydrated animals.

SIGNALMENT/HISTORY

N/A

CLINICAL PRESENTATION

- Disease caused by oxyurids is usually a secondary complication.
- Anorexia
- Lethargy
- Diarrhea
- Dehydration

RISK FACTORS

Husbandry

Inadequate husbandry may lead to stress, immunosuppression, and a myriad of secondary conditions.

Others

N/A

DIAGNOSIS

DIFFERENTIAL DIAGNOSIS

- Rule out prey items as the source of oxyurid ova.
- Oxyurid ova found in amphibian feces often originate from prey item, as they are commensals of the rodent cecum, and are also found in insect prey items.

DIAGNOSTICS

- Eggs vary in shape, can be ovoid, elongate, or D-shaped, and lack the thick wall of ascarid eggs. The eggs measure approximately 130–140 µm.
- Some eggs can be larvated
- Adult worms may be visible in fecal material.

PATHOLOGICAL FINDINGS

Intestinal impaction of the intestinal tract may be observed in sick animals with pinworm overgrowth.

TREATMENT

APPROPRIATE HEALTH CARE

Excessive numbers of these organisms in sick amphibians may require medical treatment.

NUTRITIONAL SUPPORT

- After rehydration, supportive nutrition is needed to maintain positive nitrogen balance.
- Feed small amounts more frequently.
- Use high protein and fat diets for carnivores.

CLIENT EDUCATION/HUSBANDRY RECOMMENDATIONS

- Follow proper husbandry guidelines for the species at hand.
- Environmental temperature, proper housing, and feeding regimen all play a crucial role in the wellbeing of amphibian species kept in captivity.

MEDICATIONS

DRUG(S) OF CHOICE

- Fenbendazole 50 mg/kg PO; repeat in 14 days
- Oxfendazole 5 mg/kg PO once
- Pyrantel pamoate 5-10 mg/kg PO q24h for 3 days, repeat in 3 weeks.
- Ivermectin 0.2 mg/kg topically, PO; repeat in 2 weeks.

PRECAUTIONS/INTERACTIONS

- Avoid fenbendazole and oxfendazole in severely debilitated and dehydrated animals to minimize the risk of the potential adverse effects (bone marrow suppression, intestinal cell damage) associated with these drugs.
- Ivermectin may cause flaccid paralysis in some species.

FOLLOW-UP

PATIENT MONITORING

- Evaluate hydration frequently after starting treatment.
- Make husbandry changes to provide proper environment and nutrition.

EXPECTED COURSE AND PROGNOSIS

- Oxyurids are non-pathogenic in healthy animals.
- In sick animals, treatment is aimed at decreasing the parasite load in the gut to minimize chance of impaction.
- Prognosis is good, as long as the primary source of the problem is identified and eliminated (husbandry mismanagement, primary disease process).

MISCELLANEOUS

COMMENTS

N/A

ZOONOTIC POTENTIAL

N/A

SYNONYMS

Pinworms

ABBREVIATIONS

PO = per os

Suggested Reading

Wright KM, Whitaker BR. *Amphibian Medicine and Captive Husbandry*. Malabar, FL: Krieger; 2001.

Author Sam Rivera, DVM, MS, DABVP (Avian), DACZM, DECZM (Zoo Health Management)

PENTASTOMIDS

BASICS

DEFINITION/OVERVIEW

Pentastomids are crustacean endoparasites of the respiratory system. They primarily infect carnivorous reptiles, but bufonids are also definitive hosts for *Raillietiella* spp. A variety of Australasian and neotropical frogs and toads are intermediate hosts for *Kiricephalus* and *Waddycephalus* spp. Pentastomiasis occurs on all continents except Antarctica.

ETIOLOGY/PATHOPHYSIOLOGY

- Adult pentastomids live in the lungs of toads, where they breed and feed.
- Eggs are coughed up from the lungs, or ingested and passed in feces.
- Intermediate hosts, such as insects, fish, anurans, squamates, birds, or mammals, ingest pentastomid eggs, which hatch, and go through two instars (growth periods between molts), before becoming encysted in the intermediate host.
- When the intermediate host is eaten by the definitive host, third-stage larvae emerge from the cyst and migrate to the host's lungs, where they feed on blood through the lung wall (hematophagous).
- Pentastomids damage the lungs, which may lead to secondary bacterial or fungal colonization, pneumonia, septicemia, or death.
- Heavy infestations can occlude the lungs or trachea.

SIGNALMENT/HISTORY

- Wild caught or captive toads, including cane toads (*Bufo marinus*): *Raillietiella indica* and *R. frenata*); the black-spined toad (*B. melanostictus*): *R. indica* and *R. rileyi*; Puerto Rican crested toad (*B. lemur*): *R. bufonis*, the cururu or rococo toad (*B. paracnemis*): *R. freitasi*; and Colombian, or Blomberg's, toad (*B. blombergi*): unidentified *Raillietiella* spp.
- Cockroaches are often an intermediate host.
- In Panama, 12.5% of sampled cane toads were positive for *R. frenata*.
- In Hawaii, 41% of cane toads were positive for *R. indica*.

CLINICAL PRESENTATION

Can be subclinical or have respiratory tract disease, pneumonia, dyspnea, weight loss, or poor growth, or death.

RISK FACTORS

Husbandry

Yet another compelling reason for quarantine and fecal examinations.

Others

- In wild Australian cane toads, pentastome prevalence and intensity varied seasonally.
- Male toads were four times more likely to be infected than females.

DIAGNOSIS

DIFFERENTIAL DIAGNOSIS

- Other parasites
- Viruses
- Bacteria
- Fungi
- Neoplasia
- Trauma
- Foreign bodies

DIAGNOSTICS

- Detection of pentastomid eggs on fecal flotation, lung or cloacal washes, or tracheal discharge.
- Adult pentastomids are sometimes visible on radiography, or by pulmonoscopy or ultrasound.
- Adults may also be found during exploratory surgery, necropsy, or histopathology.
- Fecal examination revealing thin-walled, large (up to 130 µm in diameter), distinct ova, containing larvae with four claw-like hooklets.
- A complete blood count might reveal anemia or eosinophilia.

PATHOLOGICAL FINDINGS

- Pentastomids are medium to large (0.25–15 cm), superficially segmented, wormlike parasites, with two compound pairs of hooks surrounding the mouth.
- Adults may be recovered from the mouth, trachea, and lungs, while encysted instars may be found throughout the body.
- Females are larger and longer lived than males.
- In tissues, pentastomids are identified histologically by the presence of acidophilic glands adjacent to the intestine, and black, sclerotized openings in the body wall.
- Inflammatory response in the lung may be mild with pentastomids because all life stages secrete surfactant very similar to host surfactant, which is thought to help them evade the host's immune system.
- Degrading molted pentastomid cuticles shed into the lung lumen may induce putrid pneumonia.
- Feed attachment sites on the lung surface can cause multiple crateriform ulcers.
- Pentastomids can be identified by morphological and molecular techniques.

TREATMENT

APPROPRIATE HEALTH CARE

Stabilize patient first with antibiotics, fluids and nutritional support as indicated.

NUTRITIONAL SUPPORT

Emeraid™ Sustain Carnivore® (EmerAid, LLC, Cornell, IL), or Oxbow Critical Care® Carnivore (Oxbow Animal Health, Omaha, NE) via stomach tube every 24 hours if anorexic or in poor body condition.

CLIENT EDUCATION/HUSBANDRY RECOMMENDATIONS

Zoonotic, wear gloves when handling amphibians.

MEDICATIONS

DRUG(S) OF CHOICE

Selamectin 6 mg/kg topically in American bullfrogs (*Rana catesbeiana*) produced higher peak concentrations than in dogs, with no clinical or histologic signs of toxicity.

PRECAUTIONS/INTERACTIONS

Living pentastomids secrete surfactant that helps them to evade the host's immune system but, on their death in tissue or lungs, a severe antigenic release, or putrefaction, with serious and potential lethal complications can occur.

FOLLOW-UP

PATIENT MONITORING

Perform serial fecal examinations post-treatment to gauge effectiveness.

EXPECTED COURSE AND PROGNOSIS

Highly variable dependent on parasitic burden, chronicity, condition of patient, and response to therapy.

MISCELLANEOUS

COMMENTS

N/A

ZOONOTIC POTENTIAL

- All pentastomids should be considered potentially zoonotic.
- Species infecting humans belong to the families Linguatulidae, Armilliferidae, Porocephalidae, and Raillietiella, with the latter reported in toads.
- Rare human cases from Raillietiella have been associated with eating raw snakes or live geckos, as part of alternative medicine therapies.
- In the intermediate hosts, pentastome larvae often hatch and bore through the stomach wall and encyst in nearby mesentery, serosa or viscera.

SYNONYMS

- Pentastomiasis
- Tongue worms

Suggested Reading

D'Agostino JJ, West G, Boothe DM, et al. Plasma pharmacokinetics of selamectin after a single topical administration in the American bullfrog (*Rana catesbeiana*). *J Zoo Wildl Med* 2007;38(1):51–54.

Jacobson ER. Parasites and parasitic diseases of reptiles. In: Jacobson ER, ed. *Infectious Disease and Pathology of Reptiles: Color Atlas and Text*. Boca Raton, FL: CRC Press; 2007:571–665.

Kelehear C, Saltonstall K, Torchink ME. An introduced pentastomid parasite (*Raillietiella frenata*) infects native cane toads (*Rhinella marina*) in Panama. *Paristology* 2015;142(5):675–679.

Pare JA. An overview of pentastomiasis in reptiles and other vertebrates. *J Exot Pet Med* 2008;17:285–294.

Author Thomas H. Boyer, DVM, DABVP (Reptile and Amphibian Practice)

PROLAPSE

BASICS

DEFINITION/OVERVIEW

A prolapse is the moving or slipping of a body part from its usual position or anatomic relation. Prolapses may be of gastric, rectal, or cloacal in origin.

ETIOLOGY/PATHOPHYSIOLOGY

- The underlying causes for prolapse of gastric, rectal, or cloacal tissue is often unknown.
- See Differential Diagnosis for a list of possible etiologies.

SIGNALMENT/HISTORY

There appears to be no specific signalment or predilections noted for the various amphibian prolapses.

CLINICAL PRESENTATION

A prolapse is easy to visualize as abnormal tissue protruding from the oral cavity or cloacal/vent region.

RISK FACTORS

Husbandry

- Several husbandry factors may lead to one of the clinical conditions listed in the Differential Diagnosis section.
- Corrections of the deficient aspects of the husbandry can lead to reversal of some of the listed conditions.
- Wild-caught amphibians may have increased stressors or parasites that may lead to increased incidence.

Others

- It should be noted that, during the physical exam, some anurans are capable of everting their stomach as a stress reaction.
- This is an extension of a normal behavior process that facilitates the use of the forelimbs to "wipe" any noxious or indigestible material from the gastric lining.

DIAGNOSIS

DIFFERENTIAL DIAGNOSIS

- Parasites
- Hypocalcemia
- Dehydration
- Impaction
- Obstruction
- Trauma
- Metabolic disease
- Gastric overload
- Bacterial infection
- Intoxication
- Neoplasia

DIAGNOSTICS

- Radiography and ultrasound may be useful in determining internal abnormalities (e.g., impactions, obstructions).
- The small size of some amphibians may lead to reduced imaging detail, which makes interpretation challenging.
- Dental radiography may be a better alternative in smaller species (< 100 g).
- A fecal examination should be performed in all cases. This can be directly from the feces, a saline cloacal wash, or direct impression smear of the prolapsed tissue may reveal the presence of parasites such as nematode larvae or eggs.
- A complete blood count and chemistry panel may assist in the determination of underlying physiologic abnormalities.

PATHOLOGICAL FINDINGS

- Protozoal infections affecting the gastrointestinal tract may be diagnosed on histopathology.
- Other findings will be consistent with the underlying cause but often no specific cause or pathology can be identified.

TREATMENT

APPROPRIATE HEALTH CARE

- Treatment often involves direct replacement of the tissue back into normal anatomic position, either by manual or surgical means, in combination with correction of the underlying etiology.
- The patient should be fully evaluated for general health status and often pre-soaked in amphibian Ringer's solution to maintain normal hydration.
- The prolapsed tissue should be evaluated for presence of necrosis, which must be surgically or medically addressed prior to prolapse reduction.
- The prolapse may be reduced in size by coating with a hyperosmotic solution such as hypertonic saline (2–5%) or dextrose (10%) solution.
- Direct application of dry salt or sugar should be performed with caution as the extreme osmolar difference could lead to direct tissue damage if not properly monitored.
- After several minutes of application, the prolapsed tissue should become less edematous and capable of reduction back into the body cavity.
- A moistened and lubricated (water soluble) cotton tip applicator or metal probe is used to gently push the tissue back inside the body cavity aligning the lumen.

NUTRITIONAL SUPPORT

- The amphibian patient may need weight and body condition monitoring to determine if additional caloric supplementation is needed.
- If required, a carnivore critical care diet or gel diets can be used to ensure caloric intake.

CLIENT EDUCATION/HUSBANDRY RECOMMENDATIONS

- If surgical correction of the prolapse was undertaken, the client should be directed on postoperative care of any surgical sites, suture, etc.
- A detailed log of activity, including food intake/defecations, should be maintained and related back to the veterinarian.
- If any changes to the husbandry are required (changes to temperature and/or humidity, increased ultraviolet lighting, etc.), the owner should correct those prior to the patient returning home.

SURGICAL CONSIDERATIONS

- Depending on the level of swelling/inflammation of the tissue, a purse string suture around the cloaca or lateral suture(s) across the lateral cloacal margins may be placed for 5–7 days to allow for the tissue swelling to resolve in place.
- An absorbable suture can be used in case the patient does not present again for re-evaluation.

MEDICATIONS

DRUG(S) OF CHOICE

- NSAIDs or opioids may be used in management of pain and inflammation associated with the physical discomfort of the prolapse or surgery.
- Depending on the determined etiology, antibiotics or antiparasiticides may be indicated.

PRECAUTIONS/INTERACTIONS

- When replacing the prolapse, extreme care must be taken not to tear or perforate the delicate, inflamed tissue.
- After the sutures are removed, the tissue may re-prolapse if swelling/inflammation are still present or the underlying etiology has not been corrected.
- Placement of additional sutures may be required.
- Hydration status of the patent must be considered before use of NSAIDs.

FOLLOW-UP

PATIENT MONITORING

- The patient should be monitored daily after replacement or surgical repair of the prolapse for reoccurrence.
- All food intake and defecations during this time should be recorded.
- Any abnormal changes from the routine should be related back to the veterinarian to determine any further changes to the therapy.

EXPECTED COURSE AND PROGNOSIS

• A pathologic gastric prolapse is often terminal unless caused by parasites or early intoxication.
• Rectal/cloacal prolapses tend to have a guarded prognosis due to the degree of underlying physical damage of the cloacal and affected tissues, and severity of the underlying etiology.
• The length of time the prolapse presents has an inverse effect on the prognosis.
• When treated early in the disease process and the tissue appears viable, cloacal prolapse replacement may lead to clinical resolution if the underlying etiology is addressed.
• Once the tissue begins to desiccate and become devitalized, there is a guarded to grave prognosis.

MISCELLANEOUS

COMMENTS

N/A

ZOONOTIC POTENTIAL

N/A

SYNONYMS

N/A

ABBREVIATIONS

NSAIDs = nonsteroidal anti-inflammatory drugs

Suggested Reading

Wright, KM. Overview of amphibian medicine. In: Mader DR, ed. *Reptile Medicine and Surgery*. 2nd ed. St. Louis, MO: Elsevier Saunders; 2006:941–971.

Wright, KM. Surgical techniques. In: Wright, KM, Whitaker, B.R, eds. *Amphibian Medicine and Captive Husbandry*. Malabar, FL: Krieger; 2001:273–283.

Author Rob L. Coke, DVM, DACZM, DABVP (Reptile & Amphibian), CVA

PSEUDOGOUT

BASICS

DEFINITION/OVERVIEW

Pseudogout is a rare condition in amphibians. It occurs due to the deposition of crystals, other than uric acid, in or around the joints.

ETIOLOGY/PATHOPHYSIOLOGY

- Crystals may be deposited for a variety of reasons. In humans, these include previous joint damage, hyperparathyroidism, or hereditary factors.
- In amphibians, the exact etiology is unclear, but deposition of calcium crystals in and around joints may be seen, especially calcium pyrophosphate dihydrate.
- This can result in an acute inflammatory response in the affected joint.

SIGNALMENT/HISTORY

- Pseudogout may be seen in amphibians with a history of inappropriate husbandry or diet.
- Signs may also be seen in combination with gout.

CLINICAL PRESENTATION

- Animals with pseudogout usually present with obvious joint swellings.
- One or more joints may be affected.
- The animal may be lame

RISK FACTORS

Husbandry

Excessive calcium and vitamin D supplementation may be a predisposing factor.

Others

Previous joint damage, previous metabolic bone disease, or renal disease are all thought to predispose to the development of pseudogout.

DIAGNOSIS

DIFFERENTIAL DIAGNOSIS

- Gout
- Septic arthritis
- Trauma
- Metabolic bone diseases

DIAGNOSTICS

- Pseudogout may be suspected based on history and clinical examination, but diagnostic testing will be necessary for definitive diagnosis.
- On radiography of affected limbs, calcified lesions may be seen in and around the joints.
- Demonstration of calcium crystals in joints or within diseased tissue is necessary for definitive diagnosis.
- Aspirates may be taken from affected joints and examined microscopically for the presence of crystals, or the whole joint may be submitted for histopathology if amputation is performed.
- Von Kossa or Alizarin red S stain may aid in the identification of calcium crystals.

PATHOLOGICAL FINDINGS

- On gross postmortem examination, pale nodules can be seen within or around joints.
- On histopathological examination, nodules are often surrounded by granulomatous inflammation.

TREATMENT

APPROPRIATE HEALTH CARE

- If signs are mild, NSAIDs can be given to reduce inflammation and pain.
- Euthanasia may be considered in severe cases.

NUTRITIONAL SUPPORT

N/A

CLIENT EDUCATION/HUSBANDRY RECOMMENDATIONS

- The diet should be reviewed to ensure that it is appropriate for the species and does not contain excessive levels of calcium or vitamin D3.
- Clients should be advised that this is a condition that will require long-term management and can potentially be very painful if allowed to progress.

SURGICAL CONSIDERATIONS

Amputation of the affected digit or limb may be considered if signs are localized.

MEDICATIONS

DRUG(S) OF CHOICE

N/A

PRECAUTIONS/INTERACTIONS

N/A

FOLLOW-UP

PATIENT MONITORING

Response to therapy is usually monitored by physical examination findings (e.g., increase in activity levels or no progression in joint swellings).

EXPECTED COURSE AND PROGNOSIS

- The prognosis for patients with severe widespread signs is poor, but if diagnosed early the condition can often be managed successfully.
- If the underlying cause is not addressed, disease can progress to affect multiple joints.

MISCELLANEOUS

COMMENTS

N/A

ZOONOTIC POTENTIAL

N/A

SYNONYMS

- Calcium pyrophosphate dihydrate (CPPD) crystal deposition disease
- Chondrocalcinosis

ABBREVIATIONS

NSAIDs = non-steroidal anti-inflammatory drugs

INTERNET RESOURCES

Veterinary Information Network: www.vin.com

Suggested Reading

Green DE. Pathology of amphibia. In: Wright KM, Whitaker BR. *Amphibian Medicine and Captive Husbandry*. Malabar, FL: Krieger; 2001:401–486.

Jones YL, Fitzgerald SD. Articular gout and suspected pseudogout in a Basilisk lizard (*Basilicus plumifrons*). *J Zoo Wildl Med* 2009;40(3):576–578.

Rosenthal AK, Ryan LM. Calcium pyrophosphate deposition disease. *N Engl J Med* 2016;374(26):2575–2584.

Author Joanna Hedley BVM&S, DZooMed (Reptilian), DECZM (Herpetology), MRCVS

RANAVIRUS

BASICS

DEFINITION/OVERVIEW

Ranavirus is a group of emerging primary pathogens known from the 1960s but with a recent exponential expansion. They have a remarkable host range, infecting fish, reptiles, and amphibians. *Ranavirus* infection in amphibians is a notifiable disease according to the OIE since 2008. Known ranaviruses include FV3, ATV, BIV, CMTV, RGV, TFV, and FEV. *Ranavirus* has been proposed as a serious threat to biodiversity of ectothermic vertebrate species.

ETIOLOGY/PATHOPHYSIOLOGY

- *Ranavirus* is a double-stranded, DNA viruses belonging to the family Iridoviridae.
- This family includes four other genera besides *Ranavirus* (*Iridovirus*, *Chloriridovirus*, *Lymphocystis* virus and *Megalocytivirus*). Recently a new genus (Hemocytivirus), has been proposed.
- Strains of the genus *Ranavirus* may infect both amphibians and reptiles.
- The outcome of *Ranavirus* infection is partially dependent on the dose of the inoculum, host characteristics (life history stage and genetic background), temperature (lower environmental temperatures associated with higher mortality), age, and host species (outbreaks more commonly occurring in larvae and recently metamorphosed animals).
- Infection route may influence the outcome of the infection.
- Hematophagus insects may play a role in *Ranavirus* transmission.
- *Ranavirus* can be efficiently transmitted by direct interaction between live animals (bumping, biting, cannibalism) as well as by necrophagy and indirectly via water and fomites.
- Waterborne FV3 infection appears to proceed through the gastrointestinal tract and disseminate to the kidney.
- *Ranavirus* spp. are found all around the world across 25 countries and detected in at least 105 species of amphibians, including 18 families.

SIGNALMENT/HISTORY

- *Ranavirus* has been detected in several species of anurans and urodeles.
- Larval stages appear to be more susceptible than adults.

CLINICAL PRESENTATION

- Clinical signs are not always present but may include lethargy in adults and a series of buoyancy, swimming and posture abnormalities, and loss of righting reflex in larval stages.
- Skin ulcers in adult anurans and caudates and necrosis of the extremities in adult caudates have also been documented.
- Multisystemic hemorrhages are common in larval stages.
- A vestibular syndrome has been observed in cultured adult bullfrogs in Brazil.

RISK FACTORS

Husbandry

- In captivity, inappropriate management, stress, temperature variation, species mixing, and contact with infected amphibians may all play a role in promoting *Ranavirus* infection and eventually the occurrence of the disease.
- High temperatures and presence of sediment contribute to the quick reduction of antibody titers.
- ATV survives during the winter and it remains infectious at 25 degrees C in water for up to 2 weeks.
- FV3 maintains infectivity after 72 days at 4 degrees C.
- Both microbial and zooplanktonic communities can rapidly inactivate *Ranavirus* in the water, minimizing environmental transmission.

Others

N/A

DIAGNOSIS

DIFFERENTIAL DIAGNOSIS

- The clinical signs associated with *Ranavirus* infection in amphibians are not pathognomonic and are similar to those associated with other significant amphibian pathogens including chytridiomycosis (*Batrachochytrium dendrobatidis* and *B. salamandrivorans*), and other fungal and bacterial dermatitis.
- The presence of hemorrhage, skin ulceration, discoloration, and abnormal sloughing should always be of concerns and a thorough set of laboratory tests should be considered for a reliable and conclusive diagnosis.

DIAGNOSTICS

- There is no gold standard test for *Ranavirus*.
- Full sampling and testing procedures are provided by the OIE.
- Available tests include conventional PCR, qPCR, DNA sequencing, ELISA (direct and indirect), bioassay, histology, cytology, immunohistochemistry, in situ hybridization, and electron microscopy.
- Antemortem samples include swabs, tail or toe clips, and blood.
- Postmortem samples include liver, kidney and spleen.
- Swabs should have plastic or wire shafts and need to be swept on the affected skin surface and/or on vent and feces especially for viral shedding.
- Tail or toe clips generally provide fewer false negatives than swabs.
- Salamanders have tail breakpoints that might facilitate the sampling procedure.
- Swabs can be kept refrigerated for a short time (less than 72 hours) prior to testing (PCR tests, isolation) or frozen if they cannot be processed quickly.
- Swabs can also be preserved in ethanol at room temperature (PCR tests) for a longer time.
- Ideally, multiple sets of tissues and swabs should be collected.
- A set of tissues should be fixed (10% buffered formalin) for histology, with a duplicate set fresh or frozen for molecular testing and virus isolation.
- Non-lethal sampling technique is useful for *Ranavirus* surveillance, although prevalence might be underestimated.
- During the diagnostic procedures is critical to use disposable gloves and sterile instruments and avoid co-housing of individuals to prevent cross-contamination.
- Trace of DNA can remain for a long time on contaminated instruments (suggested to leave them more than 12 hours in diluted 6% sodium hypochlorite).
- It is also critical to disinfect equipment, footwear and potential fomites.
- PCR is available as qualitative (positive or negative) or quantitative test.
- Internal organs provide better testing results than tail clips and swabs.
- Tail clip can underestimate the true prevalence of ATV in free-ranging amphibians.
- Kidney is considered the best tissue for ranavirus testing.
- *Ranavirus* DNA can also be recovered from formalin fixed tissues.
- Serological tests allow the determination of exposure to the virus (anti-virus antibodies) of the host.
- Blood collection can be performed from multiple sites (caudal vein, abdominal and facial veins and heart).
- Serological tests (ELISA) are available, but not widely accessible.
- Virus isolation is a laboratory test that provides the definitive proof of viral (*Ranavirus*) infection.
- Histology, immunohistochemistry, in situ hybridization and electron microscopy complement the histological investigation and are generally applied on tissues collected post mortem, or intravitam if biopsies are evaluated. Ultrastructural detection of the virus is possible by electron microscopy.

PATHOLOGICAL FINDINGS

- Gross lesions (not always present) include multisystemic hemorrhages with ecchymotic and petechial changes more frequently on the ventral aspect of the body, but also around the eye, ear drum, tongue, tail and feet, more frequently in larvae but also in the adults.

RANAVIRUS (CONTINUED)

- Ascites and subcutaneous edema can also be seen in larvae; excessive fluid in the subcutaneous lymph sacs is reported in adult anurans.
- A hemorrhagic (acute) and ulcerative (chronic) form are known in the common frog.
- Spleno- and hepatomegaly can also be observed in affected animals, along with intestinal hemorrhages.
- The histological hallmark of *Ranavirus*-associated lesions are inclusion bodies (intracytoplasmic, basophilic) in the cells of the affected tissues. Inclusions might not be present in all cases.
- Multisystemic necrosis affecting blood vessels, hemopoietic and lymphoid tissue is common.
- Spleen, liver, and kidney lesions are most commonly occurring in fatal cases.
- Degeneration, necrosis and ulceration of the epidermis, necrosis of the gastrointestinal mucosa, of the lymphoid tissue, of the neuroepithelial tissue, skeletal muscle degeneration, pancreas necrosis, multicentric hemorrhage and necrosis, and ocular malformation have been reported.
- Virus can be detected in multiple tissues beyond those affected grossly.

TREATMENT

APPROPRIATE HEALTH CARE

N/A

NUTRITIONAL SUPPORT

Assist-feeding might be necessary in case of prolonged anorexia.

CLIENT EDUCATION/HUSBANDRY RECOMMENDATIONS

- All newly introduced animals into an established collection must undergo appropriate quarantine period (at least 6 months) and molecular testing (also serological when available).
- In established colonies, always handle the animals with disposable gloves, carry out routinely diagnostic tests (at least once a year).
- Do not introduce individuals from collections that have experienced a *Ranavirus* outbreak, or in general with multiple unexplained deaths in a short period of time.
- Avoiding species mixing and overcrowding.
- Separating animals showing abnormal behavior is important.
- Clean and disinfect terraria regularly and replace bedding and water frequently.
- Disinfect gears, footwear and potential fomites.

MEDICATIONS

DRUG(S) OF CHOICE

- Vaccines are currently not available for amphibians.
- High temperature (26 degrees C) have been reported to minimize mortality.
- Acyclovir and other nucleoside analogs have been proposed as possible therapeutic agents against ranavirus. Dosage of acyclovir is derived from reptiles (80 mg/kg PO once daily); no specific pharmacology study has been carried out in amphibians.
- Antibiotic and antimycotic treatment for secondary invaders should be considered case by case.
- The aquatic environment can also be treated to reduce the viral load.
- Corexit™ 9500 (Corexit Environmental Solutions LLC, Sugar Land, TX), a dispersant used to clean up oil spills, has been shown to be able to reduce the titer of FV3 at high concentration of the product (10–0.1%).
- Nolvasan at 0.75% and 2% and bleach at 3% and 5% concentrations inactivate ranavirus both at 1 and 5 minutes' duration of contact.
- Virkon™ S (1%) is also effective at both durations. Concentrations of Nolvasan® (Zoetis Services LLC, Parsippany, NJ) bleach and Virkon S that are at least 0.75%, 3%, and 1%, respectively, are effective at inactivating *Ranavirus* after 1 minute of exposure time.

PRECAUTIONS/INTERACTIONS

N/A

FOLLOW-UP

PATIENT MONITORING

- Molecular testing during the course of the disease to assess (ideally) a progressive decrease and ultimately, the end of viral shedding is suggested.
- Testing should be repeated in survivors to monitor shedding of the virus after the end of the outbreak, in case the virus has not been completely cleared.
- Serological testing, when available, is helpful to identify exposed/Infected but not clinical individuals.
- Separation of the exposed and recovered animals from the remaining of the collection with long term monitoring is critical.

EXPECTED COURSE AND PROGNOSIS

Ranavirus can be a lethal disease, although some individuals may survive the infection.

MISCELLANEOUS

COMMENTS

Infection with a lethal dose of FV3 may be associated with neutrophilia, increase of undifferentiated blast-like cells, and reduction in the percentage of basophils and transitory reduction of lymphocytes.

ZOONOTIC POTENTIAL

There is no known zoonotic potential.

SYNONYMS

N/A

ABBREVIATIONS

- ATV = *Ambystoma* tigrinum virus
- BIV = Bohle iridovirus
- CMTV = common midwife toad virus
- ELISA = enzyme-linked immunosorbent assay
- FEV = frog erythrocytic virus
- FV3 = frog virus 3
- OIE = World Organisation for Animal Health
- PCR = polymerase chain reaction
- PO = per os
- qPCR = quantitative polymerase chain reaction
- RGV = *Rana grylio* virus
- TFV = tiger frog virus

INTERNET RESOURCES

- World Organisation for Animal Health. Aquatic Animal Health Code. Chapter 8.3: Infection with *Ranavirus* species. https://www.oie.int/index.php?id=171&L=0&htmfile=chapitre_ranavirus.htm
- Global Ranavirus Consortium. Ranavirus testing and diagnostics. April 2014. http://www.ranavirus.org/resources/testing-labs
- Gray MJ, Chinchar VG, eds. Ranaviruses: Lethal Pathogens of Ectothermic Vertebrates. Springer; 2015. http://www.springer.com/de/book/9783319137544

Suggested Reading

Duffus ALJ, Waltzek TB, Stohr AC, et al. Distribution and host range of ranaviruses. In: Gray MJ, Chinchar VG, eds. *Ranaviruses: Lethal Pathogens of Ectothermic Vertebrates*. Heidelberg: Springer Open; 2015:9–57.

Miller D, Gray M, Storfer A. Ecopathology of ranaviruses infecting amphibians. *Viruses* 2011;3:2351–2373.

Author Francesco C. Origgi, DVM, PhD, DACVM (Virology), DACVP, DECZM (Herpetology)

REGURGITATION

BASICS

DEFINITION/OVERVIEW

Regurgitationis the passive flow of minimally or undigested stomach or esophageal contents out of the mouth.

ETIOLOGY/PATHOPHYSIOLOGY

- The retrograde flow of ingesta is commonly associated with impaired swallowing, weak peristalsis, or valvular dysfunction.
- It usually occurs shortly after eating, though it may be delayed in cases where GI stasis is present.
- Regurgitation is often passive, in contrast to the active process of vomiting.
- The difference between the two may be difficult to discern.

SIGNALMENT/HISTORY

- All species, ages, sexes may be affected. The exception is juvenile anurans, which the lack anatomical features necessary for vomiting, and possibly regurgitation, prior to metamorphosis.
- Owner may report clinical signs, such as repeated opening/closing of the mouth, swallowing, body contortion, stomach eversion, expulsion of GI contents.
- Vomitus and/or mucus or blood in the enclosure may be the only finding noted.
- Associated with recent handling or feeding, changes in enclosure, substrate, or husbandry.
- Addition of new individuals to the collection may be a factor.
- Lethargy, anorexia, weight loss, respiratory distress, cutaneous lesions, coelomic distention may be seen.

CLINICAL PRESENTATION

- No clinical signs are specific to regurgitation, and physical exam may be normal.
- Presentation varies depending on the underlying cause and chronicity.
- Gastric prolapse
- Dehydration and/or emaciation/cachexia.
- Hard mass on palpation of the coelomic cavity due to an obstructive lesion.
- Skeletal abnormalities that may include pathological fractures or abnormal growth patterns.
- Lethargy and/or obtunded mentation.
- Hyperemia and petechiation/ecchymosis may be observed due to infection or in any terminal disease process.

RISK FACTORS

Husbandry

- Poor sanitation, overcrowding, hyper- or hypothermia, lack of quarantine for new individuals (increases stress, possibility of secondary infections, and disease transmission).
- Toxin exposure (cleaning chemicals, pesticides, heavy metals).
- Excessive/inappropriate handling (especially soon after feeding).
- Inadequate diet (incorrect calcium/phosphorus ratio, improper prey items, excessive feeding).
- Inappropriate substrate (may be accidentally ingested).
- Trauma (poor enclosure design, inappropriate cohabitants).

Others

- Anesthesia or motion sickness
- Concomitant infectious or parasitic disease.

DIAGNOSIS

DIFFERENTIAL DIAGNOSIS

- Gastric prolapse and vomiting/regurgitation can be associated with any terminal disease process, but are only commonly associated with *Ranavirus* and saprolegniasis in salamander species.
- Normal seasonal behavior in some anuran species.
- Handling/stress (e.g., excessive pressure to coelom, motion sickness).
- Obstructive lesions (e.g., GI foreign body, intussusception, neoplasia, abscess, granuloma).
- Metabolic disease (e.g., nutritional secondary hyperparathyroidism, hypervitaminosis A).
- Toxicoses (e.g., ammonia, chlorine, pesticides, nitrites, heavy metals).
- Hyper- or hypothermia
- Anesthesia (especially with eugenol)
- Trauma (predisposes to secondary infection)
- *Ranavirus* infection (especially in Chinese giant salamanders, *Andrias davidianus*)
- Parasites (e.g., nematodiasis, amoebiasis, coccidiosis, pentastomiasis)
- Bacteria/septicemia (e.g., *Aeromonas hydrophila*, *Salmonella*, *Mycobacterium*—[e.g., *M. marinum*, *M. fortuitum*, *M. xenopi*]).
- Fungi (e.g., saprolegniasis, *Mucor amphibiorum*, *Batrachochytrium*).

DIAGNOSTICS

- Husbandry review
- Water quality test, especially ammonia, nitrites, chlorine, heavy metals.
- Parasite evaluation of vomitus and feces (direct, flotation, cytology).
- Bloodwork, especially PCV, total solids, albumin, and electrolytes. Normal values indicate an acute process.
- Low electrolytes but other values normal indicates a chronic process.
- Elevated values suggest dehydration
- Wet mount of skin scrapings
- Bacterial and fungal cultures: *Batrachochytrium* PCR assay.
- Blood culture
- Radiography with or without contrast.
- Ultrasonography
- GI endoscopy or coeliotomy (direct tissue evaluation and biopsy).

PATHOLOGICAL FINDINGS

Dependent on underlying cause

TREATMENT

APPROPRIATE HEALTH CARE

- The primary goal is to identify and address the underlying cause.
- Non-pathologic causes are generally self-limiting and resolve without intervention.
- Supportive care may be required to correct dehydration, electrolyte imbalances, weight loss, and malnutrition.

NUTRITIONAL SUPPORT

- Correct fluid deficits and maintain hydration.
- Transdermal or intracoelomic routes are the most effective.
- Soaking in water or crystalloid (e.g., amphibian Ringer's solution) baths for 1-hour intervals once or twice daily is sufficient to maintain adequate hydration and to correct mild to moderate electrolyte imbalances.
- Tube or assist feeding liquid or gel diets such as Hill's® Prescription Diet® a/d® (Hills Pet Nutrition, Inc., Topeka, KS), Mazuri® Amphibian & Carnivorous Reptile Gel (Mazuri Exotic Animal Nutrition, St. Louis, MO), Oxbow Critical Care Carnivore™ (Oxbow Animal Health, Omaha, NE) may be beneficial during initial treatment/recovery.
- Initially feed 1% body weight daily, then gradually increase to 2–3% body weight daily or every other day.
- Gradually add normal prey items to diet as animal improves.

CLIENT EDUCATION/HUSBANDRY RECOMMENDATIONS

- Review husbandry and correct any problems.
- Feed prey items a well-balanced diet and coat with calcium supplementation when appropriate.
- Avoid large meals, overfeeding, or handling immediately following a meal.
- Institute quarantine procedures for new animals, including 30–60-day period, veterinary evaluation, and 1–3-weekly fecal exams for parasites.

REGURGITATION (CONTINUED)

MEDICATIONS

DRUG(S) OF CHOICE

- Antiemetic use has not been documented in amphibians.
- Sucralfate may be a beneficial gastroprotectant.

PRECAUTIONS/INTERACTIONS

N/A

FOLLOW-UP

PATIENT MONITORING

- Monitor clinical condition
- Recheck PCV, total solids, albumin, and electrolytes as necessary.

EXPECTED COURSE AND PROGNOSIS

- Excellent to grave prognosis depending on etiology, stage/severity of disease process at time of diagnosis, and degree of debilitation of animal at time of treatment initiation.
- Hematemesis is rare, but is associated with a grave prognosis.

MISCELLANEOUS

COMMENTS

N/A

ZOONOTIC POTENTIAL

N/A

SYNONYMS

Reflux

ABBREVIATIONS

- GI = gastrointestinal
- PCR = polymerase chain reaction
- PCV = packed cell volume

Suggested Reading

Wright KM. Overview of amphibian medicine. In: Mader DR, ed. *Reptile Medicine and Surgery*. 2nd ed. St. Louis, MO: Elsevier Saunders; 2006:941–971.

Wright KM, DeVoe RS. Amphibians. In: Carpenter JW, Marion CJ, eds. *Exotic Animal Formulary*. 4th ed. St. Louis, MO: Elsevier Saunders; 2013:53–82.

Wright KM, Whitaker BR. *Amphibian Medicine and Captive Husbandry*. Malabar, FL: Krieger; 2001.

Authors Jacqueline Serio, DVM, and Trevor T. Zachariah, DVM, MS, DACZM

RENAL SECONDARY HYPERPARATHYROIDISM

BASICS

DEFINITION/OVERVIEW

RSHP is a consequence of late-stage chronic renal failure, where calcium and vitamin D levels are depleted and PTH is overproduced. Prognosis for this disease is poor to guarded, because even if calcium imbalances can be corrected, the renal function is rarely improved by means of current treatments.

ETIOLOGY/PATHOPHYSIOLOGY

- RSHP develops in amphibians suffering from chronic renal failure.
- Reduction in renal mass results in diminished elimination of phosphorus, with a consequent increase in serum phosphate concentrations, and decreased 1,25-dihydroxycholecalciferol (vitamin D3) formation.
- Both these perturbations lead to a decrease in blood calcium, which is followed by an uncontrolled, diffuse proliferation of parathyroid cells.
- The consequent increase in PTH concentrations results in increased osteoclastic activity and bone resorption.

SIGNALMENT/HISTORY

Compared with NSHP, RSHP is more commonly seen in older animals, where a chronic decline in kidney function lead to the aforementioned metabolic disturbances.

CLINICAL PRESENTATION

- Differently from NSHP, amphibians with RSHP do not show significant bone resorption when presented for clinical examination.
- Most amphibians with RSHP are presented with clinical signs caused by renal failure, including coelomic effusion, change in urine output (anuria/polyuria); lethargy, anorexia, weight loss, and skin alterations.

RISK FACTORS

Husbandry

- Amphibians that develop RSHP during adulthood typically had improper management.
- Husbandry and dietary factors that may result in chronic renal failure and consequent RSHP include an excess in dietary protein intake.
- Low environmental humidity results in chronic dehydration, and low calcium content of the diet and water.

Others

- Toxic exposure
- Neoplasia
- Infectious disease
- Degenerative renal changes

DIAGNOSIS

DIFFERENTIAL DIAGNOSIS

Differential diagnoses for seizure-like activity and muscle tremors, include other causes of hypocalcemia, particularly NSHP and primary hyperparathyroidism.

DIAGNOSTICS

- In RSHP, a change in the normal calcium to phosphorus ratio is expected (normal around 1 : 5 to 2 : 1).
- Blood urea nitrogen and uric acid may vary depending on hydration status, seasonality, sex, age, and husbandry.
- PTH levels may be measured but reference intervals are lacking for most amphibian species.
- Radiography to evaluate the bone tissue, considering that only severe bone tissue resorption is visualized through radiography.
- Use ultrasound to evaluate renal and parathyroid gland parenchyma.
- Urinalysis and celiocentesis may also be of clinical assistance.

PATHOLOGICAL FINDINGS

- Grossly, kidneys may be enlarged and may show superficial and/or parenchymal alterations.
- Depending on the severity of the RSHP, bone softening or deformity may be observed.
- Histopathology of long bones may show thinning of cortices, with layers of osteoblasts and non-mineralized osteoid on the periosteal surface.

TREATMENT

APPROPRIATE HEALTH CARE

N/A

NUTRITIONAL SUPPORT

- Amphibians with RSHP are often anorectic.
- The anorexia is usually caused by the concurrent renal failure and may persist for weeks and even months.
- Nutritional support in form of periodic syringe feeding or force-feeding with whole prey may be needed.

CLIENT EDUCATION/HUSBANDRY RECOMMENDATIONS

Owners should be informed that, at the very first symptoms of renal failure (e.g., anorexia, decreased activity), a thorough veterinary check-up is required to limit phosphorus increase, calcium depletion, and consequent PTH increase.

MEDICATIONS

DRUG(S) OF CHOICE

- In amphibians suffering of RSHP, both the hyperparathyroidism and the renal disease should be corrected.
- Treatment of RSHP includes therapy designed to minimize the clinical and pathophysiological consequences of reduced kidney function and at correcting the primary cause of the renal impairment, including bacterial, fungal and/or parasitic disease.
- The general therapy aims to maintain appropriate calcium, phosphorus, and urea/uric acid levels.
- Dietary phosphorus should be restricted and intestinal phosphate binders administered.
- Oral administration of calcium should be supported by exposure to UVB radiation in the range 280–315 nm, depending on the species.
- Calcium gluconate 50–200 mg/kg SC, IM q12–24h; 2.3% bath
- Calcium glubionate 100 mg/kg PO q12–24h
- Other considerations: angiotensin-converting enzyme inhibitors; antihypertensive therapy; Omega-3 polyunsaturated fatty acid.

PRECAUTIONS/INTERACTIONS

Exposure to excessive ultraviolet radiation may cause detrimental effects in certain amphibian species.

FOLLOW-UP

PATIENT MONITORING

- In young amphibians with RSHP as a consequence of bacterial or viral renal infection, intensive care should be provided until the infection is resolved.
- In older animals, if the amphibian is eating on its own, a physical exam once every 7–14 days is usually adequate to assess response to therapy.

EXPECTED COURSE AND PROGNOSIS

- The prognosis for amphibians suffering RSHP is poor.
- Even if calcium and phosphorus imbalances can be corrected via exogenous supplementation and phosphate binders, there is currently no effective treatment for late-stage renal failure in amphibians.

RENAL SECONDARY HYPERPARATHYROIDISM (CONTINUED)

MISCELLANEOUS

COMMENTS

A renal carcinoma affecting amphibians, Lucke's tumor, is caused by ranid herpesvirus–1 and may theoretically lead to RSHP in entire collections.

ZOONOTIC POTENTIAL

N/A

SYNONYMS

- Metabolic bone disease
- Renal-related metabolic bone disease

ABBREVIATIONS

- NSHP = nutritional secondary hyperparathyroidism
- PO = per os
- PTH = parathyroid hormone
- RSHP = renal secondary hyperparathyroidism
- SC = subcutaneous
- UVB = ultraviolet B

INTERNET RESOURCES

- Information on nutritional values of food commonly fed to amphibians: Mack J. Nutritional Values of Amphibian Foods. Caudata Culture, July 2013. http://www.caudata.org/cc/articles/foods2.shtml
- Information on secondary hyperparathyroidism in humans: Kim L. Hyperparathyroidism. Medscape, August 18, 2020. http://emedicine.medscape.com/article/127351-overview?pa=mcKd1JF66kULHOzxxIxn2fK%2Bx5xE5kE6dUeU7dvJSrcnjyhACchqCtq5rNZR2UhkQPQxex%2Bo7mr5pATtx84gCBXKySxof3ndUJD5aivxmIc%3D#a4

Suggested Reading

Cecil TR. Amphibian renal disease. *Vet Clin North Am Exot Anim Pract* 2006;9(1):175–188.

Ferrie GM, Alford VC, Atkinson J, et al. Nutrition and health in amphibian husbandry. *Zoo Biol* 2014;33(6):485–501.

King JD, Muhlbauer MC, James A. Radiographic diagnosis of metabolic bone disease in captive bred mountain chicken frogs (*Leptodactylus fallax*). *Zoo Biol* 2011;30(3):254–259.

Authors Paolo Selleri, DMV, PhD, SpecPACS, DECZM (Herpetology & Small Mammals), and Nicola Di Girolamo, DMV, MSc (EBHC), PhD, DECZM (Herpetology)

RHABDIAS

BASICS

DEFINITION/OVERVIEW

Rhabdias is a genus of nematodes infecting the lung of amphibians and reptile. Approximately 11 species are reported to infect amphibians.

ETIOLOGY/PATHOPHYSIOLOGY

- *Rhabdias* spp. infect amphibians via free-living larvae that enter the skin and ultimately migrate into the lungs.
- The adults, typically hermaphrodites, then produce larvated eggs that move into the gastrointestinal tract to be excreted in the feces.
- The larvae hatch easily and may also migrate within the amphibian.
- The life cycle is very fast and can be completed within 2–3 days.

SIGNALMENT/HISTORY

- Primarily infects anurans but infections in urodeles and caecilians are also reported.
- Wild-caught amphibians are more prone to be infected and serve as a source of infection.

CLINICAL PRESENTATION

Varied clinical presentations from mild subclinical infections to weakness, lethargy, pneumonia, and other non-specific signs due to secondary bacterial infections.

RISK FACTORS

Husbandry

- Exposure to wild-caught amphibians
- Poor hygiene
- Overcrowding

Others

N/A

DIAGNOSIS

DIFFERENTIAL DIAGNOSIS

- *Strongyloides* infection
- Bacterial pneumonia

DIAGNOSTICS

- Fecal direct wet mount and flotation to identify the embryonated eggs or larvae. However, *Rhabdias* spp. cannot be readily distinguished from other nematodes.
- Transillumination may be used in anurans with light pigmentation, or glass frogs, to identify parasites within the lungs or in tissues, but it is not very rewarding.
- Many cases may end up being diagnosed on necropsy.

PATHOLOGICAL FINDINGS

- Little to no pathology with mild infections.
- Severe inflammation and larvae within tissues may be observed with severe infections.
- Eosinophilic pneumonia

TREATMENT

APPROPRIATE HEALTH CARE

- Overall efficacy of treatment will vary with extent of infection, severity of pathology, and number of parasites present in the lungs.
- In addition to therapeutics, the amphibians should be maintained in a simple enclosure that can be cleaned daily to remove fecal matter and minimize exposure to free larvae.
- Water must be changed daily during the course of treatment.

NUTRITIONAL SUPPORT

- Provide nutritional support to emaciated and/or anorexic animals.
- Provide fluid therapy to dehydrated animals.

CLIENT EDUCATION/HUSBANDRY RECOMMENDATIONS

- Newly acquire amphibians must be quarantined and fecal examinations performed to rule out the presence of nematode eggs or larvae.
- Strict hygiene is essential to prevent reinfection.
- Substrate and water must be changed daily during the course of treatment.
- Moist paper towels can be used as substrate during treatment.
- For aquatic amphibians, place the animal in shallow water to allow easy water changes.

MEDICATIONS

DRUG(S) OF CHOICE

- Ivermectin 0.2 mg/kg topically, PO, repeat in 2 weeks; 10 mg/l bath weekly for 12 weeks.
- Fenbendazole 50 mg/kg PO, repeat in 14 days.
- Levamisole 8–10 mg/kg ICe, topical; 100–300 mg/l weekly for 12 weeks.

PRECAUTIONS/INTERACTIONS

- Some species may be more sensitive to the indicated therapeutic drugs.
- A conservative dosing and treatment regimen is recommended for debilitated animals, critical species for conservation, or new species in which treatment has not been attempted.
- Ivermectin may cause flaccid paralysis in some species.

FOLLOW-UP

PATIENT MONITORING

Repeat fecal exams to ensure treatment is effective.

EXPECTED COURSE AND PROGNOSIS

- Good prognosis for mild infections.
- Guarded to grave for severe infections with migrating larvae through multiple tissues.

MISCELLANEOUS

COMMENTS

N/A

ZOONOTIC POTENTIAL

None reported

SYNONYMS

- Lung worms
- Rhabdiosis

ABBREVIATIONS

- ICe = intracoelomic
- PO = per os

Suggested Reading

Densmore CL, Green DE. Diseases of amphibians. *ILAR J* 2007;48(3):235–254.

Kuzmin Y, Tkach VV, Snyder SD. The nematode genus *Rhabdias* (Nematoda: Rhabdiasidae) from amphibians and reptiles of the Nearctic. *Comp Parasitol* 2003;70(2):101–114.

Wright KM, Whitaker BR. *Amphibian Medicine and Captive Husbandry*. Malabar, FL: Krieger; 2001.

Author Javier G. Nevarez, DVM, PhD, DACZM, DECZM (Herpetology)

SALMONELLOSIS

BASICS

DEFINITION/OVERVIEW

Salmonellosis is a cosmopolitan disease that can infect all vertebrates. Amphibians are also known to harbor these Gram-negative bacteria, but at a lower prevalence than reptiles. All amphibians should be considered carriers of *Salmonella* spp.

ETIOLOGY/PATHOPHYSIOLOGY

- Anaerobic, Gram-negative, straight rods, flagellated.
- Species: *Salmonella enterica* and *Salmonella bongori.*
- Subspecies: *S. enterica* [1], *S. salamae* [II], *S. arizonae* [IIIa], *S. diarizonae* [IIIb], *S. houtenae* [IV], and *S. indica* [VI].
- Amphibians patients are most likely to be carriers of *S. arizonae* [IIIa] and *S. diarizonae* [IIIb].
- There are over 2,637 extant *Salmonella* serovars. Serovars are characterized by their somatic (O) and flagellar (H) antigens. The following *Salmonella* serovars have been documented in amphibians; while none were noted to be pathogenic, all species of *Salmonella* should be considered pathogenic: *Kottbus, London, Mikawasima, Newbrunswick, Newport, Poona, Reading, Richmond, Saint-Paul, Stanley, Typhimurium, Worthington, Mendoza, Hadar, Bareilly, Weltevreden, San Diego, Thompson, Panama, Rubislaw, kaapstad.*
- The epidemiology of *Salmonella* in amphibians is primarily understood through the management of captive animals, although it is likely similar in wild species but less common because of pathogen exposure and animal density.
- Transmission of *Salmonella* spp. in amphibians can occur through direct and indirect contact with infected animals or materials in their captive environment.
- Infected animals shed the organisms through their gastrointestinal tract, contaminating the environment and directly exposing conspecifics.
- When isolated from amphibians, it is most often reported as an indigenous component of the animal's microflora and is not considered a pathogen.
- It is important to recognize that amphibians can serve as latent carriers or reservoirs.
- Stress, temperature, poor hygiene/biosecurity, and inappropriate environmental conditions (e.g., high stocking densities, low or high temperatures) can potentiate the shedding of *Salmonella.*

SIGNALMENT/HISTORY

- Many of the cases of amphibian-associated salmonellosis are from latent carriers; all animals should be considered potential carriers.
- Amphibians presenting with a *Salmonella* infection may present for anorexia, lethargy, and diarrhea, as clinical signs are typical of enteritis.
- Because *Salmonella* can enter systemic circulation by ascending through the bile duct system, multisystemic disease can develop.

CLINICAL PRESENTATION

- Amphibians that are carriers of *Salmonella* typically appear healthy on physical examination or present for another illness.
- It is important to recognize that these animals may serve as a potential source of infection to the veterinary staff working with them or that the treatment used (e.g., antibiotics) could alter the pathogenicity of the *Salmonella.*
- Amphibians presenting with primary salmonellosis may present with lethargy, anorexia, weakness, failure to thrive, weight loss, decreased body condition, neurological abnormalities, hydrocoelom, coelomic swelling or mass, or osteomyelitis.

RISK FACTORS

Husbandry

- Inappropriate husbandry conditions can potentiate the likelihood of infection for conspecifics and the human caretakers.
- Environmental temperatures should be appropriate for the species, as low or high temperatures can lead to stress and the potential for increased shedding of *Salmonella* spp.
- High organic loads can increase the potential growth of *Salmonella* so water quality and enclosure hygiene are critical aspects of proper husbandry.
- Routine cleaning and disinfection of an amphibian's enclosure is necessary to prevent dissemination of *Salmonella.*
- Increased animal density and mixing of amphibian species are additional factors that can contribute to stress and impact *Salmonella* shedding.

Others

- Source of animals: confiscated or imported animals have an increased risk associated with clinical illness and zoonotic potential because of the increased likelihood of shedding *Salmonella.*
- Stress: shipping, overcrowding and suboptimal husbandry conditions can lead to infection or increased shedding of *Salmonella.*

DIAGNOSIS

DIFFERENTIAL DIAGNOSIS

- Enteritis (other species of Enterobacteriaceae)
- Renal disease
- Liver disease
- Primary and secondary bacterial infections.
- Viral infections
- Fungal infections
- Neoplasia
- Osteomyelitis

DIAGNOSTICS

- Microbiological culture of a gastrointestinal sample or abscess can be used to confirm the presence of *Salmonella.* Positive fecal cultures in clinically normal animals are not uncommon. These animals should not be treated for *Salmonella,* as this can lead to the development of antimicrobial resistance in the *Salmonella.*
- Culture of *Salmonella* requires special consideration, as the organism can be outcompeted by other Enterobacteriaceae under standard culture methods. Thus, it is important to specifically request a *Salmonella* culture from your diagnostic laboratory if the organism is suspected. Enrichment with selenite or tetrathionate is required. Samples are then plated on to specific agars such as XLD, Salmonella–Shigella agar, or XLT-4 agar. XLD and XLT-4 agars have a hydrogen sulfide indicator system to detect lactose fermenting *Salmonella.* The sensitivity for microbiologic culture using XLT-4 in reptiles (no amphibian evidence-based comparison) is 0.67, while the specificity is 0.99.
- Factors that influence the reliability of culture include the collection method, quantity or type of sample collected, temporal variation in shedding, and culture methods. Time to perform culture can delay appropriate antimicrobial therapy and control/mitigation procedures.
- PCR testing can be used to confirm the presence of *Salmonella* in a sample. This test is considered more sensitive than culture and provides faster turnaround times for a positive diagnosis.
- One limitation of PCR is that it cannot provide an antibiotic sensitivity profile to guide treatment.
- Parallel testing with PCR and culture is recommended to increase the sensitivity and specificity of the testing methods.
- CBC can be used to evaluate an amphibian patient for an inflammatory leukogram or toxic changes that might occur in an animal that has an active *Salmonella* infection.
- Radiography can be used to examine the coelomic cavity for organomegaly and bony structures for osteomyelitis.
- Ultrasound can be used to improve visualization of the coelomic organs.
- Fine-needle aspiration of coelomic fluid and cytologic review of the sample can be used to confirm the presence of Gram-negative bacteria and inflammatory cells.

PATHOLOGICAL FINDINGS

- *Salmonella* is commonly isolated from amphibians on postmortem examinations as an incidental finding.
- Amphibians that have clinical salmonellosis will have typical inflammatory signs associated with the pathogen.

TREATMENT

APPROPRIATE HEALTH CARE

- Amphibians that are clinically normal and not showing signs of disease should never be treated for *Salmonella* sp.
- Treating animals that are latent carriers could potentiate antimicrobial resistance.
- Animals that are clinically affected by *Salmonella* sp. should only be treated if an antibiotic sensitivity profile is available. This will help to minimize the likelihood of resistance.
- Some clinicians elect to not treat affected animals with antibiotics but instead provide supportive care and allow the infection to run its course.

NUTRITIONAL SUPPORT

- Nutritional support should be implemented in patients that have concurrent weight loss, hyporexia, or anorexia; however, fluid support should be provided first to ensure the gastrointestinal tract is functioning properly.
- In animals with diarrhea, nutritional support can exacerbate the diarrhea.
- Assist feeding can support the daily nutritional requirements of these patients with a highly digestible diet, which should be based on the species life history and nutritional requirements.

CLIENT EDUCATION/HUSBANDRY RECOMMENDATIONS

- Clients should be educated on the risks of owning amphibians and should be provided information on the most appropriate husbandry and sanitation procedures for their particular species.
- Hand washing with soap and warm water is one of the simplest and most effective methods of eliminating exposure to *Salmonella* sp.
- Owners should be directed to avoid using bathroom basins or kitchen sinks to clean an amphibian or any component of its environment.
- Separate washing receptacles, such as a plastic container, are recommended.
- Dilute bleach solution can be used to clean the environment and food and water bowls; it is important that they are rinsed thoroughly to minimize the potential for toxicity.

MEDICATIONS

DRUG(S) OF CHOICE

- As with any bacterial disease, therapy should be driven by culture and antibiotic sensitivity testing. Minimum inhibitory concentration information is valuable in these cases to increase the likelihood for treatment success.
- Amikacin 5 mg/kg IM, SC, ICe q24–48h
- Enrofloxacin 5–10 mg/kg IM, PO, SC q24–48h; 500 mg/l as 6–8-hour bath q24h
- Ciprofloxacin 500–750 mg/75l as 6–8-hour bath q24h
- Oxytetracycline 50–100 mg/kg IM q48h; 100 mg/l as 1-hour bath

PRECAUTIONS/INTERACTIONS

Aminoglycosides should be used concurrently with fluid therapy to avoid adverse renal effects.

FOLLOW-UP

PATIENT MONITORING

- Serial culture and PCR testing can be done to monitor the *Salmonella* status and antimicrobial sensitivity profile of a patient or captive population of amphibians.
- CBC to monitor responses to treatment.
- Repeat radiography to monitor for progression or resolution of osseous lesions.

EXPECTED COURSE AND PROGNOSIS

- Amphibians diagnosed with salmonellosis from culture or PCR may not require any intervention.
- Many amphibians test positive for *Salmonella* spp. These animals are often latent carriers and do not show signs of disease.
- Animals that test negative for *Salmonella* sp. on a single test may still be positive because intermittent shedding is common.

MISCELLANEOUS

COMMENTS

N/A

ZOONOTIC POTENTIAL

- From 2008 to 2011, 376 cases of *Salmonella* infections in humans from 44 states originated from aquatic frogs. This outbreak was tracked to an African dwarf frog (*Hymenochirus boettgeri*) breeding facility.
- *S. Javiana* and *S. Typhimurium* represent two of the serotypes that have been diagnosed in amphibian associated salmonellosis in humans.
- To minimize the zoonotic potential of amphibians, it is important to practice strict hygiene and biosecurity.
- Individuals handling these animals, or any part of their captive habitat, should wash their hands thoroughly after working with them.
- The water removed from the enclosures should be discarded outside or down a toilet. It should never be discarded down a sink used for cooking or cleaning food or where water is obtained for drinking or a bathtub.
- The enclosure and its contents should be cleaned outside, if at all possible, and never in an area where food or drink is prepared.
- Pet owners should be made aware that it is not recommended to kiss, place in the oral cavity, or cuddle with their amphibian.

SYNONYMS

- Salmonellosis
- Typhoid fever

ABBREVIATIONS

- CBC = complete blood count
- ICe = intracoelomic
- IM = intramuscular
- PCR = polymerase chain reaction
- PO = per os
- SC = subcutaneous
- XLD = xylose lysine deoxycholate
- XLT-4 = xylose-lysine Tergitol 4

INTERNET RESOURCES

- American Veterinary Medical Association. Amphibians, Reptiles and Salmonella. 2020. https://www.avma.org/KB/Resources/Reference/Pages/Amphibians-Reptiles-and-Salmonella.aspx
- Centers for Disease Control and Prevention. Reptiles and Amphibians. October 28, 2019. https://www.cdc.gov/features/salmonellafrogturtle/index.html
- Association of Reptile and Amphibian Veterinarians: http://www.ARAV.org

Suggested Reading

Wright KM, Whitaker BR. Bacterial diseases. In: *Amphibian Medicine and Captive Husbandry*. Malabar, FL: Krieger; 2001:159–179.

Zarecki SLM, Bennett SD, Hall J, et al. US outbreak of human Salmonella infections associated with aquatic frogs, 2008–2011. *Pediatrics* 2013;131(4):724–731.

Authors Sean M. Perry, DVM, PhD, and Mark A. Mitchell, DVM, MS, PhD, DECZM (Herpetology)

SAPROLEGNIASIS

BASICS

DEFINITION/OVERVIEW

Saprolegniasis refers to mycosis caused by several species of aquatic oomycetous fungi (water molds). The genus *Saprolegnia* is most often associated with this condition.

ETIOLOGY/PATHOPHYSIOLOGY

- *Saprolegnia* spp. are typically opportunistic pathogens of traumatized or devitalized tissue.
- They are primitive fungi with a complex life cycle that includes flagellated zoospores.
- Infection is usually superficial
- Damage to the skin will result in compromised osmotic regulation.
- Primary or secondary bacterial infection may be present.
- *Saprolegnia* spp. infect egg masses and have been linked with amphibian decline along the Pacific coast of the United States.

SIGNALMENT/HISTORY

- Most *Saprolegnia* species thrive in cold, stagnant water.
- Infections are common in aquatic amphibians.

CLINICAL PRESENTATION

- A white cottony film or fuzzy growth over open lesions is suggestive of saprolegniasis.
- The cottony film is the mycelium, which may become grayish or greenish as debris and algae become entrapped in the mycelial mat.
- Saprolegniasis of egg masses also presents as a whitish cottony film covering or surrounding the eggs.
- The cottony film of fungal growth usually collapses when removed from water.
- Systemic infections are rare

RISK FACTORS

Husbandry

- Environmental and husbandry co-factors can be very important in the development of saprolegniasis.
- Water molds are primarily opportunists, often infecting open wounds.
- Water temperature is an important factor in the development of saprolegniasis, as its incidence rate decreases at water temperatures higher than 19 degrees C (68 degrees F).
- Low environmental temperatures (< 20 degrees C) enhance the growth of fungus.
- High environmental organic loads may be a predisposing factor.
- Poor water quality (ammonia) can lead to stress, immunosuppression, and skin lesions.
- Avoid skin injuries/abrasions, which are prone to become infected with *Saprolegnia* sp.

Others

N/A

DIAGNOSIS

DIFFERENTIAL DIAGNOSIS

Other oomycetes

DIAGNOSTICS

- Characteristic appearance of white to tan cotton-like material that covers skin ulcers.
- Microscopic examination of wet mounts from a skin scraping will confirm the diagnosis; may see branching non-septate hyphae and zoospores (flagellated oospore).

PATHOLOGICAL FINDINGS

- The characteristic gross appearance of white to tan cotton-like material covering skin ulcers is best appreciated when viewing the affected animal under water.
- Infections can occur anywhere, in tadpoles the oral disc (mouthparts) is commonly affected.
- Can be a primary pathogen for amphibian eggs.

TREATMENT

APPROPRIATE HEALTH CARE

- Correction of predisposing factors such as substandard water quality, inter- or intraspecies aggression, or bacterial disease.
- Elevation of water temperatures may also be useful if the patient can tolerate the higher water temperature.
- Treat skin lesions and correct for osmotic losses with appropriate fluid therapy.

NUTRITIONAL SUPPORT

- Tadpoles affected by saprolegniasis may starve if infection involves the oral disk.
- Every attempt should be made to correct underlying husbandry predisposing factors and encourage animals to eat on their own.
- Nutritional support of smaller fully aquatic amphibian species can be challenging; the stress of handling may worsen the condition.
- When absolutely necessary, a carnivorous critical care diet can be provided by mouth using a gavage needle, catheter, or pipette.

CLIENT EDUCATION/HUSBANDRY RECOMMENDATIONS

- Amphibians affected by inappropriate husbandry techniques are especially prone to fungal infections.
- Proper nutrition, sanitation, and water quality are essential for the prevention of saprolegniasis.

MEDICATIONS

DRUG(S) OF CHOICE

- Benzalkonium chloride 2 mg/l for 60 minutes daily or 0.25 mg/l as a continuous bath for 72 hours.
- Sodium chloride 10–25 g/l as a bath for 5–30 minutes.
- Malachite green 0.2 mg/liter as a bath for up to 1 hour daily.

PRECAUTIONS/INTERACTIONS

- Animals should be continuously monitored during bath treatments for any signs of distress, including agitation, tachypnea, erythema, or being unresponsive to stimuli.
- Dechlorinated water must always be used.

FOLLOW-UP

PATIENT MONITORING

- Effective treatment will eliminate the "cottony" growth on the affected area which can be assessed visually.
- Return to normal behavior is expected after resolution of lesions.

EXPECTED COURSE AND PROGNOSIS

- Prognosis is good for localized infections.
- Prognosis is guarded for severe diffuse infections throughout the body.
- Prognosis is greatly enhanced by correcting any husbandry deficiencies that may be contributing to the disease.

MISCELLANEOUS

COMMENTS

N/A

ZOONOTIC POTENTIAL

N/A

SYNONYMS

- Cotton wool disease
- Saprolegniasis
- Water mold

INTERNET RESOURCES

Lock B. Saprolegniasis in amphibians. Veterinary Information Network, July 18, 2017. https://www.vin.com/veterinarypartner/default.aspx?pid=19239&catId=102919&id=8120771&ind=1249&objTypeID=1007

Suggested Reading

Densmore CL, Green DE. Diseases of amphibians. *ILAR J* 2007;48(3):235–254.

Wright KM, Whitaker BR. Bacterial diseases. In: *Amphibian Medicine and Captive Husbandry*. Malabar, FL: Krieger; 2001:159–179.

Author Sam Rivera, DVM, MS, DABVP (Avian), DACZM, DECZM (Zoo Health Management)

SHORT-TONGUE SYNDROME

BASICS

DEFINITION/OVERVIEW

Short-tongue syndrome has been described in captive reared anurans with inability to catch prey. It is better studied in the Wyoming toad (*Anaxyrus baxteri*, a.k.a. Baxter's toad) but has been reported in other anuran species.

ETIOLOGY/PATHOPHYSIOLOGY

- Affected Wyoming toads were found to have developed of squamous metaplasia of the tongue affecting its function.
- They also had lower liver vitamin A (retinol) levels than wild toads.

SIGNALMENT/HISTORY

Juvenile to adult anurans of both sexes.

CLINICAL PRESENTATION

Animals are able to eat normally but slowly develop inability to prehend food.

RISK FACTORS

Husbandry

Inadequate intake of vitamin A

Others

N/A

DIAGNOSIS

DIFFERENTIAL DIAGNOSIS

- Hypocalcemia
- NSHP

DIAGNOSTICS

- Diagnosis is based on clinical signs consistent with this syndrome.
- Animals that were able to eat normally gradually become unable to eat and lose weight.
- Histopathology can confirm squamous metaplasia of the tongue and other organs.
- Determination of retinol in serum/plasma, liver, or whole body, can provide definitive/suggestive diagnosis if normal levels are known for the species.

PATHOLOGICAL FINDINGS

- Squamous metaplasia of the tongue, digestive tract, bladder and kidneys.
- Mostly, the dorsal aspect of the tongue is affected; evaluation should focus on this region.
- A natural progression form rostral to caudal is also reported. For this reason, longitudinal sections of the tongue are preferred over cross-sections, to allow evaluation of the entire tongue.

TREATMENT

APPROPRIATE HEALTH CARE

Treatment requires a dual approach of vitamin A supplementation of affected animals and supplementation of prey items.

NUTRITIONAL SUPPORT

- Often, amphibians must be hand-fed until response to therapy.
- Either target feeding with forceps or providing a critical care diet with a pipette can be used.

CLIENT EDUCATION/HUSBANDRY RECOMMENDATIONS

- Vitamin A supplementation is an essential part of rearing captive amphibians.
- A multimodal approach of gut loading and dusting invertebrate prey items and direct topical or oral supplementation of amphibians is recommended as part of the nutritional plan.

MEDICATIONS

DRUG(S) OF CHOICE

- Aquasol A (50,000 iu/ml): dilute to 5,000 iu/ml by using 1 part Aquasol A and 9 parts sterile water. Then apply topically at a rate of 1 drop through a 27-g needle to animals under 5g; 1 drop from a tuberculin syringe without needle for animals 5–30 g; for animals above 30 g apply 1 drop for every 10 g body weight. Apply once daily for 14 days then once weekly as needed.
- Vitamin A gel caps (10,000 iu/cap): dilute to 1,000 iu/ml by using 1 part vitamin A to 9 parts vegetable oil. Then administer 1 iu/g body weight orally once daily for 14 days then once weekly as needed.
- Preformed vitamin A (retinol) containing supplement: dust insects immediately before feeding to the amphibians.
- Use a gut loading diet with vitamin A to feed invertebrates as part of the overall supplementation of vitamin A. This is not sufficient as a stand-alone supplement or therapy.
- Cod liver oil: there are various formulations of cod liver oil available. Dosing can be based on vitamin A gel caps but must also take into consideration the vitamin D3 content of the cod liver oil to avoid hypervitaminosis D3.
- Spirulina fish flakes or meal can be used as a gut-loading supplement to dust invertebrates or for oral administration to amphibians. Can also be used to feed tadpoles.

PRECAUTIONS/INTERACTIONS

- Hypovitaminosis A is possible, especially in small animals.
- Vitamin A supplement must be calculated very carefully to avoid hypervitaminosis A.

FOLLOW-UP

PATIENT MONITORING

- While under therapy, continue to offer prey weekly to determine when clinical signs may show improvement.
- Weigh daily to very other day to monitor weight and ensure the animal is getting enough energy while being hand fed.

EXPECTED COURSE AND PROGNOSIS

Response to vitamin A supplementation is expected to result in a good to fair prognosis.

MISCELLANEOUS

COMMENTS

N/A

ZOONOTIC POTENTIAL

N/A

SYNONYMS

N/A

Suggested Reading

Clugston RD, Blaner WS. Vitamin A (retinoid) metabolism and actions: What we know and what we need to know about amphibians. *Zoo Biol* 2014;33(6):527–535.

Pessier AP. Short tongue syndrome and hypovitaminosis A. In: Mader, DR, Divers SJ, eds. *Current Therapy in Reptile Medicine and Surgery*. Saint Louis, MO: Elsevier; 2014:271–275.

Author Javier G. Nevarez, DVM, PhD, DACZM, DECZM (Herpetology)

SPINDLY LEG SYNDROME

BASICS

DEFINITION/OVERVIEW

Spindly leg syndrome, also known as skeletal and muscular underdevelopment, is characterized by abnormal development of the limbs during metamorphosis. It is invariably fatal, with tadpoles dying before metamorphosis or shortly after. There is abnormal metamorphosis characterized by abnormal development of the limbs, mostly the front, although the rear limbs can also be affected. It is primarily reported in captive reared anurans, with the majority of cases reported from dendrobatids.

ETIOLOGY/PATHOPHYSIOLOGY

- The etiology is unknown but suspected to be multifactorial.
- Different proposed etiologies include nutritional deficiencies (e.g., hypovitaminosis B), toxin exposure, genetic factors, water quality, trauma, inadequate lighting.

SIGNALMENT/HISTORY

Mostly a disease of metamorphosing anuran tadpoles with dendrobatids overrepresented.

CLINICAL PRESENTATION

- The majority of affected animals die before, during, or shortly after metamorphosis.
- Those surviving metamorphosis have abnormal limb development.

RISK FACTORS

- No single risk factor has been identified, therefore it is likely a multifactorial process.
- There is conflicting evidence supporting and disputing each of the risk factors in various species.

Husbandry

- Nutrition
- Water quality
- Inadequate lighting

Others

- Genetics
- Trauma

DIAGNOSIS

- The syndrome is diagnosed based on gross changes associated with limb development during metamorphosis.
- There is an increased need for more histopathologic evaluation of these cases.

DIFFERENTIAL DIAGNOSIS

Post-metamorphic death syndrome

DIAGNOSTICS

Based on gross observation

PATHOLOGICAL FINDINGS

- Affected animals have abnormal limb development.
- The majority of cases are described as having normal hind limb development with abnormal front limbs, but the hind limbs can then develop varus or valgus.
- The abnormalities of the limbs can present differently across species.
- Muscle atrophy, abnormal joint development.
- Missing radius, ulna, and carpal bones can occur.
- Invariably fatal in the majority of the animals.
- Animals are reported to have empty stomach upon necropsy.

TREATMENT

APPROPRIATE HEALTH CARE

- No specific treatment has been reported to reverse this syndrome.
- Supplementation of feed or water with vitamin B complex, calcium or iodine has been reported to reduce the incidence of the syndrome, but results are inconsistent.
- A study with harlequin frogs (*Atelopus* sp.) revealed a reduction in skeletal abnormalities to 10% when using water that was treated by reverse osmosis and then reconstituted by adding calcium, magnesium, potassium, and sodium. The same study did not see a significant reduction in skeletal abnormalities in animals provided increased protein and vitamin B complex supplementation.

NUTRITIONAL SUPPORT

- Vitamin B complex
- Calcium
- Iodine

CLIENT EDUCATION/HUSBANDRY RECOMMENDATIONS

- Currently, there are no confirmed techniques for preventing spindly leg syndrome.
- It appears that different factors contribute to this syndrome in different facilities and populations.
- Each facility should investigate which factors appear be pertinent for their animals and address those specifically.

MEDICATIONS

DRUG(S) OF CHOICE

N/A

PRECAUTIONS/INTERACTIONS

N/A

FOLLOW-UP

PATIENT MONITORING

N/A

EXPECTED COURSE AND PROGNOSIS

- Prognosis is grave as the disease is fatal in affected animals.
- Euthanasia is recommended for affected animals.

MISCELLANEOUS

COMMENTS

N/A

ZOONOTIC POTENTIAL

N/A

SYNONYMS

Skeletal and muscular underdevelopment

Suggested Reading

Camperio Ciani JF, Guerrel J, Baitchman E, et al. The relationship between spindly leg syndrome incidence and water composition, overfeeding, and diet in newly metamorphosed harlequin frogs (*Atelopus* spp.). *PLoS One* 2018;13(10):e0204314.

Claunch N, Augustine L. Morphological description of spindly leg syndrome in golden mantella (*Mantella aurantiaca*) at the Smithsonian National Zoological Park. *J Herp Med Surg* 2015;25(3–4):72–77.

Wright, KM. Idiopathic syndromes. In: *Wright KM, Whitaker BR. Amphibian Medicine and Captive Husbandry*. Malabar, FL: Krieger; 2001:239–241.

Author Javier G. Nevarez, DVM, PhD, DACZM, DECZM (Herpetology)

SQUAMOUS CELL CARCINOMA

BASICS

DEFINITION/OVERVIEW

SCCs are malignant epithelial cell tumors, most commonly associated with cutaneous or mucocutaneous regions of the body. In amphibians, SCCs are rarely described, and all have been associated with the skin. The amphibian SCCs described in the literature show evidence of local infiltration of adjacent tissues, and no evidence of metastatic behavior. SCCs are rare in amphibian species, and have been identified in northern leopard frogs, American bullfrogs, a European common frog, a hellbender, and a white-lipped tree frog.

ETIOLOGY/PATHOPHYSIOLOGY

- An underlying cause of SCCs in amphibians is unknown.
- Published hypotheses with respect to risk factors and etiology are based on mammalian or avian examples: overexposure to ultraviolet radiation, including exposure at higher altitudes, light skin color, chronic hypovitaminosis A, and possibly chronic viral infections.
- There is no evidence that any of these risk factors are associated with amphibian SCCs.
- No viruses have been associated with SCCs in amphibians.
- The few amphibian SCCs described in the literature tend to be locally invasive, but none is associated with metastatic behavior.

SIGNALMENT/HISTORY

- There is no clear predisposition of SCCs with respect to species, sex, or age.
- Historically, amphibians with diagnosed SCC are observed to have a focal mass or masses anywhere on the skin, most commonly extremities.
- The raised tissue may become hemorrhagic, ulcerative and/or necrotic.
- Typically, the neoplastic cells invade adjacent tissues.
- Depending on the site of the tumor, the animal may become hyporexic/anorexic, exhibit a depressed attitude, and/or favor a limb or other anatomical sites that may be involved.

CLINICAL PRESENTATION

- The clinical signs may be somewhat variable depending on the anatomic locations of the mass.
- Discrete skin lesions tend to appear raised, with erythema, hemorrhage, and/or ulceration, or appear as chronic nonhealing wounds.
- If the lesions are associated with digits, there may be more diffuse swelling and some degree of lameness.

RISK FACTORS

Husbandry

- Purely hypothetical risk factors in amphibians are based on mammalian or avian risk factors.
- In the case of husbandry, hypovitaminosis A or excessive ultraviolet light exposure could be predisposing risk factors, but there is no evidence documenting a link between these factors and SCCs.

Others

N/A

DIAGNOSIS

DIFFERENTIAL DIAGNOSIS

- Bacterial abscesses
- Mycobacterial or fungal granulomas
- Cestode larval cysts
- Chronic traumatic wounds with fibrosis.
- Rarely, other neoplastic diseases (e.g., cystadenoma, cystadenocarcinoma)

DIAGNOSTICS

- Histopathology of the lesion is the gold standard for diagnosis, through complete surgical excision or biopsy of the mass.
- A fine-needle aspirate with cytologic evaluation may or may not be diagnostic.
- Imaging modalities, such as radiography or CT may be helpful in detecting local soft tissue or bone involvement.

PATHOLOGICAL FINDINGS

- In domestic mammals, histologic subtypes of SCCs are typically described as poorly differentiated, moderately differentiated or well differentiated.
- In general, SCCs are histopathologically characterized as round to polygonal-shaped cells with varying amounts of basophilic cytoplasm, and keratinization.
- The nuclei tend to be round, with significant variation in size and chromatin pattern; from coarsely stippled to pyknotic, and commonly with perinuclear vacuoles.
- Frequently, there is marked variation in nucleus to cytoplasm ratio because the cells vary in degree of differentiation.
- In the few published cases of SCC in amphibians, the histologic description is typically of a well-differentiated SCC.
- Typically, there are anastomosing cords and nests of squamous epithelial cells with abundant eosinophilic cytoplasm, distinct intercellular bridges, and round to oval nuclei with finely stippled chromatin and multiple nucleoli, with few mitotic figures.
- Neoplastic cells are described as having differing levels of anisokaryosis, and frequently form circular keratinized foci consistent with keratin pearls and usually invade and/or replace adjacent tissues.

TREATMENT

APPROPRIATE HEALTH CARE

N/A

NUTRITIONAL SUPPORT

- Non-specific nutritional support may include regular force-feeding of an appropriate commercial diet.
- The directions on the label of the commercial diet can be followed for appropriate volume per feeding and frequency.

CLIENT EDUCATION/HUSBANDRY RECOMMENDATIONS

N/A

MEDICATIONS

DRUG(S) OF CHOICE

- There are no reports of chemotherapeutic agents or radiation therapy being used in amphibians with SCC.
- Antimicrobial drugs may be used as needed for secondary bacterial infections.
- NSAIDs may help with any discomfort, although there are no systematically derived data with respect to efficacy of NSAIDs in any amphibian species.
- Surgical excision with histopathologic evidence of clean margins is the treatment of choice.
- Depending on the species, meloxicam 0.2–0.5 mg/kg may be administered orally or subcutaneously.
- There are also no data demonstrating adverse effects such as renal impairment and/or gastrointestinal bleeding.

PRECAUTIONS/INTERACTIONS

- With surgical excision of an SCC, recurrence should be considered and discussed with the owner.

FOLLOW-UP

PATIENT MONITORING

- SCCs are likely to recur with incomplete surgical excision and may recur regardless of complete surgical excision.
- There are a few documented cases of local tissue invasion.
- The patient should be monitored for recurrence of the tumor, and contrast CT may be of some use in monitoring for local invasion or metastatic disease.
- If treatment is recommended and accepted by the owner, the treatment site should be monitored for secondary microbial infection or self-trauma.

• The owner should be instructed to report any signs of skin discoloration, discharge, or dysfunction of the anatomical region of the original tumor.

EXPECTED COURSE AND PROGNOSIS

• With complete surgical excision and clean tissue margins as evidenced by histopathology, the prognosis is good to guarded, with the possibility of recurrence.
• Promising intralesional chemotherapeutic techniques or refined radiation therapy techniques, as used in reptiles, may be applied to future cases of SCCs in amphibians, which may improve prognostic factors.

MISCELLANEOUS

COMMENTS

N/A

ZOONOTIC POTENTIAL

N/A

SYNONYMS

N/A

ABBREVIATIONS

• CT = computed tomography
• NSAIDs = nonsteroidal anti-inflammatory drug
• SCC = squamous cell carcinoma

Suggested Reading

Balls M, Clothier RH. Spontaneous tumors in Amphibia: A review. *Oncology* 1974;29:501–519.

Dombrowski DS, Vanderklok C, Van Wettere AJ. Curative surgical excision of a squamous cell carcinoma associated with the digit of an American bullfrog (*Lithobates catesbeianus*). *J Herp Med Surg* 2016;26:42–45.

Green EG. Spontaneous neoplasia in Amphibia. In: Wright KM, Whitaker BR. *Amphibian Medicine and Captive Husbandry*. Malabar, FL: Krieger; 2001:335–400.

Hiler WR, Wheeler BA, Trauth SE. The decline of the Ozark hellbender (*Cryptobranchus alleganiensis bishopi*) in the Spring River, Arkansas, USA. Herp *Conserv Biol* 2013;8:114–121.

Latney LV, Miller E, Pessier AP. Nuptial pad amputation in an American bullfrog (*Lithobates catesbeianus*) with squamous cell carcinoma. *J Zoo Wildl Med* 2015;46:941–944.

Author Kurt K. Sladky, MS, DVM, DACZM, DECZM (Zoo Health Management & Herpetology)

STOMATITIS

BASICS

DEFINITION/OVERVIEW

Stomatitis is inflammation of the soft tissues of the oral cavity, which may be caused by many different stimuli of local or systemic origin.

ETIOLOGY/PATHOPHYSIOLOGY

- Considered a secondary lesion from immunosuppression or trauma that supports abnormal bacterial or fungal colonization of oral tissues.
- Inflammation and other changes may develop in the normal oral mucosa because of the amount of vasculature in the area and its proximity to the external environment.

Infectious

- Normal bacterial flora secondarily infecting damaged oral tissue, particularly *Pseudomonas* spp., *Aeromonas* spp., *Serratia* spp., and *Providencia* spp.
- Any bacteria, particularly Gram-negatives (*Klebsiella* spp., *Salmonella* spp., *Proteus* spp., *Morganella* spp.); *Mycobacterium* spp.; *Pasteurella* spp. are implicated in tortoises; *Neisseria* spp. may be implicated.
- Any fungi, particularly *Candida* spp., *Penicillium* spp., *Aspergillus* spp., and *Mucor* spp.
- Systemic infections

Trauma

- Rostral abrasions can lead to stomatitis if not treated promptly.
- Prey injuries: bite wounds from live prey.
- Improper assist-feeding resulting in oral, pharyngeal or esophageal injuries.

SIGNALMENT/HISTORY

- Stomatitis can occur in any amphibian but is most common in frogs and toads.
- There is no age or sex predilection.

CLINICAL PRESENTATION

Systems Affected

- Alimentary: patients may approach food but ultimately not prehend or swallow it.
- Skin: may see inflammation of the skin around the lips from rubbing (either as a cause or sequela to inflammation and pain).
- Bone: osteomyelitis; infiltrating bacteria may cause lesions in liver, kidney, heart or central nervous system.

Signs

- Hemorrhage, edema, swelling of lips and oral mucosa, ulceration, plaques, tongue dysfunction, anorexia or dysphagia.
- Stages of progression: erythema, petechiation, ulceration.
- Chronic swelling of underlying tissues causing displacement of the lips and teeth.
- Rostral abrasions or callus from persistent facial rubbing or scratching.
- Osteomyelitis secondary to bacterial extension into deep tissues.
- Fungus: tenacious exudate adhering to mucosal tissues; often white and cottony with candidiasis.
- Signs of septicemia
- Signs of secondary pneumonia or gastroenteritis.

RISK FACTORS

Husbandry

- Poor hygiene, overcrowding, improper light cycles or wavelength, poor water quality, insufficient humidity (chronic dehydration), and malnutrition.
- Improper quarantine: exposure to bacteria, fungi, viruses or parasites through contaminated food, water or vectors.

Others

- Immunosuppression
- Trauma from accidental ingestion of hard substrate.
- Prolonged anorexia and cachexia
- Toxin exposure (particularly disinfectants, insecticides, PCBs, and dioxins)
- Parasitism

DIAGNOSIS

DIFFERENTIAL DIAGNOSIS

- Rule out septicemia and intoxication as cause of oral petechiation (usually ulceration and caseous lesions are observed with stomatitis).
- Ulcerated neoplasias: usually focal, whereas stomatitis is more typically diffuse.
- Consider neoplasia in cases unresponsive to supportive therapy and correction of improper husbandry.
- Tongue dysfunction from infection, trauma, inflammatory masses (heterophilic or granulomatous), neoplasia, metabolic bone disease, or hypovitaminosis A.

DIAGNOSTICS

- Thorough physical examination with particular attention to eyes, and oral/pharyngeal tissues.
- Eye loops, small otoscope, or endoscope may be necessary for complete examination and to facilitate collection of samples. Anesthesia or sedation may be required.
- Cytology and culture (aerobic, anaerobic and fungal): fine-needle aspirate of deep gingival tissues is needed to collect diagnostic samples. Sampling of superficial mucosa is non-diagnostic, as it is likely to yield contaminants. Cultures must be interpreted in conjunction with clinical signs. Bacteria and fungi associated with stomatitis are typically normal flora.
- Biopsy: articularly of recurring or persistent lesions; pre-clean tissue to collect samples for culture.
- Radiography to identify severity of bone or ocular involvement; CT or MRI may also be informative.
- Virus isolation or electron microscopy can be used to detect viral particles in tissues or secretions if viral association is suspected.

PATHOLOGICAL FINDINGS

Histologic changes may include acute necrosis, hemorrhage, inflammatory infiltrate, and granuloma formation.

TREATMENT

APPROPRIATE HEALTH CARE

- Low numbers of *Aeromonas* spp., *Pseudomonas* spp., and other Gram-negative enteric bacteria are normal oral flora and should not be treated in the absence of lesions.
- Maintain patients with suspected infectious diseases in isolation during diagnosis and treatment.
- Therapy will fail if underlying cause is not identified and corrected.
- Provide proper light quality and cycles for species.
- Oral lesions and rostral abrasions: debride, clean and treat with appropriate antimicrobial based on cytology and culture.
- Exposure gingivitis secondary to metabolic bone disease: teach client to clean tissues and keep moistened with topical ointments.

NUTRITIONAL SUPPORT

- After rehydration and correction of acid-base deficits, supportive nutrition as needed to maintain positive nitrogen balance.
- Liquid critical care diets should be used in animals with difficulty eating.
- Feed small amounts more frequently.
- Provide supplemental vitamins or minerals based on history of deficiency and specific testing.
- Provide proper, high-quality, fresh foods appropriate for the species.
- Correct dehydration and maintain normal hydration level during treatment.

CLIENT EDUCATION/HUSBANDRY RECOMMENDATIONS

- It is essential to be aggressive with the treatment regimen to prevent progression of the diseases therefore client compliance is critical.
- Husbandry deficiencies must be corrected, or treatment will not be effective.

MEDICATIONS

DRUG(S) OF CHOICE

General Considerations

- Most antimicrobial dosing in amphibians is empirical based initially on cytology and Gram staining, owing to the delay in return of culture results; disease-causing organisms may be noted on cytology that are not cultured or vice versa.
- Bactericidal drugs preferable to bacteriostatic drugs.
- Antimicrobial therapy alone is unlikely to be successful if the infection is walled off, due to poor drug penetration into exudates.
- Correct dehydration and maintain normal hydration level during treatment
- Amikacin 5 mg/kg IM, SC, ICe q24–48h
- Chloramphenicol 50 mg/kg PO, IM, SC q12–24 h; 20 mg/l continuous bath changed daily. Also been reported to treat chytridiomycosis.
- Ceftazidime 20 mg/kg IM q48–72h
- Ciprofloxacin 10 mg/kg PO q24h; 10 mg/l bath for 6–8h daily.
- Enrofloxacin 10 mg/kg PO, SC q24 h
- Metronidazole 10–20 mg/kg PO q24h; 50 mg/l continuous bath changed daily.
- Trimethoprim/sulfa 20 mg/kg PO q24h
- Amphotericin B 1 mg/kg ICe q24h
- Itraconazole 10 mg/kg PO q24–48 h; 10–25 mg/l (0.001–0.0025%) solution bath for 5–10 minutes daily.
- Miconazole: apply topical cream to lesions daily.
- Terbinafine 100 mg/l (0.01%) solution bath for 5 minutes daily.

Mild and Acute Lesions

- Acute and mild cases can be treated with aggressive topical therapy.
- Debride lesions q8–6h and flush with copious volumes of warm sterile saline followed by final flush with appropriate antimicrobial based on cytology.
- Small paintbrushes are more useful than cotton tip applicators or gauze for cleaning and debriding oral lesions, as the latter tend to snag on and further damage teeth.
- Antimicrobial preparations: mafenide acetate (Sulfamylon®, Bertek Pharmaceuticals, Inc., Research Triangle Park, NC), triple antibiotic, chlorhexidine oral cleansing solution, etc.

Deep and Severe Lesions

- Require topical treatment as well as broadspectrum systemic antimicrobials for bacteria (aerobic or anaerobic) or fungi, based on results of cytology and changed based on results of culture.
- Antimicrobials may be required for 3–4 weeks with severe soft tissue involvement.

PRECAUTIONS/INTERACTIONS

- Amphibians can have high sensitivity to a number of drugs; this sensitivity is varied across species.
- Start treatment with lower drug doses until there is evidence that no adverse effects are observed.
- Do not use iodine products, as toxicity may occur.

FOLLOW-UP

PATIENT MONITORING

- Evaluate hydration frequently after commencement of treatment.
- Make husbandry changes to provide proper environment and nutrition.
- Monitor other animals for secondary spread of infection.
- Advise client to contact veterinarian if patient shows signs of recurring disease.
- Additional diagnostics based on response to therapy.

EXPECTED COURSE AND PROGNOSIS

- Varies with underlying cause, chronicity and condition of patient.
- Lesions can progress from petechial hemorrhage to overwhelming infection and septicemia within 2–3 days.
- Acute and uncomplicated lesions usually respond to appropriate therapy.
- Untreated infections frequently progress to osteomyelitis, septicemia and death.
- Guarded to poor prognosis with osteomyelitis, depending on chronicity and severity.
- In mild cases that do not respond to traditional therapy, consider fungal, viral, untreated metabolic bone disease, neoplasia or multidrug-resistant bacteria.

MISCELLANEOUS

COMMENTS

Associated conditions include osteomyelitis, septicemia, pneumonia and/or gastroenteritis; ocular or periocular disease; permanent tongue damage resulting in dysphagia or anorexia; pharyngeal cellulitis.

ZOONOTIC POTENTIAL

- Many bacteria and fungi that infect amphibians can also cause disease in humans or other companion animals.
- Most are considered of minimal threat to immunocompetent adults.

SYNONYMS

- Infectious stomatitis
- Mouth rot
- Trench mouth
- Ulcerative stomatitis

ABBREVIATIONS

- CT = computed tomography
- ICe = intracoelomic
- IM = intramuscular
- MRI = magnetic resonance imaging
- PCB = polychlorinated biphenyl
- PO = per os
- SC = subcutaneous

Suggested Reading

Wright KM, Whitaker BR. *Amphibian Medicine and Captive Husbandry*. Malabar, FL: Krieger; 2001.

Author Sam Rivera, DVM, MS, DABVP (Avian), DACZM, DECZM (Zoo Health Management)

TICKS

BASICS

DEFINITION/OVERVIEW

Ticks are ectoparasites that feed on blood and can potentially transmit disease through their bite, along with causing local irritation, secondary infection, or rarely anemia. Ticks are rare in amphibians. They are typically only seen in wild-caught animals, so any known wild-caught animals should be closely examined for their presence. They may also be found on weak or debilitated animals.

ETIOLOGY/PATHOPHYSIOLOGY

- Ticks affecting amphibians are in the Family Ixodidae (hard ticks).
- Many are host specific and do not transmit to other species.
- Infection with *Amblyomma dissimile*, *A. fuscum*, and *A. rotundatum* have been reported.
- Hard ticks live in fields or scrub areas and attach to a host as it passes by.
- Ticks use their mouthparts to attach and feed on blood; they remain attached for several days.
- Females lay eggs after a blood meal.
- Eggs hatch as a larval stage, which feed on blood from the host.
- They progress through two or more nymph stages before becoming adults, feeding on blood between each stage.
- Larvae, nymphs, and adults can live for months without a blood meal.

SIGNALMENT/HISTORY

- No age or sex predisposition.
- Typically only seen in wild-caught animals, those that spend significant time outdoors, or those kept in unsanitary conditions with poor husbandry.

CLINICAL PRESENTATION

- Identification of tick attached to skin.
- They often attach in skin folds such as around the legs, lips, or cloaca.
- There may be swelling, erythema, or discharge at the site of attachment from local irritation or secondary bacterial infection.
- In some cases, animals may be debilitated, weak, or have other underlying problems.
- Animals may also soak frequently in an attempt to dislodge the parasites.
- If the infestation is severe, there may be signs of excessive shedding, anemia, or possible disease transmitted by the tick.

RISK FACTORS

Husbandry

- Ticks are typically only seen in wild-caught animals, and rarely in captive animals that spend significant time outdoors.
- There is no specific way to avoid infestation other than regular tick control measures, such as mowing the lawn regularly, removing debris piles or refuse, avoid overwatering or standing water, limiting access by wildlife, and using tick control pesticides on the lawn.
- Extreme caution must be taken with any pesticides around amphibians, as they will be absorbed through the skin.
- Infestations can also occur in severe cases of poor husbandry and sanitation, which also contributes to stress and other underlying medical conditions.

Others

Animals that are stressed, have underlying medical issues, or are otherwise debilitated are the most likely to harbor ticks.

DIAGNOSIS

DIFFERENTIAL DIAGNOSIS

- Diagnosis is pathognomonic
- Other ectoparasites such as mites are significantly smaller and not confused with ticks.

DIAGNOSTICS

- Diagnosis of ticks is based on physical exam alone.
- Additional tests to evaluate the animal's overall condition may be necessary if the animal is otherwise weak or debilitated.
- This may include a fecal exam, complete blood count and chemistry panel, and/or radiographs.

PATHOLOGICAL FINDINGS

- Ticks are obvious on physical exam.
- There may be evidence of inflammation, ulceration, or secondary bacterial colonization at the attachment site.
- Anemia is possible though, because ticks are large, they are often noticed and removed before significant anemia can occur.
- Other pathologic findings could include those from a pathogen transmitted by the tick.

TREATMENT

APPROPRIATE HEALTH CARE

N/A

NUTRITIONAL SUPPORT

- Not needed for this condition unless animal is otherwise debilitated.
- If clinical disease is present, and patient is not eating, weak, or lethargic, then supportive feeding may be indicated.
- Most can be fed at 1–2% of body weight once daily using a liquid carnivore diet.
- Fluid baths with electrolytes should be used if patient is dehydrated.

CLIENT EDUCATION/HUSBANDRY RECOMMENDATIONS

- Ticks must be removed from the patient and the environment for successful management.
- If tick exposure occurred in an outdoor environment, the area should be cleaned up of debris and measures taken to reduce the possibility they will colonize the area.
- Routine monitoring of animals and enclosures is needed.
- If the animal is wild caught and otherwise weak and debilitated, then husbandry needs to be ideal, to reduce stress on the animal and aid in recovery.
- Strict quarantine is necessary to avoid introducing ticks to other animals in a collection.

MEDICATIONS

DRUG(S) OF CHOICE

- Physical removal is recommended
- The tick must be grasped under the head on the mouthparts for full extraction.
- Secondary infection of the attachment site can be treated with topical antibacterial ointment, such as silver sulfadiazine cream, and systemic antibiotics if needed.
- Ivermectin applied topically may aid in tick removal, mainly for sites that are not easily accessible for physical removal.
- Additional treatments may be needed based on the animal's overall condition.
- If the animal is anemic due to blood loss, consider additional therapies such as B vitamins, iron dextran, or even a blood transfusion.
- Topical doses of ivermectin up to 2 mg/kg have been reported but one must exercise caution when using this higher dosage. Alternatively, 0.2–0.4 mg/kg PO, SC q14d.

PRECAUTIONS/INTERACTIONS

- Use caution with any drug therapy or treatment of the environment as amphibians can absorb all compounds through the skin.
- The environment must be thoroughly cleaned of all chemicals before the animal is placed back inside it.

FOLLOW-UP

PATIENT MONITORING

• None needed if ticks are physically removed.
• If secondary bacterial infection is present, resolution of clinical signs will indicate response to therapy.
• Monitor progress of any underlying medical conditions.

EXPECTED COURSE AND PROGNOSIS

• Depending on the animal's condition, the prognosis may be excellent to guarded.
• The prognosis for ticks themselves is excellent.
• Once they are removed there should be no further complications.
• The prognosis for secondary infection of the skin is good as well.
• The main concern would be in weak or debilitated animals, or if there is potential for disease transmission from the tick.

MISCELLANEOUS

COMMENTS

• One potential concern with ticks entering the country on wild-caught animals is introduction of foreign animal disease.
• This has not been reported in amphibians, but it has in ticks that can infect reptiles.
• Any tick on a wild-caught animal from another country and the animal itself should be treated with suspicion.

ZOONOTIC POTENTIAL

• Ticks can potentially attach to humans and cause irritation and pruritis at the site of a bite.
• Many can also carry and transmit disease to humans, such as tularemia, Lyme disease, and other encephalitis-causing viruses.
• Use caution during removal and kill the tick immediately.

SYNONYMS

N/A

Suggested Reading

Dantas-Torres F, Oliveira-Filho EF, Soares FA, et al. Ticks infesting amphibians and reptiles in Pernambuco, northeastern Brazil. *Brazil. J Vet Parasitol* 2008;17:218–221.

Poynton SL, Whitaker BR. Protozoa and metazoa infecting amphibians. In: Wright KM, Whitaker BR. *Amphibian Medicine and Captive Husbandry*. Malabar, FL: Krieger; 2001:196–222.

Smith RL, Schnack JA, Schaefer EF, Kehr AI. Ticks, *Amblyomma rotundatum* (Acari: Ixodidae), on toads, *Chaunus schneideri* and *Chaunus granulosus* (Anura: Bufonidae), in Northern Argentina. *J Parasitol* 2008;94:560–562.

Author Stacey Leonatti Wilkinson, DVM, DABVP (Reptile and Amphibian)

UPPER RESPIRATORY TRACT DISEASE

BASICS

DEFINITION/OVERVIEW

In amphibians, distinction between disease of the URT and LRT is complicated due to the different modes of respiration in larval and adult forms and across species. The moist skin can be responsible for up to 70% of the gas exchange in some species. Larva and neotenic species also rely on gills, while adult amphibians use lungs. Some species lack lungs. Caecilians and anurans have three modes of respiration: pulmonic, buccopharyngeal or cutaneous respiration, while adult neotenic anurans have branchial respiration from retained gill structures. In most post-metamorphic amphibians, buccopharyngeal and pulmonary respiration take place, as well as cutaneous gas exchange. Some aquatic salamanders breathe air through the nares, but some (sirens and *Necturus* spp.) take air in through the mouth. Pipid frogs commonly breathe through the mouth. If air is passed through the nostrils as external nares, air follows the narial ducts, which open via choanae (as internal nares) into the buccal cavity. In the buccopharyngeal cavity, mouth and pharynx lead to the glottis (as the beginning of the lower respiratory tract), which leads into the larynx. Male anurans, especially, fill their lungs with air to croak, making pumping movements with the bottom of the mouth, pressing the air into their vocal sack through the larynx and from thence back into their lungs. Clinical signs of URTD in amphibians include changes in the gills, nares, nasal, or oral cavity and pharynx, such as lumps or masses, larger wounds, and necrosis, as well as serous, mucous or purulent discharge within or from the oral cavity.

ETIOLOGY/PATHOPHYSIOLOGY

- Acute, subacute or chronic (unilateral or bilateral) infectious or non-infectious.
- Contact and embolic routes of infection described, depending on the amphibian species.
- Reactive inflammatory processes of the skin in amphibians may look like pseudotumors.
- Rostral abrasions, injuries and traumata of the rostrum, including the nares.
- Infection, injuries, or necrosis of the gills.
- Secondary invasion of pathogens. such as bacteria and fungi after injuries of the skin, nares, and gills.

Infectious

- Bacteria (*Mycobacteria*; *Chlamydia* spp.; Gram-negatives such as *Acinetobacter* spp., *Citrobacter* spp., *Pseudomonas* spp., *Aeromonas* spp.)
- Fungi (*Batrachochytrium dendrobatidis*, *B. salamandrivorans*; *Saprolegnia* spp.)
- *Ranavirus*: hemorrhage and necrosis throughout the body, including the gills, nasal tissue, and trachea.
- *Herpesvirus*

Parasites

- Parasites may cause physical damage to epithelium and predispose to bacterial or fungal infections (secondary invasion) and septicemia. Can infest the skin, nares, gills, oral cavity, or esophagus in amphibians.
- Myiasis: dipteran flies deposit eggs, larvae penetrate skin or migrate to the nostrils and into the nasal cavity.
- *Bufolucila* spp: maggot infestation of the nasal passage in Old World toads, occasionally infect adult anurans in North America, may be fatal for the host. Larvae cause severe ulceration of nasal mucosa and bone loss around nostrils and septum before penetrating the skull and invading the brain as well as possible infestation of conjunctiva, orbit, and tympanic region.
- Mites (*Xenopacarus africanus*) in terrestrial anurans; mite infestation in the nasal cavity of African clawed frogs (*Xenopus laevis*).
- Protozoa (ciliates)
- Gill parasites, causing gill infection, necrosis, degeneration, or adhesion: copepods, ciliates (e.g., *Trichodina* spp.), flagellates, trematodes (*Sphyranura* sp., *Aspidobothrea*).
- Nematodes (*Capillaria* in cutaneous and subcutaneous tissue)
- Trematodes in skin and gills (such as *Sphyranura* spp., *Aspidobothrea*), especially migration of larval forms.
- *Microsporidia* (causing septicemia with ulcerative dermatitis)

Non-Infectious

- Foreign bodies within the choanae, nasal or oral cavity.
- Trauma
- Neoplasia (e.g., epidermal papillomas/squamous papillomas/epitheliomas, most frequently in urodeles; melanocarcinoma of nostrils, fibropapillomas of the rostral maxilla in a Mexican axolotl; fibrosarcomas, and tumors of the neuroepithelium presumably originating from olfactory tissue)
- Intoxication through absorption or inhalation of dust, smoke, aerosols, disinfectants or other environmental toxins (algicidals, chlorine, ammonia, etc.).
- Improper husbandry or transport

SIGNALMENT/HISTORY

Some diseases appear to have predilection for certain amphibian species and/or stage of development (tadpole or adult).

CLINICAL PRESENTATION

- Dependent on the underlying cause and amphibian species.
- Nasal discharge
- Rostral abrasions
- Severe ulceration of nasal mucosa
- Bone loss around nostrils and septum.
- Obstruction of the nostrils by retained skin, mites, or blocked nostrils (sometimes due to dried nasal exudate).
- Swellings or wounds due to infections of rostral skin, possible involvement of the nares.
- Exudate (serous to mucopurulent) or obstructed external nares.
- Salivation/oral exudate/oral discharge/mucous secretion in the oral cavity.
- Severe stomatitis (labial, glossal, periglottal or general), sometimes proliferative or ulcerative.
- Foreign body within the choanae, nasal/oral cavity.
- Gill loss, (circumferential) growth of the gills, white coating, wounds and necrosis of the gills.
- Dyspnea, respiratory distress, gaping
- Nonspecific signs such as anorexia, lethargy, inactivity.

RISK FACTORS

- Depending on the underlying cause and amphibian species.
- Stressors and inappropriate husbandry

Husbandry

Improper transport conditions or husbandry (such as inadequate cage set up, ponds, tanks, or enclosures polluted with sewage, inappropriate temperatures, poor hygiene, oxygen imbalances, and high levels of ammonia and chlorine, incorrect pH, nitrogen oversaturation).

Others

Immunosuppression, which may be caused by stress, importation, overcrowding, relocation, concurrent disease or inappropriate husbandry, malnutrition and inadequate temperatures, severe endoparasitism may be a predisposing factor or even cause of the disease.

DIAGNOSIS

DIFFERENTIAL DIAGNOSIS

- Infectious diseases (bacterial, viral, fungal, parasitic)
- Neoplasia
- Foreign bodies
- Perforating foreign bodies
- Trauma
- Inhalation of irritating substances
- Retained slough or blocked nostrils (sometimes after severe infection).
- Improper husbandry with focus on water quality.

DIAGNOSTICS

- Physical examination including thorough exam of the oral cavity and choana. The use of magnification may aid in identifying subtle lesions.
- Bacterial culture and sensitivity (aerobic and anaerobic) and/or fungal culture of affected skin or gills, nasal discharge, nasal flush or inflamed tissue in the upper alimentary or respiratory tract.
- *B. dendrobatidis* and *B. salamandrivorans* are diagnosed via cytology, histopathology or PCR.
- Cytology of discharge and affected tissues.
- PCR for the diagnosis of ranavirus.
- Parasites: microscopy of oral or cloacal swab or oropharyngeal mucus examination and fecal exam.
- Viruses: PCR and histopathology
- Oral cavity examination and fecal exam.
- Diagnostic imaging (radiographs, ultrasound, CT, MRI).
- Endoscopy

PATHOLOGICAL FINDINGS

- Depending on the underlying cause signs of mild to severe inflammation, lesions and ulcerations of the rostral skin, nasal and oral mucosa and submucosa may be found.
- Histology of rostral abrasions may reveal damaged epithelium and dermal glands can contain cellular debris with markedly edematous dermis. Bacteria may be associated with necrotic epidermal cells and adnexa.
- Myiasis infestation of the nasal passage with the toad fly (*Lucila bufonivora*) larvae cause severe ulceration of nasal mucosa and bone loss around nostrils and septum before penetrating the skull and invading the brain and possible infestation of conjunctiva, orbit, and tympanic region.
- In cases of cutaneous mycobacteriosis, besides other affected regions, granulomas of the lips and mouth may be visible. Early granulomas are composed of mostly epithelioid macrophages and some lymphocytes. More chronic lesions present with dry caseous cores and thick walls of epithelioid cells. Acid-fast stains demonstrate myriad of intracellular acid-fast bacilli.
- Fungal infections of the anterior snout and gills with *Saprolegnia* spp. or *Achlya*, *Aphanomyces*, *Leptolegnia* (and others) are characterized by white cottony growth on the skin and gills. Histologically, extensive ulceration of skin with necrosis of underlying soft tissue, zoospores and hyphae can be seen. Infestation with *Ergasilus* spp. leads to inflammation and necrosis of the gills.

TREATMENT

APPROPRIATE HEALTH CARE

N/A

NUTRITIONAL SUPPORT

- Nutritional supplementation for anorexic animals is essential for recovery.
- Carnivore critical care diets can be fed until the amphibian starts eating on its own.

CLIENT EDUCATION/HUSBANDRY RECOMMENDATIONS

- Correct any husbandry deficiencies, with special attention to temperature, humidity, and ventilation.
- Isolate animal from others in collection, especially when viral etiology is suspected.
- It is important to ensure a full course of treatment to avoid recurrence of disease.

SURGICAL CONSIDERATIONS

- Parasites: in some cases, physical removal of the parasites via surgery or endoscopy may be performed.
- Neoplasia: surgical removal not feasible in most cases.

MEDICATIONS

DRUG(S) OF CHOICE

- Dependent on the underlying cause and the affected snake species.
- Bacteria: systemic or nebulized antibiotics, preferably according to sensitivity panel. Local instillation of antibiotics (injectable or ophthalmic solutions) in the nasal passage may also be effective.
- Fungi: systemic, local, nebulized antifungals.
- In case of confirmed mycobacterial infection, no treatment, euthanasia.
- In cases of severe stomatitis, local therapy including periodic debridement and removal of abscess material.
- Rostral abrasions: if these are rapidly increasing in size, gently debride with dry cotton tip applicator, antibiotic ophthalmic ointments. If saline solutions are used topically, wash off with fresh water after 10 min.
- Viral: separation, strict quarantine, and intensive supportive therapy. Antiviral therapy has had low success and euthanasia is often required depending on the state of the animal and the disease.
- Parasites: antiparasitic treatment according the species.
- Retained slough or blocked nostrils: removal of the slough and enlargement of nostrils.
- Optimization of husbandry conditions

NUTRITIONAL SUPPORT

- Nutritional supplementation for anorexic animals is essential for recovery.
- Carnivore critical care diets can be fed until the amphibian starts eating on its own.

CLIENT EDUCATION/HUSBANDRY RECOMMENDATIONS

- Correct any husbandry deficiencies, with special attention to temperature, humidity, and ventilation.
- Isolate animal from others in collection, especially when viral etiology is suspected.
- It is important to ensure a full course of treatment to avoid recurrence of disease.
- Bacteria: amikacin, doxycycline, gentamycin, enrofloxacin, oxytetracycline.
- Fungi: terbinafine, voriconazole, amphotericin B.

PRECAUTIONS/INTERACTIONS

- Many systemic antibiotics (e.g., aminoglycosides, fluoroquinolones) are excreted through the kidney or show renal toxicity, thus avoidance of those or supplemental fluid administration is recommended.
- Systemic use of itraconazole may cause severe adverse effects including death in some amphibians. Species-specific information must be researched before treatment is initiated.

FOLLOW-UP

PATIENT MONITORING

- Improvement of clinical signs should be expected within 1–2 weeks for bacterial and fungal infections when definitive diagnosis and treatment are employed.
- It is critical to continue treatment until clinical signs are fully resolved and repeating cultures to confirm resolution of infection if unsure.
- In cases that do not show any improvement or worsen during the first 1–2 weeks of treatment, it should be considered that the etiology and/or treatment are not accurate.
- Viral infections should also be considered in cases that do not respond to therapy or have chronic, intermittent recurrence of disease.
- Repeat diagnostics may be needed to assess resolution or progression of disease.

EXPECTED COURSE AND PROGNOSIS

- Dependent on the etiology
- Bacterial: good prognosis depending on response to antibiotics.
- Fungal: guarded to poor prognosis.
- Viral: poor to grave prognosis especially when showing clinical signs.
- Parasitic: good to guarded prognosis.
- Neoplastic: grave prognosis
- Others: depend on severity and involvement of other tissues.

UPPER RESPIRATORY TRACT DISEASE (CONTINUED)

MISCELLANEOUS

COMMENTS

N/A

ZOONOTIC POTENTIAL

- Depending on the causative agent.
- *Mycobacterium* spp. and *Chlamydia* spp. should be considered as possibly zoonotic, depending on the species.

SYNONYMS

Upper respiratory tract infection

ABBREVIATIONS

- CT = computed tomography
- LRT = lower respiratory tract
- MRI = magnetic resonance imaging
- PCR = polymerase chain reaction
- URT = upper respiratory tract
- URTD = upper respiratory tract disease

Suggested Reading

Baitchman EJ, Pessier AP. Pathogenesis, diagnosis, and treatment of amphibian chytridiomycosis. *Vet Clin North Am Exot Anim Pract* 2013;16(3):669–685.

Fain A, Baker RA, Tinsley RC. Notes on a mite *Xenopacarus africanus*, n. g., n. sp. parasitic in the nasal cavities of the African clawed frog *Xenopus laevi* (Ereynetidae: Trombidiformes). *Rev Zool Botan Afr* 1969;80(3–4):340–345.

Helmer PJ, Whiteside DP. Amphibian anatomy and physiology. In: O'Malley B, ed. *Clinical Anatomy and Physiology of Exotic Species*. Edinburgh, UK: WB Saunders; 2005:3–14.

Noble GK. The respiratory system. In: Noble GK, ed. *The biology of the amphibia*. New York, NY: Dover Publications; 1954:158–178.

Taylor SK. Mycoses. In: Wright KM, Whitaker BR. *Amphibian Medicine and Captive Husbandry*. Malabar, FL: Krieger; 2001:181–238.

Author Karina A. Mathes, DVM, Dr. med. vet., DECZM (Herpetology), European Veterinary Specialist in Zoological Medicine (Herpetology), Certified Specialist in Reptiles (Fachtieraerztin fuer Reptilien), Certified Specialist in Reptiles and Amphibians (ZB Reptilien und Amphibien)

VOMITING

BASICS

DEFINITION/OVERVIEW

Vomiting is the forcible ejection of partially or wholly digested contents from the stomach and small intestine through the mouth.

ETIOLOGY/PATHOPHYSIOLOGY

- Vomiting occurs due to stimulation of the emetic center in the brain.
- The emetic center can be activated by chemical stimulation via emetic compounds, vestibular input, over distention or excitation of stretch receptors in the stomach/duodenum, electrolyte imbalances, or dehydration.
- Details of the activation of the amphibian emetic center are not completely understood, but appear similar to those of mammals.
- Vomiting is a combination of reverse peristalsis and an increase in intra-abdominal pressure to expel GI contents.

SIGNALMENT/HISTORY

- All species, ages, sexes may be affected.
- The exception is juvenile anurans, which lack anatomical features necessary for vomiting prior to metamorphosis.
- Owner may report clinical signs, such as repeated opening/closing of the mouth, swallowing, body contortion, stomach eversion, expulsion of GI contents.
- Vomitus and/or mucus or blood in the enclosure may be the only finding noted.
- Recent handling or feeding
- Changes in enclosure, substrate, or husbandry.
- Addition of new individuals to the collection.
- Lethargy, anorexia, weight loss, respiratory distress, cutaneous lesions, coelomic distention.

CLINICAL PRESENTATION

- No clinical signs are specific to vomiting, and physical exam may be normal.
- Presentation varies depending on the underlying cause and chronicity.
- Gastric prolapse
- Dehydration and/or emaciation/cachexia.
- Hard mass on palpation of the coelomic cavity due to an obstructive lesion.
- Skeletal abnormalities that may include pathological fractures or abnormal growth patterns.
- Lethargy and/or obtunded mentation.
- Hyperemia and petechiation/ecchymosis may be observed due to infection or in any terminal disease process.

RISK FACTORS

Husbandry

- Poor sanitation, overcrowding, hyper- or hypothermia, lack of quarantine for new individuals (increases stress, possibility of secondary infections, and disease transmission).
- Toxin exposure (cleaning chemicals, pesticides, heavy metals)
- Excessive/inappropriate handling (especially soon after feeding)
- Inadequate diet (incorrect calcium/phosphorus ratio, improper prey items, excessive feeding)
- Inappropriate substrate (may be accidentally ingested)
- Trauma (poor enclosure design, inappropriate cohabitants)

Others

- Anesthesia or motion sickness
- Concomitant infectious or parasitic disease.

DIAGNOSIS

DIFFERENTIAL DIAGNOSIS

- Gastric prolapse and vomiting can be associated with any terminal disease process, but are only commonly associated with *Ranavirus* and saprolegniasis in salamander species.
- Normal seasonal behavior in some anuran species.
- Handling/stress (e.g., excessive pressure to coelom, motion sickness)
- Obstructive lesions (e.g., GI foreign body, intussusception, neoplasia, abscess, granuloma)
- Metabolic disease (e.g., nutritional secondary hyperparathyroidism, hypervitaminosis A)
- Toxicoses (e.g., ammonia, chlorine, pesticides, nitrites, heavy metals)
- Hyper- or hypothermia
- Anesthesia (especially with eugenol)
- Trauma (predisposes to secondary infection)
- *Ranavirus* infection (especially in Chinese giant salamanders, *Andrias davidianus*)
- Parasites (e.g., nematodiasis, amoebiasis, coccidiosis, pentastomiasis)
- Bacteria/septicemia (e.g., *Aeromonas hydrophila, Salmonella, Mycobacterium* [*M. marinum, M. fortuitum, M. xenopi*])
- Fungi (e.g., saprolegniasis, *Mucor amphibiorum, Batrachochytrium*)

DIAGNOSTICS

- Husbandry review
- Water quality test, especially ammonia, nitrites, chlorine, heavy metals.
- Parasite evaluation of vomitus and feces (direct, flotation, cytology).
- Bloodwork, especially PCV, total solids, albumin, and electrolytes. Normal values indicate an acute process. Low electrolytes but other values normal indicates a chronic process. Elevated values suggest dehydration.
- Wet mount of skin scrapings.
- Bacterial and fungal cultures
- *Batrachochytrium* polymerase chain reaction assay.
- Blood culture
- Radiography with or without contrast.
- Ultrasonography
- GI endoscopy or coeliotomy (direct tissue evaluation and biopsy)

PATHOLOGICAL FINDINGS

Dependent on underlying cause

TREATMENT

APPROPRIATE HEALTH CARE

- Primary goal is to identify and address the underlying cause.
- Non-pathologic causes are generally self-limiting and resolve without intervention.
- Supportive care may be required to correct dehydration, electrolyte imbalances, weight loss, and malnutrition.

NUTRITIONAL SUPPORT

- Correct fluid deficits and maintain hydration.
- Transdermal or intracoelomic routes are the most effective.
- Soaking in water or crystalloid (e.g., amphibian Ringer's solution) baths for 1-hour intervals once or twice daily is sufficient to maintain adequate hydration and correct mild to moderate electrolyte imbalances.
- Tube or assist feeding liquid or gel diets, such as Hill's® Prescription Diet® a/d® (Hills Pet Nutrition, Inc., Topeka, KS); Mazuri® Amphibian & Carnivorous Reptile Gel (Mazuri Exotic Animal Nutrition, St. Louis, MO); Oxbow Critical Care Carnivore® (Oxbow Animal Health, Omaha, NE) may be beneficial during initial treatment/recovery.
- Initially feed 1% body weight daily, then gradually increase to 2–3% body weight daily or every other day.
- Gradually add normal prey items to diet as the animal improves.

CLIENT EDUCATION/HUSBANDRY RECOMMENDATIONS

- Review husbandry and correct any problems.
- Feed prey items a well-balanced diet and coat with calcium supplementation when appropriate.
- Avoid large meals, overfeeding, or handling immediately following a meal.
- Institute quarantine procedures for new animals, including 30–60-day period, veterinary evaluation, and 1–3-weekly fecal exams for parasites.

VOMITING (CONTINUED)

MEDICATIONS

DRUG(S) OF CHOICE

- Antiemetic use has not been documented in amphibians.
- Sucralfate may be a beneficial gastroprotectant.

PRECAUTIONS/INTERACTIONS

N/A

FOLLOW-UP

PATIENT MONITORING

- Monitor clinical condition
- Recheck PCV, total solids, albumin, and electrolytes as necessary.

EXPECTED COURSE AND PROGNOSIS

- Excellent to grave prognosis depending on etiology, stage/severity of disease process at time of diagnosis, and degree of debilitation of animal at time of treatment initiation.
- Hematemesis is rare, but is associated with grave prognosis.

MISCELLANEOUS

COMMENTS

N/A

ZOONOTIC POTENTIAL

N/A

SYNONYMS

Emesis

ABBREVIATIONS

- GI = gastrointestinal
- PCV = packed cell volume

Suggested Reading

Wright KM. Overview of amphibian medicine. In: Mader DR, ed. *Reptile Medicine and Surgery*. 2nd ed. St. Louis, MO: Elsevier Saunders; 2006:941–971.

Wright KM, DeVoe RS. Amphibians. In: Carpenter JW, Marion CJ, eds. *Exotic Animal Formulary*. 4th ed. St. Louis, MO: Elsevier Saunders; 2013:53–82.

Wright KM, Whitaker BR. *Amphibian Medicine and Captive Husbandry*. Malabar, FL: Krieger; 2001.

Authors Jacqueline Serio, DVM, and Trevor T. Zachariah, DVM, MS, DACZM

WEIGHT LOSS

BASICS

DEFINITION/OVERVIEW

For amphibians, weight loss can take the form of body mass loss (i.e., cachexia) or fluid loss. In mammals, it is generally accepted that weight loss becomes clinically significant when the loss exceeds 10% of normal body weight (and when it is not completely due to fluid loss). From a clinical perspective, weight loss of more than 10–20% of a healthy, species-specific body weight is significant and must be systematically evaluated, with rapid weight loss being considered most urgent. Weight loss in amphibians may be a normal physiologic process (e.g., brumation/estivation, reproductive activity and behavior), and is not considered a primary disease, but, rather, a clinical manifestation of other disease processes.

ETIOLOGY/PATHOPHYSIOLOGY

- In amphibians, normal weight loss (fluid and body mass loss) will occur during times of torpor or brumation/estivation.
- Once post-torpor normal behavior returns, the amphibian will replenish lost fluids and body mass under normal circumstances or given normal access to clean, dechlorinated water and appropriate food and environmental conditions.
- Normal weight loss may be associated with reproductive behavior or gravidity as well.
- Terrestrial amphibian species also experience evaporative fluid loss normally during any 24-hour period, since they expose more wet surface directly to air, per gram of body weight, than any other terrestrial vertebrate.
- Pathologic weight loss may be associated with a variety of noninfectious and infectious disease processes.
- In pet amphibians, inappropriate husbandry is the most common underlying cause of pathologic weight loss.
- Poor husbandry may frequently lead to metabolic diseases or secondary infectious diseases due to immune system compromise of the animal.
- Infectious diseases, and debilitating non-infectious diseases, will commonly result in weight loss due to both body mass and fluid loss.
- In some cases, amphibians succumb to a nonspecific disease process referred to as "maladaptation or failure to thrive syndrome," which is characterized by the failure of a captive amphibian to adapt to its current conditions, or a wild-caught amphibian unable to adapt to the captive environment.
- Many of these animals will lose weight and die, and a specific disease process is often not diagnosed.

SIGNALMENT/HISTORY

- Weight loss in amphibians has no specific signalment, and can affect males, females, any species, and any age.
- A typical history suggests rapid weight loss of 10% or more acutely, or 20% or more chronically.
- Weight loss in amphibians typically includes some degree of dehydration, in addition to loss of body mass and/or fat stores.
- If the individual or species normally brumates/estivates, weight loss can be expected as a normal physiologic process.
- With pathologic weight loss, the husbandry and environment must be evaluated thoroughly, and infectious and noninfectious diseases must be considered as underlying causes to the weight loss.

CLINICAL PRESENTATION

- Amphibians presenting for weight loss typically show observable loss of muscle mass.
- The vertebral column, pelvic bones, and urostyle become more readily apparent, and the hind limb muscles will decrease in mass.
- Externally, the coelomic cavity may appear sunken on both sides.
- Palpation of the coelomic cavity may reveal lack of fat bodies.
- With dehydration, the eyes may sink into the bony orbits, and the skin will become more tacky, depending on the species.

RISK FACTORS

Husbandry

- Poor husbandry is the most common contributing factor to pathologic process in amphibians, including weight loss.
- Poor husbandry might include inappropriate housing type, or improper placement within a client's household or other facility; ambient temperature and humidity; poor water quality; lack of and/or appropriate maintenance of an ultraviolet light source (position, distance from amphibians, appropriate duration between bulb changes); inappropriate type, quality and quantity of food offered; intra- or inter-specific competition for food; type of substrate, cage furniture, and frequency of cleaning/replacing substrate; toxicity associated with environmental cleaning solutions; amongst others.
- Common diseases associated with inappropriate husbandry include foreign body ingestion and gastrointestinal impaction; corneal lipidosis; nutritional secondary hyperparathyroidism (metabolic bone disease); starvation due to competition for food by other individuals; and exposure to toxic chemicals (e.g., ammonia, nitrites, or chloramines in aquatic species; heavy metals; cleaning solutions).
- Maladaptation syndrome or failure to thrive syndrome should also be considered as an underlying cause of weight loss.

Others

N/A

DIAGNOSIS

DIFFERENTIAL DIAGNOSIS

Normal Behavior

- Periods of torpor, brumation and estivation are normal for some species and may be associated with weight loss (loss of body mass and fluids).
- In some species, fluid loss during brumation/estivation can contribute to more than 20% of total weight loss.
- Terrestrial amphibian species also experience a normal evaporative fluid loss during the day, and this should be taken into consideration when evaluating these species.
- Reproductive activity, behavior and gravidity may contribute to normal seasonal weight loss.

Non-Infectious Diseases

- Exposure to toxic substances or developing disease processes secondary to poor husbandry or nutrition will commonly lead to weight loss.
- Neoplasia: a number of neoplastic diseases have been identified in amphibian species, most of which would have an expected clinical sequela of hyporexia, dehydration, and weight loss.

Infectious Diseases

- Amphibians are susceptible to many infectious diseases, all of which can contribute to hyporexia, dehydration, and weight loss.
- Common amphibian diseases observed in clinical practice, include endoparasites (excessive burdens of gastrointestinal flagellates and ciliates, coccidia, nematodes, amoebae, cestode larvae, and hemoparasites); ectoparasites (trombiculid mites); Gram-negative bacterial infections and septicemia; *Chlamydia* species; atypical mycobacteriosis; chytridiomycosis and other fungal infections; and viruses (e.g., *Ranavirus*).

DIAGNOSTICS

- Since weight loss is not a specific disease, a significant clinical diagnostic workup will be necessary.
- A thorough history, will be useful, including housing, feeding practices,

WEIGHT LOSS (CONTINUED)

maintenance temperature and humidity, presence of other animals; access to UVB light spectrum, water quality.
- Comparison to conspecifics housed in the same environment may confirm individual compared with group disease.
- A complete physical examination is critical to identify obvious lesions on the skin, within the oral cavity, on the extremities, or associated with the eyes.
- A fecal sample should be evaluated by direct smear and fecal float, if possible.
- Gill clips in gilled amphibians, and skin scrapes of all amphibians may be helpful.
- A complete blood count and biochemical profile, along with imaging modalities (radiography, ultrasound, and/or CT), should be considered.
- Aerobic and anaerobic bacterial cultures of blood samples can be very useful in debilitated amphibians due to the possibility of sepsis.
- Intracoelomic or gastrointestinal endoscopy, with or without biopsy and histopathology, may help with the diagnosis.

PATHOLOGICAL FINDINGS

- Pathologic findings are non-specific for weight loss, but the underlying cause may be associated with obvious gross pathologic or histopathologic lesions.
- Gross pathology of nonspecific weight loss might include loss of intracoelomic fat bodies, lack of intracoelomic organ-associated fat, and generalized muscle wasting.

TREATMENT

APPROPRIATE HEALTH CARE

N/A

NUTRITIONAL SUPPORT

- Nutritional support using a commercial enteral feeding formula, such as Oxbow Critical Care Carnivore® (Oxbow Animal Health, Omaha, NE) or Emeraid® IC Carnivore (EmerAid, LLC, Cornell, IL) administered via feeding tube is most appropriate.
- The directions on the label of the commercial diet can be followed for appropriate volume per feeding and frequency.
- Force-feeding whole prey items (e.g., gut-loaded invertebrates, pinkie mice or small fish) may be useful.

CLIENT EDUCATION/HUSBANDRY RECOMMENDATIONS

N/A

MEDICATIONS

DRUG(S) OF CHOICE

- Based on the diagnosis of the underlying cause of weight loss, treatment should be focused on the primary disease process.
- Based on the primary underlying disease process, antimicrobial, and anti-inflammatory drugs may be warranted.
- Correct hydration status by soaking or administering appropriate fluid therapy due to fluid loss (typically an isotonic solution), as any debilitated amphibian will likely be moderately to severely dehydrated.
- In addition, vitamin and mineral supplements (e.g., calcium in the form of parenteral calcium gluconate or oral calcium glubionate) may be beneficial in cases of nutritional deficiencies.
- Oversupplementation of vitamins and minerals may need to be discontinued if this appears to be causing primary disease.

PRECAUTIONS/INTERACTIONS

N/A

FOLLOW-UP

PATIENT MONITORING

- Correction of inappropriate husbandry and/or feeding practices will significantly benefit the amphibian patient.
- If medical treatment is necessary, the body weight can be measured, and the body condition assessed daily.
- If appropriate, medical therapy can be initiated and the patient monitored for improving condition.

EXPECTED COURSE AND PROGNOSIS

- Replenishing lost fluids from normal physiologic processes, such as brumation/estivation, may be warranted and should improve the amphibian's condition and provide a good prognosis.
- Depending on the primary underlying disease process and duration, the prognosis will range from poor to good for re-establishing normal body weight and condition.
- If husbandry problems can be corrected in a relatively short amount of time, the prognosis may be good.
- If the underlying disease process is progressive and debilitating, the prognosis will be poor.
- In cases of some infectious diseases, antimicrobials can be administered for bacterial or fungal diseases using topical, parenteral, or oral solutions.

MISCELLANEOUS

COMMENTS

N/A

ZOONOTIC POTENTIAL

N/A

SYNONYMS

- Cachexia
- Wasting

ABBREVIATIONS

- CT = computed tomography
- UVB = ultraviolet B

Suggested Reading

Wright KM. Amphibians: Weight loss. In: Mayer J, Donnelly TM, eds. *Clinical Veterinary Advisor: Birds and Exotic Pets*. St. Louis, MO: Elsevier Saunders; 2013:70–71.

Wright KM, Whitaker BR. *Amphibian Medicine and Captive Husbandry*. Malabar, FL: Krieger; 2001.

Author Kurt K. Sladky, MS, DVM, DACZM, DECZM (Zoo Health Management & Herpetology)

XANTHOMATOSIS

BASICS

DEFINITION/OVERVIEW

Xanthomatosis is a lipid storage disease in anurans associated with high dietary levels of cholesterol and corneal lipid (especially cholesterol) deposition (corneal arcus or corneal lipidosis). Less commonly, deposition of cholesterol granulomas (xanthomas) elsewhere in the body can be found. Corneal arcus is the most commonly reported corneal disease of amphibians.

ETIOLOGY/PATHOPHYSIOLOGY

Experimentally, Cuban tree frogs (*Osteopilus septentrionalis*) fed diets high in cholesterol (1.7% dry matter) had significantly elevated serum cholesterol and LDL levels, which lead to significantly more corneal cholesterol deposition (13/21 frogs, 62%), than in frogs (4/26, 15%) on a lower cholesterol diet (0.7% dry matter), or wild Cuban tree frogs (0/122, no corneal arcus cases), after17 months.

SIGNALMENT/HISTORY

- Most patients are aged at least 5 years, or have been in captivity for several years.
- Females are more commonly affected than males.
- Corneal arcus has been reported in Hylidae: Cuban tree frogs, White's tree frogs (*Litoria caerulea*), red-eyed tree frog (*Agalychnis callidryas*), green and golden bell frog (*L. aurea*), Grey tree frog (*Hyla versicolor*), canyon tree frog (*H. arenicolor*), mountain tree frog (*H. eximia*), European tree frog (*H. arborea*), Microhylid: tomato frog (*Dyscophus antongilii*), banded bullfrog (*Kaloula pulchra*); Ceratophryidae: Bell's horned frog (*Ceratophrys ornata*), and toads—Colorado River toads (*Bufo alvarius*), smooth-sided toad or spotted toad (*Rhaebo* (*Bufo*) *guttatus*), and Couch's spadefoot toad (*Scaphiopus couchi*).

CLINICAL PRESENTATION

- Corneal lipidosis first appears as a haziness that progresses to opacity and blindness.
- Corneal arcus starts as perilimbal, small, white, crystalline foci, which become denser and more raised and slowly progress towards the central corneal.
- In Cuban tree frogs, lesions progressed over 8–20 months to involve 60–100% of the cornea.
- Lesions are not associated with ocular irritation early on, but as the lesions progress, the cornea becomes thickened, irregular, raised and opaque.
- In severe cases, lesions adjacent to the limbus become vascularized and pigmented.
- Eventually, the cornea may be heavily vascularized and bleed when touched, and the patient becomes blind.
- Xanthomas have been identified in the brain, some viscera (especially hepatic), peripheral nerves, periarticular soft tissues, and digital pads.

RISK FACTORS

Husbandry

- Wright speculated lack of normal biology, such as no vitellogenesis, mating behavior (males use up most of their coelomic fat reserves while calling and courting females), hibernation or estivation, lower activity and dietary diversity, as well as a lack of thermoregulation, may all predispose anurans to excess fat disposition.
- Overfeeding, and diets high in cholesterol, are thought to be contributing factors.

Others

- Cuban tree frogs and White's tree frogs are most commonly affected, with more case reports in females than males.
- There is no evidence that increased serum cholesterol in females is directly related to vitellogenesis.

DIAGNOSIS

DIFFERENTIAL DIAGNOSIS

- Corneal opacity is often diagnostic.
- Serum lipid profiles (especially cholesterol and LDL) may also contribute to diagnosis.
- Normal anuran values are summarized in Wright, 2003 (see Suggested Reading).
- Distinguish corneal arcus from corneal ulcers, old corneal scars, or anterior uveitis.
- Xanthomas should be distinguished from other granulomatous diseases, such as mycobacteriosis or chromomycosis by histopathology.

DIAGNOSTICS

- Corneal arcus can be diagnosed with ocular examination with the naked eye, an ophthalmoscope, dissecting microscope or slit lamp ophthalmoscope, the latter may help detect lesions earlier than the other methods.
- Fluorescein stain should be negative for corneal ulcers.

PATHOLOGICAL FINDINGS

- Early lesions are evident as scattered, elongate, empty clefts (presumably from vacated extracellular cholesterol crystals) running at oblique angles to the collagen lamellae of the anterior stroma, adjacent to the limbus and diminishing towards the central cornea.
- The corneal stroma may be infiltrated by lymphocytes, macrophages and fibrocytes.
- Neovascularization is most prominent adjacent to the limbus.
- Affected areas of the cornea stain positive for lipids, cholesterol and phospholipids with oil red O, Sudan black B and Schultz stains.

TREATMENT

APPROPRIATE HEALTH CARE

- Careful weight control and improved husbandry and diet may slow progression of lesions but will not reverse them.
- Vitamin A is unlikely to be effective or palliative, unknown if preventative.

NUTRITIONAL SUPPORT

- Most patients have been over fed and therefore should be fed less, no more than once a week.
- Amphibians are much more efficient (40–80%) than reptiles (4%) at converting food to body mass, and preferentially convert carbohydrates and protein to lipids.
- Wright recommended that a 50-g White's tree frog maintained at 77 degrees F, be fed no more than six adult crickets per week.
- Also, modify diet to reduce cholesterol levels and increase dietary diversity (see below).
- Avoid insect larvae, which tend to have higher lipid levels.

CLIENT EDUCATION/HUSBANDRY RECOMMENDATIONS

- Feed a wide variety of gut-loaded insects, that have been fed a diet high in calcium and vitamin A.
- Allow amphibians to thermoregulate with basking areas from 85 degrees F (29.4 degrees C), in temperate species, to 105 degrees F (40.5 degrees C), in tropical species, with ambient temperatures 15–30 degrees F lower.

MEDICATIONS

DRUG(S) OF CHOICE

N/A

PRECAUTIONS/INTERACTIONS

N/A

XANTHOMATOSIS (CONTINUED)

FOLLOW-UP

PATIENT MONITORING

• Discuss husbandry changes regularly with owner, monitor lipid profiles, if possible.
• Document ophthalmologic exams to assess response to therapy.

EXPECTED COURSE AND PROGNOSIS

• Most patients die within 18–24 months of diagnosis although some may survive as long as 48 months if hand fed.
• Frogs are highly visual so once the patient is blind, consider euthanasia, as blind frogs are reluctant to move, cannot thermoregulate, must be hand fed, and are likely highly stressed and painful.

MISCELLANEOUS

COMMENTS

N/A

ZOONOTIC POTENTIAL

N/A

SYNONYMS

• Corneal arcus
• Corneal lipidosis
• Lipid keratopathy
• Xanthomatous keratitis

ABBREVIATIONS

LDL = low-density lipoproteins

Suggested Reading

Keller CB, Shilton CM. The amphibian eye. *Vet Clin North Am Exot Anim Pract* 2002;5(2):261–274.

Russell WC, Edwards DL Jr., Stair EL, Ubner DC. Corneal lipidosis, disseminated xanthomatosis, and hypercholesterolemia in Cuban tree frogs (*Osteopilus septentrionalis*). *J Zoo Wildl Med* 1990;21(1):99–104.

Shilton CM, Smith DA, Crawshaw GJ, et al. Corneal lipid deposition in Cuban tree frogs (*Osteopilus septentrionalis*) and its relationship to serum lipids: An experimental study. *J Zoo Wildl Med* 2001;32(3):305–319.

Wright K. Cholesterol, corneal lipidosis, and xanthomatosis in amphibians. *Vet Clin North Am Exot Anim Pract* 2003;6(1):155–167.

Author Thomas H. Boyer, DVM, DABVP (Reptile and Amphibian Practice)

INDEX

This index uses letter-by-letter alphabetization.